T0176840

Dermatology Training: The Essentials

Dermatology Training
The Essentials

Edited by

Mahbub M.U. Chowdhury FRCP

Consultant Dermatologist and Honorary Senior Lecturer
Welsh Institute of Dermatology
University Hospital of Wales
Cardiff, UK

Tamara W. Griffiths FRCP

Consultant Dermatologist and Honorary Senior Lecturer
Dermatology Centre
Salford Royal Hospital NHS Trust
Manchester, UK

Andrew Y. Finlay CBE, FRCP

Professor of Dermatology
Division of Infection and Immunity
School of Medicine
Cardiff University
Cardiff, UK

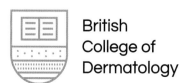

British
College of
Dermatology

WILEY Blackwell

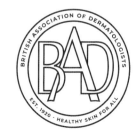

This edition first published 2022
© 2022 The British Association of Dermatologists.

All rights reserved. No part of this publication may be reproduced, stored in a retrieval system,
or transmitted, in any form or by any means, electronic, mechanical, photocopying, recording or
otherwise, except as permitted by law. Advice on how to obtain permission to reuse material from this
title is available at http://www.wiley.com/go/permissions.

The right of Mahbub M.U. Chowdhury, Tamara W. Griffiths and Andrew Y. Finlay to be identified as the
authors of the editorial material in this work has been asserted in accordance with law.

Registered Offices
John Wiley & Sons, Inc., 111 River Street, Hoboken, NJ 07030, USA
John Wiley & Sons Ltd, The Atrium, Southern Gate, Chichester, West Sussex, PO19 8SQ, UK

Editorial Office
9600 Garsington Road, Oxford, OX4 2DQ, UK

For details of our global editorial offices, customer services, and more information about Wiley
products visit us at www.wiley.com.

Wiley also publishes its books in a variety of electronic formats and by print-on-demand. Some
content that appears in standard print versions of this book may not be available in other formats.

Limit of Liability/Disclaimer of Warranty
The contents of this work are intended to further general scientific research, understanding, and
discussion only and are not intended and should not be relied upon as recommending or promoting
scientific method, diagnosis, or treatment by physicians for any particular patient. In view of ongoing
research, equipment modifications, changes in governmental regulations, and the constant flow of
information relating to the use of medicines, equipment, and devices, the reader is urged to review
and evaluate the information provided in the package insert or instructions for each medicine,
equipment, or device for, among other things, any changes in the instructions or indication of usage
and for added warnings and precautions. While the publisher and authors have used their best efforts
in preparing this work, they make no representations or warranties with respect to the accuracy or
completeness of the contents of this work and specifically disclaim all warranties, including without
limitation any implied warranties of merchantability or fitness for a particular purpose. No warranty
may be created or extended by sales representatives, written sales materials or promotional
statements for this work. The fact that an organization, website, or product is referred to in this work
as a citation and/or potential source of further information does not mean that the publisher and
authors endorse the information or services the organization, website, or product may provide or
recommendations it may make. This work is sold with the understanding that the publisher is not
engaged in rendering professional services. The advice and strategies contained herein may not be
suitable for your situation. You should consult with a specialist where appropriate. Further, readers
should be aware that websites listed in this work may have changed or disappeared between when
this work was written and when it is read. Neither the publisher nor authors shall be liable for any loss
of profit or any other commercial damages, including but not limited to special, incidental,
consequential, or other damages.

Library of Congress Cataloging-in-Publication Data

Names: Chowdhury, Mahbub M. U., editor. | Griffiths, Tamara W., editor. |
    Finlay, Andrew Y., editor.
Title: Dermatology training : the essentials / edited by Mahbub M.U.
    Chowdhury, Tamara W. Griffiths, Andrew Y. Finlay.
Description: Hoboken, NJ : Wiley-Blackwell, [2022] | Includes
    bibliographical references and index.
Identifiers: LCCN 2021023722 (print) | LCCN 2021023723 (ebook) | ISBN
    9781119715702 (paperback) | ISBN 9781119715719 (adobe pdf) | ISBN
    9781119715733 (epub)
Subjects: MESH: Skin Diseases
Classification: LCC RL74.2 (print) | LCC RL74.2 (ebook) | NLM WR 140 |
    DDC 616.50076–dc23
LC record available at https://lccn.loc.gov/2021023722
LC ebook record available at https://lccn.loc.gov/2021023723

Cover Design: Wiley
Cover Images: Courtesy of Medical Illustration Cardiff and Vale UHB, Aneurin Bevan University
            Health Board, Dr Saleem Taibjee, and Andrey_Popov/Shutterstock

Set in 8.5/11pt HelveticaLTStd by Straive, Pondicherry, India
Printed in Great Britain by Bell and Bain Ltd, Glasgow

10 9 8 7 6 5 4 3 2 1

Contents

Preface

There are plenty of excellent reference books to turn to when wanting more facts about a skin disease. This book seeks to meet a different need. At the start of training in dermatology, how does one go about making sense of such a completely new discipline? All those years of training in the broader aspects of internal medicine are essential to build upon, but this book provides an effective framework that lays down the fundamentals required to rapidly upskill and work effectively in a demanding dermatology training post.

As an introductory training textbook, it is key reading for the novice in dermatology. The contributors are actively engaged in dermatology education as trainers or trainees. This combination of experience and current insight into what a new trainee really needs to know gives the pages direct relevance to many aspects of a trainee's day. The book is packed with practical tips including, for example, how to handle common clinical situations, how to develop leadership skills, how to begin to get into research and how to gain surgical experience. It also provides insights into future directions for many aspects of our specialty, which aim to stimulate and inspire.

Key topics from the 2021 UK dermatology training curriculum are introduced in the 29 chapters. There is particular reference to the new assessment tool, Capabilities in Practice (CiPs), which evaluates the trainee's ability to deliver and perform in the workplace. Read early in training, the chapters will provide a sound foundation on which to build further knowledge and map training progression. Specialty Certificate Exam (SCE) questions aligned to each chapter are included as a separate section to be used as a learning tool and to assist exam preparation.

The sequence of chapters within the specific book sections attempts to mirror how a trainee would ideally wish to progress their own development. They will need to gain professional skills, learn the essentials for effective clinical practice, and expand general and emergency dermatology knowledge. Introduction to subspecialty elements may spark interest for consideration of further training in a post-CCT fellowship approved by the British Association of Dermatologists (BAD).

It is vital that we all acknowledge the importance of diversity and increase our understanding of issues relevant to skin of colour, in order to optimise the care of all patients without bias, whatever background and culture. In addition to a chapter dedicated to skin of colour, we have throughout the book integrated images of disease presentations in various skin types, and incorporated relevant issues relating to skin diversity within the text.

As well as being of interest to trainee dermatologists, we hope that this book will be of help to specialist dermatology nurses, to general practitioners wanting to develop their practical understanding of the subject, and to medical students or junior doctors considering the possibility of dermatology as a career. It also aims to become the 'go-to' quick reference for educational supervisors to ensure that dermatology trainees experience and complete the entire curriculum. The book may help to identify training gaps when planning future rotations, study leave or assessments.

This essential introductory training textbook, commissioned and developed by the BAD, showcases the high standard of UK postgraduate dermatology education. The 2021 training curriculum, coupled with the BAD syllabus guidance, implements pioneering educational tools to deliver the entire breadth and depth of our expanding specialty utilising evidence-based methodology.

Finally, we hope this book will contribute significantly to enhancing knowledge and skills underpinned by professional values and behaviours to ensure a well-rounded, balanced clinician with expertise in skin health and disease.

We would welcome any constructive feedback and corrections for future editions.

Mahbub M.U. Chowdhury
Tamara W. Griffiths
Andrew Y. Finlay
August 2021

About the Editors

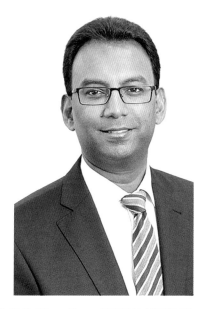

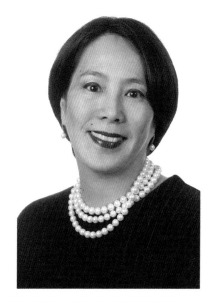

Dr Mahbub M.U. Chowdhury, MBChB, FRCP, FAcadMEd

Dr Chowdhury is Consultant Dermatologist at the Welsh Institute of Dermatology, University Hospital of Wales, Cardiff, and Honorary Senior Lecturer at Cardiff University.

He became President-elect of the British Association of Dermatologists (BAD) in July 2021, which will lead to the role of President in July 2022. As previous Academic Vice-President, he chaired the Education Subcommittee to update the new pre-CCT trainee syllabus implemented in August 2021.

He is Clinical Lead for Dermatology e-learning for Health and oversees 160 e-modules, which map to the new curriculum. He was Chair of the SCE Exam Board and Welsh Training Programme Director for 10 years. He has published over 110 papers and is co-author of the undergraduate textbook *Dermatology at a Glance* and Associate Editor for the 10th edition of *Rook's Textbook of Dermatology*.

His current interests include cutaneous allergy, and medical management and leadership. He has trained over 20 specialty registrars and supervised the first completed post-CCT cutaneous allergy fellow in the UK.

Dr Tamara W. Griffiths, BA, MD, FRCP, FAAD

Dr Tamara Griffiths is Consultant Dermatologist at the Dermatology Centre, Salford Royal Hospital NHS Trust, and Honorary Senior Lecturer at the University of Manchester.

In 2015, she was appointed Chair of the Royal College of Physicians' Dermatology Specialist Advisory Committee, responsible for all aspects of postgraduate dermatology training in the UK, including development and implementation of the 2021 curriculum. She was simultaneously elected as inaugural Director of the BAD Education Board, now recognised as the British College of Dermatology.

In addition to education, Dr Griffiths has a specialist interest in cosmetic dermatology. She was advisor to the Department of Health's Review of the Regulation of Cosmetic Interventions (2013) and Health Education England's curricula for non-surgical cosmetic interventions (2015). She is Medical Programme Director of the MSc in Skin Ageing at the University of Manchester, and Associate Editor for the 10th Edition of *Rook's Textbook of Dermatology*. Due to her commitment to education, training and standards, in 2021 she was named BAD Clinician of the Year.

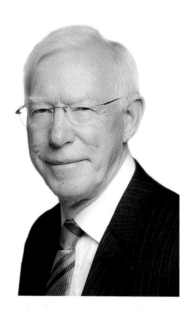

Professor Andrew Y. Finlay, CBE, MBBS, FRCP

As Professor of Dermatology at Cardiff University, Andrew Finlay created the successful international distance learning Diploma in Practical Dermatology. He co-authored the undergraduate textbook *Dermatology at a Glance* and has led dermatology training and education in Wales.

Andrew Finlay has held the positions of Director of Postgraduate Courses in the School of Medicine, Cardiff University and Chair of the RCP Specialist Advisory Committee for UK dermatology training, and was the UK representative on the European Union of Medical Specialists, with responsibility for dermatology training in Europe.

He has pioneered the use of quality-of-life measures in dermatology across the world, including creating the Dermatology Life Quality Index and other patient and family instruments. He has over 400 publications, and many of these have contributed to dermatologists and researchers being more focused on what really matters to patients.

Previously, he served as President of the BAD, and was awarded the prestigious Sir Archibald Gray Medal in 2020.

Foreword

The British Association of Dermatologists (BAD) is a charity whose vision is 'Healthy Skin for All'. To enable this, we strive to support and strengthen the education and training of all those involved in skin healthcare provision. For those starting a dermatology journey, *Dermatology Training: The Essentials* is the perfect first step.

Dermatology is very different from other medical specialties, as it not only covers adult medicine but also includes paediatrics, dermatopathology and skin surgery. There is a whole raft of new disciplines, treatments and terminologies that you may never have come across before. This book will support you in that initial steep learning curve and hopefully give you confidence and make you feel less overwhelmed!

Although it is relevant to all healthcare practitioners interested in dermatology, the book has been written to support the 2021 UK Dermatology Curriculum for specialist registrars. There are no other dermatology texts that achieve this, and the Editors, with their wealth of experience in education and training in dermatology, have more than met the brief. The 29 chapters, authored by renowned experts, cover the essential topics to support the first two years of training, with a 'how to' approach that is mapped to the new curriculum. There are also new Specialty Certificate Exam (SCE) style questions accompanying each topic.

The range of topics cover the essential building blocks and this will help produce a rounded, holistic training experience in dermatology. There are more than 4000 diagnoses in dermatology that affect the skin, hair, nails and mucosal surfaces, and all the common conditions are covered. Skin of colour has been embedded within the text, as well as in a standalone chapter, to ensure that all people with skin disease are represented equally. Practical information is covered, including advice on how to run a clinic, take a history, write a prescription, measure disease outcomes and take consent. The chapter on skin surgery is written for the novice, with advice on basic techniques, local anaesthesia, suturing and much more. Research is central to our specialty and the authors emphasise this with practical information on how to get involved and how to overcome the hurdles. At the end of each chapter there are 'pearls and pitfalls' offering excellent, practical top tips from experts. Throughout the book there are useful resource links for deeper learning.

Dermatology Training: The Essentials is the ultimate companion to someone new to dermatology. Congratulations to the Editors and authors, who have done such a superb job. I just wish that it had been available when I started my journey into this specialty.

Dr Tanya Bleiker, President,
British Association of Dermatologists

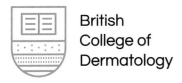

British College of Dermatology

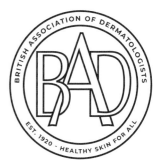

Authors

Alla M. Altayeb BMedSci (Hons), MBBS, MRCP, Pg Dip Clin Ed
Dermatology Specialist Registrar
Lauriston Building
NHS Lothian University Hospitals Division
Edinburgh, UK

Leila Asfour BSc, MBChB, FRCP (Derm)
Hair Fellow, Sinclair Dermatology Centre, Melbourne, Australia
Locum Consultant Dermatologist
The Dermatology Centre, Salford Royal NHS Foundation Trust
Manchester, UK

Ausama Atwan MBBS, MD, EBDV, FHEA, FAcadMEd
Locum Consultant Dermatologist and Honorary Senior
Lecturer
The Royal Gwent Hospital
Aneurin Bevan University Health Board
Newport, UK

Jean Ayer MBBS, BSc (Hons), MRCP, MD, FRCP
Consultant Dermatologist and Senior Honorary Lecturer
Photobiology Unit, Salford Royal NHS Foundation Trust
Manchester, UK

Sharon A. Belmo MBBS, MRCP (UK), MRCP (Derm)
Consultant Dermatologist
Croydon University Hospital
London, UK

Anthony Bewley MB ChB, BA (Hons), FRCP
Consultant Dermatologist
Barts Health NHS Trust
Honorary Professor of Clinical Dermatology
Queen Mary University London
London, UK

Raman Bhutani MBChB, MRCP (UK), MRCP (Derm),
DPD (Cardiff)
Consultant Dermatologist
The Dermatology Centre, Salford Royal NHS Foundation Trust
Royal Bolton Hospital Foundation Trust
Manchester, UK

Deirdre A. Buckley MB BCh, BAO, FRCP (Dub), FRCP (Lon)
Consultant Dermatologist
Circle Bath and Royal United Hospital
Bath, UK

Carolyn Charman BM BCh, MD, FRCP
Consultant Dermatologist
NHS England/NHSX Clinical Advisor
Royal Devon and Exeter Hospital
Exeter, UK

Mahbub M.U. Chowdhury MBChB, FRCP, FAcadMEd
Consultant Dermatologist
Honorary Senior Lecturer, Cardiff University
The Welsh Institute of Dermatology
University Hospital of Wales
Cardiff, UK

Mark Collier RGN, BA (Hons), ONC, RCNT, RNT, V300
Nurse Consultant and Associate Lecturer in Tissue Viability
United Lincolnshire Hospitals NHS Trust
Lincoln, UK

Donna Cummins MB BCh, BAO (Hons), MRCPI, MRCP (Derm)
Consultant Dermatologist
The Dermatology Centre, Salford Royal NHS Foundation Trust
Manchester, UK

Robert Dawe MBChB, MD, FRCPE
Consultant Dermatologist and Honorary Reader
Photobiology Unit, Department of Dermatology
Ninewells Hospital and Medical School
Dundee, UK

Giles Dunnill MBBS, MD, FRCP
Consultant Dermatologist
University Hospital Bristol and Weston
Bristol, UK

Andrew Y. Finlay CBE, MBBS, FRCP (London and Glasgow)
Professor of Dermatology
Division of Infection and Immunity, School of Medicine
Cardiff University
Cardiff, UK

L. Claire Fuller MA, FRCP
Consultant Dermatologist
Chelsea and Westminster Hospital NHS Foundation Trust
London, UK

Karen Gibbon MB ChB, FRCP
Consultant Dermatologist
Barts Health NHS Trust
London, UK

Kristiana Gordon MBBS, CLT, MD (Res), FRCP
Consultant and Honorary Reader in Dermatology and
Lymphovascular Medicine
St George's University Hospitals NHS Foundation Trust
London, UK

Tamara W. Griffiths BA, MD, FRCP, FAAD
Consultant Dermatologist
The Dermatology Centre, Salford Royal NHS Foundation Trust
Honorary Senior Lecturer, University of Manchester
Manchester, UK

Roderick Hay DM, FRCP, FRCPath, FMedSci
Professor of Cutaneous Infection (Emeritus)
St John's Institute of Dermatology
King's College London
London, UK

William T.N. Hunt BSc, BMBS, MSc, FHEA, MRCP
Specialist Registrar
Department of Dermatology
University Hospitals Plymouth NHS Trust
Plymouth, UK

S. Walayat Hussain BSc (Hons), MB ChB, MRCP (UK),
FRACP, FACMS
Consultant Dermatological Surgeon
Leeds Teaching Hospitals NHS Trust
Leeds, UK

Sally H. Ibbotson BSc (Hons), MD, FRCP (Edin)
Professor of Photodermatology
Honorary Consultant Dermatologist
Photobiology Unit
University of Dundee
Ninewells Hospital and Medical School
Dundee, UK

John R. Ingram MA, MSc, DM (Oxon), FRCP (Derm),
FAcadMedEd
Clinical Reader and Consultant Dermatologist
Division of Infection and Immunity
Cardiff University
Cardiff, UK

Cherng Jong MBBS, MRCP
Consultant Dermatologist
Sussex Community Dermatology Service
Worthing, UK

Manjunatha Kalavala MD, FRCP
Consultant Dermatologist and Honorary Senior Lecturer
The Welsh Institute of Dermatology
University Hospital of Wales
Cardiff, UK

Ruwani P. Katugampola BM, MD, FRCP
Consultant Dermatologist
The Welsh Institute of Dermatology
University Hospital of Wales
Cardiff, UK

Thomas King MBChB, MMedSci, MRCP
Consultant Dermatologist in Adult and Paediatric Dermatology
Sheffield Teaching Hospitals and Sheffield Children's Hospital
Honorary Senior Lecturer, University of Sheffield
Sheffield, UK

Victoria J. Lewis BMedSci, MBBS, MRCP
Consultant Dermatologist
Aneurin Bevan University Health Board
Newport, UK

Tsui Chin Ling MBBCh, BAO, FRCP, MD
Consultant Dermatologist and Honorary Senior Lecturer
Photobiology Unit, Salford Royal NHS Foundation Trust
Manchester, UK

Richard A. Logan MB ChB, FRCP
Consultant Dermatologist
Bridgend, UK

Peter Mortimer MD, FRCP (Hon), FACD
Professor of Dermatological Medicine
Molecular and Clinical Sciences Institute (Dermatology)
St George's, University of London
Honorary Visiting Professor, King's College London
London, UK

Richard J. Motley MA, MD, FRCP, FAcadMEd
Consultant in Dermatology and Cutaneous Surgery
Honorary Senior Lecturer, Cardiff University
The Welsh Institute of Dermatology
University Hospital of Wales
Cardiff, UK

Ruth Murphy MMedSci, PhD, FRCP
Professor of Dermatology, University of Nottingham
Consultant in Adult and Paediatric Dermatology
Sheffield Teaching Hospital and Sheffield Children's Hospital
Sheffield, UK

Edel A. O'Toole PhD, FRCP
Professor of Molecular Dermatology
Centre for Cell Biology and Cutaneous Research
Blizard Institute, Queen Mary University of London
London, UK

Girish K. Patel MBBS, MD, FRCP
Professor and Consultant Dermatologist
The Welsh Institute of Dermatology
University Hospital of Wales
Cardiff, UK

Jane Setterfield BDS, DCH, MD, FRCP
Professor of Oral and Dermatological Medicine
King's College London
Honorary Consultant in Dermatology
Department of Oral Medicine
Guy's and St Thomas' NHS Foundation Trust
London, UK

Manu Shah MB ChB, MD, FRCP, PGCert Med Ed
Consultant Dermatologist
East Lancashire Hospitals NHS Trust
Burnley, UK

Maulina Sharma MBBS, MMedSci, FRCP
Honorary Clinical Associate Professor
University of Nottingham
Consultant Dermatologist
Derby Teaching Hospitals NHS Foundation Trust
Derby, UK

Lindsay Shaw BSc, MB ChB, MRCPH, MRCP
Consultant in Paediatric and Adult Dermatology
University Hospitals Bristol and Weston
and Great Ormond St Hospital
Bristol, UK

Lloyd Steele MBChB, BMedSci, MRCP, FHEA
Dermatology Registrar and Academic Clinical Fellow
Barts Health NHS Trust
London, UK

Anita Takwale MBBS, MD, MRCP
Consultant Dermatologist
Gloucestershire Hospitals NHS Foundation Trust
Gloucester, UK

Sarah H. Wakelin MSc, MBBS, FRCP
Consultant Dermatologist
Imperial College Healthcare Trust
London, UK

Acknowledgements

The Presidents of the British Association of Dermatologists, Dr Tanya Bleiker and Professor Ruth Murphy, and the Chief Executive Officers, Simon Morrison and Marilyn Benham, have all encouraged and fully supported this book project from the initial proposal to final publication.

We are very grateful to the outstanding publishing team at the British Association of Dermatologists (BAD), which supported the development of this book: Shehnaz Ahmed, Director of Research and Publishing; Imogen Richardson, Journals Administrator; and David Owen, Lead Technical Editor.

We wish to thank all the authors and Editors who generously contributed to this book with no payment. Any profits from the book will go to the BAD to support further education and research.

We wish to thank the authors of the chapters in *Specialist Training in Dermatology* (Finlay AY, Chowdhury MMU, eds. Oxford: Mosby Elsevier, 2007) that have been revised for this new book: Christian Aldridge (Practical management skills), Alex Anstey (Photodermatology), Avinash Belgi (Skin cancer), Sharon Blackford (Paediatric dermatology), Peter Holt (Surgical techniques), Colin Long (Infectious diseases and infestation of the skin), Andrew Morris (Laser therapy), Nicolas Nicolaou (Contact dermatitis), Anthony Pearse (Photodermatology), Angela Steen (Dressings and wound care), Richard Williams (Systemic therapy) and Diane Williamson (Dressings and wound care). We would like to thank Mosby Elsevier for releasing their copyright on the original 2007 textbook to the editors. This copyright was subsequently given by them to the BAD.

We are grateful to the following dermatology trainees for their constructive feedback on various chapters: Faraz M. Ali, Leila Asfour, Sofia Hadjieconomou, Kate Lawlor, Ruchika Kumari and Alexandra Paolino.

We wish to thank all the patients for having given consent for their images to be published. We would like to thank the clinical photographers of the Medical Illustration Department, University Hospital of Wales in Cardiff, for taking many of the clinical images used in this book. We thank Cardiff and Vale University Health Board, the copyright owner, for permission to use these images. We thank all other individuals and institutions for permission to use their photographs. All of the clinical images used from Chowdhury MMU et al. *Dermatology at a Glance*, 2nd edn, Wiley, are copyright of Medical Illustration Cardiff and Vale UHB.

While attempts have been made to identify and credit the copyright owners of the images used within the chapters, we apologise if any have not been traced or have been overlooked. Please inform us of any errors or omissions so these can be corrected in future.

We would like to thank the Wiley publishing team: Jenny Seward, James Watson, Samras Johnson V, Sally Osborn and Lyn Nesbitt-Smith (Indexer). Thanks to the Wiley artists who created or re-created many of the excellent figures in this book.

Conflicts of interest

AYF is joint copyright owner of the DLQI and other quality-of-life questionnaires. Cardiff University receives royalties from their use: AYF receives a share under the standard university policy. AYF is on a Novartis advisory board.

MMUC has been on advisory boards for Novartis, LEO and Basilea pharmaceutical companies and was previously a paid associate editor for the Essential Evidence Plus website.

TWG is co-director of skincare company CGskin and has been on advisory boards for Walgreen Boots, Allergan and Galderma.

Abbreviations

AA	alopecia areata		DIF	direct immunofluorescence
ABPI	ankle brachial pressure index		DLQI	Dermatology Life Quality Index
ACD	allergic contact dermatitis		DMF	dimethyl fumarate
ACE	angiotensin-converting enzyme		DPD	dihydropyrimidine dehydrogenase
AD	atopic dermatitis		DRESS	drug reaction with eosinophilia and systemic
AGEP	acute generalised exanthematous pustulosis			symptoms
AIBD	autoimmune bullous disease		Dsg	desmoglein
AJCC	American Joint Committee on Cancer		EASI	Eczema Area and Severity Index
AK	actinic keratosis		EB	epidermolysis bullosa
ALA	aminolaevulinic acid		EBA	epidermolysis bullosa acquisita
AMP	antimicrobial peptide		EBD	evidence-based dermatology
APTD	argon-pumped tunable dye		EDTA	ethylenediaminetetraacetic acid
ARCP	Annual Review of Competency Progression		eGFR	estimated glomerular filtration rate
AZA	azathioprine		ELISA	enzyme-linked immunosorbent assay
BAD	British Association of Dermatologists		EM	erythema multiforme
BCC	basal cell carcinoma		EMLA	eutectic mixture of local anaesthetics
BD	Bowen's disease		ENA	extractable nuclear antigen
BMI	body mass index		EPP	erythropoietic protoporphyria
BP	bullous pemphigoid		ESCD	European Society of Contact Dermatitis
BSA	body surface area		FBC	full blood count
BSCA	British Society for Cutaneous Allergy		FDA	Food and Drug Administration
BSDS	British Society for Dermatological Surgery		FFA	frontal fibrosing alopecia
BSF	British Skin Foundation		FISH	fluorescent *in situ* hybridisation
CAT	critically appraised topic		FPHL	female pattern hair loss
CBT	cognitive behavioural therapy		FTSG	full-thickness skin graft
CCCA	central centrifugal cicatricial alopecia		FTU	fingertip unit
CD	contact dermatitis		FU	fluorouracil
CDLQI	Children's Dermatology Life Quality Index		G6PD	glucose-6-phosphate dehydrogenase
CEP	congenital erythropoietic porphyria		GCS	glucocorticosteroid
CNS	clinical nurse specialist		GMC	General Medical Council
CPSA	Cosmetic Practice Standards Authority		GP	general practitioner
CT	computed tomography		GRADE	Grading of Recommendations Assessment,
CTCL	cutaneous T-cell lymphoma			Development and Evaluation
CTLA	cytotoxic T-lymphocyte-associated protein		GVHD	graft-versus-host disease
CU	contact urticaria		HCP	healthcare professional
CXR	chest X-ray		HCQ	hydroxychloroquine
DA	dermatitis artefacta		HDU	high-dependency unit
DALY	disability-adjusted life-year		HHV	human herpesvirus
DEJ	dermoepidermal junction		HLA	human leucocyte antigen
DEXA	dual-energy X-ray absorptiometry		HPV	human papillomavirus
DHEAS	dehydroepiandrosterone sulfate		HRQoL	health-related quality of life
DHSC	Department of Health and Social Care		HS	hidradenitis suppurativa

HSV	herpes simplex virus	PCOS	polycystic ovarian syndrome
ICD	irritant contact dermatitis	PCR	polymerase chain reaction
ICDRG	International Contact Dermatitis Research Group	PCT	porphyria cutanea tarda
ICU	immunological contact urticaria	PDE	phosphodiesterase
IDQoL	Infants' Dermatitis Quality of Life Index	PDL	pulsed-dye laser
IHD	ischaemic heart disease	PDP	personal development plan
IIF	indirect immunofluorescence	PDT	photodynamic therapy
IL	interleukin	PGA	Physician's Global Assessment
IM	intramuscular	PIH	post-inflammatory hyperpigmentation
IMF	immunofluorescence	PLE	polymorphic light eruption
IPL	intense pulsed light	PNP	paraneoplastic pemphigus
IVIg	intravenous immunoglobulin	POEM	Patient-Oriented Eczema Measure
JAK	Janus kinase	PPIX	protoporphyrin IX
JRCPTB	Joint Royal College of Physicians' Training Board	PPP	pregnancy prevention programme
KA	keratoacanthoma	PUVA	psoralen with ultraviolet A
KTP	potassium titanyl phosphate	PV	pemphigus vulgaris
LAD	linear IgA disease	QS	quality-switched
LE	lupus erythematosus	RAR	retinoic acid receptor
LED	light-emitting diode	RAST	radioallergosorbent test
LMIC	low- and middle-income country	RCP	Royal College of Physicians
LP	lichen planus	RCT	randomised controlled trial
LPP	lichen planopilaris	RePUVA	retinoid psoralen with ultraviolet A
LS	lichen sclerosus	ROAT	repeat open application test
MAL	methyl aminolaevulinate	RXR	retinoid X receptor
MASI	Melasma Area and Severity Index	SAC	Specialist Advisory Committee
MCC	Merkel cell carcinoma	SALT	Severity of Alopecia Tool
MCID	minimal clinically important difference	sBCC	superficial basal cell carcinoma
MDT	multidisciplinary team	SCC	squamous cell carcinoma
MED	minimal erythema dose	SCE	Specialty Certificate Exam
MF	mycosis fungoides	SED	standard erythema dose
MHRA	Medicines and Healthcare products Regulatory Agency	SJS	Stevens–Johnson syndrome
		SLNB	sentinel lymph node biopsy
MIC	middle-income country	SPF	sun protection factor
MM	malignant melanoma	SSRI	selective serotonin reuptake inhibitor
MMF	mycophenolate mofetil	SSSS	staphylococcal scalded skin syndrome
MMP	mucous membrane pemphigoid	STD	sexually transmitted disease
MPD	minimal phototoxic dose	TB	tuberculosis
MRI	magnetic resonance imaging	TEN	toxic epidermal necrolysis
MRSA	methicillin-resistant *Staphylococcus aureus*	TGN	thioguanine nucleotide
MTX	methotrexate	Th	T helper cell
NGO	non-governmental organisation	TJ	tight junction
NHS	National Health Service	TNF	tumour necrosis factor
NICE	National Institute for Health and Care Excellence	TNM	tumour–nodes–metastasis
NICU	non-immunological contact urticaria	TPMT	thiopurine methyltransferase
NSAID	non-steroidal anti-inflammatory drug	USS	ultrasound scan
NTD	neglected tropical disease	UV	ultraviolet
NTN	National Training Number	UVR	ultraviolet radiation
ODSS	Oral Disease Severity Score	VIN	vulval intraepithelial neoplasia
P3NP	serum procollagen 3 peptide	VP	variegate porphyria
PAF	platelet-activating factor	WHO	World Health Organization
PAS	periodic acid–Schiff	XP	xeroderma pigmentosum
PASI	Psoriasis Area and Severity Index	YAG	yttrium aluminium garnet

About the Companion Website

The book is accompanied by a website:

www.wiley.com/go/chowdhury/dermatologytraining

The website features:

- Multiple choice questions
- Weblinks

Section 1

Developing professionalism

Think critically, research and publish

Girish K. Patel, Andrew Y. Finlay and John R. Ingram

Introduction

This chapter describes how you can get involved in research, publishing and writing. Crucially, it describes the key concepts surrounding evidence-based thinking and decision making in dermatology. These concepts are the essential foundations on which you can build your thinking and clinical approach during your career. This chapter is designed to help you to strengthen your academic expertise, and to gain satisfaction from investigating and contributing your ideas to the wider dermatology community.

Why undertake research?

Dermatology is a dynamic research-led specialty. Skin-related research leads the way in many spheres of scientific endeavour in relation to patient care. The dermatology training programme provides an ideal opportunity to appreciate and undertake research. So what is research?

Research is the creation of new knowledge that builds on the established foundation of our understanding. Medical research, ultimately seeking to improve individuals' wellbeing, can take many forms, including laboratory experiments, clinical studies (observation or intervention), clinical trials, quality improvement projects and evidence-based summation of findings.

Find something that genuinely interests you. The demands on your time are great, but they can be managed. Research projects do take time to complete. Moreover, if there's a chance that things can go wrong, they invariably do and the only driving force to complete a project will be your desire to succeed. Supervisors look most of all for motivated individuals, as technical skills can be taught but motivation cannot. Research success comes from a motivated person working in a supportive environment.

Dermatology Training: The Essentials. Edited by Mahbub M.U. Chowdhury, Tamara W. Griffiths and Andrew Y. Finlay.
© 2022 The British Association of Dermatologists. Published 2022 by John Wiley & Sons Ltd.
Companion website: www.wiley.com/go/chowdhury/dermatologytraining

When should I do research?

As a junior dermatology trainee, your immediate priority is to learn safe and efficient clinical competencies. But make use of the time allotted for research: as your interest in research grows you can try to expand your research sessions, for example by cross-covering with colleagues. Start on a small project that you can complete within months. You will still be surprised at how long it takes to complete a project, and to present and publish the findings. Start the journey by writing a simple case report based on an interesting clinical observation, making sure that the patient concerned has given written consent for the clinical photographs to be used for medical publication. Then take care to write it up promptly and see it through to publication; a case report is often the first step on the publishing ladder.

What type of research should I conduct?

Evidence-based medicine is the production of clinical protocols, guidelines and standards, which can inform the development of clinical care pathways. Clinical audit is used to evaluate and improve the implementation of such pathways. These approaches form the foundation for improving healthcare delivery.

Clinical audit

During your training you will be required to undertake clinical audit, preferably in cooperation with a colleague. Begin by identifying an area of clinical practice that could be improved (Table 1.1). Next identify all the key components of the process, from beginning to end (Figure 1.1).

Define standards that you can measure for each component and the acceptable benchmark for this standard that will demonstrate efficiency. The standard needs to be clearly defined so that data collection is free of ambiguity. Poorly defined standards are the main cause of failure to implement audit changes.

Next choose one simple intervention to the process pathway that will result in the greatest improvement. Discuss your proposed intervention with the staff and patients who follow the pathway. Decide on the standard for this step. Write a simple protocol for the audit and get feedback from colleagues. Seek permission from your audit committee and carry out the audit survey. Analyse the data, identify how far current practice falls short from the acceptable benchmark, and present your findings to your department, including making a credible case for the intervention.

To complete the audit cycle, you will be expected to implement your change and repeat the survey. Good-quality audit projects can often be published, either as an abstract submitted to a national or international meeting or as a short article. You should aim to carry out any audit to a standard that would potentially make it publishable so that other departments can benefit from your findings.

Medical research

Medical research may be laboratory based, 'at the bench', or clinical, 'at the bedside'. However, the boundaries between laboratory and clinical research are often blurred, with an increased emphasis on translational research. Successful research is based on ensuring that bedside observations are addressed at the bench to develop new diagnostic tools or therapies, to be evaluated once more at the bedside.

Many clinicians naturally have a clear bias towards clinical research. All trainees should ideally participate in at least one clinical trial, as this gives great insight into the reality of gathering the evidence on which we base so many of our clinical decisions. By the end of your training, you should be comfortable formulating a clinical project and taking it through to completion. In addition to taking part in clinical trials, it is important to contribute to large data registries and to understand how the data from registries can influence patient care; for some trainees this activity may constitute the majority of their research experience.

Evidence-based dermatology

Before starting a research project, you should have a good understanding of the basics of evidence-based dermatology (EBD). This knowledge is also crucial to your ability to take an informed critical approach to your reading of dermatology articles.

EBD is the process of identifying relevant evidence to inform clinical decisions. There is a science to it, in gathering evidence and assessing its quality, and an art, in applying the information to the particular patient's care and making a clinical decision in partnership with the patient. The science of EBD is based on critical appraisal of evidence, ensuring that clinicians stay up to date with new developments as part of continuous professional development and lifelong learning. The Centre of Evidence Based Dermatology at Nottingham University provides an excellent source of relevant publications.

Critically appraised topic

The EBD process is nicely illustrated by the concept of critically appraised topics (CATs). A CAT starts with a clinical decision, for example what is the most effective and safe treatment for a middle-aged man presenting with erythrodermic psoriasis? A carefully formulated question is constructed using the 'PICO' format: **p**atient (demographics), **i**ntervention, **c**omparator and **o**utcome. The components of the question ensure that only relevant medical

Table 1.1 Clinical audit categories and possible examples of the process

Clinical audit categories	Examples	Standards and benchmarks	Initiatives to improve the process
Outpatient service delivery	Number of outpatients seen	100% patient attendance	Patient-initiated telephone or text verification of appointment
Training	Research time	3-hour phone-free time per week	Internal cover timetable
Patient care	Patient satisfaction survey	All patients should know their named consultant	Create an outpatient information pack
Care pathway protocols	Surgical procedures	Every patient should sign a consent form	Consent forms available in outpatients prior to booking the procedure
Drug safety	Prescription of azathioprine	Every patient should have a thiopurine methyltransferase assay	Drug checklist and monitoring sheet available to be incorporated into medical notes
Local protocols such as shared care	Methotrexate prescribing	No interruption in treatment or its monitoring	Make available patient-held drug monitoring cards and clear protocols of care
Professional body (BAD) guidelines	Treatment of non-melanoma skin cancer	Appropriate surgical margins for excision	Make a template to document each tumour type
National professional body (RCP) guidelines	Osteoporosis	DEXA scan for all patients under 60 years of age prescribed oral corticosteroids	Clear pathway to collaborate with DEXA service
National (NICE) guidelines	Appropriate use of biologics	100% of patients should meet criteria for receiving such medication	Criteria made available to all caregivers
Health costs	Generic prescribing	No patient should be on named drug	Create a pharmacy process to intercept any new named drug prescribed

BAD, British Association of Dermatologists; DEXA, dual-energy X-ray absorptiometry; NICE, National Institute for Health and Care Excellence; RCP, Royal College of Physicians.

literature is assessed, searching databases such as PubMed. The quality of the studies is also assessed to allow a judgement about the reliability of the evidence. Then the evidence is applied back to the patient to support a clinical decision. The final element is to consider writing up and publishing the CAT, to disseminate knowledge and provide a service to other clinicians encountering the same question.

Pyramid of evidence

There are several ways to assess the quality of evidence; however, a good place to start is the 'pyramid of evidence' (Figure 1.2). While expert opinion is often very persuasive, this lies at the bottom of the pyramid if it is not based on evidence. Systematic reviews, which combine the results of multiple randomised controlled trials (RCTs) by meta-analysis, are at the top of the pyramid because they typically contain results from many more patients, providing more reliable and precise evidence.

Systematic reviews

A systematic review involves a careful and comprehensive search for all the evidence pertaining to a particular issue. The search terms and databases examined are included in the published methods to permit replication. Where results from comparable trials can be combined, they are often presented in a forest plot (Figure 1.3). Each row of the plot represents results from a single trial, with the centre of the horizontal bar representing the effect size and the horizontal line denoting the width of the 95% confidence interval (95% CI). If the 95% CI crosses the vertical line of no effect relative to the comparator intervention, then the result is non-significant. The diamond at the bottom of the plot represents the pooled results, with its vertical axis showing the pooled effect size and the width of the diamond giving the pooled 95% CI.

High-quality guidelines are typically underpinned by a systematic review. A formal system should be used to convert evidence into strengths of recommendation, such as GRADE (Grading of Recommendations Assessment, Development and Evaluation).

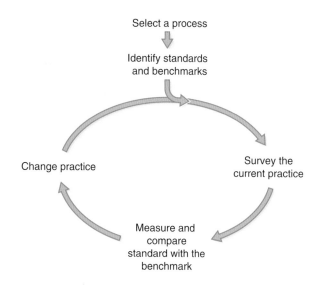

Select a process

Identify standards and benchmarks

Change practice

Survey the current practice

Measure and compare standard with the benchmark

Figure 1.1 The key components of the audit process. Finlay AY, Chowdhury MMU. *Specialist Training in Dermatology.* © 2007 Mosby Elsevier.

Randomised controlled trials

RCTs are performed to reduce the potential for bias to affect the results of a trial, so that they accurately reflect the effect of an intervention in the population being studied. Bias is defined as a systematic deviation from the truth ('moving the goalposts'), as opposed to imprecision, which usually results from small trials that can be influenced by a few outliers ('darts around the centre of a dartboard').

Randomisation is designed to minimise selection bias, giving an equal chance for the participant to enter any arm of the trial.

Performance bias, in which results can be affected by other aspects of care, are mitigated by blinding study personnel to the intervention allocated to participants. Be critical of whether blinding was really achieved in terms of the interventions being very similar in appearance, administration procedure and adverse effect profile.

Mitigation of detection bias can be achieved by blinded assessment of outcomes, for example using photos rather than assessing a participant in person. Attrition bias is the effect of dropouts from the study; extreme examples include loss to follow-up due to death or disease resolution. It is reduced by an intention-to-treat analysis and careful handling of missing data.

A CONSORT flow diagram (Figure 1.4) should be provided in any RCT report to allow readers to appreciate any loss to follow-up; the CONSORT guidelines contribute to the consistency of reporting of research studies. Reporting bias can occur due to selective reporting of the most favourable trial outcomes, and this can be assessed by reference to the registration document for the trial. All RCTs should be prospectively registered in a clinical trials database and the registration reference number should be included in the trial report and publication.

Case–control and cohort studies

Observational studies do not usually include an intervention. Case–control studies compare a variable within the target population, for example the rate of current smoking, to the same variable in another, control population. They provide information on associations, but generally cannot demonstrate causation. Cohort studies follow a group of patients over time. They can be used to assess whether exposure to a potential risk factor increases the subsequent chances of disease development compared to unexposed individuals and may provide insight into causation.

Figure 1.2 Pyramid of evidence.

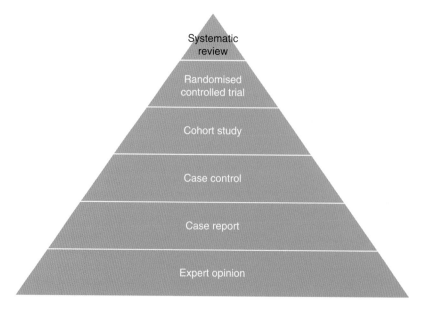

Systematic review

Randomised controlled trial

Cohort study

Case control

Case report

Expert opinion

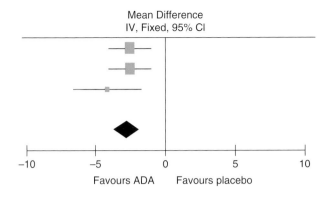

Mean Difference
IV, Fixed, 95% CI

Favours ADA   Favours placebo

Figure 1.3 Forest plot for improvement in Dermatology Life Quality Index (DLQI) scores for three trials comparing adalimumab (ADA) with placebo in hidradenitis suppurativa. Negative change scores represent an improvement in quality of life. The overall effect of adalimumab versus placebo is an improvement of 2.7 DLQI points (95% confidence interval −3.7 to −1.8 points). Modified from Ingram JR *et al.* Interventions for hidradenitis suppurativa. *Cochrane Database Syst Rev* 2015; **10**:CD010081.

Case reports

Case reports are at the bottom of the reliability pyramid for studies in humans. They are very likely to be affected by positive reporting bias, in which reports of successful treatment are more likely to be published than those in which the treatment was unsuccessful, providing an overly positive impression in the literature. Standards of reporting vary from case to case and it is important to carefully describe the patient, intervention and outcomes.

Where do I start and what are the hurdles?

Finding the hypothesis

All good research should start with a question, which can then be pared down to a yes/no answer. This is the basis of a hypothesis, a question that can be tested. Herein lies one of the great paradigms of modern research, that it is easier to refute a hypothesis than to prove it, thus favouring the setting for each study of a well-defined single research question (the reductionist approach) rather than trying to understand a system as a whole.

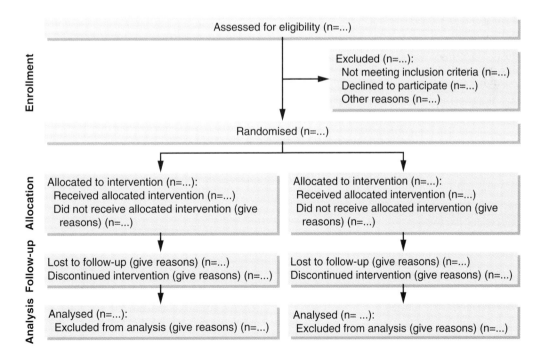

Figure 1.4 CONSORT diagram describing flow of patients through a parallel group randomised trial. Schulz KF *et al.* CONSORT 2010 Statement: updated guidelines for reporting parallel group randomised trials. *BMJ* 2010; **340**:c332.

Literature search and critical appraisal

Has anyone else thought of trying to test your hypothesis? If so, what approach did they use? To answer these questions, you need to conduct a literature search. This involves four main challenges:

- Deciding where to search.
- Using the defined research question (the hypothesis) to devise a search strategy.
- Critical appraisal of the information collected.
- Storage of references for easy access.

Searching PubMed, with or without Boolean search operations, is a minimum requirement. Limit your search by subheadings (e.g. aetiology, treatment) or language, age group or publication year. There are numerous other search engines that may be more appropriate, including Google Scholar, OVID, Web of Science, Cochrane Database and Embase. Use phrases in inverted commas and be careful to look at the URLs (e.g. .ac = academic, .edu = US university).

Do not forget the old-fashioned ways that still work: the use of an up-to-date textbook, review articles and most importantly cross-referencing (looking up the references within an article).

The hardest part of the process is to prioritise and carefully go through all the papers. Critical appraisal is a way to rationalise the papers you amass. Some basic questions to always ask yourself are listed in Table 1.2; for further guidance read the articles by Trisha Greenhalgh on how to read a paper (see Further Reading).

Writing a protocol

Even the simplest clinical study needs a clear, detailed written protocol before starting. This is essential for institutional permission, ethical review and financial planning. The intellectual process of thinking about and writing a protocol is an essential basis for ensuring that the work is successful.

Table 1.2 Critical appraisal: how to question

Critical appraisal

	Yes	No
Do I know the research group and can I trust it?		
Is there a relevant question?		
Is it clearly focused, in terms of the population, methods and outcomes?		
Is this the best or correct method to answer the question?		
Is the population studied correct and accounted for?		
Was the study randomised and blinded?		
Are the compared groups similar?		
Apart from the intervention, were both groups treated the same?		
Was the study effect large enough?		
Did they consider confounding and bias?		
Was the follow-up long enough?		
Are the data shown clearly interpretable?		
Are the statistics okay?		
Is the study funding described?		
Is it applicable locally?		

1. Protocol housekeeping

The protocol will go through several versions before it is ready to submit for review. First write the date and the draft number, '1'. Update this heading for each version: the date is the most useful as draft numbers can get muddled.

2. Title of study

Choose a clear, descriptive and preferably interesting study title. The title should include keywords that search engines are likely to use to find your article. Avoid acronyms.

3. Researchers involved

Decide who you want involved in the study, get their agreement and list their names. This list defines who you can expect to contribute. It also defines who will expect to gain authorship on abstracts and publications. Many journals now publish a description for each author of their individual contribution. Discuss and resolve all authorship issues (if any) before you submit, as these can cause problems at the publication or post-publication stage and even delay publication.

4. Background

Three or four paragraphs of background information are essential to convince the ethical and other committees that the work is worth doing. Describe how the current published work has led to a certain level of understanding about the subject, and clarify how the proposed study leads logically forward, by addressing unanswered questions (hypothesis). Reference the background, including the most relevant recent references. The work in writing the protocol background is not 'wasted', as it can be used as the basis of the introductory paragraphs of the study report, abstract or publication.

5. Decide the aims

It is essential to write down a clear aim for any proposed study. Identify as few aims as possible, preferably only one. State the main aim and the question to be answered. Document any secondary aims that provide useful confirmatory information.

6. Method (study design)

In writing the methods section, you should plan to give enough detail so that the study could be carried out successfully even without your involvement. Think through the reality of the study, imagining every step, anticipating questions that may arise and writing down the instructions. Clarify whether the study is an open study, controlled, single or double blinded.

7. Patient selection

Define the entry criteria, for instance define the disease or level of activity of disease for entry, and the sex and age range. Define exclusion criteria, such as pregnancy or presence of other diseases. Decide on the number of patients to be studied, with advice from a statistician. Consider ethnic diversity issues in your recruitment strategy. Describe how and where patients will be recruited in a timely manner. In deciding these limitations, be aware of selection biases influencing the study outcome.

8. Controls

If you are planning to include controls in the study, they need to be defined with as much care as the test group. State how you are to match the controls to the patients, and how you are going to recruit them.

9. Intervention

If a treatment or other intervention is being tested, you need to clearly define this. If you are studying a drug, you need to state the dosage and frequency. If the drug is topical, give clear definitions of how much is to be applied, and to where. Consider any techniques to be used to monitor compliance, such as patient diaries or weighing application containers. If the intervention is not licensed for the indication, you may need Medicines and Healthcare products Regulatory Agency (MHRA) approval; talk through your plans with the local research and development (R&D) department, who will guide you.

10. Assessment criteria

How will you know if the proposed intervention has worked? If there are published CORE Outcome Measures, include these if possible. All measures should be clearly defined, for example use of the Psoriasis Area and Severity Index in a study on psoriasis. The assessment methods should be as simple as possible, and you should give consideration to defining reproducibility between observers. Consider the use of objective quantitative methods if available, such as ultrasound to measure psoriasis plaque thickness.

11. Patient information sheet

The patient information sheet is an integral part of any protocol. Write it in simple English, using straightforward and non-technical terms. Be honest. Use clear paragraph headings. The Health Research Authority provides templates (see Useful websites).

12. Patient consent form

This is an integral part of the protocol. You will need to adhere to local institutional guidelines and national requirements. Usually you will require forms that are signed and witnessed.

13. Statistician

Discuss the protocol with a statistician before submitting the study for R&D approval. Advice on the number of patients, data collection and design is very helpful at this stage. It is no good going to a statistician after a study has been completed, seeking help on the interpretation of data, and discovering that there are fundamental avoidable mistakes in the study design.

14. Costing

All studies use resources. These resources need to be costed and you need to decide who will pay. Remember in costing studies that realistic estimates need to be made about how much time you and your co-workers will spend on the study. Remember to include secretarial time, nursing time and patient expenses (see Seeking support and funding).

15. Indemnity

It is essential to clarify the indemnity arrangement for any study involving patients or other volunteers. Indemnity may be provided by an NHS Trust R&D department, university and/or pharmaceutical company. Personal insurance cover is also essential. Seek advice about these matters.

16. Ethical approval

Any study involving patients or volunteers must be approved by the appropriate R&D department and ethical committee *before* it begins.

Seeking support and funding

Securing funding is a major challenge for all academic dermatologists. Government funds, such as from the Medical Research Council, are in very short supply, and so most researchers rely heavily upon charitable foundations such as the British Skin Foundation (BSF). Alternative sources of funding include grants from pharmaceutical companies or departmental funds.

Try to quickly seek and identify a senior staff member capable of getting research funding and ask for their advice. If you have decided on an academic career, consider the trainee fellowships offered by the Medical Research Council or Wellcome Trust.

The path to successful research

Learn to say 'no'

For some researchers this represents the biggest barrier to success. When undertaking research, especially in the laboratory, interruptions such as your phone can ruin your concentration and eat into your time. It is simply not possible to complete all the tasks asked of you. Hence you have to be able to prioritise and develop the ability to say 'no' with sincerity and diplomacy, within the limits of your employment contract.

Pick and choose your projects carefully. Select projects that you can see being completed in a practical timeframe. Stagger projects, so that at any one time you are not writing up two projects simultaneously. Plan some slack into your schedule, because interruptions are likely to occur in your clinical practice.

The mentor

We all need mentors to guide us through difficult career decisions. Choose your mentor carefully. A good mentor will listen and understand the issues that concern you. Most importantly, they will give you advice that you can trust even when it is unfavourable.

Clear questions, ideal methods and data analysis

Choosing the correct research question to answer is the single most important factor in defining the success of a project. The best scientific papers resolve hypotheses that everyone can understand and thus their relevance is far-reaching. The ability to identify such opportunities comes from an in-depth understanding of the subject area, experience and a creative intellect. Though you should always strive to use the best methodological approach to address the hypothesis, this has to be balanced against the time it takes to derive results. Statistical analysis provides confidence against a chance finding. There are many statistical approaches and although you should have a basic idea of statistical techniques, it is prudent to consult with a statistician before carrying out a project.

Publish or perish

A clear measure of success is the ability to publish, hence the phrase 'publish or perish'. Publications can take the form of an abstract, case report, basic science or clinical trial paper, review article or book chapter. For some people writing comes naturally, though for most of us it is a skill that we acquire by practice. Choose the journal to publish in carefully. A good measure of the strength of a journal is the number of times articles within it are cited. The journal's impact factor is also used when measuring the success of an academic department (Table 1.3). Other measures of impact include downloads, social media impact and a range of other measures as captured by Altmetrics.

The pathway to publication is often fraught with traps and delays, particularly for your first publication, but stick at it and you will prevail. The process takes much longer than may seem possible.

How to write the first draft of your article

The most common reason that clinical research studies are not published is that they are never submitted for publication. This is how to avoid that depressing outcome.

Table 1.3 Impact factors for journals (2020)

Journal	Impact factor
Scientific journals (selected)	
Nature Medicine	53
Nature	49
Science	47
Cell	42
Journal of Clinical Investigation	15
General medical journals (selected)	
New England Journal of Medicine	91
The Lancet	79
Journal of the American Medical Association	56
BMJ	40
Annals of Internal Medicine	25
PLOS Medicine	11
Dermatology journals (top five)	
Journal of the American Academy of Dermatology	11.5
JAMA Dermatology	10.3
British Journal of Dermatology	9.3
Journal of Investigative Dermatology	8.6
American Journal of Clinical Dermatology	7.4

Based on The Clarivate Analytics Impact Factor, Clarivate. Available at https://clarivate.com/webofsciencegroup/essays/impact-factor.

First, immediately a study is completed, sit down and start writing. If you have not written an article based on a clinical research study before, you may need help in overcoming the initial 'how do I start?' confusion. In fact, the task is not as difficult as it seems (Table 1.4).

Write '1st draft. Date. Your name.' On the next line give the title of the paper. Next write the names of all the authors, with your name first. Then give the institution(s) that employ the authors. Next write your contact address, telephone, email and address for correspondence. Also give your ORCID number: this is the 'Open Researcher and Contributor ID' number that is unique to you and facilitates recognition and author identification accuracy within the research community. Register for yours if you have not done so already (see Useful websites). Following this, the first heading is Abstract or Summary. After this leave a blank for the time being; this can be completed later. The next heading is Introduction. You wrote this some time ago as the 'Background' paragraphs for the protocol. Cut and paste it across; you may need to make some minor adjustments, such as in the tenses used.

The next heading is Methods. Again, all of the details are already in the protocol, so you can also copy this and make any necessary minor changes. The Results heading is next. Start to write this as completely as possible, leaving blanks where the data have not yet been analysed. Having this template also makes the process of data analysis more focused. The next heading is Discussion. You can usually write at least half of this without the final results being ready. This is where you can raise issues, difficulties or perceived weaknesses of the study – better to point these out rather than having the manuscript turned down. You should place the results in context with other previously published work, some of which you may have referred to in the Introduction.

The next heading is Acknowledgements. Here you can thank those who have contributed but whose contributions were not sufficient to warrant authorship. You can also thank patients or doctors who helped recruit participants. You can acknowledge funding here. Remember to list any conflict of interest either here or in the covering letter to the editor when the manuscript is submitted.

Each time you mention a reference in the text, add the details to the list of References. Use the Vancouver style, a numbered system also described as the 'author–number' system, as used by the *British Journal of Dermatology* and most medical journals. Although you may be using reference manager software, you may have to tweak the final version of the reference list to ensure that it complies with the journal's specific requirements.

List Tables and Figures, along with a descriptor for each. Then provide each table and figure on a separate page, or as separate files, depending on the journal's requirements.

After getting this far, you are already halfway there, and most importantly you have a first draft, which must now be reviewed and amended by the co-authors. Decide which journal you will submit the article to first and read the 'instructions for authors' for that journal. Reformat the manuscript as necessary. Now you should evaluate the data with a statistician. Put the results into a second draft and circulate it to all co-authors. Redraft, rewrite, redraft, rewrite. The main author often bears much of the burden of the work, but encourage your co-authors to contribute, and in a timely fashion. If slow responses are delaying things, politely give deadlines, stating that you will continue anyway if they are not met. The process of preparing the manuscript can often take discouraging turns, over which you must be resilient. Finally, do not rest until the manuscript has been fully submitted for publication. Remember that an important criterion for submission is that all co-authors must approve of the submitted manuscript.

You must expect either to be asked to make various changes or for the manuscript to be rejected. If you are asked to make changes, go to considerable trouble to answer and to try to meet every suggestion. This is the best way to ensure eventual acceptance. If the manuscript is rejected, do not be discouraged; rejection is normal in the academic world. Make changes

Table 1.4 Rapid guide to writing your manuscript

Title page	Write draft number, date and your name
	Title
	List of authors and institutions
	Correspondence details
Introduction	This should be a broad description leading to the question your study addresses
	Mostly derived from the protocol
Methods	Mostly derived from the protocol
Results	Give a detailed summary of all the findings in a logical order
Discussion	This should put your study findings into the context of the known literature
	Discuss perceived difficulties, weaknesses and strengths of your study
Acknowledgements	Thank those whose contribution is not sufficient to warrant authorship
	Funding sources
	Conflict of interests statement
References	Begin with the Vancouver style, though this may change depending on the journal to which you plan to submit
Legends	Should clearly describe the data presented in the figures
Figures and tables	These should consist of stand-alone data, easily interpreted with the help of the legend

based on the referees' comments, but do not give up; identify another journal and resubmit. Never be tempted to submit the same manuscript to two journals at the same time, however. Such 'duplicate publication' is forbidden by most journals (with rare exceptions such as guideline publication) and is considered a major academic offence.

Full-time research and higher degrees

If you find the challenge of research enticing, the time restraints imposed by clinical training become burdensome. A practical approach is to devote a period of your career to full-time research. Such positions are sought after and usually mean a drop in salary unless they are linked to clinical tasks. If you are committed to this kind of career change, you must seriously consider the merits of completing a higher degree, an MD or PhD. A higher degree is desirable for a successful academic career.

An important factor is the ability to retain a training post or National Training Number (NTN) during the time away from direct patient care, without which of course you cannot complete training as a dermatologist. Postgraduate deans may allow time out of programme for research, which must be pre-agreed with all relevant supervisors.

Fellowships and research abroad

If you are bitten by the research bug, completing a higher degree reinforces the need to apply for a substantive postdoctoral position in order to master the skills necessary to conduct independent research. This has major implications for developing clinical skills and also revalidation.

You should only consider a research position during your final year or after completion of specialist training, in order to allow the greatest flexibility. Do not exit a training programme and risk re-applying for training positions when returning to clinical work. There are other important considerations, such as funding (e.g. fellowships), the project and its location. Many individuals, rightly or wrongly, believe that such a post should be abroad, such as in the USA, Australia or Europe. Though many institutions will support funding applications, it is difficult to maintain one's clinical or previous level of income during research.

But in the end. . .

Whether or not you decide to pursue your academic endeavours to postdoctoral level or beyond, at the heart of your dermatology career there should remain a desire to maintain or support research. All forms of research can be continued whilst in a senior or consultant post and there are many such successful examples in the UK. It is important to realise that research offers a mindset that questions and answers the uncertainties that surround us in daily practice. By participating in research, you will enrich your own career, as well as impacting directly on the future wellbeing of your patients.

Pearls and pitfalls

- Choose your co-authors wisely: you need to work with colleagues who are interested in the project and who are committed to making it a success. Be aware that your co-authors may have other work priorities.
- The most common reason for research not getting published is the manuscript never being submitted. After completing any research work, start writing it up immediately.
- Try to be resilient when facing research difficulties. It is normal for things not to go smoothly, which makes the process eventually even more rewarding!
- Do not take it personally if your manuscript is rejected. Work hard to build on the feedback, improve the manuscript and resubmit.

SCE Questions. See questions 5 and 6.

FURTHER READING AND KEY RESOURCES

Garcia-Doval I, Albrecht J, Flohr C *et al*. European Dermato-Epidemiology Network (EDEN). Optimizing case reports and case series: guidance on how to improve quality. *Br J Dermatol* 2018; **178**:1257–62.

Garcia-Doval I, van Zuuren EJ, Bath-Hextall F, Ingram JR. Systematic reviews: let's keep them trustworthy. *Br J Dermatol* 2017; **177**:888–9.

Ingram JR. The quest for excellence (part 2): reviewing a clinical trial for the *British Journal of Dermatology*. *Br J Dermatol* 2014; **171**:1277–8.

Ingram JR, Anstey A. The evolution of clinical guidelines for dermatologists: GRADE, AGREE and occasionally consensus by experts. *Br J Dermatol* 2017; **176**:3–4.

Williams H. How to reply to referees. *J Am Acad Dermatol* 2004; **51**:79–83.

Textbooks

Brian J, Schofield J, Gerrish K *et al*. *A Guide for Clinical Audit, Research and Service Review Activities*. London: Healthcare Quality Improvement Partnership, 2011.

Greenhalgh T. *How to Read a Paper: The Basics of Evidence-Based Medicine and Healthcare*, 6th edn. Chichester: Wiley-Blackwell, 2019.

Williams HC, Bigby M, Herxheimer A *et al*., eds. *Evidence-Based Dermatology*, 3rd edn. Oxford: Blackwell Publishing, 2014.

Useful websites

Albert T, Wager E. How to handle authorship disputes: a guide for new researchers. Available at: https://publicationethics.org/files/2003pdf12_0.pdf.

Clarivate. The Clarivate Analytics Impact Factor. Available at: https://clarivate.com/webofsciencegroup/essays/impact-factor.

DORA. San Francisco Declaration on Research Assessment. Available at: https://sfdora.org/read.

Equator Network. Reporting guidelines. Available at: https://www.equator-network.org/reporting-guidelines.

Health Research Authority. Consent and participant information guidance. Available at: http://www.hra-decisiontools.org.uk/consent/examples.html.

International Committee of Medical Journal Editors. Defining the role of authors and contributors. Available at: http://www.icmje.org/recommendations/browse/roles-and-responsibilities/defining-the-role-of-authors-and-contributors.html.

International Committee of Medical Journal Editors. Preparing a manuscript for submission to a medical journal. Available at: http://www.icmje.org/recommendations/browse/manuscript-preparation/preparing-for-submission.html.

Medical Research Council. Available at: https://mrc.ukri.org.

ORCiD. Available at: https://orcid.org.

University of Nottingham. Centre of Evidence Based Dermatology. Available at: https://www.nottingham.ac.uk/research/groups/cebd/index.aspx.

2

How to lead and manage

Ruth Murphy and Mahbub M.U. Chowdhury

Introduction

Leadership in medicine is a necessary skill to acquire. A good leader has insight into their own strengths and vulnerabilities. They will understand the team they serve, building a dynamic one that supports the achievement of a common goal. A good leader is able to listen and be flexible and resilient, reflecting the shared success of the team and accountability for failure. Development of leadership skills is an essential part of training and benefits from daily practice and regular reflection.

At the start of your dermatology career there is suddenly a very steep learning curve. It may be your first exposure to the specialty, which is both exciting and daunting.

Basic dermatology consultation and common therapies are not part of internal medical training, so many new trainees have not previously prescribed creams, ointments or phototherapy or ever carried out a surgical procedure. Lacking these basic skills can be very overwhelming!

The British Association of Dermatologists (BAD) runs a course to support new dermatology registrars, which provides information and moral support to help you bridge this gap. Clinical experience, a positive mental outlook and application will do the rest, with support from your educational and clinical supervisors.

The clinical environment in dermatology

Dermatology is largely but not exclusively an outpatient-based specialty. Job plans for dermatologists reflect this, with most full-time 10-session jobs containing at least five outpatient clinics. Historically, consultations have been entirely face to face, but in

Dermatology Training: The Essentials. Edited by Mahbub M.U. Chowdhury, Tamara W. Griffiths and Andrew Y. Finlay.
© 2022 The British Association of Dermatologists. Published 2022 by John Wiley & Sons Ltd.
Companion website: www.wiley.com/go/chowdhury/dermatologytraining

the future job plans are likely to accommodate various types of remote patient interaction. During an average four-hour outpatient session, you will not only see and treat patients but will also simultaneously lead, support and train a team of allied healthcare professionals to assist you in this task.

Most of your training in dermatology will take place in an outpatient clinic setting. It is here you will learn how to manage your clinical workload, interact effectively with colleagues and perform surgical procedures. At the same time, you will be supervising nursing staff assisting in core dermatology investigations and treatments such as patch testing and phototherapy.

Acquiring leadership skills will increase your effectiveness and enjoyment of the consultant or senior role. This chapter aims to provide guidance and top tips to help you develop a positive mindset and the essential skills needed to train and function in an outpatient clinic.

The role of a dermatologist in multidisciplinary outpatient clinics

Most dermatology departments have evolved over time to be pyramidal in structure with the dermatology consultant at the apex, managing their own clinical workload as well as simultaneously supporting colleagues to do their work. It is essential to focus on time management, prioritisation, appraisal and the development and training of other healthcare professionals. Regular reflection on how your clinical and on-call sessions run allows you to identify the areas where you can make improvements. Building camaraderie and a team spirit is very important. Being excellent at work *and* having fun is a worthy aspiration.

In the early years your focus and energy will be centred on patients' diagnosis and management, but with time you will acquire the capacity to support other colleagues in clinic as well. As both a trainee and a consultant, you will need to manage ward referrals, access inpatient beds and attend relevant management meetings. Some of you may wish to become educational supervisors or engage in clinical research, and your training will provide an opportunity to develop these skills.

Each day get into the habit of asking yourself what went well and, importantly, what could the team do even better and how can the group make this change together?

Acquiring the essential skills to manage an outpatient clinic

Starting out in outpatient clinics

The outpatient clinic serves as your training ground both as a junior and beyond, and as you progress you should continue to learn from your patients and each other. Dermatology is a

specialty with a high clinical throughput and great diagnostic diversity, which means that robust clinic flow management is needed.

It is important you work closely with your supervising consultant and the wider team to ensure that you develop your skills and that the outpatient clinics run smoothly without too many delays for either patients or staff.

When you know your clinical timetable commitment, meet with the relevant consultant in person or by phone to clarify a few key points (Table 2.1):

- Will the clinic run jointly or as part of a separate list?
- How many patients do you expect to see during each clinic? (Initially you may be supernumerary, with patient numbers adjusted accordingly.)
- What are the booking rules and how do these vary when either you or the supervising consultant are on leave? When someone is away, is the clinic cancelled or is there a reduced list?
- Does the consultant expect you to discuss all the patients or only those of clinical concern? Is a run-through of the patients expected at the end of the clinic or not?
- Does the consultant want to read your clinic letters?
- Is there a preferred time for carrying out workplace-based assessments? These might be booked at the end of the clinic or arranged at another time.

As you progress through your training with different consultants, you may wish to reflect on your preferred model of supervision in various settings for when you are in charge, working and training in multidisciplinary outpatient clinics. Your experiences, both positive and negative, will shape your future management and leadership style.

Table 2.1 Running and managing your outpatient clinic

- Know exactly which clinics you are expected to attend and when

- Record the numbers of patients you can see comfortably within the allocated time and discuss this with your supervisor. This number will increase with experience

- Be punctual, arrive on time!

- Inform your consultant with good notice if you will not be available for a clinic

- Decide whether you will dictate letters after seeing each patient (preferable) or whether you will do all of them at the end of clinic

- Establish with your consultant when it is best to discuss patients. These discussions may also form the basis of workplace-based assessments

- Determine whether biopsies are performed within clinic times or on a designated biopsy list; discuss this with your supervising consultant

- Get to know the outpatient nurses and work with them to optimise clinic throughput, anticipating monitoring needs such as pregnancy tests

Planning annual leave and study leave

Most departments now require at least six weeks' notice for annual and study leave, so ensure all requests are made in good time and in writing. Check that the clinic has been cancelled before you go on leave. It is always a problem when a clinic has been booked when you are absent. Anyone can make a mistake, and identifying that a clinic needs cancelling in advance is always preferable to finding out on the day.

Running the dermatology outpatient clinic

Face-to-face outpatient clinics are a team event occurring over a four-hour period. During your training you will 'play ball' in various positions within the team, sometimes leading and sometimes following. Take five minutes to review the dynamics of each clinic and how you might be more effective, or how the clinic may become more enjoyable and less stressful.

Some of the factors to consider are detailed below.

Running clinics to booked appointment times

Starting clinics on time or slightly before time is essential, to avoid having to play catch-up and the huge stress this causes. But sitting in the clinic room is not the same as starting the clinic! Be aware that as soon as you arrive you might be distracted by emails or a telephone call, or you might be asked to do other clinical tasks such as reviewing a patient in phototherapy. While some flexibility is important, if you find yourself starting late regularly, discuss this with colleagues and adjust the clinic and your practices accordingly. Ensure that your clinic time is respected and interruptions are kept to a minimum.

Remember Parkinson's Law, that (clinical) work expands to fill the time available, so the trick is to be busy enough to keep going at a good pace over the whole clinic without falling too far behind. This pace and scale need to be reflected in the booking rules for a particular clinic and will change in accordance with clinical experience and patient mix. A remote clinic can be just as challenging as a face-to-face clinic, or even more so, despite the apparent lack of patients sitting outside the door. Think about putting a 'clinic in progress' sign on your door.

Configuring the booking rules

Clinics are often built to a template that does not allow flexibility in the time allocated to each patient. Early on in your training you are likely to need more time to evaluate each patient and may be supernumerary for a short period, but this will quickly change.

In the first year, it is a good idea to keep a record of the number of patients you feel you can comfortably see in clinic and then gradually increase this after discussion with your clinical and educational supervisors. By the end of training, you should be able to see as many patients in an outpatient clinic as the consultant. If your clinic is always running late, consider whether you could be more efficient, or whether the booking rules need

to be changed. Getting the booking rules correct is an important part of professional happiness throughout your career.

Considerations when deciding on clinic numbers

Not every consultation requires the same time or resources. However, giving each patient your undivided attention, even for a very short period, will make them feel that they are valued and that their voice has been heard. By achieving this, a positive doctor–patient relationship is formed and in most cases it is invaluable and time well spent. Doing so quickly and efficiently is an acquired skill.

Being actively aware of those patients who need more of your time (and those who need less) is a skill you need to develop to avoid constantly running late. It is worth reflecting each day which patients have taken you longer and why. Dictating after each patient is preferable to dictating at the end of clinic and is more likely to accurately reflect the consultation. Feeling in control of your workload is important and key to reducing stress, increasing job satisfaction and maximising enjoyment at work, which in turn promote professional longevity and reduce risk of burn-out.

Think about the role of other members of the team and the part they can play in helping the clinic flow better. For example, could a junior colleague or medical student clerk and present new patients to you to maintain clinic flow when there are delays? Could nursing staff help with pregnancy tests or blood pressure measurement? Could parallel clinics be run by senior nurse practitioners or physician associates for skin biopsy or follow-up appointments such as drug monitoring?

The type of consultation the patient needs

In line with technological innovation and to meet the objectives of the NHS Long Term Plan, there is an increasing trend to use remote consultation techniques instead of face-to-face consultation (Figure 2.1). Chapter 6 explains image-based triage, consultation and advice and guidance. It is important to choose the type of consultation most acceptable to the patient that still allows you to practise safely. Use of appropriate non-face-to-face consultations can be discussed with the patient and their GP if necessary. Be aware that remote consultations are not necessarily easier, and often require decision making with less information than a face-to-face consultation. If doing regular teletriage and/or teledermatology consultations, your training programme should ensure good educational and clinical supervision, as well as ensure a robust governance process for this training and service need.

Overbooked clinics and complicated patients

There is high demand for dermatology services, so overbooking in clinics frequently occurs. It is best to see additional 'extra' patients in a formal clinic setting, as all clinical work needs to be clearly documented and managed appropriately. Think about

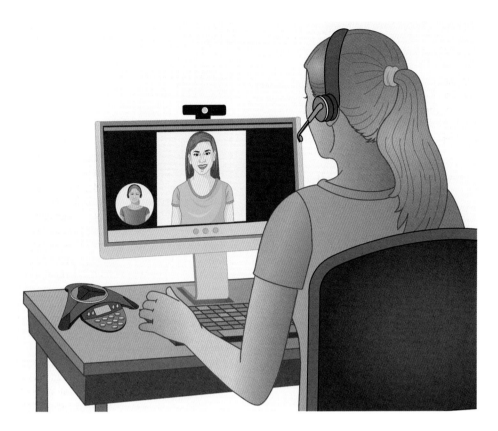

Figure 2.1 Remote virtual consultations can complement face-to-face meetings when appropriate equipment is available.

the most suitable time in your clinic to add an urgent patient. Overbooking at the beginning of the clinic means that the rest of the clinic will almost always run late. Booking extra patients at the end will allow clinic flow to be maintained, but the clinic may extend beyond the allocated four hours. A patient who is known to be complicated is better scheduled at the end of a clinic; if possible, schedule a double clinic slot. Relying on patients who do not attend to accommodate compensatory overbooking is not recommended. It is better to improve booking and patient reminder methods to reduce rates of non-attendance.

A repeated need to overbook clinics may mean that your booking rules would benefit from adjustment and you should consider this in the interests of both patient safety and your own and the wider team's wellbeing. An overbooked clinic on a regular basis probably means that more clinical sessions (and staff) are needed to accommodate the patient need.

How to approach the consultation

Regardless of the type of consultation (remote or face to face), after the initial introductions there should be three key components: the patient agenda, summary of the consultation and the agreed next steps. From the start, it is helpful to determine the patient's expectations and whether these can be managed in the time available or whether a further appointment will be needed. Most patients appreciate clarity and honesty in their consultation,

and sometimes benefit from time to reflect if a complicated consultation needs to be truncated and re-booked at a later date.

You will gain more professional satisfaction if you enhance the doctor–patient experience. This can be achieved by three key factors: managing clinical expectations, explaining disease prognosis and describing the anticipated time interval before a likely response to therapy.

At the end of the consultation, summarise these key components, check understanding and ensure that there is a clearly agreed plan for the next steps between you and the patient. Decide whether all the investigations you might be requesting are really necessary and explain this rationale to the patient. Always ask yourself whether these investigations will alter your management plan or just confirm what you already know. The next question to consider is whether a follow-up is necessary and, if so, by whom, and whether this should be face to face or done remotely.

Follow-up appointments: when, how and by whom?

There are various reasons why a patient might need to be seen for review and not discharged. These could include:

- Breaking bad news for skin cancer of metastatic potential, such as malignant melanoma and squamous cell cancer.
- Ongoing surveillance for skin cancer with metastatic potential.

- Commencing or monitoring systemic therapies.
- Assessing disease response to a therapeutic intervention, such as response of blistering disease to immunosuppressive therapy.
- Patient-triggered urgent follow-up due to disease flare or surgical complication.

If you have decided that a follow-up is necessary, then consider whether any other members of the dermatology team might be able to help with this. Specialist nurses can run drug monitoring clinics for isotretinoin and immunosuppressive therapies, and many perform surgical biopsies and excisions. Some patients with stable disease may be more than happy to take over monitoring their own disease and prefer discharge back to primary care (see the next section).

For patients stabilised on systemic therapies, actively use any shared-care arrangements between primary and secondary care to help minimise follow-up appointments. A patient-initiated follow-up or open appointment can be very useful and avoid routine consultation when there is no clinical need for it on a regular basis.

Think about which clinic appointments need to be held face to face and which might be more suitable for remote virtual consultation. Patient preference and equity of access will form part of this decision, as not all patients will have the necessary digital access or literacy. Disability may make use of a telephone or computer for an effective consultation challenging. Always ask yourself why you are arranging follow-up and who in the team is best placed to deliver this and why. Can the patient be discharged?

What to consider when discharging patients from an outpatient clinic

Whether to discharge a patient can be a taxing decision even for senior clinicians. Appropriate discharge decision making is a complex process and competence in leading a satisfactory discharge process for each patient is an essential aspect of clinical care. Outpatient discharge decisions affect the quality of patient care and the efficiency of clinical services. The process of discharge needs to be clear and may include advance patient discussions, patient training for self-care and liaising with GPs.

You can discuss individual cases with your supervisor regarding how appropriate it is to discharge them; some strategies are useful to consider (Table 2.2). A 'traffic-light design' dermatology outpatient discharge information checklist is useful to give some structure to discharge training (Table 2.3).

When to ask for assistance

During your training and consultant years, colleagues will provide formative feedback about your communication skills, time management and leadership, as well as your clinical acumen and communication. As a consultant you will need 360-degree multisource feedback prior to revalidation. You will continue to learn and develop clinically, and you will gradually learn to teach, train and assess others.

Table 2.2 How to discharge outpatients appropriately

- Have discharge in mind during all consultations
- Set expectations for discharge at the first appointment
- Where appropriate, prime patients by flagging 'possible discharge at the next visit'
- Ask patients directly if they want to come back
- Ask patients what they were hoping for from the consultation
- Be honest if you have nothing more to offer
- Allow extra time to explain reasons and plan the discharge with a patient
- Inform and summarise events and investigation results in a positive manner
- Prepare patients to self-manage
- Provide patients with a safety net for re-accessing the service
- Provide the general practitioner with a clear management plan

---

Table 2.3 Questions to ask yourself when considering discharge (traffic-light design)

Disease-related questions
- Can the patient be managed in primary care?
- Will the patient benefit from my follow-up?

Patient-related questions
- Have I explained a clear plan of management?
- Does the patient understand how to self-manage?

Addressing patient concerns
- Can the patient re-access secondary care easily?
- Is the patient happy to be discharged?

One of the most difficult questions for a trainee in outpatient clinics is whether or not to ask for assistance. Most consultants are happy to discuss any issues you have about patient care. Consultants expect less experienced trainees to need a significant amount of help, and clinic numbers are adjusted accordingly. It is in your interest and that of the patient to take every opportunity to discuss any areas of doubt, interest or clinical concern at your earliest chance, preferably during the session in real time.

Patients with unusual clinical presentations or with therapeutic dilemmas may lead to case-based discussions, clinically appraised topics, case reports or presentations at national meetings. Try to be proactive to maximise learning opportunities. Even as a consultant there will be times when you need to ask for help and seek the opinions of your colleagues on challenging cases.

Acute dermatology

Practising acute dermatology can be very rewarding for both the clinician and the patient. It is an opportunity to hone diagnostic skills and learn to manage risk and uncertainty in the clinical setting. Given the diagnostic diversity within the specialty, it is

Table 2.4 On-call cover: best practice

- Have a well-organised diary system for recording on-call commitments
- Ensure that the switchboard is aware of any changes in the rota
- Ensure that both parties fully understand any swap
- Record all swaps in writing
- The department should have accurate contact details readily available

Table 2.5 Ward referrals

- Try to attend to these on the day of referral
- ICU and paediatrics will expect prompt assessment
- Biopsies are best performed during normal working hours
- Write a concise and informed management plan in the notes
- If unsure, seek consultant advice
- Patients may need reviewing after initial assessment, as this provides service, valuable learning and an opportunity for a workplace-based assessment

also an essential part of demonstrating capability in practice for entry onto the GMC dermatology specialist register. Currently dermatology registrars are not required to undertake unselected medical on call, but they are on call for their specialty. Acute or urgent referrals can come from primary care and other colleagues, usually during the day. However, the clinical need to attend to them has to be prioritised around other daily clinical commitments, which means that some of the referrals are seen after clinic in the early evening. Tips to help you deal with on-call patients and ward referrals are detailed in Tables 2.4 and 2.5.

Good communication is needed for on-call rota swaps: the switchboard, wards, colleagues and secretaries should all be informed. When on call as a non-resident doctor, it is particularly essential to be contactable at all times. You can be sure that the one time you are temporarily unavailable will be the occasion when a serious patient-related event will need your urgent input. Some training programmes require you to be on call and conduct a clinic simultaneously; effective prioritisation can be challenging and strategies to optimise clinic flow may be best discussed with your supporting consultants.

Inpatient care

Not all dermatology departments have a dedicated ward with protected beds. It is common for dermatology units to compete with acute medicine for available bed occupancy. Inpatient dermatology care is undoubtedly more focused and productive when performed by trained dermatology nurses who have the experience, expertise and time to treat and educate patients on self-care. Where there is a dermatology ward, it is likely to be staffed by foundation doctors responsible for the day-to-day running

of the ward, and they can be supervised by a specialist registrar who leads their own ward rounds and makes management decisions under the guidance of the responsible consultant. It is the trainee's role to support the consultant on their ward round with accurate up-to-date information. It is essential to ensure that all decisions from previous consultant ward rounds have been actioned and all available investigations are to hand.

Nursing staff and day case treatments

Day case treatment is an intermediate form of management, falling between inpatient and outpatient care. As the name implies, this part of the overall care plan is designed to offer specialist treatment without the need to admit the patient. The unit is typically staffed by senior experienced nurses who can provide one-to-one care, and give informed advice and educational support to patients. There are advantages to using this service (Table 2.6).

It is important to identify in clinics which patients would be suitable for day care treatment and to liaise with senior staff running the unit to ensure full cooperation. It is essential that expectations from the treatment are realistic and are explained to the patient at the point of referral. With the increased use of immunosuppressive and biologic therapies, day case treatment attendances have reduced, but they still have a place for certain patients.

Table 2.6 Advantages of day case treatment

- Can avoid unnecessary admissions to hospital
- Allows for controlled, supervised application of treatment
- Reinforces learning points for patients and carers
- Allows for initial regular review without the need for outpatient appointments

How to demonstrate capability for inclusion in the specialist register

Capabilities in Practice

These are discussed in the Dermatology training section (page 429) and details can be found in the dermatology curriculum.

Workplace-based assessments

The Joint Royal College of Physicians Training Board (JRCPTB) has developed various methods of performance assessment, and all of these are important ways in which you will demonstrate capability in practice. These include:

- Mini-clinical evaluation exercises (mini-CEX).
- Case-based discussion.
- Directly observed procedural skills.
- Multisource feedback or 360-degree assessment.

Mini-CEX

The skills that are being assessed during the mini-CEX include:

- Medical interviewing skills.
- Physical examination skills.
- Consideration for the patient and professionalism.
- Clinical judgement.
- Counselling and communication skills.
- Organisation and efficiency.
- Overall clinical competence.

A mini-CEX is a supervised learning event used to evaluate a clinical encounter with a patient to indicate the trainee's clinical skills, and can be carried out in both outpatient and inpatient settings. It is recommended that trainees should be assessed by several consultants during their course of training using the Multiple Consultant Report assessment tool. The JRCPTB suggests that each mini-CEX should take approximately 15 minutes.

The outpatient clinic provides many opportunities to demonstrate these skills. Ask your supervising consultant when the best time to do this will be. Sometimes opportunities just arise and if they do, take them! Often it will be at the end of a clinic; at other times it might be scheduled for another day.

The mini-CEXs provide an important learning opportunity for both you and your consultant and can be great fun and provide affirmation of your ongoing progress. Never be afraid to do them and always seize the learning opportunity. Emergency patients with acute dermatology conditions and ward referrals can also provide cases for clinical assessment. As a consultant, you can record the number of work-based assessments you have performed to evidence your educational role within appraisal.

Case-based discussion

This is another form of supervised learning event used for assessing management of a patient, providing feedback on clinical reasoning, decision making and application of medical knowledge in relation to patient care. It focuses on active cases seen directly or managed by the trainee. Discussions can be completed easily throughout training if organised in advance, as the patients do not need to be present. Ideally, the medical notes should be available for a full retrospective discussion of the care provided.

Directly observed procedural skills

This focuses on the core skills that trainees require when undertaking a clinical practical procedure, which can be surgical or non-surgical. The trainee and consultant decide on a particular procedure. The consultant then directly observes the trainee performing the task. Let your assessor know in good time if you wish for a procedure to be observed. Take opportunities to free up time during clinic or surgery if they arise, for example if a patient cancelled or did not attend.

Multisource feedback or 360-degree assessment

This is a method of assessing generic skills such as communication, leadership, team working, teaching, punctuality and reliability. It allows objective, systematic collection and feedback of performance data that is derived from several stakeholders, for example nurses, other doctors, secretaries, clerical staff and other allied health professionals. The data from an average of 20 forms is collated to provide structured anonymous feedback. Try to obtain feedback from a range of colleagues, even those you feel you are not getting on well with. Multisource feedback is an opportunity for personal development and growth, as well as being used for assessment during your training and consultant post for appraisal and revalidation.

Teaching

As a specialist registrar, you will be expected to undertake teaching duties. Your heart should not sink at this prospect! Teaching can often be very rewarding. Medical students are attached to dermatology for only a short period of time, usually one or two weeks. With this brief exposure to the subject, it is imperative that learning experiences are maximised, as delivering a consistent minimum standard of dermatology teaching to all undergraduates is important to upskill the healthcare workforce.

Teaching a subject is one of the best ways to learn it. In dermatology this can take the form of bedside learning, slide tutorials, case histories, outpatient instruction and online e-learning modules and discussion sessions. There is an increasing use of webinars to teach at all levels.

If as a trainee you deliver a lecture, ask for a teaching observation assessment to be completed. As a consultant, always ask for feedback on any of the lectures you give, to add to your annual appraisal documentation. Try to embrace teaching and fit the teaching to the learning needs of the audience. Always encourage timely feedback and respond to this appropriately.

Personal development plans

Continuing professional development is a move from unstructured, traditional continuing medical education to the accreditation of structured personal development plans (PDPs). A PDP is a tool to encourage lifelong learning and identify any areas for further development. A similar model is applied as part of the appraisal and revalidation process of consultants.

The basis of a PDP is to reflect on your previous year and identify your educational and training needs to meet your goals over the next 12 months. The PDP is considered by trainees when they meet up with their educational supervisors and as a consultant within the annual appraisal process.

During dermatology training, it is recommended that trainee and trainer should meet at least three times a year. The initial session is to outline a PDP for the forthcoming year, which is important to identify learning needs mapped to the curriculum. The subsequent meetings are to assess progress and the success of this training plan.

Working with other colleagues

Primary healthcare

GPs are aware of the huge prevalence of skin disease, which accounts for up to 20% of all GP consultations, and this heavy workload is compounded by the deficiencies in their dermatological training. It is useful for trainees to develop an understanding of the pressures faced in primary care and to attend some clinics with GPs.

In the future, it is likely that primary and secondary care teams will work more closely together. In these new models of integrated and intermediary care, the roles of the consultant dermatologist and GP are both likely to change.

It is essential to be aware of the dermatology pathways of care between primary and secondary care in your area and to discuss how they may be optimised via local management and clinical governance structures.

Secondary and tertiary healthcare

When making referrals to other consultant teams, make sure you clearly document the main reasons for the referral. It is a good idea to inform and discuss with your consultant prior to sending a referral for advice and/or a second opinion. Miscommunication or wrong information passed between teams can lead to confusion, poor management decisions and dissatisfied patients.

The transition to the consultant role

Management skills

Newly appointed consultants often describe the transition from trainee to consultant as 'dramatic', and the hallmark of an effective training period is when this progression is described as 'natural'. As a group, new dermatology consultants commonly state that they have been poorly prepared for seniority, particularly regarding management issues.

Over the last decade the political landscape of the NHS has changed dramatically and will continue to do so, as articulated in the NHS Long Term Plan. The management courses available to the trainee are mandatory for completion of training; however, this limited preparation is only a starting point. Throughout your professional career, it is advisable to keep abreast of the wider political agenda in healthcare and local trust policies and management structures. Handling complaints, clinical risk management, clinical governance, PDPs and appraisal are all part of learning healthcare management. Job planning skills and business case development are other useful skills to acquire.

Appraisal

Specialty training relies on reports from supervising clinicians and educational supervisors to inform the annual assessment of progression. The PDP is the cornerstone of this annual progression and is good training for the annual consultant appraisal process. This is an essential component of a consultant's development throughout their career. It currently forms the main foundation for GMC revalidation, which is required every five years.

Appraisers should provide careful and constructive feedback, backed up with specific examples. Appraisees should be encouraged to give their perceptions of their consultant role without fear of reprisal. They should suggest realistic ways in which difficult areas of their jobs could be improved. At the end of the appraisal, the appraisee should have a set of written learning needs and objectives for the next year, and these should form part of their appraisal documentation (Tables 2.7 and 2.8).

Complaints

Receiving a complaint can be a distressing and upsetting experience. Patients are no longer passive consumers of the care that their doctors provide. Improved education, increased expectations, the internet, blanket media coverage of rare and extreme cases and a desire for compensation may explain the increasing number of complaints. Most doctors will face at least one complaint during their professional lifetime and many will come across several. Poor communication is the most important aspect of most complaints referred to the medical defence societies (Table 2.9).

Table 2.7 Learning needs

These may arise from:

- Clinical incidents and complaints
- Awkward moments with colleagues
- Important events, e.g. British Association of Dermatologists annual meetings
- External priorities, e.g. clinical governance
- Educational appraisal with tutor

Table 2.8 Appraisal points

- Appraisal is an integral part of working as a specialist
- It should be used constructively by both appraisee and appraiser
- Setting objectives is a key to success
- Appraisees must be able to discuss their development
- Appraisal requires time and should be undertaken in protected time, set aside and identified in advance
- Use of personal development plans should be encouraged
- Appraisal is a confidential process

Table 2.9 Minimising communication misunderstandings

- Set out what you intend to do in clear and simple language
- Avoid medical jargon when communicating with patients
- Make sure the patient understands – ask them to repeat what you have told them
- Obtain informed consent
- Write clearly in medical notes
- Provide information leaflets where appropriate (and record in notes)
- Make referrals with clear aims to other consultants
- Do not criticise other doctors or practitioners for patient care provided to date – even informal comments may trigger a formal complaint

Once you have received a complaint, it is vital to adopt the basic approach to handling this situation correctly:

- Do not take criticisms personally.
- Act very quickly and efficiently.
- Be willing to listen and sympathise.
- Provide an apology where appropriate.
- Give assurance that steps have been taken to prevent a recurrence.

If you are unsure how to proceed when a complaint arises, get in touch with your medical defence organisation. The hospital complaints teams are usually very helpful. If you are asked to respond to a complaint in writing, use the medical records to form the basis of a factual account only. It is important to respond in a rational manner and not with emotional reactivity, though this may be challenging. Do not give an opinion or view unless it is specifically asked for. It is important to remember that apologising for what happened is not an admission of guilt or liability, and a rapid apology may be very important to the person making the complaint.

Clinical governance and clinical risk management

Clinical governance is defined by the Department of Health and Social Care as 'a framework through which NHS organisations are accountable for continuously improving the quality of their

Table 2.10 Quality improvement activities

- Clinical guidelines and evidence-based practice
- Continuing professional development and lifelong learning
- Clinical audit
- Effective monitoring of clinical care
- Research and development

services and safeguarding high standards of care, by creating an environment in which excellence in clinical care will flourish'.

Thus, clinical governance aims to ensure that patients get effective safe treatment and that the risks associated with clinical care are prevented or minimised. Improvement of the quality of services can be undertaken through various activities (Table 2.10).

Healthcare risk is the probability of a patient suffering harm from a clinical activity. The risk may be clinical (wrong diagnosis, wrong treatment, faulty equipment), environmental (slippery floors, falling objects) or organisational (poor supplies, inadequate staff). Risks are minimised by recognition and prevention and by adhering and responding to good-quality audit at local and national levels. Familiarise yourself with risk registers within your trust and how these relate to areas of clinical concern.

Time management and its importance

Time is something we value increasingly as the years pass. However, it is a non-renewable resource and the most precious gift we can give to ourselves and one another. Whenever you make a decision to trade your time for something, first ask yourself whether the transaction is worth it: what is the opportunity cost? Make sure that you reflect regularly on how you spend your time at work and outside.

Procrastination and perfection are the thieves of time, so it is worth putting time boundaries around any projects and prioritising them accordingly. These are skills that require constant practice. Even as an experienced practitioner, make people aware of your time limits and protect yourself from unwanted interruptions. You can delegate appropriate tasks based on a planned strategy rather than 'dumping' or offloading work at the last minute.

Regularly reflect on whether you are achieving your goals and whether you are feeling generally fulfilled and happy. Try to achieve the balance you seek in your private and professional life and this should lead to you continuing to enjoy being a specialist in dermatology.

Conclusions

Learning leadership skills may seem very daunting at the outset. Most of us are not born leaders; we need to listen to, act on and learn from feedback from previous and continued experiences.

Be brave and consider volunteering for specific leadership roles that interest you and ensure you have sufficient time and support to perform the role properly with full commitment. There are many opportunities available via the BAD and its affiliated specialist societies and within training programmes and local departments.

Pearls and pitfalls

- Always check that your clinics have been cancelled in advance of planned leave.
- Ensure that your clinic time is respected and interruptions are kept to a minimum.
- Discuss with the patient (and their GP) whether a virtual consultation might be appropriate.
- Overbooking patients at the beginning of the clinic means that the rest of the clinic will almost always run late.
- Discuss follow-up and discharge plans with the patient, making sure that good support structures are in place.
- Patients may often prefer to be discharged back to their GP: ask them directly whether this is the case.
- Always ask for a colleague's support for any challenging clinical cases and maximise opportunities for learning.
- For a complaint, it is important to remember that an apology for what happened is not an admission of guilt or liability.

SCE Questions. See questions 55–57.

FURTHER READING AND KEY RESOURCES

Goldie J, Dowie A, Goldie A *et al*. What makes a good clinical student and teacher? An exploratory study. *BMC Med Educ* 2015; **15**:40.

Harun A, Finlay AY, Salek MS, Piguet V. How to train to discharge a dermatology outpatient: a review. *Dermatology* 2017; **233**:260–7.

Harun NA, Finlay AY, Salek M, Piguet V. The development and clinical evaluation of a 'traffic-light design' dermatology outpatient discharge information checklist. *Br J Dermatol* 2016; **175**:572–82.

Rimmer A. How do I prepare a personal development plan? *BMJ* 2018; **363**:k4725.

Textbooks

Abib-Pech M. *The Financial Times Guide to Leadership: How to Lead Effectively and Get Results*. London: Pearson Education, 2013.

Adair J. *Develop Your Leadership Skills*, 4th edn. London: Kogan Page, 2019.

Finch B. *How to Write a Business Plan*, 6th edn. London: Kogan Page, 2019.

Forsyth P. *Successful Time Management*, 5th edn. London: Kogan Page, 2019.

Useful websites

BMA. Medical appraisals. Available at: https://www.bma.org.uk/advice-and-support/career-progression/appraisals/medical-appraisals.

British Association of Dermatologists. A guide to job planning for dermatologists. Available at: https://www.bad.org.uk/shared/get-file.ashx?itemtype=document&id=6127.

British Association of Dermatologists. Delivering care and training a sustainable multi-specialty and multi-professional workforce. Available at: https://www.bad.org.uk/shared/get-file.ashx?id=6569&itemtype=document.

British Association of Dermatologists. Writing a business case for success. Available at: https://www.bad.org.uk/shared/get-file.ashx?itemtype=document&id=1885.

Faculty of Medical Leadership and Management (FMLM). Available at: www.fmlm.ac.uk.

General Medical Council. Continuous professional development. Available at: https://www.gmc-uk.org/-/media/documents/cpd-guidance-for-all-doctors-0316_pdf-56438625.pdf.

Joint Royal Colleges of Physicians Training Board (dermatology curriculum and SCE details). Available at: www.jrcptb.org.uk.

Kogan Page. Creating Success book series. Available at: https://www.koganpage.com/listing/creating-success.

National Health Service. Medical Leadership Curriculum. Available at: https://www.leadershipacademy.nhs.uk/wp-content/uploads/2012/12/NHSLeadership-Leadership-Framework-Medical-Leadership-Curriculum.pdf.

National Health Service. NHS Long Term Plan. Available at: www.longtermplan.nhs.uk.

NHS Employers. Consultant job planning. Available at: https://www.nhsemployers.org/jobtoolkit.

3

Ethical dilemmas

Leila Asfour and Andrew Y. Finlay

Introduction

This chapter is about those awkward or embarrassing situations that we all encounter as part of a clinical team. Ethical issues are rarely discussed and often not even acknowledged. But being aware of them, and knowing that you are not the only one who finds them difficult, may make it easier for you to handle them. In most circumstances there is no absolute right or wrong way to react, but different responses may lead to different outcomes, not all of which may be optimal. As a trainee, the ethical issues you encounter fall broadly into six groups (Table 3.1).

This chapter describes 18 hypothetical ethical situations. The scenarios are all inspired by real situations and illustrate the range of difficulties that you may encounter. There are several issues intermingled into each scenario; this is usual in real life. It is important for you to develop the insight to look beyond the 'presenting problem' and reflect on the wider picture.

You can use these scenarios to stimulate thinking about ethical issues, or even as an icebreaker to initiate discussion with colleagues. They may also help you to consider and reflect on issues you experience in your own practice.

How should you approach these sometimes baffling and worrying situations? Just as in the clinic, where you follow a plan, take a structured history, do a physical examination and develop a management strategy, you similarly need a clear framework to help you think logically and systematically about ethical problems (Table 3.2).

Dermatology Training: The Essentials. Edited by Mahbub M.U. Chowdhury, Tamara W. Griffiths and Andrew Y. Finlay.
© 2022 The British Association of Dermatologists. Published 2022 by John Wiley & Sons Ltd.
Companion website: www.wiley.com/go/chowdhury/dermatologytraining

Table 3.1 Areas of ethical dilemmas

Relationships with patients
Relationships with friends/chance encounters
Relationships with colleagues
Relationships with mentors/trainers
Professional standards
Conflicts of interests

Table 3.2 Structured thinking about ethical problems

1. Ensure that you have all the relevant information. Do not necessarily rely on just one source: it may be biased or inaccurate
2. Try to view the issue from the perspective(s) of each individual involved
3. Identify the different possible responses, including doing nothing
For each possible response:
a. Consider the practical consequences
b. Try to imagine how you would feel
c. Try to imagine how the other individuals involved would feel
d. Consider the unintended consequences that might occur

'Your mother should know'

(Figure 3.1)

A 15-year-old girl with severe acne arrives in clinic accompanied by her mother. You think isotretinoin is indicated and start to tell them about the teratogenicity risks. The mother rapidly butts in, saying that it's not relevant. The girl looks embarrassed.

What issues arise here?

- Gillick competence.
- Informed consent (see definition in Table 3.3).

How do you handle this?

This is a common scenario, both with isotretinoin and with other teratogenic systemics used in children. You must establish that you have a duty of care to the child. However, it is important to ensure that you maintain rapport with both child and parent in order to support the girl through her treatment. You can ask to examine her, to find a private

Figure 3.1 Your mother should know.

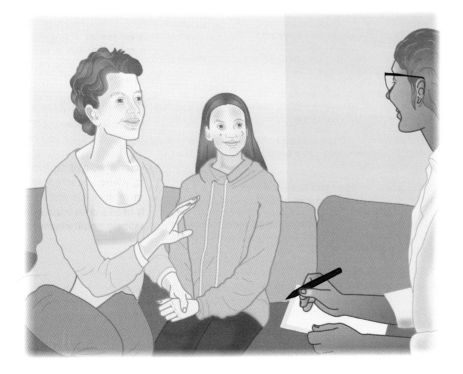

Table 3.3 Important definitions

Informed consent	• The process by which a healthcare provider educates a patient about the **risks, benefits and alternatives of a procedure or intervention** • The patient must be competent to make a **voluntary decision** about whether to undergo the intervention • Informed consent is **an ethical and legal obligation** of medical practitioners, upholding the core value of patient autonomy
Best interest	If a person 'lacks capacity' in relation to a matter, then other people can make decisions for them in their 'best interests' Based on Section 4 of the Mental Capacity Act, they must: • Consider the **person's past and present wishes and feelings, values and beliefs** • Consult, as practicable and appropriate, with others engaged in caring or interested in their welfare
Professionalism	The Royal College of Physicians' definition of professionalism in healthcare is: **'A set of values, behaviours, and relationships that underpins the trust the public has in doctors'** In day-to-day practice, doctors are committed to: • Integrity • Compassion • Altruism • Continuous improvement • Excellence • Team working
Probity	• Probity means being **honest and trustworthy and acting with integrity** • Be honest about your experiences, qualifications and position • You must be open and honest about any financial arrangements with patients and employers
Moonlighting	A secondary job worked in addition to one's main, primary job. For trainees, **moonlighting** may mean working as an independent **physician** outside of their training programme
Confidentiality	The right of an individual to have personal, identifiable **medical** information kept private. Such information should be available only to the physician and other healthcare and insurance personnel
Caldicott Guardian	A Caldicott Guardian is a senior person responsible for protecting the confidentiality of people's health and care information and making sure it is used properly
Negligence	Medical negligence is a **three-part test** whereby a **duty of professional care** is owed to a patient and as a **consequence of a breach of that duty**, the patient **suffers harm.** All parts of the test must be satisfied
Duty of candour	It is a legal duty to be **open and honest** with patients or their families, when something goes wrong that appears to have **caused or could lead to significant harm**
Duty of care	Healthcare workers owe a **duty of care to patients, colleagues, employers and themselves**. The duty of care to a patient exists from the moment the patient is accepted for treatment or a task is accepted and the patient begins to receive services
Gillick competence	• Gillick competence is concerned with determining a child's capacity to consent • **Children under 16 years can consent** if they demonstrate capacity to fully understand what is involved in a proposed treatment, including its **purpose, nature, likely effects and risks, the chances of success and the availability of other options**. However, as with adults, this consent is only valid if given voluntarily and not under undue influence or pressure by anyone else

moment to ask her if she is sexually active and on any contraceptive. This enables you to assess her capacity without external pressures. It is important to stress the risks of treatment and being open regarding measures that can be taken for her safety with both her and her mother present. It is vital to explain the concerns and outcomes if that treatment is not given. Of course, it is essential to record these points in the notes.

'You're my first'

You started your dermatology training post six weeks ago. You introduce yourself as a 'trainee dermatologist'. Your patient, a 52-year-old male engineer, has attended for an incisional biopsy on the face, which you have never performed before. Your supervising consultant has called in sick and you are running the theatre list on your own. The patient has been told that he may have Brunsting–Perry pemphigoid and he asks you about the prognosis. You really have no idea.

What issues arise here?

- Professionalism.
- Working within limitations and seeking help.
- Truth telling and duty of candour (see the definition in Table 3.3).
- Training versus patient safety.

How do you handle this?

Although you are keen to progress your surgical skills and logbook, it is important to be honest with patients about your skill set in order for them to weigh up this information during their consent. If you are not comfortable with undertaking a procedure, you should seek help or postpone it. Within the context of professionalism and probity, you must be honest with regard to your knowledge and experience. A possible approach would be to tell the patient you cannot answer their questions, but you will try to find out and can then address them personally or in a letter directed to the patient at a later stage.

'A picture's worth a thousand words. . .' (Figure 3.2)

A 23-year-old man presents with an odd annular lesion on his forearm; you are not sure what it is. You ask the patient if he minds you taking a photo with your smartphone; he agrees. Later, you text the photo around to three dermatology trainees who you recently met at a British Association of Dermatologists (BAD) meeting. Two suggest the same diagnosis, and you discuss this with the patient at the next consultation.

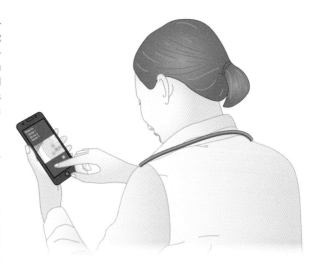

Figure 3.2 A picture's worth a thousand words.

What issues arise here?

- Confidentiality and information governance.
- Data Protection Act (important legal documents are outlined in Table 3.4).
- Social media and professionalism.
- General Medical Council (GMC) social media guidance and BAD digital software guidance (guidance documents outlined in Table 3.5).

How do you handle this?

It is crucial that the patient gives written informed consent to having a photograph taken with any device unless they have taken it themselves. Taking images with a device that is not organisational or securely configured is fraught with pitfalls. Before you take the photos, you need to be honest about who the images are being sent to and the benefit it may have to the patient's care. Consider using the images to obtain advice from your senior, who also has a duty of care to this patient. It is best that images are anonymised or pseudonymised. If a patient is sending images to you, they need to be aware that the transfer may not be secure.

Table 3.4 Key legal documents

Mental Capacity Act 2005
Human Rights Act 1998 (Article 8: Respect for your private life)
Data Protection Act 2018
Human Tissue Act 2004
Female Genital Mutilation Act 2003

Table 3.5 Key guidance documents

General Medical Council (GMC) Ethical Guidance

    Good clinical practice

    Confidentiality

    Consent and shared decision making

    Maintaining professionalism

    Candour and raising concerns

    Cosmetic interventions

    Research

British Association of Dermatologists Digital Software Guidance

GMC Social Media Guidance

Confidentiality: National Health Service (NHS) Code of Practice

Cosmetic Practice Standards Authority: Clinical and Practice Standards

Table 3.6 The 'four principles': a medical ethics framework used for decision making

Beneficence	Requires that the procedure be provided with the intent of doing good for the patient
Non-maleficence	An obligation not to harm others: 'First, do no harm'
Autonomy	Requires that the patient has autonomy of thought, intention and action when making decisions regarding healthcare. Therefore, the decision-making process must be free of coercion
Justice	The idea that the burdens and benefits of new or experimental treatments must be distributed equally. The healthcare provider must consider four main areas when evaluating justice: fair distribution of scarce resources, competing needs, rights and obligations, and potential conflicts with established legislation

'Can't get you out of my head'

A 62-year-old woman is very distressed as she tells you about the insects that are biting her, causing her great itchiness and sleeplessness. She shows you an envelope containing what she says has come out of her skin. You realise that this is primarily a psychiatric disorder and tactfully suggest that it might be helpful to see one of your colleagues in the psychiatry department. Three days later the hospital management informs you that the patient has made a complaint about you.

What issues arise here?

- Autonomy (an ethical framework is outlined in Table 3.6).
- Non-maleficence and beneficence.
- How to deal with a complaint.

How do you handle this?

This scenario is extremely challenging, as the doctor–patient rapport can be irreversibly affected. Apart from the management of delusional disorder, there are core principles that a clinician needs to be aware of. Supporting the patient's autonomy in decision making is vital regarding their ongoing management, including decisions over who should be involved in their care. If drugs such as antipsychotics are prescribed, there is a responsibility to be honest about their nature and to balance their benefit and risks to the patient and to the doctor–patient relationship.

    The key to handling patient complaints is very rapid and clear communication with the complainant. This should demonstrate acknowledgement of the patient's concerns and show that a

transparent investigation leads to a review of local policies and procedures. This includes drawing conclusions from the information obtained, discussing the conclusions within the team and drawing up an action plan.

'What doesn't meet the eye'

A 35-year-old woman tells you that she is very worried about severe itchiness 'down there' between her legs. You explain that you will need to examine the area in order to help her, but she refuses to allow the genital area to be examined.

What issues arise here?

- Addressing cultural barriers.
- Ensuring the patient receives high-quality treatment and care.
- Awareness of the mandatory duty to report female genital mutilation and of safeguarding.

How do you handle this?

An initial approach would be to assess what the patient's concerns are regarding the examination and how you can address these. Offering a female doctor may alleviate some anxiety, or it may be that there are underlying anxieties regarding diagnosis and treatment or societal expectations. Language, cultural or behavioural barriers should not have an impact on the standard of care you provide, even if it requires more time or extra resources such as a chaperone or interpreter. It is also important to address your own underlying cognitive biases during these types of consultations.

    When examining a female patient's genital area, be aware that all healthcare professionals have a mandatory duty to report any type of female genital mutilation in girls under 18 years old and to raise safeguarding concerns.

'Please pass the peppermints'

You have been assigned to train with the consultant who runs the biologics clinic. When the consultant sees a new patient with hidradenitis suppurativa, it is clear to you that your knowledge about this is more up to date than that of the consultant. She then advises a course of action that you think may not be in the patient's best interests. Another day, during the morning clinic, you notice a distinct smell of alcohol on the consultant's breath and you think her manner is overly cheerful. The consultant is in charge of assessing your performance during the attachment.

What issues arise here?

- Trainee–trainer relationship.
- Patient safety.
- GMC duties of a doctor: staying up to date.
- Evidence-based medicine.

How do you handle this?

The dynamics between a trainer and a trainee can be complex, but this should never adversely influence the treatment of a patient. There are subtle ways to direct the trainer to new guidelines or recent literature in the spirit of promoting evidence-based medicine within the team.

There is a high prevalence of alcohol dependency amongst doctors. On a pragmatic level, it may be very difficult or impossible to raise your concerns directly with your consultant without causing friction. You do however have a responsibility to ensure patient safety at all times. You can ask for advice from any other consultants in the department during that clinic in order for them to ensure appropriate assessment and immediate action. This might even include your consultant being sent home and alternative arrangements being made for the patients. This situation needs to be escalated in confidence to the clinical director.

'Love, sex and. . . drama'

You get suspicious that your registrar colleague is having an affair with the newly appointed consultant: there are significant looks, furtive behaviour and unexplained absences. It is announced that the registrar is going to be allowed to go to a major meeting abroad, even though you had previously been promised that it was going to be your turn.

What issues arise here?

- Relationships with colleagues.
- Probity and professionalism.

How do you handle this?

Issues of this sort are more common than you might think and can be very difficult to handle. These situations can negatively influence the team and department dynamics; having insight into this can help prevent patient care being compromised, but unfortunately working relationships can be impacted. When promises have not been fulfilled, there is a certain degree of betrayal of trust. If there is a concern that patient care or the team's work is affected, then there is a responsibility to raise it with your educational supervisor.

'Spotted in the lift' (Figure 3.3)

You are in the lift going to a ward referral. On the third floor an orthopaedic surgeon gets in, notices that you are from dermatology and immediately asks you 'What do you think of this?', drawing up his trouser leg to reveal a highly suspicious black lesion. He is about to get off at the next floor.

What issues arise here?

- Duty of care: when is that established?
- There is case law on 'corridor consultations' gone wrong.
- The three-part test involved in negligence liability (the three-part test is outlined in Table 3.3, and see Table 3.7 for influential negligence case law).
- Medical documentation.

How do you handle this?

We can all recognise an appropriate setting for patient consultation (good illumination, privacy, unhurried atmosphere); we can also recognise an inappropriate one: a supermarket aisle or the proverbial kerbside. Requests often come from colleagues, friends or even strangers for a 'quick look' that takes the form of a peek at their skin, in poor lighting, along with a hasty history that is usually not recorded anywhere. These consultations are frequently inaccurate.

Merely answering a colleague's question or performing a corridor consultation may not give rise to a doctor–patient relationship; hence, there is no liability. However, if a problem arises from advice given, circumstances may be examined to review

Table 3.7 Influential negligence case law: one example

Montgomery *v* Lanarkshire case (March 2015) drew fresh attention to **informed consent**	A patient should be told whatever they want to know, not what the doctor thinks they should be told

Figure 3.3 Spotted in the lift.

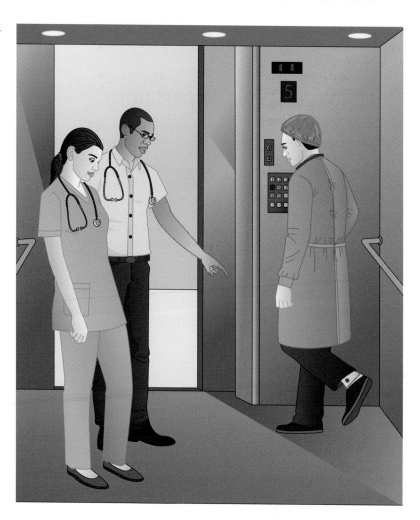

whether a doctor–patient relationship existed and, therefore, if duty of care can be established, for which a physician may be liable for medical malpractice.

In general, you should encourage formal consultation when expert advice is sought because a more reliable and complete exchange of information will occur. Most importantly, a written record of the interaction can then be kept. You need to get out the lift with the surgeon and advise a proper review!

'Workhorse, not training?'

Two of your trainee colleagues are on maternity leave. The dermatology clinical director, also your trainer, asks you to cover an extra two clinics per week for the next six months, on top of your already clinic-heavy schedule. You know that this will make any chance of taking forward any research impossible.

What issues arise here?

- Relationship between trainee and trainer.
- Clinical service and research commitment.
- Contractual rights.
- Trainee's voice.

How do you handle this?

These issues are extremely common within the NHS training setting. Diplomacy is key here. There needs to be a level of flexibility from both parties. It can be very challenging for trainees to raise these concerns, as they fear how they might impact their relationship with their seniors or clinical director. Trainees should try to address the problem by offering solutions. For example, suggest supporting the service during this difficult time, but ask for more research time when staffing is back to normal.

If training is persistently affected, then this should be escalated to the training programme director or Specialist Advisory Committee (SAC) lead. The BAD and SAC trainee representatives may help to identify issues that are consistently not being addressed. Remember that the local training programme director and the SAC are there to ensure that training is appropriately delivered, so do seek their advice.

If there are concerns about working hours and contractual rights not being upheld, then it may be helpful to seek advice from a trade union such as the British Medical Association. The report 'Being a junior doctor' addresses some of these issues (see Further reading).

'Nightmare on Derm Street'

During a follow-up appointment, you review a patient for the first time and on examination you see that the scar is on the opposite side from where the naevus was stated on the referring letter. You confirm with the clinical photographs that the wrong lesion has been removed.

What issues arise here?

- Never event.
- Duty of candour.
- Relationship with colleagues.

How do you handle this?

Removal of the wrong lesion classifies as wrong-site surgery and therefore is considered a 'never event'. This is a serious adverse event, for which there are national guidance and protective measures in place to try to ensure that such situations do not ever occur. It is important to be honest with the patient regarding what has happened (duty of candour) and to immediately offer an apology and full support. You need to inform them that a detailed root-cause investigation will be carried out to find out why this has occurred and to ensure that measures are in place to prevent it from happening again.

You should immediately inform the clinicians involved, formally report the clinical incident and alert the complaints department. A 'never event' will trigger a cascade of actions by the NHS Trust, so be sure to gather the support of your clinical and educational supervisors, who can help you navigate this process. Urgent plans should be made for the patient's further management and support.

'Does he take lidocaine?'

You are working in a very busy clinic where an elderly man from a residential home attends with a 10-week history of a lesion on his eyebrow that may need to be excised. He has a history of mild-to-moderate dementia. His carer mentions that he was given a sedative before attending the appointment.

What issues arise here?

- Autonomy and mental capacity.
- Best interest.
- Non-maleficence and beneficence.

How do you handle this?

Such a scenario is becoming more common in view of the increasing elderly population. It is important not to make any assumptions about a person's mental capacity in the decision-making process. In the first instance one must assume capacity: capacity is decision and time specific. Despite behaviour changes resulting from dementia, the patient may still have capacity to consent to treatment, but sedation may be impairing capacity and undermining his autonomy. His capacity must be formally assessed (Table 3.8).

If he lacks capacity and does not regain it when sedation wears off, then a decision must be taken in his best interests. You will need to weigh up the benefits versus the risks, after consulting family and carers who know his likely wishes, and plan how to undertake the procedure. Even if he lacks full capacity to consent, he must still be involved as much as possible at every step.

Table 3.8 Steps to assess capacity

To make a decision, can the person (when supported):
1. Understand the information (tailored for the person)?
2. Retain the information (for long enough)?
3. Weigh up the information (pros and cons)?
4. Communicate their decision (using any support needed)?

'I want whatever he is having. . .'

A consultant obstetrician attends the clinic with a recent history of plaque psoriasis affecting parts of her arm and significant involvement of her scalp. She has no previous history of skin problems. She is aware of the use of biologics and is keen to have only this treatment.

What issues arise here?

- Justice: resource allocation.
- Informed consent: patient can refuse but cannot demand treatment.

How do you handle this?

Mainstream media have influenced the way the public perceives access to targeted therapies with 'miracle' drugs. The main ethical principle raised here is that of justice. As clinicians we have a responsibility to consider how we allocate our resources and cost-effectiveness. You can explain NHS guidance and the importance of using standard therapies first prior to proceeding with more expensive treatment. As established by case law, autonomy does not entitle patients to the right to demand a treatment. A court has ruled that doctors could not be forced to give treatment that they believed was 'clinically unnecessary, futile or inappropriate'.

'The rep rap!'

A pharmaceutical company representative is visiting your dermatology department and providing a free lunch for trainees who attend a short lecture. She mentions that their drug has not been prescribed often in recent months and enquires why that might be. She starts asking about what treatments are currently used and how these decisions are made.

What issues arise here?

- Patients' best interests and confidentiality.
- Justice.
- Physician relationship with industry.

How do you handle this?

It is easy to blur the lines in a physician–pharmaceutical representative relationship, and it is important as clinicians to be conscious of this. It is crucial always to have the patient's best interests at the forefront of our decision making.

The pharmaceutical industry has immensely benefited patients through the development of new and effective drugs. However, the world of industry has different motivations from the NHS, and priorities may not be aligned. Clearly, it is in the interests of pharmaceutical companies that their drugs are prescribed and they therefore, within legal constraints, seek to influence doctors.

Provided doctors have insight into the nature of the influences on them, a healthy relationship with the pharmaceutical industry can be achieved. There are benefits to this with regard to supporting education and the development of new treatments. Feedback on how treatments are being used in real-life practice (compared to trials) is also of importance. However, the relationship needs to be transparent and honest, with patients' care as the core principle.

'Liar, liar. . .'

A final-year medical student attends your clinic, where he takes and presents a clinical history. A few days later, you receive an email from a medical school administrator that states you have signed off a clinical history and also a surgical procedure that actually never took place.

What issues arise here?

- Professionalism and probity.
- Supervisor's responsibility: integrity.

How do you handle this?

As a clinical supervisor you have a responsibility, specified by the GMC, to promote and raise any concerns regarding professionalism or probity. You should first contact the medical student and obtain all the relevant information. The email may have been written in error. If it was the student's intention, or they ask you to lie on their behalf, then this should be raised with their educational supervisor in the medical school to review if there has been a pattern of behaviour and to plan appropriate action. As a supervisor you have a responsibility to act with integrity and to demonstrate accountability for actions taken.

'Show me the money!'

One of your dermatology trainee colleagues has been on sick leave for several weeks. When doing a weekend on call, you saw him carrying out a shift as a medical locum. You are also aware that he is taking on extra evening theatre lists. As you are the trainee organising the rota, your training programme director tells you that this doctor is having a phased return from sick leave and has needed his training extended. The programme director asks you to complete multisource feedback for him and to plan the rotation with adequate support in the clinics, as he has been identified as a 'trainee in need'.

What issues arise here?

- Moonlighting and professionalism.
- Relationship with colleagues.
- Welfare.
- Probity.

How do you handle this?

It is important to state that carrying out any paid work during sick leave may be considered fraud and risks being investigated by the GMC. If registrars are working outside their main employment, their clinical director needs to be aware and to have approved this additional work. If, as a registrar, you suspect that a colleague is conducting such work, then you should highlight these concerns to the clinical director. In this situation, it would be best not to complete the multisource feedback until the issues have all been resolved. However, we should always bear in mind the welfare needs of this individual and whether there are other underlying circumstances that are having an impact on their decision making and pattern of behaviour.

'Kitchen table surgery'

You come across the social media page of one of the new dermatology juniors, which is advertising non-surgical cosmetic procedures performed by them. The address stated on the page for their 'clinic' is actually their home.

What issues arise here?

- Professionalism.
- False advertising.
- Cosmetics Practice Standards Authority (CPSA) standards and Joint Council for Cosmetic Practitioners (JCCP) register for cosmetic practitioners.

How do you handle this?

Non-surgical cosmetic procedures are not regulated in the UK, which means that anyone (including hairdressers) can perform them. This leads to several safety concerns. The CPSA has developed professional standards to which practitioners engaging in non-surgical cosmetic practice should adhere. The JCCP has developed a voluntary register of those who adhere to these standards, and helps members of the public to identify practitioners adhering to the agreed standards. Affiliated false and misleading advertising is illegal in the UK. In this particular case it is important for the junior doctor's educational supervisor to be informed in order for them to advise the doctor of the professionalism concerns and risks associated with their work outside of training.

'Round 'em up'

You are in a very busy specialist clinic, which the research nurses attend to recruit patients to a study. You shadow one of the senior trainees, who consents a patient for a clinical trial with a new targeted treatment. In order to be eligible for the study, the trainee suggests to the patient that he repeats the quality-of-life questionnaire to increase the score. When discussing the risks and benefits, you realise that some of the side-effects and risks have not been fully disclosed. The patient agrees to go ahead with the clinical trial.

What issues arise here?

- Informed consent.
- Human rights in research.
- Ethical research in human subjects.

How do you handle this?

This scenario implies that informed consent may not have been achieved and that the trainee is behaving dishonestly. Research ethics and legislation have been revised over the years, building on the Nuremberg Code, which is a set of ethical principles set out as a response to crimes of human experimentation. The three fundamental principles of research ethics are respect for persons, beneficence and justice. In this case, it would be important to highlight to the senior trainee regarding the side effects and risks that have not been explained to the patient, and to ensure that the patient is subsequently appropriately informed. It is clearly unethical

and dishonest to manipulate patient-reported outcome data; the trainee needs to be given the opportunity to reflect on this.

'Hello, is it me you're looking for?'

You perform a follow-up telephone consultation with an 80-year-old man who is partially deaf, has psoriasis and is on methotrexate. Carers visit him four times a day and one of them is present during the consultation. The patient asks you to speak louder. You assess the situation and it sounds as if he needs to change his systemic agent. You try to counsel him over the phone about changing to acitretin. He agrees to everything you say, but you are not sure whether he is retaining the information or hearing everything. You mention that he needs to attend hospital to be reviewed in person and to discuss his treatments again, but he is too scared to come to hospital and wants the new treatment posted out to him.

What issues arise here?

- Virtual consultation: technical difficulties, impact on communication and confidentiality.
- GMC guidance on remote consultation.

How do you handle this?

Telemedicine consultations are on the rise and are becoming increasingly more common in daily practice. Technical difficulties can be an added issue in virtual consultations, especially with some elderly patients. Be aware of several pitfalls: documentation, confidentiality, standard of care and ethical principles all need to be upheld to the same level during a virtual consultation as for a face-to-face one. Consider the setting in which the consultation takes place, the people present and whether the patient has complete understanding of the plans for their care. Be prepared to switch from a video to a telephone or in-person consultation, depending on technical, patient or clinical factors.

Conclusions

The discussion points in this chapter are not the only aspects that you need to consider for these scenarios. Try to think through, for each scenario, other insights into the thinking and behaviour of the various participants. If you disagree with any of the suggestions given, consider how you would act and what the consequences might be.

It can sometimes be a useful exercise to try to imagine the issue happening in a different cultural or historical context. Then consider whether responses might be the same or different.

All ethical issues usually concern behaviours, involve more than one person and pose dilemmas about what action to take. At the core of all ethical dilemmas and complaints is communication. Having the opportunity to work through these types of scenarios may facilitate you having discussions with your colleagues and your supervisors, and enable you to acquire a reflective approach in managing challenging ethico-legal situations.

Pearls and pitfalls

- In any clinical dilemma, always consider what is in the best interests of the patient.
- When concerned about a situation, share your worries with a colleague or your supervisor.
- Try to develop some critical insight into your own behaviour: none of us are perfect.
- Do not turn a blind eye to things that you think are going wrong: take advice and tackle the issues.
- Remember that you work in a framework that is governed by ethical principles, legal constraints and employment law. Be cautious!

SCE Questions. See questions 7 and 8.

Conflicts of interest. The authors do not claim that they actually behave more (or less) ethically than the readers. These issues are difficult for us all. And by the way, awareness of and declaration of conflicts of interest is another important ethical issue.

FURTHER READING AND KEY RESOURCES

Car J, Koh GC-H, Foong PS, Wang CJ. Video consultations in primary and specialist care during the covid-19 pandemic and beyond. *BMJ* 2020; **371**:m3945.

Fickweiler F, Fickweiler W, Urbach E. Interactions between physicians and the pharmaceutical industry generally and sales representatives specifically and their association with physicians' attitudes and prescribing habits: a systematic review. *BMJ Open* 2017; **7**:e016408.

Gillon R. Medical ethics: four principles plus attention to scope. *BMJ* 1994; **309**:184–8.

Muzumdar S, Grant-Kels JM, Feng H. The ethical conundrum of writing a recommendation letter for someone you would not recommend. *J Am Acad Dermatol* 2020; **82**:1270–1.

Stoff BK, Grant-Kels JM, Brodell RT *et al*. Introducing a curriculum in ethics and professionalism for dermatology residencies. *J Am Acad Dermatol* 2018; **78**:1032–4.

J.M. Grant-Kels has written many challenging and novel publications on ethics in dermatology. You are strongly recommended to do a PubMed search on her name.

Useful websites

British Association of Dermatologists. UK guidance on the use of mobile photographic devices in dermatology. Available at: https://www.bad.org.uk/shared/get-file.ashx?itemtype=document&id=5818.

Cosmetic Practice Standards Authority. Available at: www.cosmeticstandards.org.uk.

General Medical Council. Remote consultations. Available at: https://www.gmc-uk.org/ethical-guidance/ethical-hub/remote-consultations.

Royal College of Physicians. Being a junior doctor: experiences from the front line of the NHS. Available at: https://www.rcplondon.ac.uk/guidelines-policy/being-junior-doctor.

Section 2

Fundamentals
of clinical practice

4

Basic science of the skin

Lloyd Steele and Edel A. O'Toole

Introduction

As dermatologists we are privileged to spend our working lives thinking about, observing and trying to sustain one of the most amazing human organs – the skin. Its anatomy and physiology reflect a range of functions that have evolved to allow us to survive in a hostile environment. Our understanding of the complex cellular functions of the skin is rapidly developing, but we can be fairly sure that our current knowledge will be overtaken during our careers ahead. This is a frontier of science that to skin scientists is just as exciting as the science of space exploration or of artificial intelligence.

It is really important for dermatologists to understand the basic science of skin. This is so that we can comprehend in depth the pathogenesis of diseases (for example pemphigus or epidermolysis bullosa) and why current therapies work (such as biologics), as well as to provide clues as to how therapies in the future might be developed and targeted. It differentiates us from a multitude of other practitioners who address skin conditions, positioning dermatologists as leaders to drive forward practice, training and research to ultimately improve skin health for our patients and the public.

The skin: overview and functions

The skin consists of three layers – the epidermis, the dermis and the subcutaneous tissue ('subcutis' or 'hypodermis'). It also contains cutaneous appendages including hair follicles, sebaceous glands and sweat (eccrine and apocrine) glands (Figure 4.1).

The skin is life preserving, performing crucial functions, namely:

- An 'inside-outside barrier': preventing loss of water and other components of the body to the environment.
- An 'outside-inside barrier': protecting the body from environmental toxins, antigens and pathogens.
- Antimicrobial protection: from both innate and adaptive immunity.
- Protection against damage from ultraviolet (UV) radiation.
- Regulation of body temperature.

Dermatology Training: The Essentials. Edited by Mahbub M.U. Chowdhury, Tamara W. Griffiths and Andrew Y. Finlay.
© 2022 The British Association of Dermatologists. Published 2022 by John Wiley & Sons Ltd.
Companion website: www.wiley.com/go/chowdhury/dermatologytraining

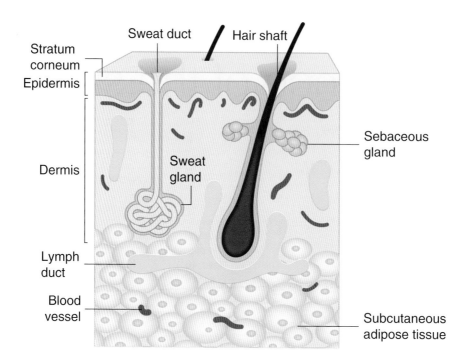

Figure 4.1 An overview of the skin structure demonstrating the epidermis, dermis and subcutaneous tissue, as well as associated cutaneous appendages. Kabashima *et al. Nat Rev Immunol* 2019; **19**:19–30.

- Somatosensation: detecting sensory stimuli from the external world, which are perceived by the brain as touch, temperature, position, pain and itch.
- Vitamin D production.
- Stimulation and enhancement of intimate and sexual human relationships, through its appearance, its feel and pheromone production.

The skin has an amazing ability to rapidly repair itself when injured to maintain these functions, coupled with rapid mechanisms for self-repair of DNA damaged by radiation. We benefit every day from, and can only survive because of, the way our skin has evolved to provide the critical interface between our bodies and the external hostile environment in which we live.

Epidermis

Layers of the epidermis

The most superficial layer of the skin is the epidermis. This is formed predominantly (90–95%) of keratinocytes. These cells are named after their main cytoplasmic protein, 'keratin', which

organises into intermediate filaments to provide cells with structural integrity and resilience.

Keratinocytes are integral to the self-renewal of the epidermis, which turns over every 28–40 days in a finely balanced process. During this process, keratinocytes pass through sequential stages of differentiation, programmed death and desquamation. The reprogramming of gene expression during differentiation causes essential changes in cell morphology and function. These changes can be used to divide the epidermis into four distinct layers: the stratum basale, the stratum spinosum, the stratum granulosum (SG) and the stratum corneum (Figure 4.2). In reality, the upward flow of keratinocytes, perpetuated by new cells forming in the basal layer, is a gradual process, and these 'layers' (a historical construct of histopathologists) are really descriptions of phases in a dynamic process.

Stratum basale (basal layer)

The stratum basale is the deepest (basal) layer of the epidermis. This is a single layer of cells attached to the underlying basement membrane zone via hemidesmosomes. Keratinocytes in this layer express keratins 5 and 14 (Figure 4.2) and produce various components necessary for the formation of the

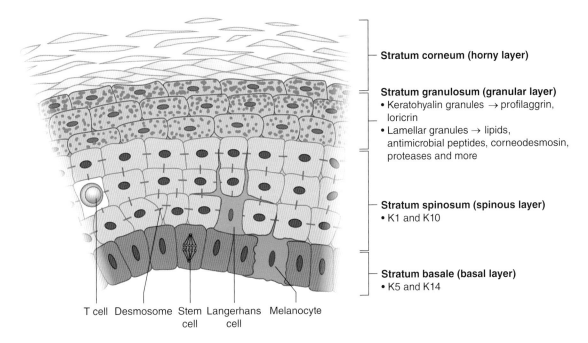

Stratum corneum (horny layer)

Stratum granulosum (granular layer)
- Keratohyalin granules → profilaggrin, loricrin
- Lamellar granules → lipids, antimicrobial peptides, corneodesmosin, proteases and more

Stratum spinosum (spinous layer)
- K1 and K10

Stratum basale (basal layer)
- K5 and K14

T cell Desmosome Stem cell Langerhans cell Melanocyte

Figure 4.2 Layers of the epidermis. Basal cells express keratin 5 (K5) and/or K14, stratum spinosum cells express K1 and/or K10, and stratum granulosum cells express K2. Modified from Bikle D, Christakos S. New aspects of vitamin D metabolism and action – addressing the skin as source and target. *Nat Rev Endocrinol* 2020; **16**:234–52.

underlying basement membrane (see 'Basement membrane zone and dermoepidermal junction').

The stratum basale is the only part of the epidermis that is proliferative, with approximately 15% of cells dividing at any one time, and the remainder in a resting or quiescent state. Cells that migrate from the stratum basale are replenished by pools of transit-amplifying cells, which are generated from a smaller number of long-lived, slow-cycling stem cells present in both the stratum basale and hair follicles. These pools of proliferative progenitor cells are not only able to replenish migrating cells, but can also make short-term contributions to wound healing, when needed. The use of pools of finite progenitor cells, rather than lifelong stem cells directly, allows the stem cell population to remain small and minimises the number of cell replications they are required to undertake, which limits the numbers of somatic mutations they acquire.

Stratum spinosum (spinous/prickly layer)

When basal cells detach from the basal layer, they stop proliferating and start differentiation. Their keratin expression changes to keratins 1 and 10, and they also begin to produce involucrin and transglutaminase in the stratum spinosum, which are important later for stratum corneum formation.

The stratum spinosum ('prickly layer') is given its name from the prominent appearance of intercellular junctions, particularly desmosomes. Desmosomes are one of four intercellular junctions present in the epidermis, along with adherens junctions, gap junctions and tight junctions (TJs) (Figure 4.3). Desmosomes and adherens junctions maintain epidermal integrity by linking the cytoskeletons of keratinocytes. Skin blistering can result if desmosomes are damaged (Figure 4.4). Gap junctions facilitate small-molecule transfer across cell membranes and are composed of connexins. TJs are found in the SG and are discussed below.

Stratum granulosum (granular layer) and the process of cornification

The SG consists of at least three layers, named SG3 (the layer immediately above the stratum spinosum), SG2 (which contains TJs) and SG1 (the layer immediately beneath the stratum corneum; Figure 4.3). Together these layers are important in maintaining epidermal barrier function and in providing the constituents necessary for stratum corneum formation ('cornification') through keratohyalin and lamellar granules (hence the name, 'granular layer').

While barrier function is typically associated with the wall-like structure of the stratum corneum, SG2 also has an important role. TJs present in SG2 form a seal of the intercellular space (Figure 4.3), preventing the entry of large molecules from the external environment. These channels are also ion and size selective, and thus the selectivity of the barrier can vary. The importance of TJs is shown when their predominant structural protein (claudin) is absent: in mouse models this is lethal within one day of birth because of tremendous water loss, and in humans it results in a form of ichthyosis.

Keratinocytes in the SG produce profilaggrin, which aggregates within cells to form keratohyalin granules. These granules become increasingly abundant as cells near the stratum

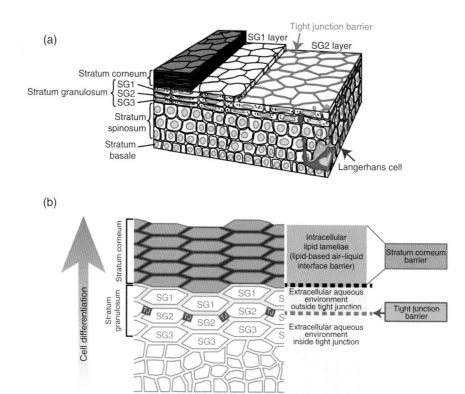

Figure 4.3 Tight junctions (TJs) between cells in the second layer of the stratum granulosum (SG2) form an important part of the skin barrier, in addition to the overlying stratum corneum. This is shown in (a) the three-dimensional structure of the epidermis and (b) a vertical section. Yokouchi M, Kubo A. Maintenance of tight junction barrier integrity in cell turnover and skin diseases. *Exp Dermatol* 2018; **27**:876–83.

corneum (Figure 4.5). Up to this point, keratin filaments within keratinocytes have provided structural integrity to keratinocytes. However, as keratinocytes of the SG approach the acidic skin surface, the keratohyalin granules disperse. Profilaggrin is cleaved to filaggrin (*fil*ament *aggr*egation prote*in*), which then acts to aggregate the keratin filaments within keratinocytes into tight bundles. This aggregation ultimately breaks the internal 'scaffolding' structure of keratinocytes and results in their collapse into a flattened shape (Figure 4.5). All cellular organelles are lost at this point, and thus keratinocytes are rapidly transformed into flattened, dead 'corneocytes' or 'squames'. Filaggrin degradation products contribute to pools of amino acids, which retain water in the skin, collectively termed 'natural moisturising factor', and they are also suggested to contribute to the process of acidification of the stratum corneum (to a pH of 4.1–5.8), although this latter role is questioned. Various other mechanisms for acidification are reported, including sodium/hydrogen exchanger 1 (NHE1), which selectively acidifies the SG–stratum corneum interface.

Keratohyalin granule dispersal also releases loricrin, which becomes the major constituent of the 'cornified envelope' that develops around corneocytes. Loricrin is cross-linked with other constituents of the cornified envelope, such as involucrin and filaggrin fragments, in a reaction catalysed by transglutaminases that renders corneocytes resilient and highly impermeable structures (Figure 4.5).

Other products needed for cornification are provided by lamellar granules. These release lipids, antimicrobial peptides (AMPs), proteases, protease inhibitors – including lympho-epithelial Kazal-type-related inhibitor (LEKTI) – and corneodesmosin. Corneodesmosin binds to desmosomes (Figure 4.4) to form corneodesmosomes, which bind neighbouring corneocytes. The released lipids seal the intercellular space between corneocytes. Particularly important are ceramides, which also form a monolayer around corneocytes (the 'lipid envelope'; Figure 4.5). The formation of ceramides is dependent upon two acidic pH-dependent enzymes (acidic sphingomyelinase and β-glucocerebrosidase), further demonstrating the importance of acidification of the stratum corneum.

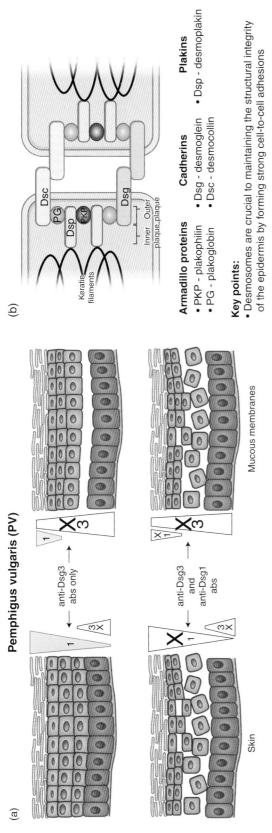

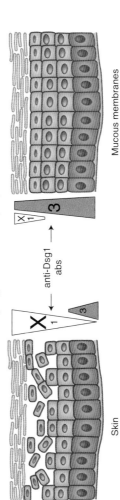

Armadillo proteins
• PKP - plakophilin
• PG - plakoglobin

Cadherins
• Dsg - desmoglein
• Dsc - desmocollin

Plakins
• Dsp - desmoplakin

Key points:
• Desmosomes are crucial to maintaining the structural integrity of the epidermis by forming strong cell-to-cell adhesions

Pemphigus vulgaris (PV)

anti-Dsg3 abs only

anti-Dsg3 and anti-Dsg1 abs

Skin

Mucous membranes

Pemphigus foliaceus (PF)

anti-Dsg1 abs

Skin

Mucous membranes

Key points:
• Dsg1 and Dsg3 are expressed differently in the skin than in the mucous membranes. The important point here is that knocking out Dsg3 (as can be seen with the autoantibodies of pemphigus vulgaris) causes more damage (including mucosal membrane involvement) than knocking out Dsg1 alone (as can be seen in pemphigus foliaceus).

Figure 4.4 (a) Desmoglein is a key component of desmosomes, and the expression of the desmogleins 1 (Dsg1) and 3 (Dsg3) varies by both location (skin vs. mucous membrane) and depth in the epidermis. This is clinically relevant as Dsg1 is targeted in pemphigus foliaceus, hence superficial skin-only blisters occur (often resulting in erosions), whereas Dsg1 and Dsg3 can both be targeted in pemphigus vulgaris, causing mucous membrane involvement as well as deeper skin blisters. (b) Desmosomes form important intercellular junctions by linking the keratin filaments of adjacent cells. The desmosome structure contains cadherins – desmoglein (Dsg1–4) and desmocollin (Dsc1–3) – attached to inner and outer plaques formed of armadillo proteins – plakoglobin (PG) and plakophilins (PKP1–3) – and plakins (desmoplakin, periplakin and envoplakin). (a) Modified from Hammers CM, Stanley JR. Recent advances in understanding pemphigus and bullous pemphigoid. *J Invest Dermatol* 2020; **140**:733–41. (b) Modified from Ishida-Yamamoto A et al. Clinical and molecular implications of structural changes to desmosomes and corneodesmosomes. *J Dermatol* 2018; **45**:385–9; and McMillan JR, Shimizu H. Desmosomes: structure and function in normal and diseased epidermis. *J Dermatol* 2001; **28**:291–8.

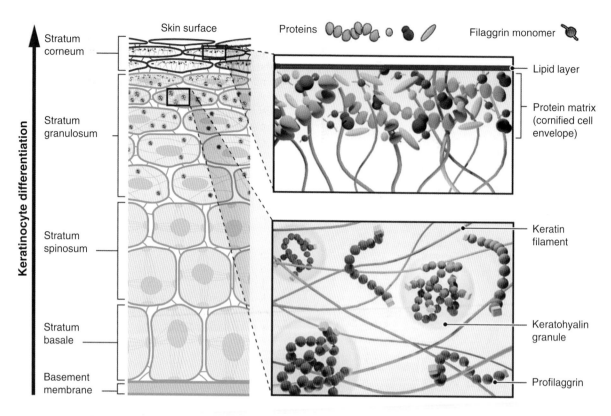

Figure 4.5 As profilaggrin accumulates in keratinocytes in the stratum granulosum, keratohyalin granules form. As cells approach the acidic stratum corneum, these granules disperse and filaggrin collapses the keratin network within keratinocytes (lower inset), forming flattened cells in the stratum corneum. Filaggrin fragments can also become part of the cornified envelope, which is surrounded by an outer lipid layer (upper inset). Rai A, Pelkmans L. Liquid droplets in the skin. *Science* 2020; **367**:1193–4.

Stratum corneum (horny layer)

The result of 'cornification' is the stratum corneum. This is the unique anatomical feature of the epidermis, consisting of flattened, anuclear corneocytes surrounded by intercellular lipid lamellae (Figures 4.2 and 4.3). This structure has been compared to a hydrophobic 'brick-and-mortar' wall.

This 'wall' is largely responsible for the protective functions of the epidermis. The required protection varies by site, with some sites subject to repetitive mechanical trauma, such as palmoplantar epidermis, whereas others are not, such as the eyelid. Substantial variations in the thickness of the stratum corneum are thus seen to meet these requirements. At areas with a very thick stratum corneum, an extra stratum lucidum ('clear layer') may be seen at the base of the stratum corneum.

A criticism of the 'wall' model is that it understates the dynamic nature of the stratum corneum. In order to allow self-renewal, superficial corneocytes must be shed from its outermost surface. This is a finely regulated process: the exact details of this regulation remain one of the mysteries of cutaneous biology. However, it involves proteases, such as kallikrein-related peptidases (KLKs), which cleave the corneodesmosomes holding corneocytes

together, as well as protease inhibitors, such as LEKTI, which inhibit protease activity in the lower stratum corneum, preventing premature epidermal detachment. The acidic environment is also important as it prevents protease overactivity. When performed correctly, this process results in corneodesmosomes being degraded first on the apical and basal surfaces, leaving lateral intercorneocyte connections intact. This results in the classic 'basket-weave pattern' on histological examination (Figure 4.6).

Drug delivery

The efficacy of the epidermal barrier is such that few drugs can be successfully delivered transdermally. This is because such drugs need to have a low molecular weight and be lipophilic in order to penetrate the epidermis, as well as highly potent as so little is absorbed.

The role of the epidermis in immunity and the microbiome

The epidermis is the most superficial layer of the skin and so is constantly exposed to a range of pathogens. In addition

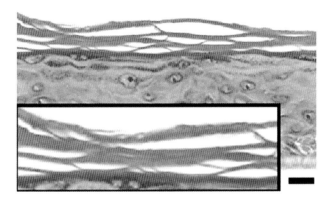

Figure 4.6 In formalin-fixed and paraffin-embedded normal skin, the stratum corneum can be seen to have two layers: a lower compact layer and an overlying 'basket-weave pattern' layer. This basket-weave pattern is frequently considered a hallmark of normal epidermis, as it reflects the normal process of corneodesmosomes generally being degraded on apical and basal surfaces (in non-palmoplantar epidermis) first – a pattern that is often lost in inflammatory disease. Bar = 25 μm. Goto H *et al.* Basket-weave structure in the stratum corneum is an important factor for maintaining the physiological properties of human skin as studied using reconstructed human epidermis and tape stripping of human cheek skin. *Br J Dermatol* **2020**; 182:364–72.

to it being a physical barrier, AMPs, such as defensins and cathelicidins, accumulate in the stratum corneum and exhibit broad-spectrum killing activity against a range of microorganisms. The epidermis also contains immune cells, of which the most prevalent are Langerhans cells. Derived from bone marrow dendritic cells, Langerhans cells have an important role in antigen presentation, and may also be significant in eliciting tolerance. Finally, keratinocytes below the level of TJs can also have an immune function as they can recognise pathogens and communicate with resident leukocytes.

Despite the antimicrobial mechanisms of the epidermis and its dry, acidic surface, it is home to more than 10^{10} bacteria on an individual's total body skin surface area. This diverse skin microbiome has an essential role in the education of the immune system and in preventing colonisation by pathogens ('colonisation resistance'). While implicated in both health and disease, the forces that shape and maintain these complex communities remain poorly understood, but it is an exciting area of research.

Other epidermal functions

Melanocytes are found in the stratum basale of the epidermis. They produce melanin, which is transferred to neighbouring keratinocytes in melanosomes to protect their cell nuclei from UV damage. While numbers of melanocytes are similar between different skin types, the amount and type of melanin produced differ. Eumelanin is associated with darker colours, whereas phaeomelanin is associated with lighter colours. Differences in skin types are thought to reflect their previous evolutionary advantages,

with darker skin protecting cell nuclei and folate stores from UV damage at high UV exposures, and lighter skin maximising UV conversion of 7-dehydrocholesterol to vitamin D at low UV exposure. Variations in skin colour can also occur pathologically when mutations affect melanin synthesis and transfer, such as tyrosinase null mutations in oculocutaneous albinism type 1 (OCA1).

Finally, neural cells can be found in the epidermis. These include Merkel cells and intraepidermal free nerve endings. These have a sensory role, which is detailed in the 'Dermis' section.

Basement membrane zone and dermoepidermal junction

Given the crucial functions of the epidermis, it needs to be firmly adhered to underlying structures to prevent loss. This is achieved by the basement membrane, which anchors the epidermis to the underlying dermis through a range of different components (Figure 4.7). Abnormalities in this structure can cause various, often severe diseases (Table 4.1).

Dermis

The dermis is connective tissue of variable thickness (0.5–5 mm) that confers mechanical resistance and elasticity to the skin. The epidermis forms invaginations into the dermis known as rete ridges, which can divide it into an upper 'papillary' dermis and a lower 'reticular' dermis. The papillary dermis has a dense meshwork of thin, poorly oriented collagen fibres, whereas the reticular dermis has thick, highly organised collagen fibre bundles.

Fibroblasts are responsible for the synthesis and renewal of the acellular component of the dermis, the extracellular matrix (ECM). The predominant ECM component is fibril-forming collagen: mainly type I, but with contributions from types III and V. These fibrils provide tensile strength to the dermis. Type VI collagen, a microfibrillar collagen, is also present in the upper papillary dermis. This has a role in regulating assembly of the matrix through interacting with other ECM elements such as glycosaminoglycans, proteoglycans and fibronectin.

The elasticity and tear resistance of the dermis are provided by elastic fibres, which are composed of an amorphous elastin core with surrounding fibrillin-rich microfibrils. In normal healthy skin, the elastic fibre system adopts a characteristic highly ordered architecture, with three types of fibres: oxytalan, elaunin and mature elastic fibres. Fine, oxytalan fibrillin-rich microfibrils orient perpendicularly in the upper papillary dermis, abutting the dermoepidermal junction, and have a 'tent peg' effect, mitigating shearing force between the epidermis and dermis. Intermediate-sized elaunin fibres lie in a parallel direction deeper in papillary dermis. Larger-diameter, mature elastic fibres, composed primarily of elastin, form in the reticular dermis. The copper-dependent enzyme lysyl oxidase mediates the cross-linking of both elastic and collagen fibres.

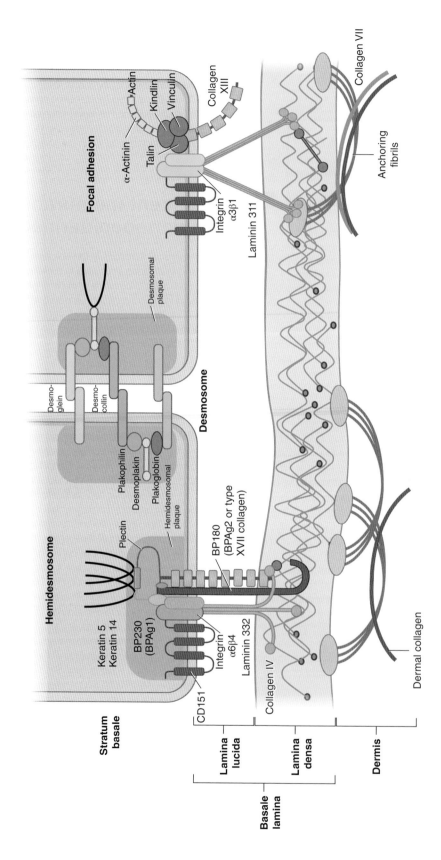

Figure 4.7 Basement membrane zone, where keratinocytes of the stratum basale are connected to the underlying dermis. Stationary keratinocytes attach to the basement membrane via hemidesmosomes, and migrating keratinocytes move, for example during wound healing using focal adhesions. Adapted from Has C et al. Clinical practice guidelines for laboratory diagnosis of epidermolysis bullosa. *Br J Dermatol* 2019; **182**:574–92.

Table 4.1 Components of the basement membrane and how abnormalities in these components, either genetic or acquired, can result in severe disease

Basement membrane component	Genetic disease	Acquired antibody-mediated disease
BP180/collagen 17	Junctional epidermolysis bullosa	Bullous pemphigoid, mucous membrane pemphigoid
		Lichen planus pemphigoides
		Pemphigoid gestationis
		Paraneoplastic pemphigus
BP230		Bullous pemphigoid, mucous membrane pemphigoid
		Lichen planus pemphigoides
		Paraneoplastic pemphigus
Laminin 332	Junctional epidermolysis bullosa	Mucous membrane pemphigoid (can be associated with solid malignancies)
Alpha 6 integrin	Junctional epidermolysis bullosa (± pyloric atresia)	
Beta 4 integrin	Junctional epidermolysis bullosa (± pyloric atresia)	Mucous membrane pemphigoid (pure ocular)
Alpha 3 integrin	Junctional epidermolysis bullosa (± nephrotic syndrome and pulmonary fibrosis)	
Keratin 5	Epidermolysis bullosa simplex with mottled pigmentation	
	Migratory circinate erythema epidermolysis bullosa simplex	
	Dowling–Degos disease	
Keratin 14	Epidermolysis bullosa simplex	
Collagen VII	Dystrophic epidermolysis bullosa	Epidermolysis bullosa acquisita
		Bullous lupus erythematosus
Kindlin-1 (fermitin family homolog 1)	Kindler syndrome	
Plectin	Epidermolysis bullosa simplex with pyloric atresia/muscular dystrophy	Paraneoplastic pemphigus

The dermis contains a range of cell types beyond fibroblasts. Resident immune cells include dendritic cells, macrophages, mast cells and innate lymphoid cells. These cells are involved in eliciting an immediate, non-specific response against a wide range of invading microorganisms, including the release of alarm signals. These signals can recruit more immune cells to the region, such as neutrophils, lymphocytes, plasmacytoid dendritic cells and eosinophils. Of these, lymphocytes are particularly important for their persistence after the event, affording the immune system 'memory'. Resident memory cells increase with increasing immunological events and exposures during early life, and there are an estimated 20 billion effector lymphocytes in healthy adult skin. Lymphocytes carry out diverse functions depending on their cell type ($\alpha\beta$ and $\gamma\delta$ T cells, B cells, plasma cells), cell subset (e.g. T cells can be subdivided into CD4+ and CD8+ T cells) and cell state [e.g. T-helper (Th) states include Th1, Th2 and Th17].

The recruitment of immune cells to the skin is permitted by mesh-like networks of blood vessels in the dermis (Figure 4.1). As well as being able to vasodilate and vasoconstrict to regulate temperature control, dermal blood vessels, specifically post-capillary venules, can increase their vascular permeability to allow T cells, immunoglobulins, albumin and water into the dermis.

Exudate is drained by lymphatic vessels, the failure of which can result in marked swelling ('lymphatic failure') (Chapter 26).

Finally, the dermis is innervated by a wide variety of sensory neurone subtypes, rendering the skin a sensitive organ able to detect pain, itch, temperature, position, pressure and touch. Touch mechanisms on glabrous sites (i.e. skin without hairs) such as the palms have been particularly well defined, with Merkel discs, Pacinian corpuscles, Meissner's corpuscles and Ruffini endings recognised (Table 4.2). These glabrous skin receptors are innervated by fast-conduction velocity neurones (i.e. Aβ, which are thickly myelinated) (Table 4.2), but Aδ (thinly myelinated) and C nerve fibres (unmyelinated) also innervate the skin, with the latter particularly associated with itch.

Subcutaneous tissue and hypodermis

The subcutis contains adipose tissue surrounded by septa (containing blood vessels, lymphatics and nerves). It provides padding, an energy reserve and insulation for thermoregulation. It also has a role in host defence. However, immune cells can function aberrantly in obesity, leading to an excessive release of inflammatory mediators termed adipokines.

The pilosebaceous unit and sweat glands

Hairy skin covers > 90% of the body surface and is characterised by the presence of hair follicles. Hair follicles form pilosebaceous units along with sebaceous glands and arrector pili muscles (Figure 4.8). Arrector pili muscles can move the hair off the skin surface, and sebaceous glands release lipid-rich sebum, which lubricates and provides an antibacterial shield to the hair and skin. These structures can also be used to divide the hair follicle into three regions:

- The infundibulum: from the follicular ostium to the opening of the sebaceous gland duct.
- The isthmus: from the sebaceous gland duct to the insertion site of the arrector pili muscle.
- The lower portion (bulb and suprabulbar region): below the insertion site of the arrector pili muscle.

The stratum basale of the epidermis extends to form the outer root sheath of the hair follicle. However, unlike interfollicular epithelium, hair follicle epithelium has no stratum corneum and is an immune-privileged site (in other words, it is able to tolerate the introduction of antigens without eliciting an inflammatory immune response).

The lower portion (below the level of the isthmus) is also able to repeatedly grow and regress in hair follicle cycles that are characteristic of hair growth. At any one time, approximately 80–90% of hair follicles are growing (anagen), around 1% are being destroyed (catagen) and 10–20% are resting (telogen).

To start the growth stage, the dermal papilla at the base of the bulb acts as an instructive signalling niche (the concept of a 'niche' of stem cells refers to a specialised microenvironment that includes supporting cells along with their secreted trophic factors that influence stem cell phenotype). This dermal papilla niche triggers progenitor cells in the hair/follicular matrix to proliferate, migrate upwards and differentiate, forming the inner root sheath and the hair shaft itself, which is composed of an outer cuticle, a cortex and an inner medulla. When hair follicles move to the catagen state, this newly developed lower portion of the follicle regresses. Contraction of the dermal sheath then returns the dermal papilla to a position closer to the hair bulge. This is important as the bulge is a stem cell reservoir, and thus the dermal papilla can replenish its store of progenitor cells in preparation for restarting the cycle.

Melanocyte stem cells are also present in the hair bulge. The melanocytes present in hair follicles are responsible for determining the production of eumelanin and phaeomelanin, which determine hair colour. Hair type, which can be terminal (longer and thicker), vellus (shorter and finer) or lanugo hair (usually shed before birth and seen only in abnormal states), varies by site. Whereas most primates have a densely pigmented terminal hair coat, humans have terminal hairs covering only small portions of the body, including the scalp, eyebrows and axilla.

A suggested reason why humans do not have widespread terminal hair (a fur coat) like other primates is that this absence permitted an evolutionary advantage through excellent thermoregulation. Humans have an extraordinary sweating capacity relative to other mammals, with three million eccrine glands widely distributed over the body surface (particularly abundant on the palms, soles, axillae, forehead and cheeks). In exceptional conditions, these can produce up to 10 litres of odourless, clear, thin hypotonic secretion per day. This cools the body surface, permitting increased exercise capacity in extreme heat, which would have been advantageous to early humans reliant on exercise capacity for hunting and survival.

The skin also contains apocrine glands, but these are far less numerous than eccrine sweat glands. They are also restricted to certain sites, namely the axillae, anogenital region, areolae, eyelids (Moll glands) and ear (a specialised form called ceruminous glands). Apocrine glands become active during puberty and result in viscid, odorous sweat, containing pheromones. These glands are under the control of adrenergic nerves, whereas eccrine sweat glands are innervated by cholinergic nerves.

Nails

The most visible part of the nail structure is the nail plate. This is a laminated keratinised structure that overlies the nail matrix (15–25%) and the nail bed (75–85%) (Figure 4.9). Fine longitudinal ridges are visible in the nail plate, corresponding to complementary ridges on the underlying nail bed.

Table 4.2 The four major mechanoreceptors of glabrous skin

Receptor	Meissner	Merkel disc	Pacinian corpuscle	Ruffini corpuscle
Diagram	Meissner's corpuscle	Merkel cells	Pacinian corpuscle	Ruffini endings
Superficiality	Superficial dermis	Basal epidermis	Deep dermis and subcutaneous fat	Dermis
Innervation	Aβ rapidly adapting type I	Aβ slow adapting type I	Aβ rapidly adapting type II	Aβ slow adapting type II
Sensation	Movement across the skin	Touch	High-frequency vibration	Skin stretch

Images modified from Kim Sweeney, *Introduction to Physiological Psychology*, Regents of the University of California.

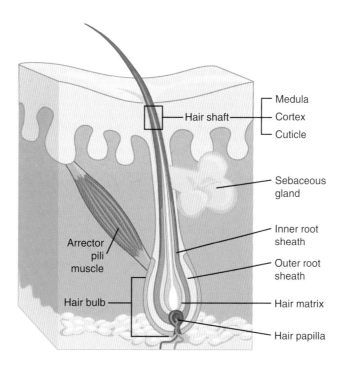

Figure 4.8 Hair follicle anatomy. FancyTapis/iStock/Getty Images.

The nail plate is synthesised by the nail matrix, which is found at the proximal part of the nail. It may be partially visible as the 'lunula', characterised by its half-moon shape (Figure 4.9), but sometimes it is fully covered by the proximal nail fold. Protection of the nail matrix by the proximal nail fold is important as it is the germinative part of the nail and thus damage can result in permanent nail scarring. The proximal nail fold also extends onto the superficial surface of the nail plate as the 'cuticle' (Figure 4.9) to create a seal, further protecting the matrix. The nail matrix is the only subungual location of functioning melanocytes.

The nail bed, on which the nail plate lies, is richly supplied with glomus bodies. These neurovascular bodies act as arteriovenous anastomoses, bypassing the intermediary capillary bed and ensuring that blood supply is preserved to the peripheries in cold conditions. However, glomus bodies can be the site of disease, with glomus tumours being particularly common on the nail bed (as well as on the palms).

Embryology

This chapter has detailed the extraordinary complexity of the skin. How this organ develops in the human embryo is a fascinating process. This section briefly overviews the embryological origins of the main skin structures.

The epidermis first exists shortly after 'gastrulation', a process in which the embryo changes from a single-layered blastula to a multilayered gastrula. Derived from ectoderm, the epidermis starts as a single layer of unspecified epithelial progenitor cells. These cells divide and asymmetrical divisions contribute to stratification and differentiation. This division is still poorly understood, but clinical presentations of cutaneous mosaicism provide some insights into how these divisions occur.

Hair follicles form from the germinative layer of the epidermis, typically between weeks 8 to 10 of gestation. Wnt (an abbreviation of 'Wingless' and 'Int-1') signalling is important in this

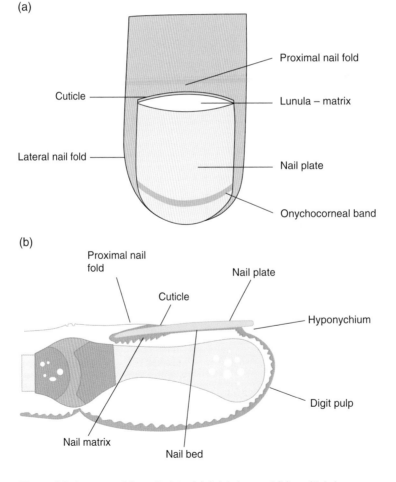

Figure 4.9 Anatomy of the nail plate. (a) Axial view and (b) sagittal view. de Berker D. Nail anatomy. *Clin Dermatol* 2013; **31**:509–15.

process. Signalling involved in hair follicle formation prompts the underlying mesenchyme to organise into a dermal condensate, and 'cut-and-paste' tissue recombination experiments also indicate that the underlying mesenchyme/dermis signals to the epidermis and hair follicles. In these experiments, when epidermis from hairy skin is grown over dermis from glabrous sites, no hair follicles grow. However, when epidermis from glabrous sites is grown over dermis from hairy skin, hair follicles form.

Melanocytes are derived from neural crest cells (neuroectoderm). This migratory cell population can differentiate into a broad range of cell types. Melanocytes migrate not only to the epidermis but also to other structures, including the eye and the meninges. More recent data has also suggested the existence of a novel population of melanocyte precursors, derived from mesoderm.

Dermal fibroblasts have two embryonic origins: mesodermal cells (body and scalp skin) and cranial neural crest cells (facial skin). Recent research has shown that fibroblasts are not homogeneous, and that there are subpopulations of fibroblasts with distinct functional identities.

Ageing

With time, the skin is subject to intrinsic changes, arising from telomere shortening and natural DNA replication errors, as well as to environmental insults. In intrinsically aged skin, these manifest as thinning of the epidermis, flattening of the dermoepidermal junction and degradation of dermal ECM, including elastin, fibrillin-containing oxytalan fibres and collagens I and III. These changes result in dermal atrophy and reduced adhesion between the epidermis and the dermis, which manifests as fragility with easy bruising and tearing – which are often problematic in old skin. Thinned epidermis and altered proteoglycan composition impact on the ability of skin to retain moisture and to act as an effective barrier, increasing the risk of infection, irritant dermatitis and xerosis (Figure 4.10). Other functional skin changes in the older patient population include impaired vitamin D production and altered sensory perception, resulting in intractable itch. Extrinsic ageing, from sunlight radiation or cigarette smoking, further compounds these problems, and the phenotypes of intrinsic and extrinsic ageing are discussed further in Chapter 21.

Carcinogenesis

Cancer is inextricably linked with the ageing process. Genetic and epigenetic mutations accumulate with age and can lead to activation of growth-promoting genes (oncogenes) and/or inhibition of growth-suppressing genes (tumour suppressor genes), shifting the homeostatic balance of a tissue towards uncontrolled proliferation. As previously mentioned, UV radiation can also cause mutations. This is particularly pertinent to cancers

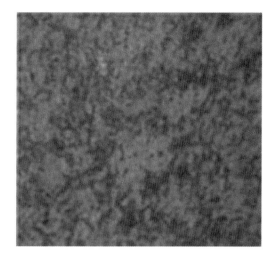

Figure 4.10 Asteatotic eczema (eczema craquelé), induced by erlotinib. This is particularly common in older patients due to loss of effective barrier function with age, resulting in significant xerosis of the skin. This can be exacerbated in the winter, when it is most commonly seen. Chiu HY *et al.* Erlotinib-induced generalized eczema craquelé and follicular rash sparing the previous radiation field. *Clin Exp Dermatol* 2012; **37**:912–24.

derived from keratinocytes, namely basal cell carcinomas (BCCs) and squamous cell carcinomas (SCCs), which characteristically occur on sun-exposed sites. It is also relevant to melanoma, which can be broadly categorised into chronically sun-damaged (CSD) and non-CSD melanoma.

Cells acquire mutations and epigenetic changes with surprising frequency, and thus it is remarkable that cancer in the first 50 years of life is relatively rare. In addition to maintaining a small, largely quiescent population of stem cells (limiting mutations in stem cells to approximately 10 per year), this reflects the efficient mechanisms that the body has to repair DNA damage. Moreover, if DNA repair is not possible, DNA damage surveillance mechanisms exist to eliminate genetically unstable cells. These include removal by immune cells, such as natural killer cells, as well as by apoptosis (a form of programmed cell death). A good example of successful p53-dependent apoptosis can be observed after sunburn, in which sheets of epidermis slough off after damage from high doses of UV radiation. Populations of mutant cells can also be eliminated by a 'neighbourhood watch-like' mechanism, in which mutant cells are recognised, surrounded and eliminated by non-mutant keratinocytes.

The efficiency of these regulatory mechanisms falls with time, reflecting the absence of evolutionary pressure after reproductive age. Somatic mutations in genes involved in repair pathways, such as *TP53* (which encodes p53), are frequently observed in sun-exposed skin, resulting in abundant somatic mutations in 'normal' skin with advanced age and thus a predisposition to skin cancer.

Immunosuppression (such as the immunosuppressive regimens used after organ transplantation) also increases the risk of skin cancer significantly, including SCC (100–250 times higher), Merkel cell carcinoma and melanoma. This occurs not only because immunosuppression impairs the previously described immune-cell-mediated mechanisms to clear mutant cells, but also because immunosuppression predisposes to oncogenic infections such as Merkel cell polyomavirus (responsible for most cases of Merkel cell carcinoma) and certain human papillomaviruses.

Regulatory mechanisms can also fail prematurely from germline mutations in genes involved in DNA repair mechanisms. These can be observed in xeroderma pigmentosum, Muir–Torre syndrome, Bloom syndrome and Werner syndrome, which are all associated with a predisposition to cancer.

The future

Interestingly, a nearly complete three-dimensional skin was assembled *in vitro* from human pluripotent stem cells, including epidermis, dermis and hair follicles (Figure 4.11). The only missing component was immune cells. This exciting development may offer the opportunity to further understand the embryology of the skin, as well as facilitating functional genomic studies. This is an important advance in stem cell biology, but advances are also being seen in the fields of genomics, including single-cell RNA sequencing and gene editing, as well as artificial intelligence. The future thus offers significant promise of further understanding of skin diseases and new therapeutics.

Pearls and pitfalls

- Filaggrin is crucial in collapsing keratinocytes into flattened corneocytes. Mutations in the filaggrin gene can thus result in abnormal corneocytes and a dysfunctional skin barrier, which clinically can manifest as ichthyosis vulgaris or atopic dermatitis.
- Eccrine sweat glands are innervated by cholinergic nerves, therefore anticholinergic drugs can be effective in primary hyperhidrosis.
- The number of mutations in epidermal stem cells is around 10 per year, per person. However, regular UV exposure increases mutations, leading eventually to large areas of 'field change'.

- Variations in stratum corneum thickness result in differing rates of drug absorption. Potent topical corticosteroids are therefore required for inflammatory conditions affecting the palms and soles, but are not appropriate at thin stratum corneum sites, such as the eyelid.
- A diagnostic skin biopsy of the proximal nail matrix (the germinative part of the nail) can cause scarring and permanent deformity. This is essential to discuss pre-operatively.
- Immunosuppressant regimens after organ transplant increase skin cancer risk through reduced immune surveillance and by a predisposition to oncogenic infections.

SCE Questions. See questions 1 and 2.

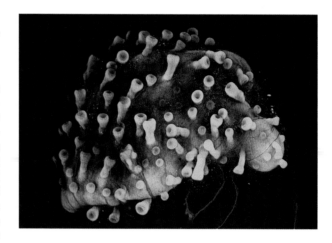

Figure 4.11 This is human skin – complete with hair follicles – that has been grown from scratch using 'pluripotent' stem cells that can develop into any cell type. Researchers hope that this kind of lab-grown skin will aid in disease research and improve reconstructive surgery such as skin grafts. Credit: Jiyoon Lee and Karl R. Koehler, Springer Nature Limited. (https://www.nature.com/immersive/d41586-020-03436-5/index.html)

FURTHER READING AND KEY RESOURCES

de Berker D. Nail anatomy. *Clin Dermatol* 2013; **31**:509–15.

Brettmann EA, de Guzman Strong C. Recent evolution of the human skin barrier. *Exp Dermatol* 2018; **27**:859–66.

Brown S, Pineda CM, Xin T *et al*. Correction of aberrant growth preserves tissue homeostasis. *Nature* 2017; **548**:334–7.

Byrd AL, Belkaid Y, Segre JA. The human skin microbiome. *Nat Rev Microbiol* 2018; **16**:143–55.

Haniffa M, Gunawan M, Jardine L. Human skin dendritic cells in health and disease. *J Dermatol Sci* 2015; **77**:85–92.

Ishida-Yamamoto A, Igawa S, Kishibe M. Molecular basis of the skin barrier structures revealed by electron microscopy. *Exp Dermatol* 2018; **27**:841–6.

Jeggo PA, Pearl LH, Carr AM. DNA repair, genome stability and cancer: a historical perspective. *Nat Rev Cancer* 2016; **16**:35–42.

Kabashima K, Honda T, Ginhoux F, Egawa G. The immunological anatomy of the skin. *Nat Rev Immunol* 2019; **19**:19–30.

Kinsler VA, Larue L. The patterns of birthmarks suggest a novel population of melanocyte precursors arising around the time of gastrulation. *Pigment Cell Melanoma Res* 2018; **31**:95–109.

Lai-Cheong JE, Arita K, McGrath JA. Genetic diseases of junctions. *J Invest Dermatol* 2007; **127**:2713–25.

Martincorena I, Roshan A, Gerstung M *et al*. Tumor evolution. High burden and pervasive positive selection of somatic mutations in normal human skin. *Science* 2015; **348**:880–6.

McGrath JA, Uitto J. The filaggrin story: novel insights into skin-barrier function and disease. *Trends Mol Med* 2008; **14**:20–7.

Tsakok T, Woolf R, Smith CH *et al*. Atopic dermatitis: the skin barrier and beyond. *Br J Dermatol* 2019; **180**:464–74.

Ziegler A, Jonason AS, Leffell DJ *et al*. Sunburn and p53 in the onset of skin cancer. *Nature* 1994; **372**:773–6.

Zimmerman A, Bai L, Ginty DD. The gentle touch receptors of mammalian skin. *Science* 2014; **346**:950–4.

Useful websites

BioInteractive. Available at: www.biointeractive.org.

European Academy of Allergy and Clinical Immunology. Global Atlas of Skin Allergy. Available at: https://www.eaaci.org/images/Atlas/Global_Atlas_IV_v1.pdf.

Journal of Investigative Dermatology. Skin Biology Lecture Series. Available at: https://www.jidonline.org/content/skinbiologyarchive.

NCBI. GeneReviews. Available at: https://www.ncbi.nlm.nih.gov/books/NBK1116.

Jonathan Rees. Skin biology and skin science. Available at: https://vimeo.com/showcase/3914207.

5

Dermatopathology

Richard A. Logan

Introduction

The teaching and study of histology and histopathology no longer enjoy the position of importance in undergraduate medical curricula that they once did. Consequently, most young doctors starting their training in dermatology have little or no experience in the use of a microscope, or much idea of what they are looking at down it. Therefore, the learning curve is steep when a new trainee is first exposed to dermatopathology.

A sound working knowledge of dermatopathology is of fundamental importance to the practising dermatologist. It assists the development of a logical approach to clinical diagnosis. It helps to decide when, where and how to take a skin biopsy. Furthermore, it allows a more productive working relationship between dermatologist and histopathologist. Many dermatological surgeons, particularly Mohs surgeons, regularly interpret histology (frozen) sections in their routine work.

Whether consciously or not, dermatologists choose their specialty because they have an aptitude for visual pattern recognition. Histopathologists share this skill, so it is not a surprise that significant numbers of dermatologists are interested and skilled in dermatopathology.

In this chapter, the basic concepts of dermatopathology are introduced, along with a suggested methodical approach to histological diagnosis of skin disease.

The magnification hierarchy

Diagnosis may be achieved by examining the skin at increasing degrees of magnification.

- Naked eye: most clinical diagnoses are made without further investigation.
- Dermoscopy: recent introduction of handheld devices allows instant magnification up to ×10. This is useful in assessing pigmented lesions in particular, but requires practice to learn a complete new range of pattern recognition (Chapter 7). Its principal advantage is to increase diagnostic confidence concerning the need for surgical excision.

Dermatology Training: The Essentials. Edited by Mahbub M.U. Chowdhury, Tamara W. Griffiths and Andrew Y. Finlay.
© 2022 The British Association of Dermatologists. Published 2022 by John Wiley & Sons Ltd.
Companion website: www.wiley.com/go/chowdhury/dermatologytraining

- Light microscopy: this remains the gold standard in the diagnostic process. The high-power ×40 lens is used regularly, which, combined with the ×10 eyepiece lenses, gives a magnification of ×400. A ×100 oil immersion lens can further increase magnification to ×1000.
- Electron microscopy: this is now seldom used in diagnostic dermatopathology because newer and simpler immunohistochemical techniques are often able to provide sufficient information, for example in the field of epidermolysis bullosa diagnosis.

Although skin histopathology is the technique most relied upon for accurate diagnosis, not infrequently a pathology report is received along these lines:

'Skin showing a moderate degree of irregular epidermal acanthosis with patchy parakeratosis. There is a mild perivascular lymphocytic infiltrate but no true vasculitis. The changes are mild and non-specific.'

Thus, histopathology does not always provide a specific diagnosis. However, even when a report is not diagnostic, it often helps to eliminate some diagnoses.

It is vital that the pathological appearances are correlated with the clinical impression. Thus, corroboration between clinician and pathologist is of paramount importance.

Help your pathologist

It is said of computers, 'Rubbish in, rubbish out'. In much the same way, to get the most helpful report from our pathologists, it is essential to assist them in several important ways:

- Choosing the most appropriate lesion to biopsy.
- Using the correct biopsy technique.
- Collecting and labelling the specimen accurately.
- Providing enough information on the pathology request form.
- Discussing difficult cases.

The most appropriate lesion to biopsy

- As a general rule, the newer the lesion, the more appropriate it is for biopsy. Older lesions are more likely to have been modified, for example by scratching or secondary bacterial infection. This is particularly true for inflammatory bullous diseases such as bullous pemphigoid.
- For eruptions on the legs such as suspected vasculitis, biopsy the highest lesion, because gravitational effects on the cutaneous vasculature are more marked lower on the leg and these can cause diagnostic confusion.
- Do not biopsy the middle of a scarring condition such as morphoea or cicatricial alopecia. Take an ellipse of skin from the actively inflamed edge of the lesion to include normal skin for comparison.

The correct biopsy technique
Punch biopsy

This delivers a small cylinder of skin, usually 3–4 mm in diameter. Its main uses are as follows:

- To establish the diagnosis of a tumour, e.g. basal cell carcinoma, where further definitive treatment will follow.
- To investigate inflammatory diseases where there is unlikely to be major variation in pathological changes in different parts of the lesion, e.g. discoid lupus erythematosus, vasculitis or Jessner's lymphocytic infiltrate.
- To remove very small lesions.
- To produce minimal scarring in cosmetically important areas such as the face.
- To obtain specimens for immunofluorescence (see later).

Punch biopsy has important disadvantages relevant to pathological assessment:

- The specimen is small, which may lead to it not being sectioned perpendicular to the epidermis.
- Small size can lead to sampling error in lesions where there is a gradation of pathological changes in different parts of the lesion, e.g. bullous conditions, suspected lentigo maligna and the edge of ulcers.
- In conditions where the pathology is suspected to be deep in the skin (e.g. panniculitis), the punch may not remove sufficient deep material.

Curettage

This is widely used for removing superficial lesions such as seborrhoeic warts, viral warts and solar keratoses, and also for debulking tumours prior to excision of the base. Because the curettage specimen is fragmented and variably orientated (Figure 5.1), the pathologist can only comment on the likely nature of the pathology and is unable to offer an opinion on the adequacy of tumour removal. It is common, for example, for reports on curetted Bowen's disease to include a caveat regarding the possibility of foci of invasive squamous carcinoma. Keratoacanthoma is a special case in point. If the lesion is fragmented during the process of curettage, as seen in Figure 5.1, the overall architectural arrangement of the tumour is lost (Figure 5.2). This makes it even more difficult for the pathologist to differentiate between keratoacanthoma and squamous cell carcinoma.

Shave excision

With this technique, superficial skin is removed using either a scalpel blade or a razor blade cutting horizontally, parallel to the skin surface. Its main application is in the removal of cellular naevi, when almost always the lower intradermal parts of the naevus are left behind. This does not usually matter clinically unless the naevus was pigmented. In this case the wound may heal with an unusual pattern of re-pigmentation. This can cause

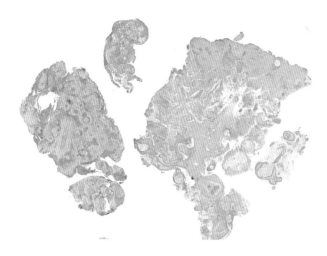

Figure 5.1 Fragmented curettings from a suspected keratoacanthoma (magnification ×4). The pathologist will not be able to give a definitive report on diagnosis or adequacy of removal. Courtesy of Dr Saleem Taihjee.

clinical concern about the possibility of malignant melanoma, and if the area is subsequently re-excised it may show atypical melanocytic changes (pseudo-melanoma). In other situations,

sampling only the superficial part of a lesion may lead to misdiagnosis, where characteristic and diagnostic pathological changes are seen more deeply. This is especially true for malignant tumours such as angiosarcoma and dermatofibrosarcoma protuberans, where the superficial changes may seem banal.

Ellipse biopsy

This is the standard and most widely used technique. It is appropriate for the removal of tumours in that it allows the pathologist to examine the periphery of the excised specimen and thus comment on the likelihood of the adequacy of removal. It should be employed if the pathology is likely to be in the dermis. It should also be used for diagnostic biopsies where there is likely to be a gradation of pathology from the normal skin into the centre of the lesion, for example in ulcers, scarring and blistering disorders. In this case the long axis of the biopsy should be at right angles to the margin of the lesion to include normal skin (Figure 5.3).

Collecting and labelling the specimen

Regardless of the type of biopsy, it is important to minimise trauma to the excised skin. The local anaesthetic should be injected into the fat under the skin to be removed, to avoid

Figure 5.2 Architecture of keratoacanthoma. The lesion shows symmetry, which is only apparent to the pathologist if it is removed intact. Finlay AY, Chowdhury MMU. *Specialist Training in Dermatology.* © 2007 Mosby Elsevier.

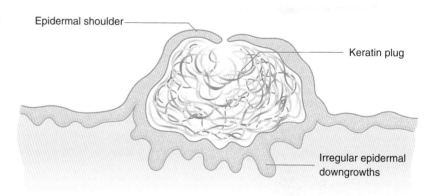

Epidermal shoulder

Keratin plug

Irregular epidermal downgrowths

Figure 5.3 The correct way to biopsy a blister or an ulcer. Finlay AY, Chowdhury MMU. *Specialist Training in Dermatology.* © 2007 Mosby Elsevier.

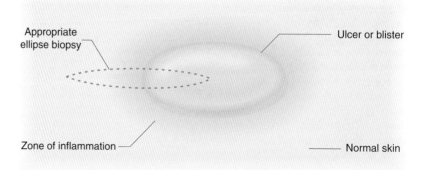

Appropriate ellipse biopsy

Ulcer or blister

Zone of inflammation

Normal skin

haemorrhagic changes and other distortions in the dermis from the passage of the injecting needle. If urticaria pigmentosa is suspected, the local anaesthetic should be injected around rather than under the lesion to reduce the risk of degranulating the mast cells. Crush artefact (Figure 5.4) is very common, especially in lymphocyte-rich pathologies such as lymphoma. It is due to the skin being gripped by dissecting forceps. This can be avoided by holding the skin at one end (preferably the normal skin) or, better, by the use of a skin hook.

In some situations, it is wise to take more than one biopsy, especially if lesions have different morphology at separate sites. This is especially true if cutaneous T-cell lymphoma is suspected.

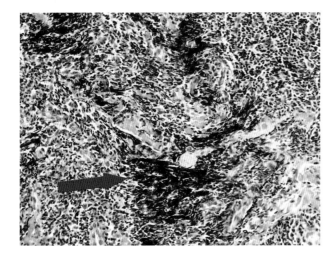

Figure 5.4 Crush artefact. The arrow indicates an area where lymphocytes have been crushed during biopsy of follicular lymphoma (×20). © Cwm Taf Morgannwg University Health Board.

In this condition, even when there is strong clinical suspicion of the diagnosis, it can take many biopsies, sometimes over years, before the diagnosis is confirmed histologically.

Punch biopsy for alopecia should be taken parallel to the direction of hair growth. It is often beneficial to submit two punch biopsies to allow processing of one biopsy for standard vertical sections and the second for horizontal sections. The latter allows for assessment of multiple hair follicles or follicular units in cross-section, and is particularly important in assessment of counts and ratio of anagen compared to telogen or catagen follicles in differential diagnosis of non-scarring alopecia (Figure 5.5).

For routine histopathology, the excised skin specimen is placed into a specimen pot containing 10% neutral buffered formalin. Specimens for immunofluorescence and molecular biological techniques such as polymerase chain reaction (PCR) should be placed in Michel's transport medium, which preserves antigens and antibodies in the specimen for up to six months. This avoids the need for such specimens to be snap-frozen and transported in liquid nitrogen.

Occasionally it is also necessary to send parts of a biopsy for additional tests such as bacteriological or fungal culture. It is tempting to remove a skin ellipse and then divide this up into smaller pieces. This should be avoided, as it traumatises the main specimen and may make histological assessment more difficult. It is preferable to take two samples and divide the second into halves for further tests.

It is vitally important that the details of the patient tally on the histology request form and the specimen pot. If more than one specimen has been removed, then they should be put into separate pots and the forms and pots labelled with an identifying letter and the site of the biopsy. This is to avoid confusion at a later date when one biopsy may turn out to be malignant and the other benign. Consider a simple line drawing to clarify the site of lesions on the pathology form and in the medical notes.

(a)   (b)

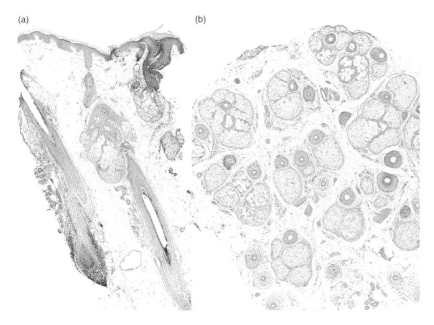

Figure 5.5 Scalp biopsies (×4). (a) Vertical section (alopecia areata); (b) transverse section (androgenetic alopecia). Courtesy of Dr Saleem Taibjee.

What happens to my biopsy in the laboratory?

It is important to know how a skin biopsy is processed in the laboratory. This aids in the understanding of some of the limitations, artefacts and delays inherent in the system.

For routine histopathology skin biopsies are initially placed into formalin fixative. From receipt in the laboratory to the specimen being ready for histopathological assessment takes on average about 48 hours, although occasionally it is possible to have a result in 24 hours. Frozen sections are rarely used in dermatology apart from the assessment of micrographic (Mohs) sections (Chapter 19), but these specimens can be assessed in 20 minutes.

Depending on the size of the biopsy and when it is received in the laboratory, the specimen will remain in formalin for between 3 and 18 hours (longer at weekends). The formalin 'fixes' the specimen, making it sufficiently firm to facilitate cutting up into a size small enough to allow the process of paraffin wax embedding.

For curettings, the pieces are processed 'all in'. It follows that they will be orientated in many different directions. This means later that the pathologist will not be able to make any statement on the adequacy of excision of, for example, a curetted basal cell carcinoma. A small punch biopsy or shave biopsy will also be processed 'all in'. However, here it is usual for the technician to be able to orientate the specimen so that the epidermis and dermis are correctly positioned for later sectioning. 'Ellipse' biopsies are usually sectioned longitudinally before processing. However, for larger specimens (e.g. removal of malignant melanoma) the biopsy may be divided as shown in Figure 5.6. A narrow transverse section will be taken from the middle of the biopsy, with up to six to nine further transverse sections (or levels known as 'bread-loafing') for more detailed analysis (e.g. Breslow tumour thickness assessment). The remnants of the original four quarters of the biopsy may be sectioned longitudinally. Increasingly, laboratories rely solely on the simpler bread-loaf technique (Figure 5.6, sections A–L only). Examination of several levels may lead to a delay in receipt of the report on a suspicious pigmented lesion.

Malorientation of the specimen at the 'cut-up' stage will lead later to the sample being sectioned at an angle that is not perpendicular to the skin surface. This can make the epidermis look thicker than it actually was and also leads to inaccurate assessments of tumour thickness. The process of fixing and subsequent dehydration causes shrinkage artefact. Thus, histological assessments of the measurement of excision margins are not exactly the same as the true surgical margins, which should be measured at the time of biopsy.

After 'cut-up', the pieces of the biopsy are then placed in 3-mm-thick cassettes to allow the process of wax embedding. This takes up to 16 hours and involves progressive dehydration of the specimen through several alcohol baths, 'clearing' in xylene (to remove the alcohol) and then embedding in paraffin wax to form a block. Sections of 4-μm thickness are then cut from the block with a microtome and floated onto a warm water bath, from which they are picked up onto glass slides for staining.

Staining techniques

The standard technique for routine histology is haematoxylin and eosin staining (H&E). This process is automated and takes about 20 minutes. Nuclei stain blue-purple, while connective tissue and red blood cells stain pink-red. This stain is sufficient for most diagnostic purposes, but does have some limitations. It cannot differentiate between different pigments and does not show some structures such as elastic fibres very well. Microorganisms such as bacteria will require additional staining techniques.

Some suspected diagnoses prompt additional stains to be carried out immediately, for example periodic acid–Schiff (PAS) for fungi (Figure 5.7). More often, additional stains may be carried out after the slides have been examined by the pathologist, for example Ziehl–Neelsen for acid-fast bacilli, if the pathology is granulomatous. Some of the stains used more commonly for dermatopathology are listed in Table 5.1.

Figure 5.6 Method of taking step sections (levels) through a biopsy of a suspicious pigmented lesion. Finlay AY, Chowdhury MMU. Specialist *Training in Dermatology.* © 2007 Mosby Elsevier.

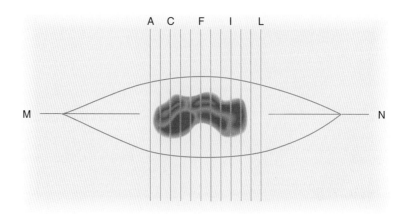

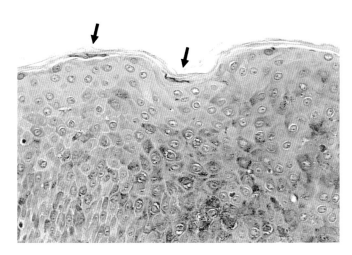

Figure 5.7 Periodic acid–Schiff stain highlighting fungal hyphae (black arrows) in the stratum corneum (×40). Courtesy of Dr Saleem Taibjee.

Table 5.1 Histochemical stains commonly used in dermatopathology

Stain	Tissue	Colour reaction
Periodic acid–Schiff (PAS)	Glycogen (e.g. Degos acanthoma)	Magenta
	Mucopolysaccharide (e.g. basement membrane; fungal walls – see Figure 5.7)	
Grocott methenamine silver (GMS)	Fungal wall	Black
Gram	Gram-positive bacteria	Blue/violet
	Gram-negative bacteria	Red/pink
Ziehl–Neelsen	Acid-fast bacilli	Red
Wade–Fite	Leprosy bacilli	Red
Alcian blue	Acid mucopolysaccharides, e.g. mucinoses; extra-mammary Paget's	Blue
Toluidine blue	Acid mucopolysaccharides, e.g. mast cell granules	Purple metachromasia
Giemsa	Mast cells	Purple metachromasia
	Leishmania	Blue
Van Gieson	Collagen	Red
	Muscle/nerve	Yellow
Acid orcein–Giemsa	Collagen	Pink
	Elastic fibres	Brown/black
	Mast cell granules	Purple
	Melanin	Black
Perl's (Prussian blue)	Iron (usually in haemosiderin)	Blue
Congo red	Amyloid (best to confirm using additional technique such as thioflavin T or CK5)	Red (with green birefringence under polarised light)
Gomori's silver	Reticulin (especially for assessing growth pattern in melanocytic lesions)	Black
Chloroacetate esterase	Mast cells	Red

Examining the slide

There are several steps in the microscopic assessment of a histology slide and each practitioner will develop their own method. Briefly these steps are as follows:

Naked eye

- Check that the label on the slide matches the details on the request form.
- Hold the slide up to the light: how many sections are there? How big are they? Are they from the same specimen?
- Is there more than one specimen from the patient and, if so, which one are you looking at?
- What is the dominant staining colour?

Low power (scanning magnification: ×2.5–4 objective lens)

- Is there any obvious pathology?
- Where is the pathology? Is it in the epidermis, the dermis or both? Is it in the fat?
- What is the pattern of the pathology (see later)?
- Look at all the sections on the slide – do they differ significantly?

Higher power (×10–100 objective lens)

- Study the cellular detail.
- Are the cells homogeneous or a mixed population?
- Is the process inflammatory, neoplastic or otherwise?
- If neoplastic, is it benign or malignant?
- Are further techniques (e.g. immunocytochemistry or immunofluorescence) needed to clarify either the type of cells or the immunopathology?

Return to low power – have you missed anything?

Regional variations of normal skin structure

Normal skin has significant variations according to body site, which can be summarised as follows:

- Face: this shows smaller hair follicles and prominent sebaceous glands. The epidermis is thinner than on the scalp, with a less well-developed rete ridge pattern. Striated muscle fibres may be seen in the upper dermis in biopsies taken from around the mouth and eye.
- Axilla: hair follicles and apocrine glands are evident and the epidermis may be folded (papillomatous).
- Trunk: the dermis is much thicker than in other parts of the body, especially on the back.
- Mucous membranes: the cells of the Malpighian layer of the epidermis are large and pale. There is very little stratum corneum, which usually retains its nuclei (physiological parakeratosis).
- Scrotum and nipple: the epidermis is papillomatous and smooth muscle fibres can be seen in the superficial dermis.
- Lower leg: in older patients, especially in the presence of venous hypertension, the dermal capillary network becomes dilated and tortuous. This can lead to a histological appearance of increased numbers of small capillaries in the papillary dermis.
- Palms and soles: the epidermis is thick with a well-marked rete ridge pattern. The stratum corneum is considerably thickened (Figure 5.8a).
- Scalp: this has large hair follicles with sebaceous glands. The hair bulbs are often in the subcutaneous fat (Figure 5.8b).

Common dermatopathology terms

There is a large vocabulary used in the description of skin histopathology. It is perhaps easiest to consider these terms 'from the outside inwards', or from superficial to deep. An overview of normal skin histopathology is given in Figure 5.9.

(a)

(b)

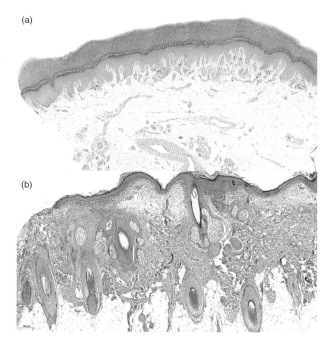

Figure 5.8 Anatomical comparison. (a) Acral skin showing thick stratum corneum (×2). (b) Scalp skin showing numerous pilosebaceous follicles with hair bulbs in the fat (×2). Courtesy of Dr Saleem Taibjee.

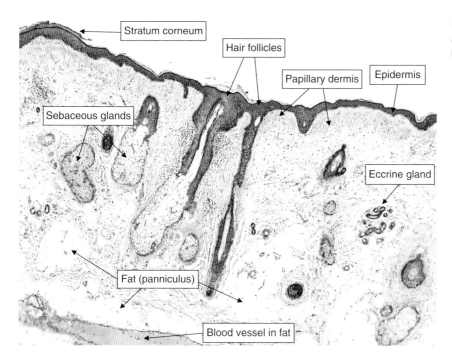

Figure 5.9 Normal skin showing some anatomical features (×4). © Cwm Taf Morgannwg University Health Board.

Epidermis

Acanthosis is thickening of the epidermis. It may be even and regular as in psoriasis (Figure 5.10), or uneven as in chronic eczema or prurigo nodularis. Thinning of the epidermis is *atrophy*, seen for example in lichen sclerosus or after topical steroid therapy. When the epidermis is thrown into folds it is known as *papillomatosis*. This can be physiological as in the axilla or pathological (e.g. viral wart).

Stratum corneum

The normal pattern is 'basket-weave' *orthokeratosis*, where the nuclei have been shed from the corneocytes. *Hyperkeratosis* describes any condition where the stratum corneum is thickened. In *parakeratosis*, nuclei are retained in the corneocytes. A large range of disturbances can produce parakeratosis, especially inflammatory diseases such as eczema and psoriasis. It is physiological on mucous membranes. The collection together of serous exudates, bacteria and inflammatory cell debris on the surface is *crust*.

Stratum granulosum

Hypergranulosis is thickening of this layer. It is typical of, but not exclusive to, lichen planus. *Epidermolytic hyperkeratosis* is a striking appearance where the granular layer is thickened and shows increased coarse granulation and perinuclear vacuolation.

Stratum spinosum

Widening of the gap between keratinocytes with oedema fluid is *spongiosis*, typically seen in acute forms of eczema. Coalescence

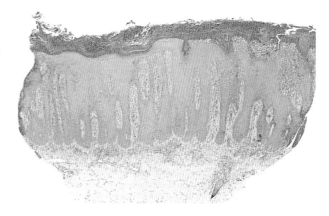

Figure 5.10 Psoriasis, low-power view showing regular acanthosis and parakeratosis (×4). Courtesy of Dr Saleem Taibjee.

of this fluid may lead to *vesicles* or even *bullae*. When the cells lose their intercellular adhesion and fall apart from each other it is known as *acantholysis*, a change typical of pemphigus, Darier's disease and Hailey–Hailey disease. *Dyskeratosis* is an abnormal pattern of premature keratinisation of keratinocytes. The cytoplasm is pinker than normal and nuclei are usually small and dark (*pyknosis*). It is typical of squamous carcinoma and Bowen's and Darier's diseases. *Exocytosis* is the term used when inflammatory or other cells permeate from the dermis into the epidermis, for example lymphocytes in eczema and psoriasis. Atypical lymphocytes may collect in the epidermis in cutaneous T-cell lymphoma by a process known as *epidermotropism*, where they may coalesce to form small *Pautrier microabscesses*.

Necrolysis is death of all or part of the epidermis as in erythema multiforme or toxic epidermal necrolysis.

Basal layer

This is damaged in conditions such as lichen planus and lupus erythematosus. The cells may initially show *vacuolar degeneration* and later die to form *colloid (Civatte) bodies*, which are rounded and eosinophilic. The shape of the rete ridges may be altered to a '*saw-tooth*' *pattern* in lichen planus. Increased numbers of melanocytes are seen in *lentigo*. A *villus* (pl. *villi*) is an upwards projection of dermal papilla retaining a single layer of basal cells. It may be seen in various blistering disorders such as pemphigus.

Dermis

Papillary

This is often the site of inflammatory changes. An intense band-like concentration of lymphocytes in this area and the adjacent upper dermis is called *lichenoid infiltration*. It is seen in lichen planus, other lichenoid conditions and cutaneous T-cell lymphoma (Figure 5.11). Collections here of polymorphonuclear cells with oedema are called *papillary tip microabscesses* and are typical of dermatitis herpetiformis. The absence of inflammation in this area with abnormalities deeper in the dermis is called a *grenz zone*. Collections of melanocytic naevus cells in this area are called *nests* or *theques*, and are seen in junctional and compound melanocytic naevi. *Pigmentary incontinence* is the presence in the upper dermis of melanin, either free or phagocytosed in melanophages. It usually signifies previous damage to the basal layer, as in lichen planus.

Reticular

Elastotic degeneration affects the papillary and upper reticular dermis due to damage from ultraviolet or less commonly ionising radiation. *Fibrinoid change* is the deposition of eosinophilic material around dermal blood vessel walls, most commonly due to necrotising vasculitis. *Hyaline change* is amorphous pale pink material, seen for example in the upper dermis in lichen sclerosus and around blood vessels in porphyria. *Nuclear dust (leucocytoclasis)* is fine stippled basophilic material near blood vessels, seen typically in small vessel vasculitis (leucocytoclastic vasculitis). *Storiform (curlicue) patterning* is the description of the way cells in dermatofibroma and dermatofibrosarcoma protuberans twist amongst collagen fibres to resemble the interwoven pattern of fibres as seen in a doormat. *Desmoplasia* is sclerosis of dermal connective tissue in reaction to tumours such as morphoeic basal cell carcinoma or desmoplastic malignant melanoma. *Necrobiosis* arises from granulomatous disorders leading to the death of dermal connective tissue. There is a zone of pale homogenised tissue usually surrounded by a 'palisade' of mixed histiocytic cells. This change may be seen in granuloma annulare, necrobiosis lipoidica and rheumatoid nodules.

Subcutis (fat)

Panniculitis is the term used to describe inflammation of the fat, which can be either in the fat lobules (*lobular panniculitis*) or in the intervening fibrous septa (*septal panniculitis*). In practice both patterns are often seen together. Panniculitis has a wide range of causes, the most common being erythema nodosum (Figure 5.12).

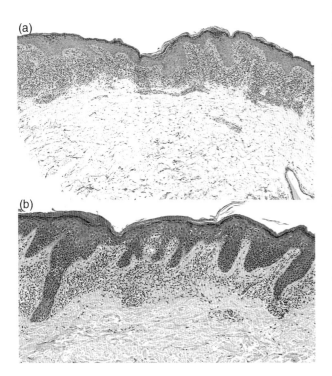

Figure 5.11 Bandlike (lichenoid) infiltrates (×4): (a) lichen planus; (b) cutaneous T-cell lymphoma. Courtesy of Dr Saleem Taibjee.

High-power cytology

After studying the slide at low and high power and observing the overall pattern of pathology, it is usually necessary to look carefully at the appearance of the individual cells. Of course, the most important decision to be made is whether the condition is benign or malignant.

Inflammatory conditions may contain a variety of different cell types (polymorphism) such as lymphocytes, histiocytes, plasma cells and eosinophils. Alternatively, the infiltrate may be monomorphic and consist of almost pure populations of one cell type, for example lymphocytes or neutrophils. Some of the important features of these commoner cells are shown in Table 5.2.

Features suggesting malignancy are:

- Variable size and shape of cells (pleomorphism) (Figure 5.13).
- Variation in nuclear size and staining pattern; increase in nucleoli.

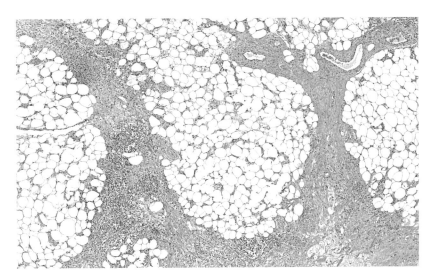

Figure 5.12 Panniculitis. Septal pattern in erythema nodosum (×10). Courtesy of Dr Saleem Taibjee.

- Increased number of mitotic figures: the caveat is that some inflammatory conditions such as psoriasis, and some benign tumours such as pilomatrixoma, can show increased cell turnover and mitoses. Thus mitoses per se do not equate to malignancy.
- Abnormal mitoses.
- Loss of polarity of epidermal cells. The normal, orderly arrangement of epidermal cells becomes haphazard and chaotic. This is seen particularly in pre-malignant epidermal dysplasias such as solar keratoses and Bowen's disease, as well as in frank malignancy such as squamous cell carcinoma.
- Invasion of neurovascular bundles.
- Single-cell infiltration between collagen bundles.

Further laboratory tests

Having examined the slide at low and high power, the histological appearances may suggest the need for additional tests. These include:

- Deeper (step) sectioning: there is a lot of truth in the adage 'the best stain is a deeper section'. Sometimes a diagnostic feature such as a scabies mite is revealed by cutting further into the block, obviating the need for further techniques.
- Examination of the slide under polarised light (see later).
- Histochemical stains (Table 5.1).
- Immunopathological examination: (i) immunofluorescence; (ii) immunoenzyme methods.
- Molecular biological studies.

Polarised light examination

Most light microscopes are equipped with a polarising filter that can be turned to examine the specimen under polarised

light. Refractile foreign material such as starch powder, suture material, plant fragments or urate crystals will shine brightly under these conditions. The technique is also used with Congo red staining to look for amyloid. Polarisation should always be included in the assessment of a granulomatous tissue reaction.

Immunofluorescence

This is used to detect the presence and position of antigens in skin biopsies (direct immunofluorescence). It can also be used to detect the presence of circulating antibody in serum (indirect immunofluorescence). Its main application in dermatology is the evaluation of immunobullous diseases.

For direct immunofluorescence, a small skin biopsy (usually 3–4 mm punch) is best taken from skin that is not usually exposed to sunlight (e.g. inner arm). Alternatively, it may be taken from non-lesional skin at least 2 cm away from the edge of a lesion. The specimen should preferably be placed in Michel's medium or snap-frozen in liquid nitrogen. It should *not* be placed in formalin, which can degrade the antigens in question and make their retrieval more difficult. After sectioning, the specimen is incubated with a rabbit-derived antihuman antibody labelled with fluorochromes that fluoresce when examined under ultraviolet. Fluorescein is used to locate antigen and gives apple-green fluorescence, and rhodamine glows orange-red and is used as a 'counterstain' to show the position of epidermal nuclei. The patterns of fluorescence seen in various immunobullous diseases are described in Table 5.3.

This technique can also be used as a prognostic indicator in the evaluation of cutaneous lupus erythematosus (lupus band test). The presence of one or more immunoreactants (other than IgM) on the basement membrane zone of non-sun-exposed skin increases the likelihood of systemic involvement.

In indirect immunofluorescence the patient's serum is incubated with an epidermal substrate (e.g. monkey oesophagus,

Table 5.2 Common cell types in inflammatory conditions

Cell type	Size	Cytology	Examples	Comments
Lymphocyte	7–12 μm	Small, round, darkly staining nucleus with thin rim of cytoplasm	Predominant cell in many inflammatory skin diseases; lymphomas and leukaemias	T and B lymphocytes indistinguishable on light microscopy but distinguished by immunohistochemical techniques
Neutrophil	10–15 μm	Multilobed nucleus; more cytoplasm than lymphocyte containing lysosomal granules; cytoplasm appears pink	Pus-forming infections, e.g. *Staphylococcus* abscesses; sterile pyodermas, e.g. pyoderma gangrenosum; leucocytoclastic vasculitis	Phagocytic cells – cytoplasmic granules not visible on light microscopy
Eosinophil	12–17 μm	Nucleus has only two lobes; cytoplasm is eosinophilic and appears orange	Drugs and bugs, i.e. insect bites, infestations and drug reactions; pemphigoid and pemphigus	Phagocytic cells – often seen in allergic reactions
Plasma cell	10 μm	Eccentric nucleus with 'clock face' pattern of chromatin; perinuclear pale halo in cytoplasm	Inflammatory conditions of hair-bearing skin and mucous membranes; late stage of granulomata; syphilis	Plasma cell is a specialised B lymphocyte dedicated to immunoglobulin production. Remember the rule of thumb: one plasma cell = infection; two plasma cells = syphilis; more plasma cells = plasmacytoma or myeloma
'Histiocytes' (tissue macrophages)	15–25 μm	Very variable. Fairly large cells, with a pale elongated nucleus. Cytoplasm pale. Shape varies from spindle-shaped to dendritic or epithelioid	Wide range of inflammatory, granulomatous, chronic infectious and neoplastic disorders, e.g. granuloma annulare; lupus vulgaris	Derived from circulating blood monocytes. Function is phagocytosis
Giant cells (GC). Three main types occur	40–120 μm	1. Langhans' GC have a horseshoe arrangement of nuclei	Tuberculosis and other mycobacterial diseases, but not specific to these	
		2. Foreign body GC have a random arrangement	Foreign body: may contain ingested foreign material	
		3. Touton GC have a central ring	Touton: xanthomata and juvenile xanthogranuloma	

human foreskin, rat bladder) to allow any antibody present to bind to epidermal substrate. Any bound human antibody is then detected by a second incubation with fluorochrome-labelled antihuman antibody and examined as above. The main application of this technique is in the evaluation of bullous pemphigoid and pemphigus. The titre of antibody present correlates with disease activity in pemphigus but not in pemphigoid. To distinguish between bullous pemphigoid and its rarer, troublesome 'variant' epidermolysis bullosa acquisita, patients' serum can be incubated with salt-split skin as the substrate (Table 5.3).

In many smaller hospitals it is common practice for immunofluorescence studies to be carried out on 'batched' specimens. This is because reagents are expensive, and the technique may only be carried out every 2–4 weeks. Thus the results of immunofluorescence tests are often received later than the initial histopathology report.

Immunoenzyme methods

The principle of this technique is like that of immunofluorescence. The difference is that instead of conjugating a diagnostic antibody to a fluorochrome, it is conjugated to an enzyme, usually horseradish peroxidase (occasionally alkaline phosphatase). When the enzyme substrate is added, the substrate is broken down into coloured reaction product (brown for peroxidase, blue for alkaline phosphatase) at the site of binding of the antibody on the section (Figure 5.14).

The advantage of this technique is that it can be used on paraffin-embedded sections and the reaction product does not

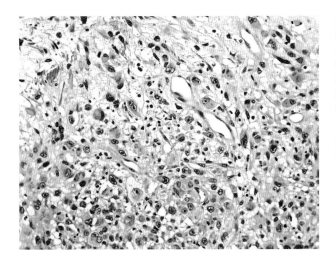

Figure 5.13 Pleomorphism. Variable cell size and shape seen in a high-power view of atypical fibroxanthoma (×20). © Cwm Taf Morgannwg University Health Board.

decay with time. It is used to categorise the likely cell type on a section, and is particularly useful in diagnosing tumours. Many antibodies to different cell types have been developed in recent years, some of which are listed in Table 5.4.

Molecular biological studies

Increasingly, mutations associated with malignant diseases are being characterised. This allows tissue specimens to be analysed using a variety of techniques, such as Southern blot analysis, PCR, fluorescent in situ hybridisation (FISH) and flow cytometry. These tests are highly specialised and carried out in only a few reference

laboratories. Although the results may take several weeks to obtain, this is not always the case and some labs are able to turn around results quickly. These techniques have particular application in dermatopathology for characterising, for example, malignant melanoma (BRAF status), lymphomas (T- and B-cell receptor gene rearrangement) and sarcomas. Some techniques such as BRAF analysis will work on fixed specimens, but others require fresh tissue.

Although the demonstration of the presence of a clonal T-cell receptor gene re-arrangement can help in the diagnosis of cutaneous T-cell lymphoma, this cannot be regarded as the sole

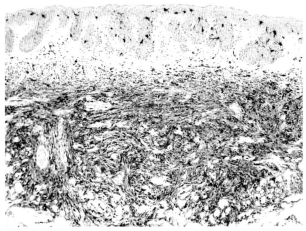

Figure 5.14 Biopsy of an epithelioid blue naevus stained for S100 (immunoperoxidase technique ×10). Naevus cells stain brown, as do the normal epidermal melanocytes and Langerhans cells. © Cwm Taf Morgannwg University Health Board.

Table 5.3 Results of direct immunofluorescence

Disease	Immunoreactant(s)	Site	Pattern
Bullous pemphigoid	IgG and C3	Dermoepidermal junction (DEJ) (epidermal side on salt-split skin)	Linear
Epidermolysis bullosa acquisita	IgG and C3	DEJ (dermal side on salt-split skin)	Linear
Cicatricial pemphigoid	IgG and C3	DEJ	Linear
Pemphigoid gestationis	C3	DEJ	Linear
Linear IgA disease	IgA	DEJ	Linear
Pemphigus	IgG and C3	Around epidermal cells	Net-like
Paraneoplastic pemphigus	IgG (occasionally C3)	Around epidermal cells	Net-like
	IgG, C3 (occasionally IgM)	DEJ	Linear and granular
Dermatitis herpetiformis	IgA	Papillary tips	Granular and focal
Bullous lupus erythematosus	Many immunoglobulins, C3 and fibrin	DEJ	Linear homogeneous or non-homogeneous

Table 5.4 Selection of cell markers used in immunocytochemistry

Diagnostic group	Marker	Cell or tumour type
Epidermal tumours	BerEP4	Basal cell carcinoma
	CK5/6 (cytoplasmic), p63/p40 (nuclear), EMA	Squamous cell carcinoma
	Ki67 proliferation marker	Widely used as an indicator of tumour growth and prognosis
Poorly differentiated malignancy	Cytokeratins: AE1/AE3, CAM 5.2	Carcinoma
	S100, melan-A, HMB-45, MART-1, SOX10 (nuclear)	Melanoma
	LCA, CD45	Lymphoma
Lymphoma	CD2–5, CD7, CD8	T-cell markers
	CD20	B-cell marker
	Ber-H2 (CD30)	Lymphomatoid papulosis, transforming T-cell lymphoma and anaplastic large cell lymphoma
Soft-tissue neoplasms	S100	Neurofibroma; schwannoma
	Factor XIIIa	Dermal dendrocyte (dermatofibroma)
	Desmin, SMA	Leiomyoma; glomus tumour
	CD-34	Dermatofibrosarcoma protuberans
Small, blue cell tumours	LCA, CD45	Lymphoma
	CD56, CK20, synaptophysin	Merkel cell tumour
	S100	Benign melanocytic tumours (naevi) and melanoma
	Neurone-specific enolase	Neuroblastoma
	TTF-1	Metastatic small cell carcinoma
Vascular tumours	ERG, factor VIII-related antigen	Endothelium
	HHV-8	Kaposi's sarcoma

HHV, human herpesvirus; LCA, leucocyte common antigen; SMA, smooth muscle actin; TTF, thyroid transcription factor.

diagnostic test, as certain benign diseases such as lymphomatoid papulosis, pityriasis lichenoides and cutaneous lymphoid hyperplasia may occasionally show such abnormalities.

Low-power pattern recognition

This is a vital skill for a dermatopathologist. First championed by the late Dr Bernard Ackerman of New York, it has become enshrined in literature and subsequently adapted many times. On first looking at a slide, it is usually possible to put it into one of the low-power patterns, as shown in the algorithm in Figure 5.15. These main categories can be further expanded, as shown in the list in Table 5.5. For each subcategory there is a wide differential

diagnosis, for example for an apparently 'normal' slide (Table 5.6). It should also be remembered that life is not always so straightforward and overlapping patterns may be seen.

Some illustrative case examples for low-power pattern recognition:

- Case 1. Figure 5.16 is an example of epidermally derived neoplasia. There is a collection of basophilic cells growing down from the epidermis, with surrounding retraction artefact. This is the histology of a typical superficial basal cell carcinoma.
- Case 2. The appearance in Figure 5.17 shows regular, psoriasiform epidermal hyperplasia with hyperkeratosis and parakeratosis. This was from a case of pityriasis rubra pilaris.
- Case 3. In Figure 5.18 there is hyperkeratosis, follicular plugging, vasodilation and a lymphocytic infiltrate around hair

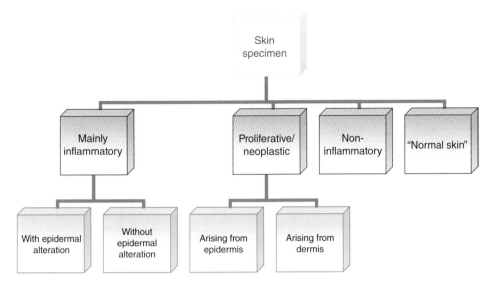

Figure 5.15 Skin pathology algorithm. Adapted from Barnhill RL, ed. *Textbook of Dermatopathology.* New York: McGraw-Hill, 1998.

Table 5.5 List of low-power patterns seen in dermatopathology

- **'Normal'-appearing skin**
- **Inflammatory patterns**
  - Spongiotic dermatitis
  - Vacuolar (cell-poor) interface dermatitis
  - Lichenoid (cell-rich) interface dermatitis
  - Psoriasiform dermatitis
  - Intraepidermal vesicular or pustular dermatitis
  - Subepidermal bullous dermatitis
  - Superficial perivascular infiltrate
  - Nodular dermal infiltrate
  - Diffuse dermal infiltrate
  - Panniculitis (lobular/septal)
- **Non-inflammatory**
- **Neoplasia**
  - Epidermal
  - Dermal

---

follicles and blood vessels. This pattern is highly suggestive of lupus erythematosus.
- Case 4. Figure 5.19 shows both a diffuse and, predominantly, a nodular pattern of dermal inflammation. Eosinophils were conspicuous on high power. This was an example of an insect bite reaction.
- Case 5. In Figure 5.20 at first glance there is not much going on. This is an example of a normal-looking or 'quiet slide', (Table 5.6) for which many potential diagnoses need to be considered. The diagnosis here was macular amyloidosis, confirmed by Congo red staining.

Conclusions

As an intermediate step in learning histopathology, it is recommended to try to develop a visual correlation between the clinical and histopathological appearance of skin conditions. This can be done by studying one of several dermatological atlases that include histology, such as the latest edition of Du Vivier's atlas (see Further reading).

To obtain more information from the web, there are numerous excellent online resources. However, any student of dermatology should invest early in their career in a full reference text on dermatopathology.

Pearls and pitfalls

- There is no substitute for practice. Look regularly at the slides of your own cases.
- Study the 'teaching slides' in your training institution.
- Attend meetings with your histopathologists. Do not discuss just skin cancer cases in multidisciplinary team meetings, but also inflammatory skin diseases.
- Make an effort to get to know and be on good terms with your histopathologists and discuss tricky cases directly with them (not only by email). Go and visit their labs!

SCE Questions. See questions 43 and 44.

Table 5.6 Causes of a 'quiet' section with little or no obvious histological abnormality

Category	Features	Solution or further tests
Technical error	Too small a sample including normal skin only, or an immunofluorescence biopsy of normal skin sent for histology by mistake	Repeat the biopsy and take a larger specimen
Epidermal conditions		
• Ichthyoses	Compact hyperkeratosis	
• Fungal infection	Patchy spongiosis and parakeratosis	Periodic acid–Schiff (PAS) or Grocott stain
• Porokeratosis	Cornoid lamellae easy to miss	Take more sections from block
• Atrophic solar keratoses	May show little dysplasia	Ellipse biopsy to include normal skin for comparison
Dermal conditions		
• Urticaria	Slight oedema with a few inflammatory cells (especially neutrophils) around blood vessels	
• Morphoea	Collagen bundles: coarse, compact and hyalinised	Ellipse biopsy to include normal skin for comparison
• Diffuse granuloma annulare	Collagen bundles dissected by mononuclear cells	
• Anetoderma	Loss of elastic fibres	Elastic stain
• Pseudoxanthoma elasticum	Dystrophic clumped elastic fibres	Elastic stain
• Urticaria pigmentosa	Adult forms show fewer, rather dendritic mast cells	Chloroacetate esterase; toluidine blue; alcian blue
• Blue naevi	Dendritic melanocytes in dermis	Melan-A (S100 may be paradoxically negative)
• Amyloid	Expanded dermal papillae may contain pink-staining bodies	Congo red; thioflavin T
• Iron deposition		Perl's stain
• Argyria	Silver granules seen near basement membrane of eccrine sweat glands	

FURTHER READING AND KEY RESOURCES

Calonje E, Bhogal BS. Histopathology of the skin: general principles. In: *Rook's Textbook of Dermatology* (Griffiths CEM, Barker J, Bleiker T, Chalmers R, Creamer D, eds), 9th edn. Chichester: Wiley, 2016; 3.1–3.41.

Textbooks

Ackerman AB, Boer A, Bennin B, Gottlieb GC. *Histologic Diagnosis of Inflammatory Skin Diseases*, 3rd edn. New York: Ardor Scribendi, 2004.

Barnhill RL, ed. *Textbook of Dermatopathology*. New York: McGraw-Hill, 1998.

Billings, SD, Cotton J. *Inflammatory Dermatopathology: A Pathologist's Survival Guide*. New York: Springer International, 2016.

Calonje JE, Brenn T, Lazar A, Billings S, eds. *McKee's Pathology of the Skin*, 5th edn. Amsterdam: Elsevier, 2019.

Du Vivier A. *Atlas of Clinical Dermatology*, 4th edn. London: Churchill Livingstone, 2012.

Patterson J. *Weedon's Skin Pathology*, 5th edn. Elsevier: Amsterdam, 2020.

Useful websites

DermNet NZ. Offers good, concise clinicopathological correlation for most conditions. At the right level for the non-pathologist. Available at: www.dermnetnz.org.

DermpathPRO. As the name suggests, this is aimed at high-level dermatopathologists. However, there is a daily Spot Diagnosis where new cases are posted that are available free to view. This is an excellent way to practise your pathological analytical skills, and also to see the erudite

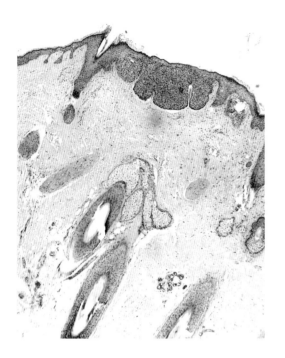

Figure 5.16 Superficial basal cell carcinoma (×4). © Cwm Taf Morgannwg University Health Board.

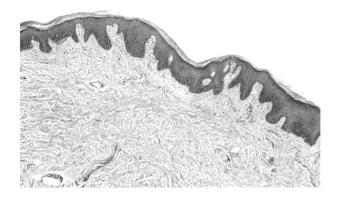

Figure 5.17 Psoriasiform (psoriasis-like) epidermal hyperplasia in a case of pityriasis rubra pilaris (×2). © Cwm Taf Morgannwg University Health Board.

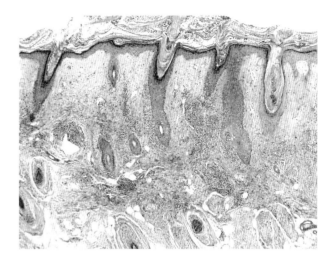

Figure 5.18 Lupus erythematosus (low power, ×4). © Cwm Taf Morgannwg University Health Board.

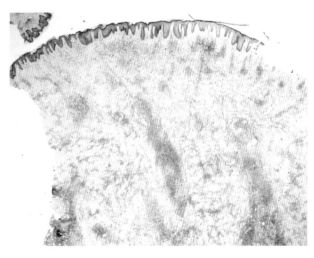

Figure 5.19 Insect bite reaction (low power, ×2). © Cwm Taf Morgannwg University Health Board.

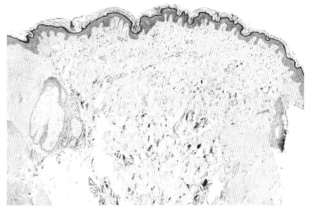

Figure 5.20 Macular amyloidosis (low power, ×2). © Cwm Taf Morgannwg University Health Board.

case discussions from world experts around the globe. Available at: https://dermpathpro.com.

e-Learning for Healthcare. An online programme developed jointly between Health Education England and the British Association of Dermatologists. Every registrar should make sure they have completed the interactive dermatopathology modules. Available at: https://www.e-lfh.org.uk/programmes/dermatology.

Leeds Virtual Pathology. A freely accessible, very large slide library. Available at: www.virtualpathology.leeds.ac.uk.

PathologyOutlines.com. A US-based definitive source of information, especially for rarer conditions and special stains. Available at: www.pathologyoutlines.com.

Acknowledgements

I am very grateful to Dr Nadine Burke for her helpful critique of the manuscript and to Dr Saleem Taibjee for his expert advice and also for providing many of the photomicrographs.

6

Teledermatology

William T.N. Hunt and Carolyn Charman

Introduction

Teledermatology can be defined as the practice of dermatology remotely. It uses digital technology to exchange clinical information and images to support patient care. The applications of teledermatology are wide, although a primary aim is to support the management of the patient by the right person in the right place at the right time. Teledermatology can be used to support all stages of the patient journey, ranging from self-care and community management to triage to the correct hospital service, tertiary care, and long-term monitoring and follow-up. It can be used as an effective tool to increase the efficiency of services, but it must be acknowledged that it is not a panacea, and the potential risks and benefits must be fully understood (Table 6.1). This chapter focuses on its use in the UK, but many of the principles discussed are universal.

Digital technology is a rapidly advancing and integral part of daily life, and telemedicine is transforming the delivery of healthcare. Teledermatology will form an increasing part of dermatologists' work schedules. Many events, including the COVID-19 pandemic, have accelerated the implementation of teledermatology pathways within dermatology departments and across healthcare organisations worldwide, with optimisation and mobilisation of teledermatology services playing a vital role in the restoration of elective care. As teledermatology is such a rapidly evolving area, dermatologists are advised to refer to the British Association of Dermatologists' (BAD) teledermatology guidelines and online resources, which link to the National Teledermatology Roadmap and are regularly updated in line with national guidance.

Teledermatology is a multidisciplinary discipline that requires close collaboration between clinicians, patients, commissioners, managers, administrative staff and information technology teams from primary, community and secondary care. National teledermatology guidelines should be tailored to local needs to support effective implementation.

Dermatology Training: The Essentials. Edited by Mahbub M.U. Chowdhury, Tamara W. Griffiths and Andrew Y. Finlay.
© 2022 The British Association of Dermatologists. Published 2022 by John Wiley & Sons Ltd.
Companion website: www.wiley.com/go/chowdhury/dermatologytraining

Table 6.1 Teledermatology for inflammatory skin disease

Benefits	Risks and limitations
Teledermatology is effective for photographing localised areas of skin disease or rashes, including the most severely affected areas	It can be time consuming and technically challenging for primary care teams to take photographs of widespread skin disease, particularly if there is scalp or mucosal involvement
Teledermatology can support rapid diagnosis and management of a wide range of inflammatory skin diseases, such as eczema, psoriasis and urticaria	Asynchronous teledermatology does not allow dialogue with the patient in order to readily assess symptoms, concerns and expectations; these factors need to be communicated indirectly through the general practitioner or referring healthcare professional
Teledermatology may enable patients to be triaged to the most appropriate clinic first time, including directly to specialist services such as patch testing or phototherapy	It is vital that patients receive adequate information about tests and treatments if being triaged directly to specialist services. This may require a telephone consultation with a dermatology healthcare professional prior to the specialist service appointment
Face-to-face appointments can be reserved for patients who are likely to benefit, enabling patients who have not yet received adequate first-line topical therapy to be prescribed appropriate treatment in the community	The quality of dermatological care in the community will depend on the quality of the digital advice provided by the dermatology specialist, and the resources and experience of the primary care team to provide and maintain care in the community

Teledermatology can be broadly divided into two models, which will be discussed in context through the chapter:

- **Asynchronous teledermatology**. Patient information and images are transmitted to dermatology healthcare professionals using secure web-based platforms, using either mobile or desktop devices. Information can be reviewed by the clinician and responded to flexibly, within mutually agreed timeframes. Asynchronous teledermatology (sometimes called store and forward) is the most commonly used form of teledermatology.
- **Synchronous teledermatology**. Teledermatology consultations are carried out in real time using secure video-consultation technology or video-conferencing platforms, with real-time exchange of clinical information between patients and clinicians. Synchronous teledermatology is less frequently used for advice and guidance and referral triage, but can be used to replace face-to-face outpatient consultations where appropriate.

A combination of synchronous and asynchronous teledermatology can be used to support clinical teaching and multidisciplinary case discussion between healthcare professionals locally, regionally, nationally or internationally, using platforms approved by the National Health Service (NHS) (such as Microsoft Teams® and Zoom®).

Teledermatology and the patient journey

Patient-facing teledermatology

Patients are increasingly taking their own skin images and submitting these electronically to their general practitioner (GP) – with a clinical history – through secure digital primary care triage platforms. Some apps and triage platforms designed to support patient-facing teledermatology are described in the NHSX Dermatology digital playbook. These include mobile phone apps to enable patients to store their own images conveniently, or record patient outcome measures of disease severity in graphical form to share with their healthcare professionals electronically or in person.

The availability of scaled-up web-based teledermatology platforms to directly link patients with dermatologists remains limited, with GPs still retaining the role as gatekeepers for images; this is an area for future teledermatology expansion.

Web-based portals allow more effective audit and data access by all healthcare professionals involved in patient care, compared to email-based teledermatology.

Images emailed directly to dermatologists by the patient may provide direct access to secondary care, but patients should be advised that those sent from personal email addresses to centralised addresses are not encrypted.

Teledermatology between primary and secondary care (including intermediate care)

Digital technology is increasingly allowing dynamic discussion and exchange of clinical images between primary and secondary care healthcare professionals (usually but not exclusively GPs and dermatology consultants) at the point where an outpatient referral would traditionally have been required. Teledermatology at the primary–secondary care interface enables GPs and dermatologists to collaboratively support and prioritise patients, bypassing the need for secondary care clinicians to see every patient face to face. This approach can build relationships between clinicians and support digital case-based clinical education around common skin conditions, treatment pathways and clinical guidelines.

The most common form of asynchronous teledermatology is the 'advice and guidance' (A&G) model, where images are taken by the GP or other member of staff within primary care and uploaded to digital platforms for assessment by dermatology. Asynchronous A&G digital platforms include the NHS e-Referral Service (e-RS) (described in the NHS A&G Toolkit and Advice and Guidance high impact intervention guides) or other commercial A&G platforms. These offer both telephone and asynchronous advice through mobile devices where there is agreement from all stakeholders. These A&G models allow audit and data access by all healthcare professionals involved in patient care, with significant benefits over email-based teledermatology.

Clinical images can also be attached to standard electronic outpatient referrals. This can enable dermatology specialists to either return the referral with advice or triage the referral to the correct outpatient service. If the quality or uptake of primary care photography is low, teledermatology models using medical photographers (based in community hubs or in the hospital) can be beneficial, particularly in skin cancer teledermatology pathways (where high-quality dermatoscopic images are recommended).

Teledermatology within secondary care

Within secondary care, teledermatology has a wide range of applications, including remote outpatient consultations, on-call referrals, multidisciplinary team meetings, undergraduate and postgraduate teaching, and inter-hospital digital referral. Remote consultations should aim to provide a comparable level of care to face-to-face assessment, taking into account patient choice and access to digital technology. Flexibility to convert to a face-to-face consultation is needed, alongside the provision of safety netting and treatment escalation plans.

Synchronous teledermatology outpatient consultations

Teledermatology can be used to deliver new or follow-up consultations to patients who have been referred and accepted for outpatient review, as an alternative to face-to-face consultation if appropriate. A remote consultation is a synchronous appointment that takes place between a patient and a clinician over the telephone or using a secure web-based video consultation platform (see Further reading). A wide range of factors should be taken into account when assessing the suitability of patients for digital consultation, as described in the NHS England guidance 'Setting up remote consultation services for people with skin conditions'. Synchronous video consultations cannot always provide sufficient image resolution for dermatology diagnosis and management, due to patient movement, connectivity restrictions, inadequate lighting and difficulty focusing on close-up lesions or certain body sites.

Asynchronous teledermatology can be used to supplement both phone and video consultations.

Teledermatology for inter-speciality and on-call referral

Within the hospital setting, clinicians can discuss the management of dermatology patients and exchange images using a range of digital technologies, depending on the hospital IT system.

Several hospitals have advanced electronic patient records that support teledermatology using personal mobile phones via integrated secure apps, which automatically upload images to the central electronic patient record, avoiding the risk of inadvertent storage of clinical images on personal devices. This allows dermatologists to securely document rashes and skin lesions or surgical procedures, and to exchange this information with other teams within the hospital.

Other hospitals may use commercial A&G platforms that are external to the electronic patient record to support secure in-hospital telephone and asynchronous teledermatology through mobile devices and personal phones. Images can be exchanged within various apps or downloaded from a secure password-protected cloud into the patient record.

Secure clinical communication apps developed primarily for hospital communication allow clinical messaging and exchange of images between individual healthcare professionals or hospital teams, and the creation of patient lists and tasks to support in-patient care.

NHS emails can be used to securely exchange images and clinical dialogue within the hospital setting, but images should ideally be uploaded to the patient electronic record in order to be accessible by all of the healthcare professionals involved in the patient's current or future care.

Teledermatology for tertiary patient care between hospitals

Synchronous and asynchronous teledermatology are both increasingly being used to support patients with complex or rare skin conditions (e.g. epidermolysis bullosa) who require care from national tertiary specialist dermatology teams. It creates a 'virtual' hub-and-spoke network to provide tertiary-level care without the usual geographical and demographic limitations. This important advancement facilitates standardisation of high-level care for patients with rare and complex diseases.

Benefits, risks and limitations of teledermatology

Teledermatology provides many potential benefits for patients, clinicians, carers and the environment compared to face-to-face referral. However, it is important that the risks and benefits are assessed for each patient, retaining the option for the patient to receive face-to-face care if appropriate and required.

Teledermatology benefits

- Rapid GP access to specialist teledermatology advice on individual patients, including diagnosis, recommended primary care investigations, interpretation of results, treatment, and appropriateness or route for onward referral if required.
- Reduced risk of redirection or rejection of a referral.
- Potential to allow the patient to be managed in a community setting, with no need to refer to secondary care.
- Reduction in unnecessary travel and time off work for patients and relatives, with beneficial effects on climate change and the environment.
- Improved access to dermatology care for those living in geographically remote areas.
- Image exchange and digital dialogue between healthcare professionals can improve education and awareness of common skin conditions.
- Builds relationships between primary and secondary care clinicians.
- Ensures most effective use of face-to-face clinical capacity.
- Provides a digital record of advice and guidance communication for patient care, service evaluation and audit, providing advantages over telephone, paper and email advice and guidance.
- Flexibility in service delivery as asynchronous teledermatology can be provided remotely and at any time (within agreed turnaround times), including working from home (where appropriate).
- Can provide a rich source of data in the form of enquiries and reports, and inform future practice.

Teledermatology risks and limitations

- Loss of face-to-face interaction and communication between patient and clinician.
- Loss of ability to palpate the skin.
- Some patients prefer a face-to-face consultation, with the ability to discuss treatment options with relatives or carers present.
- Variation in patient access to digital technology and usability can impact on the value of teledermatology in different patient groups.
- Issues around educational governance: trainees without adequate experiential learning with face-to-face consultations may find teledermatology consultations challenging.
- Issues around digital poverty and digital literacy may put some patient groups at a disadvantage.
- May have an unintended consequence of increasing unrecognised workload.

Tables 6.1 and 6.2 list the benefits, risks and limitations relating to teledermatology for inflammatory skin disease and skin cancer.

Table 6.2 Teledermatology for skin cancer and lesions

Benefits	Risks and limitations
High-quality macroscopic and dermoscopic images may allow rapid diagnosis of benign lesions such as seborrhoeic keratoses, avoiding the need for a face-to-face referral in patients with no risk factors for skin cancer	High-quality macroscopic and dermoscopic images require the referring healthcare professionals to have access to dermatoscopes and be trained in dermoscopy and dermoscopic photography
Teledermatology with dermoscopy can support rapid diagnosis of melanoma, and ensure the patient is referred to the correct clinic urgently	The teledermatology reporting clinician may misdiagnose a skin cancer using images alone, and appropriate safety netting should be in place, including patient information to report any change
Face-to-face appointments can be reserved for patients who are likely to benefit most from total skin examination, particularly those with risk factors for skin malignancy	No total skin examination by a specialist trained in the diagnosis of skin malignancy. Incidental skin cancer (non-index lesions not detected by the patient or referring clinician) may be missed
Images may allow patients to be triaged directly to the most appropriate service such as skin biopsy, surgical excision or photodynamic therapy, avoiding unnecessary travel to appointments where treatment facilities might not be available on the same day	Patients require informed consent around the range of treatment options available before being triaged to a procedure. Therefore teledermatology triage to surgery or procedure usually requires a telephone consultation to allow two-way dialogue and discussion
Teledermatology can redirect patients to more appropriate services such as community dermatology skin surgery, plastic surgery or maxillofacial surgery	Clear teledermatology pathways between providers should be in place to ensure rapid and safe digital transfer of care, ensuring the patient is kept informed about their treatment pathway
Teledermatology provides a bank of macroscopic and dermoscopic images that in the appropriate setting may be used for teaching and research, including artificial intelligence (AI)	Clinically identifiable teledermatology images should not be used for teaching without patient consent. AI algorithms based on secondary care images should not be used to implement skin cancer diagnostic and triage pathways in primary care without being appropriately tested in a primary care setting

Taking patient images

Teledermatology can be most effectively performed using smart-phones or other mobile devices with internet connectivity to capture and transfer images. A range of commercial secure clinical image apps are available on NHS frameworks for commissioning by healthcare organisations (see Further reading).

In their simplest form these commercial apps allow images to be transferred from healthcare professionals' mobile phones to a secure cloud for downloading by clinicians or administrative staff into NHS clinical systems. No clinical information is stored on the mobile device. More advanced commercial apps and platforms can provide bespoke communication platforms linking patients directly to their dermatologist and into the electronic patient record.

Traditional cameras without internet connectivity can be used to capture images, but limitations with both portability and the complexity of transferring images to NHS systems can reduce teledermatology uptake and digital productivity compared to use of mobile phones and devices.

Obtaining high-quality medical images

The quality of images will depend primarily on the resolution and quality of the camera and the skills of the photographer, rather than on the platform used to send the image. The camera resolution and capability of the current generation of smart-phones far exceed the technical requirements for capturing high-quality dermatological images. Photography skills are most effectively acquired by practice and familiarity with a device. Basic principles for medical photography are as follows:

- Before taking images, ensure you have received informed consent from the patient (see below).
- Backgrounds should be plain and dark if possible (particularly in skin of colour). Light and plain-coloured backgrounds can be useful when photographing skin of colour.
- To avoid shadows, ideally the skin should be in contact with a background surface.
- Use good overhead lighting or flash (except with dermoscopy images). It can help to have the light source coming slightly from the side, to highlight any change in skin texture. Natural light may be more effective when taking images of skin of colour.
- When photographing lesions in particular, if possible include a scale to illustrate the size.
- Focus on the lesion or area of interest. Most smartphone cameras have a built-in autofocus feature, and you can touch the part of the screen you want the camera to focus on.
- For close-up images move the camera 10–12 cm from the skin in order to achieve a sharp focus. If you get too close the camera will not be able to focus.
- Check that the images are an accurate representation of the skin condition in real life and are crisply in focus. If the photos are not representative or are out of focus, then do not use them.

Teledermatology for inflammatory skin disease, lesions and skin cancer generally requires a minimum of three or four photos:

- A 'localising' distanced image showing the distribution and location of the lesion or rash on the body, allowing the size to be assessed in the context of the surrounding anatomy.
- A close-up view of the lesion or rash showing the configuration and morphology.
- If the lesion is raised, then a sideways photo can be very helpful to show the shape and height of the lesion.
- A dermoscopic image is required for accurate diagnosis of pigmented lesions, and can be helpful for a wide range of skin disease including haemangiomas, basal cell carcinoma and pre-cancerous skin lesions.

Taking a dermoscopic image

- A wide range of dermatoscopes have adaptors that allow attachment to smart devices and cameras (see Further reading). Most dermatoscope manufacturers provide step-by-step video guidance tutorials on connecting and using dermatoscope adaptors for teledermatology – refer to the manufacturer's website.
- Adaptors have a magnetic ring to attach the dermatoscope to the smart device and are very easy to use. A wide range of magnetic adaptors are available, including integrated phone case adaptors and universal smartphone adaptors, which can be secured onto any smartphone and have a mobile magnetic arm that can be positioned over the camera.
- Focus the dermatoscope for use in contact dermoscopy and attach the smart-device camera. Use a liquid interface and press the dermatoscope lightly against the skin; do not press too hard or you may compress the blood vessels. Take images with both polarised and non-polarised light.
- Include the measuring graticule (if the dermatoscope has one) in the image.
- If using a smart-device camera without an adaptor, when you hold the camera up to the eyepiece it is important to make sure the device is level compared with the scope. If it is on an angle it will be impossible to focus. Focusing the smart-device camera down the dermatoscope eyepiece (often by tapping the smart-device screen) will assist with obtaining a clear and crisply focused image.

More information is provided in Further reading.

Teledermatology for inflammatory skin disease

Teledermatology can be used for almost any form of skin disease, in both adults and children. Digital images can be particularly useful in supporting GPs to diagnose less common conditions such as granuloma annulare, lichen planus, tinea incognito and lichen striatus, or to support the management of common conditions such as eczema or psoriasis.

Where a patient has a widespread rash or skin condition, they should be referred via teledermatology only if it is physically appropriate and practical to take images that provide a representative view of all the affected areas. The accurate diagnosis of many inflammatory skin conditions requires a review of the whole body, including scalp, nails and mucosal surfaces. Certain body sites, such as dense hair-bearing skin, darkly pigmented skin, mucosal surfaces and genitalia, may be difficult to image accurately.

Asynchronous teledermatology does not generally allow two-way interactive dialogue between patient and dermatologist; therefore, teledermatology will only be effective if the referring clinician (usually the GP) has the facilities and clinical experience to provide ongoing patient support and review based on the diagnosis and management plan provided by the skin specialist.

Teledermatology for skin cancer

Teledermatology has significant potential to support the diagnosis and triage of patients with suspected skin cancer, and in addition artificial intelligence (AI) is likely to play an increasing role in future skin cancer teledermatology pathways. However, virtual skin cancer diagnosis carries risk, and robust safety standards and quality control, including audit and service evaluation, are required to ensure patient care is streamlined and not compromised by implementation of teledermatology skin cancer services. Patients with suspected malignant melanoma, squamous cell carcinoma or basal cell carcinomas at high risk of causing significant morbidity should be referred urgently to skin specialists who are part of a skin cancer multidisciplinary team (Figure 6.1).

Virtual skin cancer dermatology pathways should:

- Maintain the ability for referring clinicians and patients to choose to access urgent face-to-face appointments if required.
- Maintain the ability for provider clinicians to request to see patients face to face if required.
- Use all reasonable diagnostics to exclude cancer (with high-quality macroscopic and dermoscopic images).
- Provide direct communication with the patient (written or verbal) and referring GP.
- Provide patients with all suitable management options and explain their benefits and material risks as they would in a face-to-face process.
- Record the point where the patient is discharged back to their GP.

All healthcare professionals taking dermoscopic images should be trained in dermoscopy and dermoscopic photography. Teledermatology may be used outside of the skin cancer pathway to triage patients with suspected malignant skin lesions (usually basal cell carcinomas) and direct them to the most appropriate skin cancer service. This provides scope for the dermatologist to upgrade or downgrade referrals, triage directly to skin surgery (with a pre-operative phone consultation to discuss

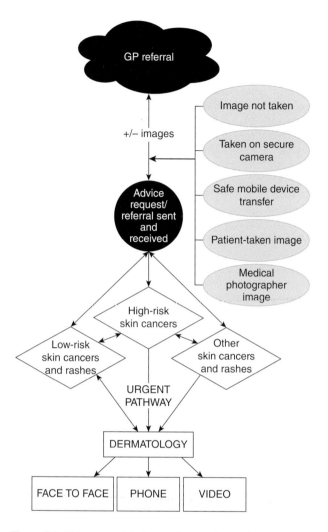

Figure 6.1 Skin cancer teledermatology patient pathway.

all treatment options), or redirect to other specialties such as plastic surgery if appropriate.

Teledermatology of individual skin lesions should only be used as an alternative to face-to-face consultation in cases where the referring clinician feels the patient does not require a total skin examination by a skin specialist (the patient should be informed of this limitation). This is particularly relevant in immunosuppressed patients, where tumours may be multiple and more aggressive.

Information governance and medicolegal aspects

Teledermatology should be used as a means of improving access to accredited dermatologists 'to provide high-quality, high-value diagnostic care'. The British Association of Dermatologists' position statement on teledermatology specifies essential criteria to ensure that any commissioned teledermatology service is of high quality, contributes to the management of patients (rather than fragmentation), meets National Institute for Health and Care Excellence guidance and quality standards, and protects patient privacy and choice.

Dermatologists should refer to the BAD teledermatology website and contact the BAD Clinical Services Unit, available at teledermatology@bad.org.uk, for any questions relating to information governance or concerning the medicolegal aspects of teledermatology.

Clinical risk

Teledermatology involves shared risk between the referring clinician and the dermatologist providing advice on diagnosis, management or onward referral. For asynchronous teledermatology, clinical decisions can only be made within the boundaries of the clinical information and images provided, as direct dialogue with the patient is not usually involved. For synchronous teledermatology, the quality of care may be limited by the inability to examine the entire skin accurately through video consultation, even though verbal dialogue with the patient is possible. Patients and clinicians should be aware of these limitations and there should be clear safety netting to allow face-to-face review within an appropriate and safe timeframe if required, particularly for suspected skin cancer.

Educational risk

Teledermatology requires the practitioner to make clinical decisions based on less overall information, for example the reduction or absence of non-verbal communication, lack of family interactions and inability to complete a total-body skin exam, elements that enrich face-to-face assessments. For trainees, adequate experiential learning and training in the face-to-face setting are required to develop the fundamental skill set to draw upon during virtual consultations. Without these underlying capabilities, it will be a challenge for the trainee to function safely and effectively in a virtual consultation setting. Adequate support and supervision from senior colleagues are required for effective learning and development.

Data storage and transfer

The core principles of teledermatology information governance, including data storage and consent, are described in two BAD documents:

- UK guidance on the use of mobile photographic devices in dermatology.
- Quality standards for teledermatology.

The General Medical Council regularly updates guidance on general data protection regulation (see Further reading).

Consent for teledermatology

Consent is required for patient images to be used for patient care, including diagnosis or triage. Written consent is recommended and specimen consent forms are available on the BAD teledermatology website.

Photographic consent policies should be discussed with the local healthcare organisation information governance and medical photography teams, as policies may vary across organisations.

The consent process:

- Informs the patient that there may be a difference between the accuracy of clinical care using photographs compared to face-to-face clinical assessment.
- Explains how the images will be used, transmitted and stored in the healthcare organisation.
- Obtains wider consent for teaching, publication or research if relevant.

If written patient consent is not possible or practical and only verbal consent is given, the healthcare professional should document this. Verbal consent would not extend beyond direct provision of care. Written consent is required for the use of identifiable images for teaching.

When patients take and transfer their own images

If patients send images to dermatologists from personal email accounts or mobile messaging, they should be informed that this constitutes a non-secure transfer, and that images are not subject to information governance and data protection until they have been received by the healthcare professional. There is risk in the transfer, although extremely low, that such information could be intercepted.

Once the image has been received by a healthcare professional, any onward data transfer and storage should meet the NHS data protection and information governance requirements of the healthcare organisation, and be accessible by healthcare professionals involved in the patient's care. It is recommended that images are retained when they have been used to make clinical judgements on patient care.

Integrated teledermatology

Dermatologists delivering teledermatology services should ideally be working in the region in which the patient receives services (except for tertiary services), in order to have an understanding of local and regional referral pathways.

Some commercial teledermatology platforms provide GPs with access to a national consultant network to address imbalances in capacity and demand for dermatology services across the country. It is vital that robust governance and transparent evidence-based commissioning mechanisms are in place when teledermatology extends beyond locally integrated services, to ensure patient safety and stability of local services.

Audit and service evaluation

In order to ensure teledermatology services are streamlining patient care effectively, regular audit and service evaluation are recommended, every 6–12 months. The Quality Standards for Teledermatology include guidance on audit and quality control.

Audit and service evaluation can identify variation in the quality of teledermatology referral information from primary care (clinical history and image quality) and teledermatology care provided by the dermatology team (quality of advice and turnaround time). Quantitative and qualitative data should be provided by the healthcare organisation to support optimisation and improvement of teledermatology pathways:

- **Quantitative** data on the monthly number of teledermatology requests at the GP and commissioning organisation level can support mobilisation of services and resource allocation in primary care. Monthly assessment of the number of teledermatology requests requiring further information (including inadequate images or insufficient clinical history) can identify where targeted teledermatology training in primary care may be beneficial. Quantitative monthly provider data on the number of teledermatology requests managed with advice, and the number of teledermatology requests converted to referral, at the level of dermatologist, department and hospital, can support job planning and resource allocation in secondary care. Long-term data on the number of teledermatology patients requiring an outpatient appointment within six months (or a locally agreed timeframe) can provide a more accurate overview of the impact of teledermatology on patient pathways.
- **Qualitative** feedback on the user interface and effectiveness, accuracy and educational value of teledermatology can be measured using clinician questionnaires and regular clinical review of cases within clinical teams.

Artificial intelligence and the future

Artificial intelligence (AI) is the science of developing computer systems to perform tasks that normally require human intelligence. There is immense potential to improve the diagnosis and precision management of skin diseases through AI interventions, particularly in the diagnosis of skin cancer. This is provided that AI interventions are adopted through a robust evidence-based and regulatory framework.

Events such as the COVID-19 pandemic have accelerated the adoption of digital technologies to reduce the need for face-to-face contact with patients and created a sense of urgency to implement AI in dermatology. AI interventions in dermatology have focused on differentiating between benign and malignant skin lesions, with a particular emphasis on melanoma diagnosis (convoluted neural networks). Despite this rapidly advancing field and the commercial drive to integrate AI algorithms into clinical practice, the current evidence base for the effectiveness and safety of dermatology AI in primary care is not yet sufficient to support widespread mobilisation, although this is likely to be an area of rapid change in the future. Current potential applications involve assisting decision making regarding referral in primary care and stand-alone mechanisms.

Conclusions

Teledermatology is a rapidly evolving area and therefore all resources are dynamic and web based. All the resources described in this chapter are accessible through the 'healthcare professional' section of the BAD website under teledermatology, and in the NHSX and NHS digital resources. It is critical that those engaged in teledermatology services have a good understanding of governance structures and national guidance, as well as potential risks and unintended consequences.

The practice of teledermatology requires dermatologists to get actively involved in regular teledermatology advice and guidance reporting and referral triage with consultant colleagues. Dermatology trainees should have supervised and supported exposure to teledermatology to acquire the necessary knowledge, skills and behaviours. Fully integrating teledermatology into clinical service models and pathways is likely to be the future of dermatology across healthcare settings globally.

Pearls and pitfalls

- Teledermatology can be defined as the practice of dermatology remotely. It is either asynchronous, whereby patient information and images are transmitted securely to dermatologists and assessed remotely, or synchronous, with real-time remote assessments employing secure video-consultation platforms.
- Teledermatology can be employed to assess inflammatory dermatology or skin cancer and lesions. The underlying provision and infrastructure regarding each of these teledermatology applications differ, and each approach carries its own benefits, risks and limitations.
- Teledermatology can be used directly between patients and healthcare providers, between primary care and secondary care, in secondary care, or between secondary and tertiary care. There are a number of applications involving synchronous and asynchronous approaches supported by different NHS and commercial platforms.
- A number of technologies are in development to enhance teledermatology. The integration of AI is readily being investigated to improve teledermatology pathways. Use of AI within teledermatology must be employed within existing regulatory frameworks, enhance patient safety and improve clinical efficacy.

SCE Questions. See questions 53 and 54.

FURTHER READING AND KEY RESOURCES

Lester JC, Clark L Jr, Linos E, Daneshjou R. Clinical photography in skin of colour: tips and best practices. *Br J Dermatol* 2021; **184**:1777–9.

Useful websites

British Association of Dermatologists. COVID-19: clinical guidelines for the management of dermatology patients remotely. Available at: https://www.bad.org.uk/healthcare-professionals/covid-19/remote-dermatology-guidance.

British Association of Dermatologists. COVID-19: guidance for dermatology patients for remote consultations. Available at: https://www.skinhealthinfo.org.uk/wp-content/uploads/2020/07/FINAL-BAD-Guidance-for-dermatology-patients-for-remote-consultations-.pdf.

British Association of Dermatologists. Dermatoscopes comparison. Available at: https://www.bad.org.uk/library-media/documents/FINAL%20Version%20of%20the%20Dermatoscope%20Comparison%20table.docx.

British Association of Dermatologists. Teledermatology. Available at: https://www.bad.org.uk/healthcare-professionals/teledermatology.

British Association of Dermatologists. UK guidance on the use of mobile photographic devices in dermatology. Available at: https://www.bad.org.uk/shared/get-file.ashx?itemtype=document&id=5818.

General Medical Council. Confidentiality: good practice in handling patient information. Available at: https://www.gmc-uk.org/ethical-guidance/ethical-guidance-for-doctors/confidentiality.

National Health Service. Advice and guidance: high impact intervention guides. Available at: https://www.england.nhs.uk/publication/advice-and-guidance-high-impact-intervention-guides.

National Health Service. Advice and guidance toolkit for the NHS e-Referral Service (e-RS). Available at: https://digital.nhs.uk/services/e-referral-service/document-library/advice-and-guidance-toolkit.

National Health Service. A teledermatology roadmap for 2020–21. Available at: https://www.imperial.nhs.uk/~/media/website/services/dermatology/gp-referral/notp-teledermatology-roadmap-202021-v10-final.pdf.

National Health Service. Health Systems Support Framework. Available at: https://www.england.nhs.uk/hssf.

National Health Service. Setting up remote consultation services for people with skin conditions. Available at: https://future.nhs.uk/OutpatientTransformation/viewdocument?docid=99385349&done=OBJChangesSaved.

NHSX. Clinical communications procurement framework. Available at: https://www.nhsx.nhs.uk/key-tools-and-info/procurement-frameworks/clinical-communications-procurement-framework.

NHSX Dermatology. Dermatology digital playbook. Available at: https://www.nhsx.nhs.uk/key-tools-and-info/digital-playbooks/dermatology-digital-playbook.

Primary Care Commissioning. Quality standards for teledermatology. Available at: https://www.bad.org.uk/shared/get-file.ashx?itemtype=document&id=794.

Primary Care Dermatology Society. Photography for the patient – how to take a good photograph of a skin condition/skin lesion. Available at: http://www.pcds.org.uk/clinical-guidance/photography-for-the-patient-how-to-take-a-good-photograph-of-a-skin-conditi.

Primary Care Dermatology Society. Photography – how to take a good dermoscopic photograph. Available at: http://www.pcds.org.uk/clinical-guidance/photography-how-to-take-a-good-dermoscopic-photograph.

Royal College of General Practitioners. Dermatology toolkit. Available at: https://www.rcgp.org.uk/dermatologytoolkit.

7

Dermoscopy

Ausama Atwan

Introduction

This chapter describes the 'dermatologist's stethoscope'. The stethoscope is a very simple device, enhancing hearing, and the dermatoscope is also very simple, enhancing vision. For both devices the challenge and interest lie in the interpretation of the signs.

Attempting to visualise details of skin structures is not a new ambition. It can be traced back to 1655, when 'surface microscopy' was used to investigate the small vessels in the nail unit. However, further significant development did not occur until two centuries later. In 1893, Unna recognised that the upper layers of the epidermis blocked light from entering the skin and that it could be made more translucent with water-soluble oils and other fluids. In the early 1900s, several monocular and binocular capillary microscopes were made. The term 'dermatoscopy' was coined in 1920 by Saphier, who applied dermoscopy mainly to evaluate skin capillaries in normal and pathological skin conditions. Advances in technology eventually led to the development of the smaller, more practical tools that are currently used in clinical practice.

What is dermoscopy?

Dermoscopy, also called 'dermatoscopy', is the application of a handheld non-invasive tool, the dermatoscope, to visualise skin structures and colours not normally seen with naked-eye examination. The dermatoscope has a light source for illumination and a magnifying lens. Some dermatoscopes are also equipped with polarising filters and are called polarised dermatoscopes (see Types of dermatoscopes).

Dermoscopy has become increasingly popular in clinical practice over the last few decades, mirrored by a rapid increase of related publications. In 2003, the International Dermoscopy Society was founded as a clinically orientated organisation to promote dermoscopy clinical research and to improve education in dermoscopy.

Why is dermoscopy important?

The incidence of skin cancers is on the rise. Morbidity and mortality are well-known risks with such cancers, especially when diagnosed late. Moreover, the clinical presentations of skin lesions, both benign and malignant, are widely variable, and can be deceiving or non-specific. Excising increasing numbers of lesions to detect the cancerous ones is obviously not a practical or cost-effective solution. Similarly, monitoring equivocal skin lesions until they develop overt clinical features of invasive malignancy can lead to harm and worse outcomes. Therefore, there is a need for a fast, reliable, cheap and non-invasive tool to aid clinicians'

Dermatology Training: The Essentials. Edited by Mahbub M.U. Chowdhury, Tamara W. Griffiths and Andrew Y. Finlay.
© 2022 The British Association of Dermatologists. Published 2022 by John Wiley & Sons Ltd.
Companion website: www.wiley.com/go/chowdhury/dermatologytraining

decision making. The aim is to detect and treat suspicious lesions at an early stage to improve the outcome, and to diagnose benign lesions with confidence to avoid unnecessary excisions.

Multiple studies including systematic reviews have revealed the added benefits of dermoscopy in the diagnosis of melanoma and non-melanoma skin cancers, compared with naked-eye examination alone. This has led to the recognition of dermoscopy as an essential tool in several skin cancer guidelines and in the National Institute for Health and Care Excellence (NICE) recommendations. It is a requirement in the current dermatology curriculum that every healthcare professional involved in the diagnosis of skin lesions should be trained in dermoscopy.

The applications of dermoscopy are not limited to skin lesions. Now it is commonly used to aid in the diagnosis of inflammatory skin conditions, hair disorders, nail disease, and skin infections and infestations. Dermoscopy for skin lesions will be the main focus in this chapter.

Types of dermatoscopes

Normally most light falling on the skin surface is reflected and scattered by the stratum corneum, so only very superficial skin can be seen by the naked eye (Figure 7.1a). However, applying a contact medium between the dermatoscope glass plate and the skin surface alters the light reflectance, enhancing light penetration and allowing reflection of light from deeper in the skin. This results in visualisation of skin structures within the epidermis, down to the dermoepidermal junction. This technique uses 'contact dermatoscopes', also called 'non-polarised dermatoscopes' (Figure 7.1b). The contact medium can be liquid paraffin, oil, ultrasound gel or medical alcohol (70% ethanol). Use of ethanol is advised as it forms fewer air bubbles under the lens and acts as a disinfectant to minimise cross-contamination.

An alternative approach is to use a dermatoscope equipped with two polarised filters that can achieve cross-polarisation, hence called 'polarised dermatoscopes'. They enhance the transmission of directed and reflected light, allowing better visibility of deeper skin structures to the level of the dermoepidermal junction and upper dermis (Figure 7.1c). Unlike non-polarised dermatoscopes, polarised dermatoscopes do not require direct contact with the skin surface or a contact medium.

Dermatoscope users should be aware of some other differences between types of dermatoscopes (Table 7.1). Some dermatoscopes have both polarised and non-polarised modes (hybrid dermatoscopes), where the user can toggle between the two with the press of a button. The use of these hybrid tools is recommended as each mode can provide different useful information.

Starting dermoscopy practice

Dermoscopy must be used in conjunction with, not instead of, detailed history taking and clinical examination. The patient's age, the duration of the lesion and its evolution over time, and associated symptoms (e.g. bleeding, tenderness, itching) are very helpful information in making a diagnosis. Dermoscopy adds extra information to aid in the diagnosis.

Although interpretation of dermoscopy images can be confusing at first, it is relatively easy to get to grips with the most important features. As you gain experience in using a dermatoscope, your attitude may progress from initial bafflement to finding it useful and then becoming a keen advocate, enthusiastically enjoying and propagating its use. It is helpful to have an experienced colleague to guide you. However, do not relax your critical attitude: insist on finding out the evidence base for the usefulness or specificity of dermoscopic signs, and keep an open mind about developments in this rapidly expanding field.

Some general points to consider are as follows:

- Melanocytic skin lesions refer to lesions arising from melanocytes. However, not every melanocytic lesion is pigmented. For example, amelanotic melanoma, non-pigmented Spitz naevus and intradermal naevi are 'melanocytic', but they lack pigmentation.
- Remember that not every pigmented skin lesion is melanocytic. For example, seborrhoeic keratoses and dermatofibromas can be pigmented, but they do not develop from melanocytes.
- Dermoscopy terminology has its own set of nomenclature. Specific dermoscopy terms used in this chapter are presented in *italics*.

Melanocytic lesions

Melanocytic lesions include benign and atypical naevi, Spitz naevi, lentigo maligna and melanoma.

Pigmented melanocytic lesions

These typically show one or more of the following patterns:

- ***Pigment network (reticular pattern)***: this is formed by lines of pigment (histologically representing rete ridges) and holes between the lines (representing dermal papillae). This pattern represents junctional activity of melanocytes.
- ***Globules (clods)***: these are round pigmented structures. They represent the 'nests' of melanocytes. Globules at the periphery of a reticular naevus indicate growth.
- ***Streaks***: peripheral radial lines emerging from the centre, a sign suggestive of growth.
- ***Homogeneous blue***: a blue featureless blotch. This represents pigment within the dermis, which appears blue because of the Tyndall effect (scattering of a light beam by a medium containing small particles).

Benign versus suspicious moles

When examining pigmented lesions, one should scrutinise the overall 'global' appearance of the lesion and the details of the components. Table 7.2 compares these patterns in benign and suspicious pigmented melanocytic lesions (Figures 7.2–7.9).

Figure 7.1 How dermoscopy works.
(a) Normally, most light rays falling on the skin's surface will be deflected and scattered by the stratum corneum. Only a fraction can penetrate the epidermis.
(b) Applying a contact medium (e.g. medical gel) on the skin's surface increases light penetration, allowing better visualisation of deeper structures. (c) Cross-polarised dermatoscopes enhance the transmission of directed and reflected light. Chowdhury MMU *et al. Dermatology at a Glance*, 2nd edn. Chichester: Wiley, 2019.

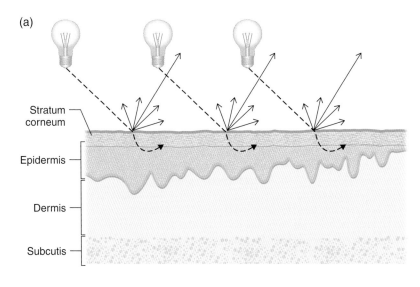

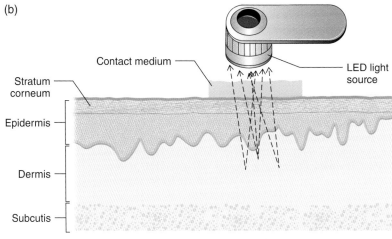

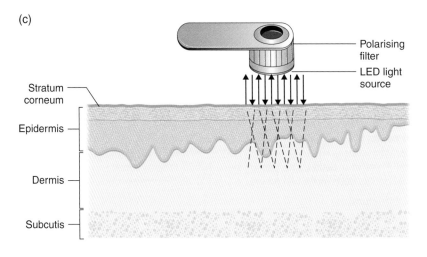

Table 7.1 Differences between polarised and non-polarised dermoscopy

	Contact dermatoscope (non-polarised)	Polarised dermatoscope
Vascular lesions	Pressing on the lesion can make vascular structures blanch, which may hinder the diagnosis	No contact required so pressure can be avoided
Patients with multiple lesions	Time consuming as application of contact medium is required for each lesion	Quicker for screening patients with multiple lesions
Structures seen only with certain dermoscopy modes	Milia-like cysts and comedo-like openings	Chrysalis structures (also called crystalline structures or shiny short white lines)

Table 7.2 Comparison between benign and suspicious pigmented melanocytic lesions

	Benign pigmented melanocytic lesion	Suspicious pigmented melanocytic lesion
Network	Symmetrical in colour and structure where the network tends to fade away at the periphery (e.g. benign junctional naevus; Figure 7.2)	Asymmetrical network (Figure 7.3)
		Featureless brown/black blotches (Figure 7.3)
		Sharp cut-off at periphery (Figure 7.3)
Globules	Similar in size and symmetrically distributed (e.g. benign compound naevus; Figure 7.4)	Various sizes and colours, and irregularly distributed (Figure 7.5). Note: peripheral globules can be a sign of growth (Figure 7.3)
Streaks	Radial lines emerging from a central structureless black blotch are characteristic of a pigmented Spitz naevus, called 'starburst pattern' (Figure 7.6)	Irregular streaks emerging from a reticular lesion should raise suspicion, suggestive of growth
Blue colour	The whole lesion is a structureless uniform blue blotch 'homogeneous blue' (e.g. benign blue naevus; Figure 7.7)	The blue colour is seen in part of the lesion, often with a white/grey hue (called a 'blue-white veil') (Figure 7.8)
Other features		Vascular structures (can be dotted, linear irregular, coiled or polymorphous)
		Multichromatic (multiple colours in the same lesion)
		Chrysalis structures (short white lines) (Figure 7.9)
		Scar-like white area (represents regression) with or without grey 'pepper-like' granules (represent melanophages)

Normal variations in benign melanocytic lesions

- **Structural variations**. It is common to see benign moles with more than one pattern (e.g. central globules and peripheral network). The symmetry in colour and structures is a reassuring finding. However, a lesion with multiple patterns in asymmetrical arrangements should be considered suspicious for an atypical naevus or even melanoma.
- **Phenotypic variations**. It is expected to see benign melanocytic lesions with central hyperpigmentation in skin of colour and central hypopigmentation in lighter skin types. In benign moles the overall appearance of the lesion will be symmetrical. Asymmetrical variation in pigment, on the other hand, can be a suspicious feature.
- **Age-related variations**. Peripheral arrangements of monomorphic globules can be a normal finding in a benign naevus of an adolescent child, where naevi tend to evolve. However, peripheral globules in a naevus of an adult can be an indication of unexpected growth. This should raise suspicion, particularly if the globules are of various sizes and irregular distribution.

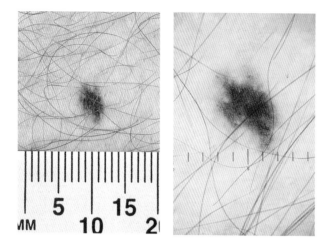

Figure 7.2 A benign junctional naevus on the leg of a 32-year-old man. The network looks symmetrical in colour and structure, fading at the periphery. © Aneurin Bevan University Health Board.

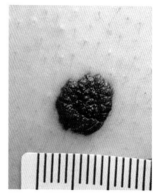
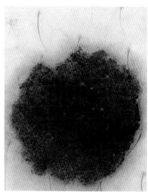

Figure 7.4 The globules in this naevus are similar in size and symmetrically distributed, in keeping with a benign compound naevus. Chowdhury MMU *et al. Dermatology at a Glance*, 2nd edn. Chichester: Wiley, 2019.

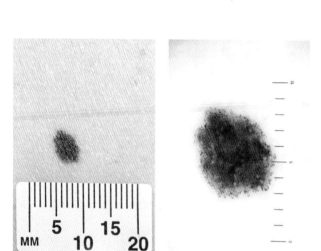

Figure 7.3 A dark naevus on the back of a 46-year-old woman. Dermoscopy shows irregular pigment network and peripheral globules (a sign of growth). Histology confirmed moderately atypical naevus. © Aneurin Bevan University Health Board.

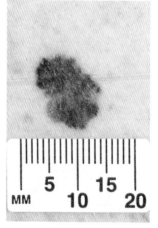
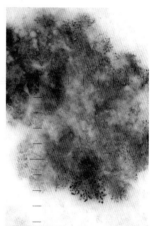

Figure 7.5 A melanoma on the lower back. On dermoscopy, irregularly distributed globules of various sizes can be seen, in addition to other melanoma features (featureless brown/black blotches and grey granular structures). © Aneurin Bevan University Health Board.

Facial pigmented lesions

A range of pigmented skin lesions can be seen on the face, such as pigmented actinic keratosis, pigmented basal cell carcinoma, seborrhoeic keratosis, solar lentigo, benign naevus, lentigo maligna and of course invasive melanoma.

Unlike in the skin on other body sites, the dermoepidermal junction in facial skin is flattened, and the interdigitation between rete ridges and dermal papillae is blunted. As a result, the typical 'network' pattern is not seen in pigmented melanocytic facial lesions. Instead, the pigment will be diffuse but interrupted by follicular openings, yielding a pattern known as *pseudo-network*.

Lentigo maligna

Unlike a simple lentigo, lentigo maligna (LM) appears asymmetrical in colour and structure under the dermatoscope. The abnormal melanocytes proliferate within the basal layer and extend down some hair follicles. This results in an appearance of grey *rings* at follicular openings (Figure 7.10). These rings can be fine, irregular or semicircular.

Another sign of LM is dark *polygonal lines* (also called *angulated lines*) around and between adnexal openings (Figures 7.10 and 7.11). As these lines get thicker and darker, they can coalesce to form *rhomboidal structures*. Finally, a dark featureless blotch can also be seen, which eventually obliterates the follicular openings. The presence of these *hyperpigmented blotches* (which do not have any specific pattern) is a good indicator for LM.

Melanocytic lesions in acral sites

The skin on the palms and soles has a unique structure formed of furrows and ridges, which create individualised dermatoglyphics (fingerprints). The *furrows* are the thin invaginations, whereas the *ridges* are the wider lines that also contain the openings of the eccrine ducts.

In benign acral naevi, the pigment lies within the furrows, giving a *parallel furrow pattern* (Figure 7.12). If the pigment is noted on the ridges (*parallel ridge pattern*) the mole should be considered suspicious (Figure 7.13).

There are several other dermoscopic variants of acral melanocytic lesions that are worth learning about (see Further reading).

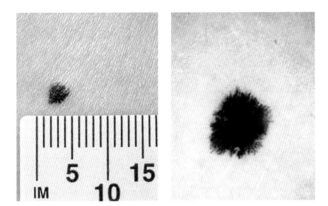

Figure 7.6 Radial lines emerging from a central structureless black blotch are characteristic of a pigmented Spitz naevus, called 'starburst pattern'. Chowdhury MMU *et al. Dermatology at a Glance*, 2nd edn. Chichester: Wiley, 2019.

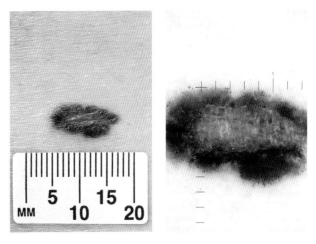

Figure 7.8 This melanoma with a Breslow thickness of 0.7 mm shows a blue-white veil in the centre, which also contains short white lines and grey granular dots. The surrounding featureless brown/black pigment and irregular globules also indicate a melanoma. © Aneurin Bevan University Health Board.

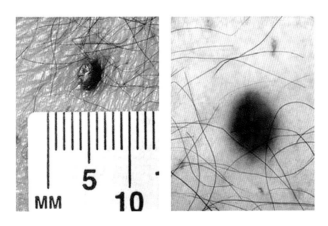

Figure 7.7 The whole lesion is a structureless uniform blue blotch of 'homogeneous blue' (e.g. benign blue naevus). Chowdhury MMU *et al. Dermatology at a Glance*, 2nd edn. Chichester: Wiley, 2019.

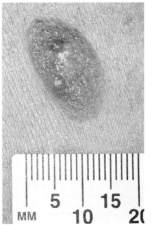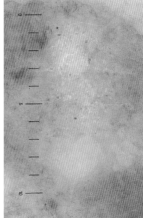

Figure 7.9 A hypomelanotic melanoma with Breslow thickness of 2.5 mm lacks clear melanoma features. The short white lines, along with the subtle dotted and short linear blood vessels seen in the centre of the lesion, raised suspicion for urgent excision. © Aneurin Bevan University Health Board.

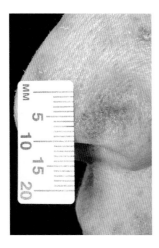
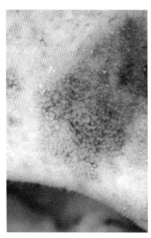

Figure 7.10 A lentigo maligna on the nasal ala. Dermoscopically the adnexal openings are of various colours and sizes, with dark grey angulated lines observed. © Aneurin Bevan University Health Board.

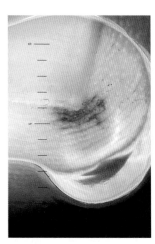

Figure 7.12 A benign acral naevus on the great toe shows pigment predominantly in the furrows (the thin lines between the ridges). Also note the eccrine duct openings in the ridges, seen as small white dots. © Aneurin Bevan University Health Board.

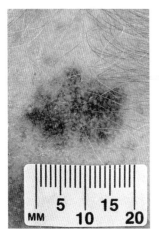
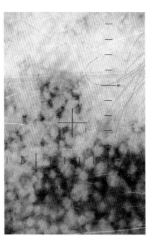

Figure 7.11 A lentigo maligna on the upper forehead shows adnexal openings of various sizes, semicircles (left side) and dark polygonal lines forming rhomboid-shaped structures. © Aneurin Bevan University Health Board.

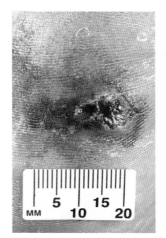
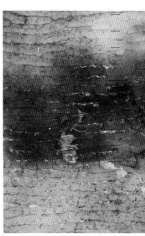

Figure 7.13 An acral melanoma on the heel of a 52-year-old woman. Pigmentation is noted in the ridges. Also note the scaling compacted in the furrows. ©Aneurin Bevan University Health Board.

Non-pigmented melanocytic lesions

These can be benign (e.g. benign intradermal naevi) or malignant (e.g. amelanotic melanoma). Differentiating such lesions relies on the vascular structures, in addition to any extra features.

- **Benign intradermal naevi**. In such naevi, *comma-shaped* vessels are seen, occasionally with traces of subtle pigment (Figure 7.14).
- **Non-pigmented Spitz naevi**. These show *dotted vessels* throughout the lesion intersected by white network-like lines, often described as a *negative network* (Figure 7.15).

- **Amelanotic malignant melanoma**. These can be easily missed or diagnosed late because of the lack of suspicious pigmented structures. Amelanotic melanoma can have one or more of the following features:

  - Polymorphous vascular structures (dotted, coiled, linear irregular, hairpin vessels).
  - Milky-red colour.
  - Short white lines, also called *chrysalis structures* (only seen with polarised dermoscopy) (Figure 7.9).

o Granular structures: minute grey dots that give the impression of *black-pepper sprinkles* (Figure 7.8). These are formed by melanophages (macrophages engulfing melanocytes).

Some melanomas only have traces of non-specific pigment, called 'hypomelanotic melanomas'. These traces can be a helpful clue, when seen with one or more of the above features.

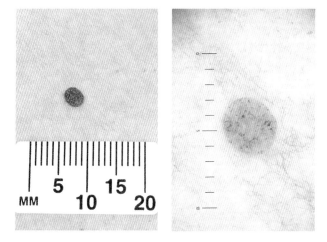

Figure 7.14 A papillomatous naevus on the upper chest shows short curved (comma-shaped) blood vessels with minimum pigment, in keeping with a benign intradermal naevus. © Aneurin Bevan University Health Board.

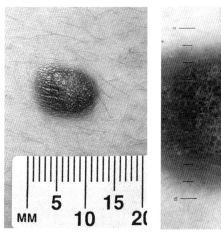
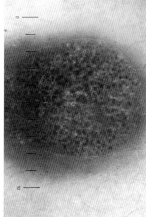

Figure 7.15 A dark red lesion on the posterior thigh of a young female patient shows numerous dotted blood vessels and intersected white lines forming a negative network, confirmed to be atypical Spitz naevus. © Aneurin Bevan University Health Board.

Non-melanocytic skin lesions

These lesions develop from skin cells other than melanocytes.

Actinic keratosis

The key dermoscopic features of actinic keratoses (AKs) are *background pink erythema* and *surface scaling*. On the face, the redness will be interrupted by white follicular openings (indicating keratin plugs in the follicles), which gives the appearance of strawberry skin, hence called *strawberry pattern*.

It is also possible to see *rosettes* (four white dots grouped in the follicular opening) in some AKs (Figure 7.16). This sign is not pathognomonic for AK as it is seen in other conditions caused by sun damage.

In hypertrophic AK, the lesion is hyperkeratotic and this can obscure the dermoscopic features of the base. The differential diagnosis can include Bowenoid AK or perhaps squamous cell carcinoma (SCC), and so a biopsy may be required.

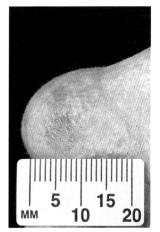
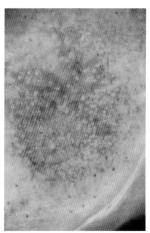

Figure 7.16 A flat red scaly patch on the nose. Dermoscopy shows a red background and rosettes, in keeping with a patch of actinic keratosis. © Aneurin Bevan University Health Board.

Basal cell carcinoma

The dermoscopic features of basal cell carcinoma (BCC) depend on the type:

- **Superficial BCC**. Red with small areas of ulceration, called *micro-erosions* (Figure 7.17). Occasionally, areas of pigment can be seen at the periphery in a *leaf-like* pattern.
- **Nodular BCC**. The hallmark of nodular BCC is the sharply focused branching telangiectasia, called *arborising vessels* (Figure 7.18).
- **Pigmented BCC**. It is common to see areas of pigment in nodular BCCs. However, the pigment is not of a melanocytic pattern. The pigment here appears as large and discrete blue-grey ovoid areas called *ovoid nests*. Occasionally, these can be multiple and smaller blue-grey dots or globules.

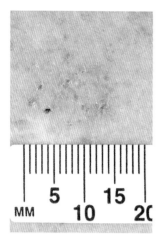
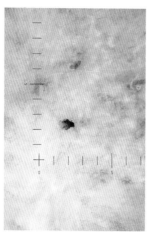

Figure 7.17 A flat scaly pink patch on the shoulder of an elderly patient shows micro-erosions on dermoscopy, a sign of superficial basal cell carcinoma. © Aneurin Bevan University Health Board.

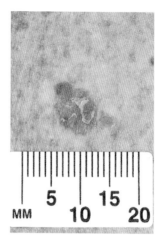
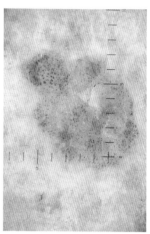

Figure 7.19 A scaly red plaque on the shoulder of an elderly woman with significant sun damage. Dermoscopy shows the coiled (glomerular) vessels and areas of keratinisation (scaling), consistent with Bowen's disease. © Aneurin Bevan University Health Board.

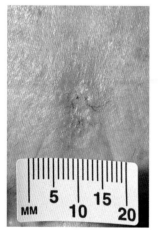
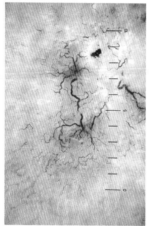

Figure 7.18 A smooth plaque on the glabella shows branching (arborising) vessels. The white scar-like areas suggest fibrosis, which can be seen in sclerosing basal cell carcinomas. © Aneurin Bevan University Health Board.

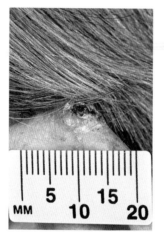
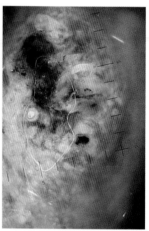

Figure 7.20 A tender crusted nodule on the ear helix suggests squamous cell carcinoma. Dermoscopy shows the yellow/brown keratin mass in the centre, white circles and some linear vessels. © Aneurin Bevan University Health Board.

Bowen's disease (squamous cell carcinoma *in situ*)

Bowen's disease presents as well-demarcated scaly pink to red patches and/or plaques with a scalloped edge. On dermoscopy, clusters of coiled vessels (called *glomerular vessels*) and superficial keratinised areas can be seen (Figure 7.19).

Squamous cell carcinoma

The clinical features of invasive SCC depend on the degree of keratinocyte differentiation. Well-differentiated cells are capable of producing keratin. Hence, well-to-moderately differentiated SCC presents as keratotic nodules or plaques. In contrast, the keratinocytes in poorly differentiated SCC are not keratinising and so lesions are often non-specific fleshy red nodules or plaques.

Dermoscopy is less helpful in SCC as the patterns are variable and depend on the degree of SCC differentiation and whether it is at an early or advanced stage of invasion.

In well-to-moderately differentiated SCC the usual features include (Figure 7.20):

- A structureless yellow to light brown keratin mass in the centre.
- A pale pink or white background interrupted by white rings at follicular openings.
- Blood vessels surrounding the central keratin mass. These can be dotted, hairpin and/or irregular linear vessels.

In poorly differentiated SCC the keratinisation process is lacking so one can see featureless redness with polymorphous blood vessels (dotted, linear, looped). This is not a specific pattern as it can also be seen in other conditions such as pyogenic granuloma and amelanotic malignant melanoma.

Solar lentigo

This is seen as a flat, well-demarcated brown patch. The pigmentation in solar lentigo is due to enhanced melanin production and retention in basal keratinocytes, rather than melanocytic proliferation. Dermoscopically, the pigment is usually homogeneous, with concave areas at the edge giving the appearance of a *moth-eaten* border (Figure 7.21). Importantly, the shape and size of the follicular openings interrupting the pigment are uniform and they are not hyperpigmented. Sometimes one can see a fine network in solar lentigo, representing elongated and pigmented rete ridges in histology, which gives the appearance of *fingerprint*-like pigmentation.

Several dermoscopic features of seborrhoeic keratosis have been described, reflecting the variable clinical morphology:

- **Comedo-like openings**. Round to oval-shaped dark holes (craters) give the appearance of comedo-like plugs (Figure 7.22).
- **Milia-like cysts**. Small white-yellow round structures, which look bright against the lesion's pigmented background (Figure 7.22). These are visualised with non-polarised dermoscopy.
- **Fissures and ridges**. Fissures are depressed invaginations (sulci). They are linear and curved forms of the comedo-like openings. Ridges are the raised papillomatous structures (gyri). The combination of these gyri and sulci gives the lesion a *cerebriform* or *brain-like* appearance (Figures 7.23 and 7.24).
- **Fat fingers**. This term is used to describe linear, curved or circular ridges, seen without the fissures (Figure 7.25).
- **Hairpin vessels**. These U-shaped vessels are the typical vascular pattern in seborrhoeic keratosis. They are more noticeable in the non-pigmented variant, where the vessels are conspicuous and symmetrical (Figure 7.26). One must note that hairpin vessels can also be seen in SCC and melanoma, but usually along with other features of melanoma or SCC.

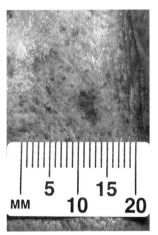
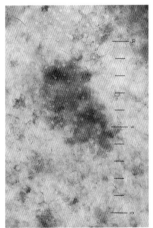

Figure 7.21 A pigmented patch on the nasal wall shows a moth-eaten border on dermoscopy (noticed at the 11–12-o'clock margin) consistent with a solar lentigo. © Aneurin Bevan University Health Board.

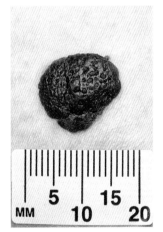
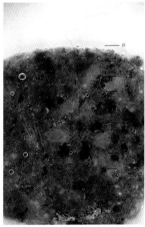

Figure 7.22 A dark seborrhoeic keratosis on the lower abdomen. Dermoscopy shows the round/oval craters (comedo-like openings). A few small white/yellow clods (milia-like cysts) can also be seen. © Aneurin Bevan University Health Board.

Seborrhoeic keratosis

This benign growth can be either pigmented or non-pigmented. It can present in various sizes and degrees of thickness, ranging from flat to a raised warty plaque. Dermoscopy is often helpful to diagnose seborrhoeic keratosis with confidence. However, occasionally seborrhoeic keratosis can present as a warty black blotch with no other dermoscopic features, which can be difficult to distinguish from a warty melanoma.

Clear cell acanthoma

This benign epithelial lesion is seen on the legs in older age groups. It presents as a raised smooth plaque or nodule, which can be pink, red or pigmented. It can therefore be confused clinically with BCC, seborrhoeic keratosis, SCC or amelanotic malignant melanoma.

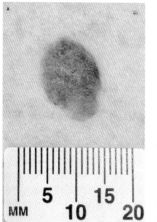 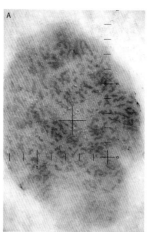

Figure 7.23 A keratotic plaque of seborrhoeic keratosis on the back. On dermoscopy the fissures and ridges show a cerebriform appearance. © Aneurin Bevan University Health Board.

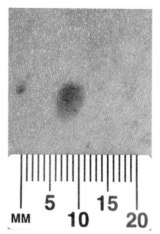 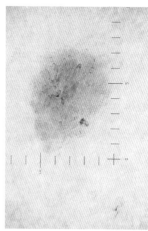

Figure 7.25 A uniform plaque of seborrhoeic keratosis on the shoulder shows broad parallel finger-like projections, so-called fat fingers. © Aneurin Bevan University Health Board.

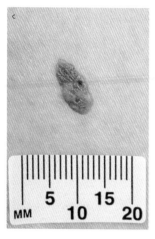 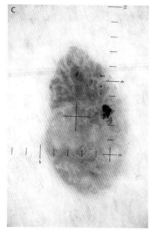

Figure 7.24 Another seborrhoeic keratosis, on the flank, where the ridges and fissures look prominent under the dermatoscope. © Aneurin Bevan University Health Board.

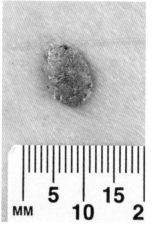 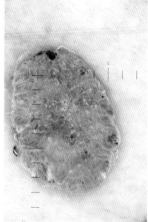

Figure 7.26 A warty non-pigmented plaque of seborrhoeic keratosis on the lower back. Dermoscopically, conspicuous hairpin-shaped vessels can be seen. © Aneurin Bevan University Health Board.

Under the dermatoscope, clear cell acanthoma has a fascinating characteristic pattern that helps to establish the diagnosis and avoid unnecessary excision. The pattern is described as a *string of pearls*. This sign is made up by numerous dotted vessels arranged in linear and serpiginous patterns (Figure 7.27). Occasionally, these 'strings' intersect to form a network of dotted vessels.

Sebaceous hyperplasia

Enlarged sebaceous glands are seen as single or multiple papular lesions on the forehead, cheeks and nose in middle-aged and elderly individuals. Clinically they appear as yellowish papules with central umbilication. Clinically, they can be difficult to distinguish from BCC. Dermoscopy can reassure by showing classical dermoscopic features.

The two main structures seen in sebaceous hyperplasia are (Figure 7.28):

- White-yellow aggregated lobules.
- Crown vessels: these are radial vessels, sometimes with little branching, sitting at the periphery of the lesion, like a crown. Unlike the arborising vessels seen in BCC, crown vessels normally do not cross the midline of the lesion.

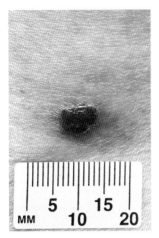
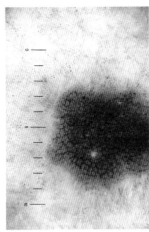

Figure 7.27 A non-specific dusky red plaque on the calf of an elderly patient. Dermoscopy demonstrates dotted blood vessels in linear and serpiginous arrangements, forming what looks like a network, a characteristic pattern for clear cell acanthoma. © Aneurin Bevan University Health Board.

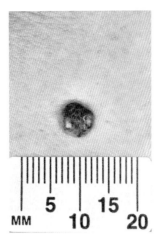
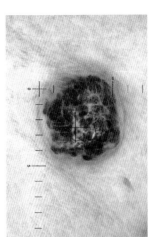

Figure 7.29 A dusky red lesion on the arm. Dermoscopy shows the lacunae in multiple sizes intersected by the septa, a typical pattern of a harmless angioma. © Aneurin Bevan University Health Board.

Dermatofibroma

These are benign fibrosing cutaneous lesions characterised by an increased number of fibrocytes in the dermis and occasionally the subcutis. The clinical morphology of dermatofibroma (DF) is variable, and so is the dermoscopic appearance.

The typical dermoscopic pattern is:

- Central scar-like white area (Figures 7.30 and 7.31).
- Peripheral delicate pigment network (Figure 7.30). Although 'pigment network' is a feature of 'melanocytic' lesions, there are exceptions. As we know, DF is not a melanocytic lesion.

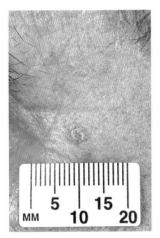
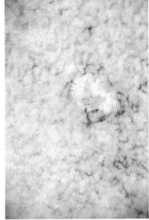

Figure 7.28 A shiny papule on the temple of a middle-aged man shows white/yellow lobules and radial crown blood vessels, consistent with a sebaceous hyperplasia. © Aneurin Bevan University Health Board.

Angioma and haemangioma

There are many vascular anomalies, of which haemangioma and cherry angioma are the most common. Dermoscopically, these benign vascular lesions show:

- **Lacunae**: sharply demarcated round red areas, so-called lagoons. These can be of various sizes in the same lesion and are void of other vascular structures (Figure 7.29).
- **Septa**: white lines separating the lacunae.

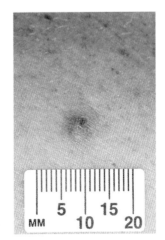
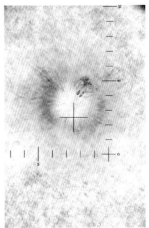

Figure 7.30 A firm lesion on the arm of a young adult. Under the dermatoscope, a central white scar-like area is seen with a subtle delicate pigment network at the periphery, in keeping with a pigmented dermatofibroma. © Aneurin Bevan University Health Board.

The pigment in DF is a result of basal layer hyperpigmentation, rather than melanocyte proliferation. Also, the pigment in DF is arranged in fine delicate lines and is usually more subtle than in a melanocytic lesion.

This typical pattern is observed in about 70% of DFs. The other 30% can show an atypical pattern or a pattern of other DF variants. Any equivocal features should raise suspicion and the lesion should be removed for histology to exclude malignancy.

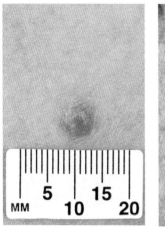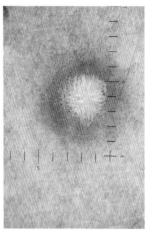

Figure 7.31 A pink dermatofibroma on the thigh of a young adult. Dermoscopically no pigment can be seen, but the central featureless white area and monomorphic dotted blood vessels at the periphery indicate the diagnosis. © Aneurin Bevan University Health Board.

Approach to dermoscopic examination of skin lesions

Several algorithms have been established to aid in making a diagnosis of pigmented skin lesions. Examples include the Menzies method, 7-point checklist, 3-point checklist, chaos and clues, and pattern analysis. These were designed primarily to diagnose suspicious melanoma.

Another algorithm, called the 'Prediction Without Pigment' decision algorithm, was developed to make decisions about non-pigmented skin lesions. This depends on whether the lesion has ulceration or white clues (white structureless areas, white lines and white circles). If the answer is yes, a biopsy should be performed to exclude malignancy. A lesion should also be biopsied if the lesion has polymorphous vascular structures, even in the absence of ulceration and white clues.

It is beyond the scope of this chapter to discuss each of these algorithms individually. However, one suggested approach with dermoscopic examination is summarised in Figure 7.32.

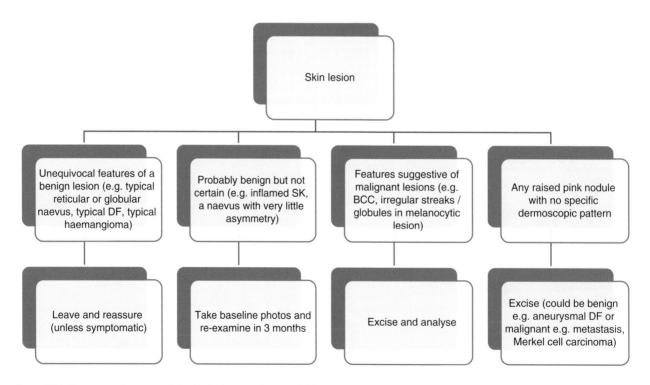

Figure 7.32 Dermoscopic approach in skin lesion examination. BCC, basal cell carcinoma; DF, dermatofibroma; SK, seborrhoeic keratosis.

Use of dermoscopy in non-lesional skin conditions

Applications of dermoscopy are no longer limited to skin lesions. Several pivotal studies have described the dermoscopic features in inflammatory conditions, hair and nail disorders, and skin infections and infestations. Dermoscopy is now widely used in dermatology practice and hence all dermatologists will require training in the use of these applications.

Studies have demonstrated the usefulness of dermoscopy in aiding in the diagnosis of inflammatory rashes that can be challenging to differentiate clinically. Examples include differentiating psoriasis from pityriasis rosea and eczema, morphoea from lichen sclerosus, and rosacea from sarcoidosis. One example where dermoscopy can be very helpful to ascertain the diagnosis is lichen planus, where Wickham's striae can be easily observed under the dermatoscope as white short lines (Figure 7.33). Another example is in the diagnosis of scabies, where a small dark triangular structure (the anterior section of the mite) can be seen at the tip of a linear structure (the burrow), together resembling a jet with contrail (Figure 7.34).

Similarly, dermoscopy can be helpful in differentiating hair disorders. Several dermoscopic signs have been described to aid the diagnosis of tinea capitis, alopecia areata, lichen planopilaris, trichotillomania and other conditions. Awareness of such features can reduce the need for invasive diagnostic biopsies.

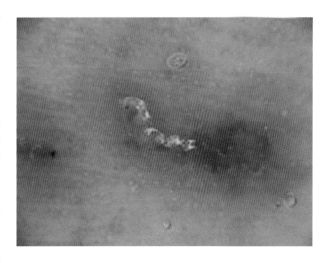

Figure 7.34 The pathognomonic 'jet with contrail' of scabies. Lallas A *et al. Br J Dermatol* 2014; **170**:514–26.

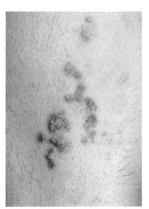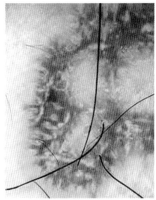

Figure 7.33 Wickham's striae can be easily observed under the dermatoscope as white short lines. Chowdhury MMU *et al. Dermatology at a Glance*, 2nd edn. Chichester: Wiley, 2019.

Conclusions and the future

In the current era of fast-paced technology developments, artificial intelligence (AI) is being employed to analyse dermoscopic images. Some studies have shown promising results, but like most technologies there are limitations. More data and scrutiny are needed to be able to draw conclusions about the full potential of AI.

A few other skin imaging devices are being studied. Reflectance confocal microscopy has attracted much attention in recent years, and several studies have explored its accuracy and usefulness in the diagnosis of skin tumours. Interpretation of normal and pathological structures seen in reflectance confocal microscopy requires additional training and regular updates of the emerging studies. Other tools such as optical coherence tomography and electrical impedance spectroscopy have been studied in some skin lesions, but it is still too early to determine their potential.

Gaining experience in using a dermatoscope is essential, and it is helpful to have an experienced colleague to guide you. Your knowledge can expand gradually with practice and multiple resources may need to be used to supplement your clinical hands-on training.

Pearls and pitfalls

- 'Grey circles' and 'hyperpigmented blotches' obliterating follicular openings are ominous signs in pigmented facial skin lesions. Lentigo maligna or lentigo maligna melanoma should be considered.
- In acral pigmented lesions, remember **F**urrows: **F**ine but **R**idges: **R**emove.

- Individuals with multiple naevi (e.g. atypical naevus syndrome) tend to have a similar pattern (signature) of their moles. A naevus that shows a different dermoscopic pattern from others should be biopsied.
- Melanocytic naevi change throughout life. Be aware of the age-related variations in their dermoscopic patterns.
- Any pink nodular lesion with a non-specific dermoscopic pattern should be biopsied to exclude malignancy.

SCE Questions. See questions 46–48.

FURTHER READING AND KEY RESOURCES

Fried LJ, Tan A, Berry EG *et al*. Dermoscopy proficiency expectations for US dermatology resident physicians: results of a modified Delphi survey of pigmented lesion experts. *JAMA Dermatol* 2021; **157**:189–97.

Lallas A, Giacomel J, Argenziano G *et al*. Dermoscopy in general dermatology: practical tips for the clinician. *Br J Dermatol* 2014; **170**:514–26.

Saida T, Koga H, Uhara H. Key points in dermoscopic differentiation between early acral melanoma and acral nevus. *J Dermatol* 2011; **38**:25–34.

Vestergaard ME, Macaskill P, Holt PE, Menzies SW. Dermoscopy compared with naked eye examination for the diagnosis of primary melanoma: a meta-analysis of studies performed in a clinical setting. *Br J Dermatol* 2008; **159**:669–76.

Zalaudek I, Kreusch J, Giacomel J *et al*. How to diagnose non-pigmented skin tumors: a review of vascular structures seen with dermoscopy: part I. Melanocytic skin tumors. *J Am Acad Dermatol* 2010; **63**:361–74.

Textbooks

Marghoob A, Malvehy J, Braun RP, eds. *An Atlas of Dermoscopy*, 2nd edn. Boca Raton, FL: CRC Press, 2012.

Rosendahl C, Marozava A, eds. *Dermatoscopy and Skin Cancer: a Handbook for Hunters of Skin Cancer and Melanoma*. Banbury: Scion Publishing, 2019.

Useful website

Dermoscopedia. Available at: www.dermoscopedia.org.

Acknowledgements

Thanks to the Medical Illustration Unit at Aneurin Bevan University Health Board for providing the teledermoscopy service and the images, and to Professor Iris Zalaudek, President of the International Dermoscopy Society, for commenting on the first draft of this chapter.

8

Clinical measurement methods

Andrew Y. Finlay

Introduction

Dermatology was late in appreciating the value of objective measurement. Our immediate ability to see and touch diseased skin perhaps made clinical measurement seem unnecessary. However, for any field to develop into a science, there need to be validated measurement methods. You need to know about them, as they will be used in the clinic for patient assessment and to inform management decisions. This chapter describes some of the most widely used measurement methods, but it is not exhaustive. Novel techniques, mostly disease specific, are frequently being published, and in order to deliver the best quality of care you should try to keep up to date.

Apart from the basic (but important) use of a ruler to measure the size of lesions, the first major measurement development came in the assessment of psoriasis. Multiple methods to measure clinical severity were proposed and used in the 1960s and 1970s, from which the Psoriasis Area and Severity Index (PASI) evolved as the frontrunner: an imperfect technique that remains pre-eminent. Other methods for use in a variety of skin diseases have been created, supplemented by highly pertinent patient-reported outcome tools, including questionnaires that measure quality of life.

There is no international body overseeing these measurement methods; they follow an evolutionary path with survival of the fittest but not necessarily the 'best'. Many (often incompatible) measurement techniques are published in dermatology, reminiscent of the days before the adoption of the metric system across world science. Another complication is that very detailed validated methods may be scientifically sound, but impractical for use in busy routine clinics.

There is a problem with some measurement methods, as they are not applicable across all skin types. Early efforts at developing techniques to score skin and skin disease were mostly by white researchers, and were developed, evaluated and used in

Dermatology Training: The Essentials. Edited by Mahbub M.U. Chowdhury, Tamara W. Griffiths and Andrew Y. Finlay.
© 2022 The British Association of Dermatologists. Published 2022 by John Wiley & Sons Ltd.
Companion website: www.wiley.com/go/chowdhury/dermatologytraining

their mostly white local populations. For example, the authors of PASI created this method for use in a clinical study that was carried out in Sweden; it was only later that others began to use the method more widely.

Applying such techniques to people with skin of colour can result in several inaccuracies. When the skin is inflamed, there is increased blood supply near the surface of the skin, and the inflammation may also result in increased pigmentation. In white skin the most obvious sign is redness, whereas in dark skin the most obvious sign is accompanying increased pigmentation. An assessment of redness, such as in PASI, Simplified Psoriasis Index (SPI), Eczema Area and Severity Index (EASI) and Scoring Atopic Dermatitis (SCORAD), may therefore not be an appropriate sign to be measured in dark skin. We need new techniques to be developed (and validated) that are sensitive to the need for universal applicability across all skin types. Perhaps as an interim, older methods could be modified: for example, questions about erythema could be changed from 'degree of erythema' to 'degree of colour change', but even this suggestion needs validating.

Core outcome measures

This unregulated environment leads to different measurement methods being used by different clinicians or researchers, with resulting lack of compatibility or ability to compare results. However, there are now several organisations focused on recommending 'core outcome measures', initially in psoriasis and atopic dermatitis (Table 8.1), but also now for acne, hidradenitis suppurativa and other conditions. These are the measurement methods recommended for use as a minimum standard in all research projects, while researchers remain free to add other techniques should they wish. If in the future all studies use the core outcome measures, there will be huge benefits in being able to compare and combine study data.

Table 8.1 The core outcome set and core outcome instruments for eczema clinical trials, recommended by the Harmonising Outcome Measures for Eczema (HOME) group

Clinical signs: Eczema Area and Severity Index (EASI)

Patient-reported symptoms: Patient-Oriented Eczema Measure (POEM) and Numerical Rating Scale (NRS)-11 (for peak itch over the past 24 hours)

Long-term control: Recap of Atopic Eczema (RECAP) or Atopic Dermatitis Control Test (ADCT)

Quality of life: Dermatology Life Quality Index (DLQI) (adults), Children's DLQI (CDLQI) (children), Infants' Dermatitis Quality of Life Index (IDQoL) (infants)

Why measure?

Measurement techniques may be useful clinically in patient assessment and monitoring and to inform management decisions. The traditional clinical process of a doctor 'gaining an impression' of change in disease severity from memory or by guesswork (where a different doctor previously saw the patient) is still widespread, but hard to defend in an age of evidence-based medicine. Clinical practice is moving to becoming truly 'personalised medicine', and national guidelines are increasingly dependent on accurate assessment of disease severity. Accurate measurement and recording are therefore becoming essential.

Which methods should you try to understand first?

Some measurement techniques have become so widely accepted that they are incorporated in national guidelines or registries. These are the key techniques that you should first become familiar with, for example PASI, SCORAD, EASI, Physician's Global Assessment (PGA) and Dermatology Life Quality Index (DLQI). It is also useful to know about the flaws of the techniques currently in use, how they were created, the extent to which they have been validated and any practical aspects of their use.

Reliability

There is no such thing as a perfect scoring system, at least in medicine. Errors can creep in because of doctor or patient bias, mistakes in calculation of score or variation in the way the operator undertakes the measurement. On top of this, most things that are measured in medicine are not static, there is variation from minute to minute, and there are diurnal variations and fluctuations in disease states themselves. Measurement techniques can be assessed for their reliability, for example test–test reliability to assess how consistent operators are in measuring the same parameter. For a measure to be useful in medicine it also has to be seen to respond to clinical change in an appropriate direction.

How to interpret scores

If the 'output' of a measure is presented as a score (as is usual), the score needs to mean something to the clinician. We are used to learning 'normal ranges' for blood parameters and we need to develop an understanding of the scores of measures used in dermatology. Equally importantly, we need to be able to interpret change in score. We apply the concept of 'minimal clinically important difference (MCID)' without thinking about it, say when interpreting a change in haemoglobin level. However, there are research techniques that make it possible to prospectively calculate the MCID for different measures. For example, the MCID for the DLQI is a score change of 4; a smaller change may be statistically 'significant', but is not clinically relevant.

This is an important point for you to remember when interpreting score change in published clinical trials. The same concept is, or should be, applied to all clinical scoring systems but the MCID has not been calculated for most, due to lack of motivation or knowledge.

Psoriasis

Psoriasis Area and Severity Index (PASI)

PASI was created, almost by chance, by Fredriksson and Pettersson in 1978 for one of the first studies of systemic retinoids in psoriasis. There were already quite a few different published methods, but these researchers decided to create a new technique. They very briefly described it and used it, without any attempt to validate it. It was mostly ignored for the next 10 years, but in the 1990s it gradually gained popularity. The concept must have seemed fairly simple and logical when it was initially designed, but in practice it is virtually impossible to accurately and repeatably clinically assess psoriasis area, and the definition of the grading of redness, thickness and scaling is unclear.

Designed for use in research, PASI remains a clumsy technique when used in clinical practice. It has nevertheless evolved into the central measure of psoriasis and so you must understand how to use it.

Knowing PASI's flaws, several authors have proposed other systems that have much better validation; however, PASI remains the dominant measure used.

How to use PASI (Table 8.2)

First ask the patient to undress. Consider each of the four specified areas separately: head, arms, trunk and legs. For each area examine the psoriasis lesions and give an 'average score' for redness, scaling and thickness (each 0–4). For each area add the three scores together and multiply by either 0.1 (head), 0.2 (arms), 0.3 (trunk) or 0.4 (legs) to give B1, B2, B3 and B4.

Then for each of the four areas record the percentage area affected by psoriasis. This is a difficult process that challenges you to try to imagine the lesions in each area coalesced together. Then convert the approximate percentage into the grade, as shown in Table 8.2.

Multiply B1 by its area grade, B2 by its grade, B3 by its grade and B4 by its grade, then add these four figures together to give the PASI score (range 0–72). Although the maximum score is 72, the vast majority of patients with psoriasis in the community have a score of less than 10, and a score of 10 or above is often considered a criterion for considering systemic therapy.

Simplified Psoriasis Index (SPI)

The SPI is a summary measure of psoriasis with separate components of (a) current severity, (b) psychosocial impact and (c) past history and interventions.

Table 8.2 Psoriasis Area and Severity Index (PASI)

Four regions of the body are evaluated:

Head (H)
Arms (A)
Trunk (Tr)
Legs (L)

For each region, the area of psoriasis involvement is given a numerical value (area):

< 10%	= 1
10–29%	= 2
30–49%	= 3
50–69%	= 4
70–89%	= 5
90–100%	= 6

For each region:

Redness (R)	is scored 0–4 (0 = none, 4 = maximum)
Scaling (S)	is scored 0–4
Thickness (T)	is scored 0–4

The PASI score (range 0–72) is calculated thus:

PASI score = [AreaH × 0.1 × (R + S + T)] + [AreaA × 0.2 × (R + S + T)] + [AreaTr × 0.3 × (R + S + T)] + [AreaL × 0.4 × (R + S + T)]

a. Current severity: the body is divided into 10 unequal areas; the involvement with psoriasis for each area is scored 'clear', 'obvious' or 'widespread'. The current 'average severity' describing redness, scaling, thickening, inflammation and pustulation is scored from 0 to 5.
b. Psychosocial impact: this is scored on a 10-cm visual analogue scale.
c. Past history and interventions: four questions concerning the patient's psoriasis history and six concerning past treatment, scored out of 10.

There are two versions of the SPI, one for use by healthcare professionals and the other for self-assessment by patients.

The SPI score consists of three figures, one for each component, a, b and c. The first two figures are able to alter with changes in the patient's condition, but the figure for past history and interventions is fixed, at least in the short term.

Body surface area (BSA) involvement

To measure BSA involvement with psoriasis, the patient needs to be fully undressed. The area of disease involvement can be roughly calculated using the 'Rule of Nines', whereby the head

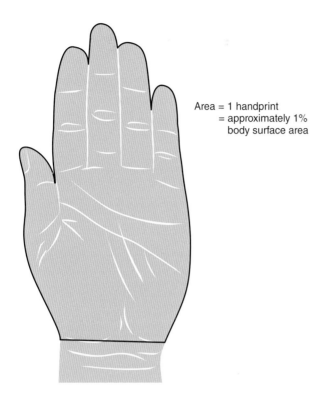

Area = 1 handprint
= approximately 1% body surface area

Figure 8.1 The handprint.

and neck is considered to be 9% BSA, each arm 9%, each leg 18%, anterior trunk 18%, posterior trunk 18% and genitalia 1%. Another way is to use your 'handprint'. This is the area of your palm and fingers, which roughly equals 1% (more accurately 0.8%) of adult total body surface area (Figure 8.1). By placing your handprint over the affected areas you can count up (roughly) the percentage of involvement.

Eczema

Eczema Area and Severity Index (EASI)

The EASI scoring system for atopic dermatitis (AD) is obviously based on the PASI concept. The same four areas are considered, but for each area four (not three as in PASI) signs are scored 0–3 (not 0–4 as in PASI): redness, oedema/papulation, excoriation and lichenification. The same methods for assessing and recording area are used, and the same multipliers are applied for each area. The final score range (0–72) is the same as for PASI. Slightly different multipliers are used when children aged under 8 years old are assessed.

EASI scores are interpreted as 7–21 = 'moderate AD' and > 21 = 'severe AD'; these bands can be used to inform decisions to consider systemic therapy.

Patient-Oriented Eczema Measure (POEM)

POEM is a validated, reliable and simple tool to measure atopic eczema in adults and children. It is a questionnaire completed by the patient or, for young children, by the parent or guardian (Figure 8.2). There are seven questions, each with five answer choices, scored 0–4. Each question asks how many days over the last week specific symptoms or signs occurred. The score (range 0–28) is interpreted as 0–2 (clear/almost clear); 3–7 (mild); 8–16 (moderate); 17–24 (severe); 25–28 (very severe).

Scoring Atopic Dermatitis (SCORAD)

SCORAD has three components, recording the extent of AD, the intensity of the signs and the severity of symptoms.

The extent of the AD is measured according to the Rule of Nines (0–100% = A).

The intensity of each of six signs (redness, oedema/papules, effect of scratching, oozing/crust formation, lichenification and dryness) is given a grade of 0–3 (total 0–18 = B).

The severities of itch and sleeplessness are each measured on separate 10-cm (0–10) visual analogue scales (total 0–20 = C).

The three component scores are combined using the formula A/5 + 7B/2 + C to give a score range of 0–103. It is clear that while SCORAD may be appropriate for use in a research setting, its design makes it difficult to use in a busy clinical setting. There is also an 'objective' version of SCORAD that omits the itch and sleeplessness scores.

Acne

Despite the very high prevalence of acne and the apparent simplicity of recognising the key signs of comedones, pustules, papules and scars, there has been great difficulty in establishing a simple validated measure of the clinical signs. This is partly because of challenges posed by incorporating various areas, such as the face, back or chest, which may be affected to widely differing degrees in the same person. Multiple methods have been proposed and used, some based on counting lesions, but most using global severity rating scales. The 'Leeds technique', popular in the late twentieth century, was based on comparison with a standard set of photographs, but the photographs were from the pre-isotretinoin era and were heavily biased towards very severe acne, which is seldom seen today.

The Global Evaluation Acne (GEA) scale, described by Dreno et al. (2011) to record acne severity, is a simple method that can be used in the clinic (Table 8.3). It is an example of one of the better techniques available to measure acne. However, there is still no agreed single standard method.

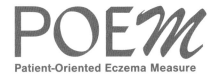

POEm
Patient-Oriented Eczema Measure

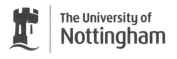

The University of
Nottingham

UNITED KINGDOM · CHINA · MALAYSIA

POEM for self-completion

Patient Details: ....

....

.... Date: ....

Please circle one response for each of the seven questions below about your eczema. Please leave blank any questions you feel unable to answer.

1. Over the last week, on how many days has your skin been itchy because of your eczema?

   No days   1-2 days   3-4 days   5-6 days   Every day

2. Over the last week, on how many nights has your sleep been disturbed because of your eczema?

   No days   1-2 days   3-4 days   5-6 days   Every day

3. Over the last week, on how many days has your skin been bleeding because of your eczema?

   No days   1-2 days   3-4 days   5-6 days   Every day

4. Over the last week, on how many days has your skin been weeping or oozing clear fluid because of your eczema?

   No days   1-2 days   3-4 days   5-6 days   Every day

5. Over the last week, on how many days has your skin been cracked because of your eczema?

   No days   1-2 days   3-4 days   5-6 days   Every day

6. Over the last week, on how many days has your skin been flaking off because of your eczema?

   No days   1-2 days   3-4 days   5-6 days   Every day

7. Over the last week, on how many days has your skin felt dry or rough because of your eczema?

   No days   1-2 days   3-4 days   5-6 days   Every day

Total POEM Score (Maximum 28): ....

© The University of Nottingham

Figure 8.2 The Patient-Oriented Eczema Measure (POEM) tool to measure atopic eczema in adults and children. Reproduced with permission from the Centre of Evidence Based Dermatology, Nottingham.

Table 8.3 The Global Evaluation Acne (GEA) scale

0 Clear. No lesions. Residual pigmentation and erythema may be seen

1 Almost clear. Almost no lesions. A few scattered open or closed comedones and very few papules

2 Mild. Easily recognisable: less than half of the face is involved. A few open or closed comedones and a few papules and pustules

3 Moderate. More than half of the face is involved. Many papules and pustules, many open or closed comedones. One nodule may be present

4 Severe. Entire face is involved, covered with many papules and pustules, open or closed comedones and rare nodules

5 Very severe. Highly inflammatory acne covering the face with presence of nodules

Table 8.4 The six stages of the hidradenitis suppurativa Physician's Global Assessment (PGA)

Clear: no inflammatory or non-inflammatory nodules

Minimal: only the presence of non-inflammatory nodules

Mild: fewer than 5 inflammatory nodules or 1 abscess or draining fistula and no inflammatory nodules

Moderate: fewer than 5 inflammatory nodules, or 1 abscess or draining fistula and 1 or more inflammatory nodules, or 2–5 abscesses or draining fistulas and fewer than 10 inflammatory nodules

Severe: 2–5 abscesses or draining fistulas and 10 or more inflammatory nodules

Very severe: more than 5 abscesses or draining fistulas

Hidradenitis suppurativa

The most widely reported measures for hidradenitis suppurativa (HS) are the Hurley, Sartorius and modified Sartorius techniques. A simpler 'Physician's Global Assessment' with six categories (Kimball *et al*. 2012) has been used in several clinical studies (Table 8.4). With the great growth of interest in HS over the last few years, it is hoped that a consensus will emerge for the core outcome measures for HS and for the method most appropriate for routine clinical use.

Table 8.5 The Severity of Alopecia Tool (SALT)

The scalp is divided into four areas:	
The top of the scalp	40% of scalp surface area
The right-side view of the scalp	18% of scalp surface area
The left-side view of the scalp	18% of scalp surface area
The back of the scalp	24% of scalp surface area

The percentage of hair loss in each of the four areas is estimated and multiplied by the proportion of scalp of that scalp area, i.e. 0.4, 0.18, 0.18 or 0.24

These four products are then added up to give the SALT score. This score represents the percentage of hair loss

Alopecia

The severity of alopecia can be measured by the Severity of Alopecia Tool (SALT), devised by the National Alopecia Areata Foundation (Table 8.5). Another version of SALT incorporates details of hair density.

Melasma

The Melasma Area and Severity Index (MASI) (Table 8.6) is based on a PASI-like structure, assessing area, darkness and homogeneity in four regions of the face. The simpler 'modified MASI' omits homogeneity and is only based on area and darkness.

Physician's Global Assessment (PGA)

This is perhaps the simplest method of recording overall skin disease severity. A mark is made on a visual analogue scale; that is, a straight line divided usually into 10 (Figure 8.3). One end of the line represents 'no disease' and the other end of the line represents 'the worst possible disease severity'. It may in theory be useful in the clinic, but it is seldom used outside the research setting: the lack of specificity gives little confidence that different doctors would score the same patient similarly.

Table 8.6 The Melasma Area and Severity Index (MASI)

The face is divided into four regions:

Forehead (f)	
Malar right (mr)	
Malar left (ml)	
Chin (c)	

In each facial region, the percentage area of melasma involvement is assigned a numerical value (A):

None	0
1–10%	1
10–29%	2
30–49%	3
50–69%	4
70–89%	5
90–100%	6

In each facial area, the darkness (D) is scored:

Absent	0
Slight	1
Mild	2
Marked	3
Severe	4

In each facial area, the homogeneity (H) is scored:

Minimal	0
Slight	1
Mild	2
Marked	3
Maximum	4

The MASI score (range 0–48):

MASI score = $[0.3 \times (Df + Hf) \times Af] + [0.3 \times (Dmr + Hmr) \times Amr] + [0.3 \times (Dml + Hml) \times Aml] + [0.1 \times (Dc + Hc) \times Ac]$

The modified MASI score (range 0–24):

Modified MASI score = $(0.3 \times Af \times Df) + (0.3 \times Aml \times Dml) + (0.3 \times Amr \times Dmr) + (0.1 \times Ac \times Dc)$

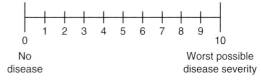

The physician or patient is asked to make a mark on the scale to represent their view of the disease severity.

Figure 8.3 A visual analogue scale (VAS).

Quality of life

There are a large number of quality-of-life questionnaires created for use in dermatology. These include disease-specific measures and generic dermatology ones that can be used across all skin diseases, including the DLQI and Skindex (several versions).

Dermatology Life Quality Index (DLQI)

The DLQI has become the most widely used patient-reported outcome measure in clinical dermatology (Figure 8.4). It consists of 10 simple questions about the quality of life of the patient over the last week. It can be used easily in the clinic as it is short and self-explanatory.

Each question is answered on a 0–3 scale, and the scores are summed. The DLQI is useful to inform clinical decisions because it is possible to interpret what the score means (Table 8.7). A score change of 4 is required to denote it as being clinically important (the MCID).

If the score is > 10 this indicates that the skin disease is having a very large effect on the quality of life of the patient. This should act as a warning sign to the clinician that more needs to be done to help this patient and to consider different or more effective therapy. The use of the DLQI can therefore give the clinician more insight into an individual patient, enhancing communication. It is also useful for the clinician to have evidence in the patient record of the patient's quality-of-life impairment, to justify the use of expensive therapy or of drugs with side-effects. Having a DLQI > 10, PASI > 10 or BSA > 10% (the 'Rule of Tens') was suggested as a way to define 'current severe psoriasis'; this influenced the criteria set in many national guidelines for using biologics.

DERMATOLOGY LIFE QUALITY INDEX

Hospital No: Date:

Name: Score:

Address: Diagnosis:

DLQI

The aim of this questionnaire is to measure how much your skin problem has affected your life OVER THE LAST WEEK. Please tick one box for each question.

1.	Over the last week, how **itchy**, **sore**, **painful** or **stinging** has your skin been?	Very much ☐ A lot ☐ A little ☐ Not at all ☐	
2.	Over the last week, how **embarrassed** or **self conscious** have you been because of your skin?	Very much ☐ A lot ☐ A little ☐ Not at all ☐	
3.	Over the last week, how much has your skin interfered with you going **shopping** or looking after your **home** or **garden**?	Very much ☐ A lot ☐ A little ☐ Not at all ☐	Not relevant ☐
4.	Over the last week, how much has your skin influenced the **clothes** you wear?	Very much ☐ A lot ☐ A little ☐ Not at all ☐	Not relevant ☐
5.	Over the last week, how much has your skin affected any **social** or **leisure** activities?	Very much ☐ A lot ☐ A little ☐ Not at all ☐	Not relevant ☐
6.	Over the last week, how much has your skin made it difficult for you to do any **sport**?	Very much ☐ A lot ☐ A little ☐ Not at all ☐	Not relevant ☐
7.	Over the last week, has your skin prevented you from **working** or **studying**?	Yes ☐ No ☐	Not relevant ☐
	If "No", over the last week how much has your skin been a problem at **work** or **studying**?	A lot ☐ A little ☐ Not at all ☐	
8.	Over the last week, how much has your skin created problems with your **partner** or any of your **close friends** or **relatives**?	Very much ☐ A lot ☐ A little ☐ Not at all ☐	Not relevant ☐
9.	Over the last week, how much has your skin caused any **sexual** **difficulties**?	Very much ☐ A lot ☐ A little ☐ Not at all ☐	Not relevant ☐
10.	Over the last week, how much of a problem has the **treatment** for your skin been, for example by making your home messy, or by taking up time?	Very much ☐ A lot ☐ A little ☐ Not at all ☐	Not relevant ☐

Please check you have answered EVERY question. Thank you.

©AY Finlay, GK Khan, April 1992. This must not be copied without the permission of the authors.

Figure 8.4 The Dermatology Life Quality Index (DLQI). Reproduced with permission. https://www.cardiff.ac.uk/medicine/resources/quality-of-life-questionnaires/dermatology-life-quality-index. Finlay AY, Khan GK. *Clin Exp Dermatol* 1994; **19**:210–16.

Table 8.7 How to interpret Dermatology Life Quality Index (DLQI) scores

DLQI score range is 0–30
0–1 = no effect on quality of life
2–5 = small effect
6–10 = moderate effect
11–20 = very large effect
21–30 = extremely large effect
The minimum clinically important difference in score change is 4 points

Although it is widely used, there are some criticisms of the validation of the DLQI, which was developed before the advent of more recent validation methodology. However, it remains very useful clinically, it is embedded in national guidelines in over 45 countries and its use is a requirement in many National Institute for Health and Care Excellence (NICE) guidelines, especially relating to the use of biologics in psoriasis, AD and urticaria.

There is a children's version, the Children's DLQI (CDLQI), which is also available with added cartoons, much liked by younger children (Figure 8.5). The impact of a skin disease in a patient (of any age) on the quality of life of adult family members can be measured using the Family DLQI: this often reveals a major secondary burden of skin disease. A generic family measure, the Family Reported Outcome Measure (FROM-16), can be used across all specialties, including dermatology.

The future

It is highly likely that advances in image analysis and objective measurement of physical properties of the skin, combined with artificial intelligence techniques, will dramatically improve the ability to measure, record and monitor skin disease severity. Better measurement techniques will be essential to fully develop delivery of care and therapy optimised for individual patients. Perhaps in the future, the 2020s will be perceived to have been in a short-lived transition phase between no measurement and high-quality automated objective measurement, with this chapter's current methods discarded.

There are competing business interests promoting measurement techniques. It is the responsibility of the new generation of dermatologists to ensure that the techniques that are created and used are well validated. Development of a national or international body to assess (and possibly even regulate) the quality of novel measurement techniques would help standardise and quality assure these important and increasingly relevant clinical tools.

Pearls and pitfalls

- Even if you do not want to use a questionnaire to assess quality of life, consider routinely asking your patients: 'How is your skin problem affecting your life?'
- To roughly estimate surface area involvement, think of a handprint as approximately 1% BSA (in adults).
- When interpreting published score changes, do not just look for 'statistically significant' change, but consider the minimal clinically important difference.
- A DLQI score > 10 should ring alarm bells to indicate significant impact on a patient's quality of life.

SCE Questions. See questions 9 and 10.

Trouble with Skin

The aim of the questionnaire is to measure how much your skin problem has affected you OVER THE LAST WEEK. Please tick ✔ one box for each question

OVER THE LAST WEEK

OVER THE LAST WEEK

Very much ☐
Quite a lot ☐
A little ☐
Not at all ☐

1

How **itchy**, **'scratchy'**, **sore** or **painful** has your skin been?

Very much ☐
Quite a lot ☐
A little ☐
Not at all ☐

2

How upset or **embarrassed, self-conscious** or **sad** have you been because of your skin?

Very much ☐
Quite a lot ☐
A little ☐
Not at all ☐

3

How much has your skin affected your **friendships**?

Very much ☐
Quite a lot ☐
A little ☐
Not at all ☐

4

How much have you changed or worn **different** or **special clothes/shoes** because of your skin?

Very much ☐
Quite a lot ☐
A little ☐
Not at all ☐

5

How much has your skin trouble affected **going out**, **playing** or **doing hobbies**?

Very much ☐
Quite a lot ☐
A little ☐
Not at all ☐

6

How much have you avoided **swimming** or **other sports** because of your skin trouble?

Children's Dermatology Life Quality Index

Figure 8.5 The cartoon version of the Children's Dermatology Life Quality Index (CDLQI). Reproduced with permission. https://www.cardiff.ac.uk/medicine/resources/quality-of-life-questionnaires/childrens-dermatology-life-quality-index.

OVER THE LAST WEEK

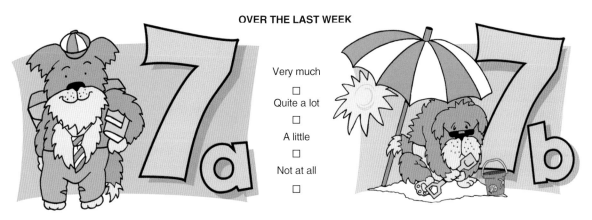

Very much ☐
Quite a lot ☐
A little ☐
Not at all ☐

If school time: How much did you skin affect your **school work**?

If holiday time: How has your skin problem interfered with your **holiday plans**?

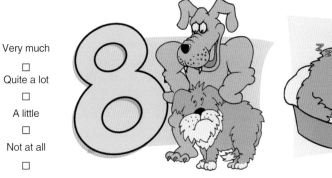

Very much ☐
Quite a lot ☐
A little ☐
Not at all ☐

How much trouble have you had because of your skin with other people **calling you names, teasing, bullying, asking questions** or **avoiding you**?

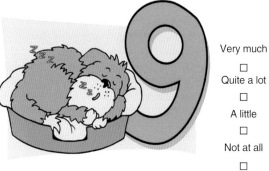

Very much ☐
Quite a lot ☐
A little ☐
Not at all ☐

How much has your **sleep** been affected by your skin problem?

Very much ☐
Quite a lot ☐
A little ☐
Not at all ☐

How much of a problem has the **treatment** for your skin been?

Hospital No:
Name:
Age:
Address:

CDLQI. © MS Lewis-Jones, AY Finlay June 1993.
Illustrations © Media Resources Centre, UWCM December 1996

Please check that you have answered EVERY question. Thank you.

Figure 8.5 (Continued)

FURTHER READING AND KEY RESOURCES

Charman CR, Venn AJ, Williams HC. The Patient-Oriented Eczema Measure: development and initial validation of a new tool for measuring atopic eczema severity from the patients' perspective. *Arch Dermatol* 2004; **140**:1513–19.

Dreno B, Poli F, Pawin H *et al*. Development and evaluation of a Global Acne Severity Scale (GEA Scale) suitable for France and Europe. *J Eur Acad Dermatol Venereol* 2011; **25**:43–8.

Finlay AY. Current severe psoriasis and the Rule of Tens. *Br J Dermatol* 2005; **152**:861–7.

Finlay AY, Khan GK. Dermatology Life Quality Index (DLQI) – a simple practical measure for routine clinical use. *Clin Exp Dermatol* 1994; **19**:210–16.

Finlay AY, Salek MS, Abeni D *et al*. Why quality of life measurement is important in dermatology clinical practice. An expert-based Opinion Statement by the EADV Task Force on Quality of Life. *J Eur Acad Dermatol Venereol* 2017; **31**:424–31.

Fredriksson T, Pettersson U. Severe psoriasis – oral therapy with a new retinoid. *Dermatologica* 1978; **157**:238–44.

Kimball AB, Kerdel F, Adams D *et al*. Adalimumab for the treatment of moderate to severe hidradenitis suppurativa: a parallel randomized trial. *Ann Intern Med* 2012; **157**:846–55.

Puzenat E, Bronsard V, Prey S *et al*. What are the best outcome measures for assessing plaque psoriasis severity? A systematic review of the literature. *J Eur Acad Dermatol Venereol* 2010; **24** (Suppl. 2):10–16.

Useful websites

Cardiff University School of Medicine. Quality of life questionnaires. Direct access to 11 quality of life questionnaires and translations, including DLQI and CDLQI. Available at: https://www.cardiff.ac.uk/medicine/resources/quality-of-life-questionnaires.

Harmonising Outcome Measures for Eczema (HOME). Centre of Evidence Based Dermatology, University of Nottingham. Available at: www.homeforeczema.org.

Conflicts of interest

A.Y.F. is joint copyright owner of several quality-of-life measures, including the DLQI, CDLQI, Infants' Dermatitis Quality of Life Index (IDQoL), Family DLQI and FROM-16. Cardiff University and A.Y.F. receive royalties.

9

Global and public health

Thomas King and L. Claire Fuller

Introduction

The chapter introduces the basic concepts of global and public health dermatology and explains why it is relevant to the dermatologist in training in the UK and worldwide. It is important to understand what concepts and challenges are encompassed by global and public health issues and how these can affect our perception of and interactions with the wider world of dermatology. Furthermore, key skills gained in this arena are likely to be required in your local department, depending on patient demographics in your area. Particularly relevant may be issues relating to cultural norms and communication challenges. Attitudes and approaches are changing and are dynamic, and dermatologists are in a key position to influence this.

What is global health dermatology?

'Global health' has been defined succinctly as a discipline that advances efforts to improve the wellbeing of people and the planet. Focusing on issues that transcend national borders, it is an area of study, research and practice that places a priority on improving health and health equality for all people worldwide. It requires and promotes interdisciplinary collaboration, including extension beyond health sciences, in order to address health issues that combine population-based health prevention with individual-level medical intervention. Practically this can be considered as a global health 'approach' comprising three strands:

- **Equitable partnerships**, encompassing principles of respect and trust, planned together and carried out together with measurable outputs. More recently an emphasis on the 'decolonisation' of global health interventions has been raised. Initiatives often involve partnerships between institutions in low- and middle-income countries (LMICs) that have previously been colonised by high-income countries (HICs). The influence of this legacy of historical colonial relationships on current health education partnerships has not been critically addressed. Should knowledge and practices generated in HIC settings be 'imposed' on the LMIC? Are their content and approach location appropriate? Techniques for reviewing attitudes and methods and achieving this 'decolonisation' include agreeing to a matrix of Fair Trade Learning developed by the Campus Connect Consortium, which prioritises reciprocity in partnership relationships through cooperative, cross-cultural participation in learning, service and civil society efforts (see Further reading).

Dermatology Training: The Essentials. Edited by Mahbub M.U. Chowdhury, Tamara W. Griffiths and Andrew Y. Finlay.
© 2022 The British Association of Dermatologists. Published 2022 by John Wiley & Sons Ltd.
Companion website: www.wiley.com/go/chowdhury/dermatologytraining

- **Capacity strengthening** to support trainers, health systems and institutions based in LMICs.
- **Sustainability**, whereby the capacity built, and skill generated, remains and continues once a partnership arrangement has reached its conclusion.

For the purposes of this chapter, 'global health dermatology' represents the medical contribution to this theme, focusing on skin health.

What is public health dermatology?

Skin disease causes substantial morbidity worldwide, affecting almost one-third of the world's population. All skin conditions combined were the fourth leading cause of non-fatal disease burden noted in the Global Burden of Disease 2010 study. Common conditions that we see in our clinics, which are also prevalent worldwide, include atopic dermatitis, psoriasis, acne, urticaria, skin cancers and infections such as HIV and scabies (see Further reading). The impact of skin conditions on life quality, commonly expressed in disability-adjusted life-years (DALY), was high across both high- and low-income countries.

'Public health' has been usefully explained as:

- The science and the art of preventing disease, prolonging life, and promoting physical health and mental health and efficient healthcare systems.
- Being achieved through organised community efforts towards a sanitary environment, the control of community infections and the education of the individual in principles of personal hygiene.
- The organisation of medical and nursing services for the early diagnosis and treatment of disease.
- The development of the social machinery to ensure that every individual in the community has a standard of living adequate for the maintenance of health.

How can this be done in reality? There are four key areas:

- Preventing disease and promoting health.
- Improving medical care.
- Promoting health-enhancing behaviour.
- Modifying the environment.

Public health dermatology focuses on overall skin health and continues to be relatively underdeveloped. The majority of our training directs us towards helping individual patients rather than concentrating on population health.

What is important in global health dermatology?

Stigma and disability in relation to skin disease

Skin disease is typically highly visible and potentially stigmatising, particularly in the context of neglected tropical diseases (NTDs). Understanding the stigma and how it worsens disability is a key part of addressing the health burden of these disorders.

Different types of stigma exist. An enacted stigma is the experience of unfair or discriminatory treatment by others, whereas an anticipated stigma is a fear of being stigmatised or discriminated against. Both enacted and anticipated stigma can lead to similar consequences, including feeling shame, being rejected, isolation and experiencing anxiety and depression. There are many different causes of stigma, but they include fear, unease, association with being 'undesirable' or 'infectious', and lack of education and understanding.

Historically, leprosy has been one of the most stigmatised diseases. Biblical passages refer to leprosy and the need for isolation. Leprosariums and leprosy colonies, where people with leprosy were isolated from the general public, feed into stigma that continues to this day. The stigma often stems from the general public's misconceptions about leprosy being a highly contagious disease, when in fact it is not easily transmitted and we have very effective treatments that are readily available. Common phrases in general use exacerbate stigma, such as 'I was treated like a leper.'

To find out more, go to the tools provided in Guides on stigma and mental wellbeing, developed by the International Federation of Leprosy Associations. Details can be found in the resources section at the end of the chapter.

Neglected tropical diseases

NTDs are a group of predominantly infectious diseases that affect the poorest and most marginalised communities in the tropical regions of the world. The World Health Organization (WHO) list of NTDs includes 20 diseases affecting more than 2 billion people, and many of these diseases have cutaneous manifestations (Table 9.1).

Dermatologists are well placed to contribute to the early diagnosis of NTDs. It is also a duty of the dermatology community to make efforts to grow the capacity of dermatology services, to reduce the overall burden of skin disease in endemic countries. Increasing basic dermatology expertise in areas affected with a high burden of NTDs is a strategy supported by the WHO.

Ensuring high-level advocacy with appropriate governments and international agencies is critical to generate political will and advance global health dermatology interventions.

The Neglected Tropical Disease Non-Governmental Organization (NGO) network is a global forum for NGOs to contribute to the global control, elimination and management of consequences of NTDs, outlined within the internationally agreed WHO NTD Roadmap (see Further reading).

Integrated approaches

The WHO now promotes an integrated approach to diagnosing and controlling skin-related NTDs, rather than disease-specific methods, recognising that failure to diagnose and treat these early can lead to long-term disfigurement, disability and stigmatisation, as well as socioeconomic disadvantage. It acknowledges the cost-effectiveness of combined interventions concentrating around non-specialist skin descriptor groupings

Table 9.1 List of neglected tropical diseases

Diseases with known skin manifestations

Buruli ulcer

Chagas disease

Dengue and chikungunya

Dracunculiasis (Guinea worm disease)

Foodborne trematodiases

Human African trypanosomiasis (sleeping sickness)

Leishmaniasis

Leprosy

Lymphatic filariasis

Mycetoma, chromoblastomycosis and other deep mycoses

Onchocerciasis (river blindness)

Scabies and other ectoparasites

Schistosomiasis

Snake bite envenoming

Soil-transmitted helminthiases

Taeniasis/cysticercosis

Yaws (endemic treponematoses)

Diseases less likely to have skin manifestations

Echinococcosis

Rabies

Trachoma

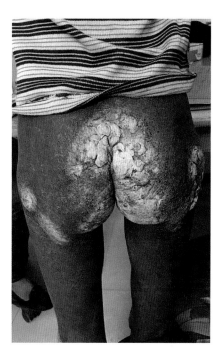

Figure 9.1 Crusted scabies. © Dr Richard Weller.

staphylococcal and streptococcal infections lead to systemic consequences such as glomerulonephritis and bacterial endocarditis, with the potential long-term sequelae of chronic renal impairment, hypertension and cardiac valve disease.

The International Alliance for the Control of Scabies is a global multidisciplinary network committed to the control of human scabies and the promotion of the health and wellbeing of all those living in affected communities (see Further reading).

such as ulcers, lumps, patches and swollen limbs. Dermatologists have been instrumental in progressing this initiative, which is leading to the acknowledgement that additional focus is required to improve the diagnosis and management of background common skin disease in NTD-endemic communities and countries.

The WHO Rationale highlights opportunities and factors underlying successful integration in skin NTDs.

Neglected tropical disease case study: increasing the influence of dermatology and skin health in global health

Human scabies, caused by infestation with the *Sarcoptes scabiei var hominis* mite, is included in the classification of NTD. This small mite, only just visible to the naked eye, burrows into the epidermis, lays eggs and triggers an immune host response. This can lead to severe itching with the presence of even a few mites. In the tropics, scabies, including crusted scabies (Figure 9.1), is frequently complicated by secondary bacterial infection resulting in significant skin pyoderma. These

Examples of schemes to increase dermatology skills in a resource-limited setting

Tropical dermatology: a syndrome-based approach

For many years the WHO has endorsed a syndromic approach to the management of sexually transmitted infections, in settings where aetiological diagnoses may be problematic (e.g. urethral discharge, genital ulcer disease, scrotal swelling). The rationale for this approach includes constraints on time, resources, costs, access to treatments and accuracy of available tests. In many parts of the world dermatologists are dermatovenereologists, so some knowledge of this area is relevant to training, especially when thinking about global health practice.

Building on experience from sexual health practices, using the 'syndromic approach', the University of Minnesota has developed an online course providing an overview of skin diseases in the tropics, with an emphasis on diagnoses that are common and/or of medical or public health importance. The approach is organised by presenting complaint, reflecting how the clinician evaluates the patient, rather than by aetiology. The course is aimed at primary healthcare doctors and is divided into seven sections including itch in the tropics, pigmentary disorders, nodules, rashes and ulcers.

One-day training for primary healthcare workers: the Mali approach

A one-day course was devised focusing on just a few conditions that local data indicated were most important: pyoderma, scabies, tinea capitis, other superficial mycosis and contact dermatitis. Guidance was also provided on the referral of suspected cases of early leprosy. Over a period of three years, 400 healthcare workers were trained in groups of 20. Assessment of the efficacy of this training showed that the proportion of patients who presented with skin diseases and who benefited from a clear diagnosis and appropriate treatment increased from 42% before the training to 81% after. This was associated with a 25% reduction in prescription costs. Improved levels of knowledge and practice persisted for up to 18 months after training and were achieved at a cost of just $40 per trainee.

Transferable skills gained in global health settings

Traditional medicine: understanding local cultural norms

The WHO defines traditional medicine as 'the sum total of the knowledge, skill, and practices based on the theories, beliefs, and experiences indigenous to different cultures, whether explicable or not, used in the maintenance of health as well as in the prevention, diagnosis, improvement or treatment of physical and mental illness'. The term 'complementary medicine' or 'alternative medicine' refers to a broad set of healthcare practices that are not part of that country's own tradition or conventional medicine and are not fully integrated into the dominant healthcare system. This section primarily addresses traditional medicine, but some common themes also apply to use of complementary medicine.

Traditional medicine is wide ranging and could include herbal medicine, or spiritual or religious practices. It is thought that healing with medicinal plants is as old as humankind itself, with the earliest written evidence going as far back as 5000 years. Traditional medical practices and treatments of skin disease have been used all over the world in various cultures, including in China, India and Africa. In developing countries including Ethiopia, it is thought that up to 80% of people rely on traditional

medicine for primary healthcare services. The reasons for this are very complex, but include modern medicine being too expensive or not accessible. On the other hand, traditional medicine has advantages of acceptability, affordability, perceived efficacy and accessibility, as well as providing psychological comfort. With increasing travel and multiculturalism, traditional skin treatments from all over the world are ever more likely to be encountered in clinical practice in the UK. For example, a questionnaire study of 100 consecutive children with atopic dermatitis in Leicester found that 46% of patients had used, or were currently using, complementary medicine.

The risks of using certain traditional medicines and treatments are well documented. For example, herbal drugs have been documented as containing unlabelled corticosteroids, and can also cause allergic skin reactions, photosensitisation, arsenic dermatoses and mercury poisoning (Table 9.2). Substances that kill unwanted tissue ('escharotics') made from plants have been used to treat skin cancers in various cultures historically, including by Native Americans. These types of treatments are not evidence based, and there are reports of very advanced and neglected skin tumours that had been treated in this manner, including basal cell carcinomas that have metastasised. Regulation of traditional herbal medicines is another concern: standardisation for herbal drugs is being developed, but currently regulation is not uniform across different parts of the world in terms of active ingredients, purity and concentration. Additional concerns include regulation about claims made for alleviation of specific symptoms by herbal medicines.

Addressing the practice of traditional medicine or complementary medicine in a standard clinical setting can be challenging. Data suggest that only 40% of complementary medicine usage is actually discussed with physicians. It is important for you to be aware of cultural norms and belief systems not aligned to contemporary evidence-based practice, and to approach these in a non-judgemental and open-minded manner.

There is a risk that differences in beliefs and attitudes between healthcare professionals and patients represent a divide preventing safe and effective treatment, both at home and abroad. Advice will be ignored if it is not culturally acceptable. Healthcare-seeking behaviour from patients is subject to a complex

Table 9.2 Reported adverse drug reactions to herbal medications

Allergic skin reactions
Stevens–Johnson syndrome
Photosensitisation
Sweet's syndrome
Pellagra
Arsenic dermatoses
Mercury poisoning

sociocultural belief paradigm. A study of healthcare-seeking behaviour in Ghana indicated that choosing traditional medicine is heavily influenced by illness perceptions, cultural beliefs, norms and traditions. These shape health beliefs in the form of personal philosophies and include a desire to be part of the healing process with holistic and natural healing approaches. This, factored against displeasure with the pure medicalisation of Western medicine, pushes individuals into or keeps them using traditional medicine. For these reasons, patients who believe in traditional medicine may be less compliant with modern medicine. A study in Uganda found that patients who think that traditional medicine can treat onchocerciasis are less likely to be compliant with ivermectin treatment.

To summarise, the role of an effective dermatologist is to understand and encapsulate all of the above factors in your consultation to:

- Identify whether traditional medicine is relevant to your consultation: this is not always obvious, and you might need to ask directly.
- Manage any risks to your patient posed by traditional medicines.
- Engage your patient to be concordant (adherent) with evidence-based treatment.
- Ensure you allow your patient to meet their health, sociocultural, psychological and holistic healthcare needs, which may involve aspects of traditional medicine.

Communication challenges

Migrants often do not speak the language of their host country. These language barriers can cause major health disparities, including inappropriate diagnosis, poorer adherence to treatment and follow-up, medication complications, longer hospitalisations and poorer patient satisfaction.

Unfortunately, despite the evidence of the importance of interpreters, professional interpreters are used in less than 20% of consultations with patients of limited English proficiency. Barriers to the use of interpreters include time constraints and availability of appropriately trained personnel (Table 9.3). Some doctors have described 'getting by' using untrained interpreters, family members or the patient's limited second language.

The General Medical Council's Good Medical Practice document states that doctors 'must give patients the information they want or need to know in a way they can understand. You should make sure that arrangements are made, wherever possible, to meet patients' language and communication needs.'

Family members should not be used as interpreters for many reasons, including lack of confidentiality, tangential conversations, embarrassment and unfamiliarity with medical terminology.

Improving cultural competence

The UK population is becoming more diverse. In England and Wales the percentage of the population identifying as White British decreased from 87.4% in 2001 to 80.5% in 2011. There

Table 9.3 Tips for using a medical interpreter

Identify patients who may benefit from an interpreter
Allow extra time
Document the name of the interpreter in the medical notes
Most patients understand some English, so do not make comments you do not want them to understand
Sit the interpreter next to or slightly behind the patient
Speak directly to the patient, using first-person statements
Speak in short sentences and one question at a time
Prioritise and limit key points
Insist on sentence-by-sentence interpretation
Do not use acronyms, jargon or humour
Check patient understanding

were increases in other ethnic populations, including 'other white' groups such as people born in Poland, and in black African ethnic groups. It is therefore vital that as doctors we build our skills in cultural competence to help us manage all patients optimally.

Culture can be defined as 'patterns of human behaviour inherent in the lives of a racial, ethnic, religious, or social group'. Cultural competence is 'an acknowledgment and incorporation of the importance of culture, assessment of cross-cultural relations, vigilance toward the dynamics that result from cultural differences, expansion of cultural knowledge, and adaptation of services to meet culturally unique needs on the part of clinicians and health-care systems'.

Cultural competence is important for many reasons, including understanding different illness and healthcare beliefs and the ways patients might present to a doctor. This understanding increases patient satisfaction and potentially compliance with treatment, and will help eliminate racial and ethnic healthcare disparities. In the USA, five-year melanoma survival is much better in white patients than in African Americans: 93.6% versus 69%, respectively. Although melanoma is less common in ethnic minorities, these patients often present later, and have worse outcomes. There are many reasons for this disparity, including poor access to healthcare and mistrust of the healthcare system.

Consequences of where communication and cultural competencies start breaking down are illustrated in *The Spirit Catches You and You Fall Down: A Hmong Child, Her American Doctors, and the Collision of Two Cultures*, a book written by Anne Fadiman. It tells the story of Lia Lee, a little girl with epilepsy living in a migrant Hmong family in the USA. There is a clash between the Hmongs' spiritual and cultural beliefs about illness and healing, and the Americans' scientific medical approach, failing to empathise and understand the Hmong culture. This leads to mistrust on both sides, with poor compliance with prescribed treatments, eventually leading to disastrous consequences despite the best intentions of a loving family and highly trained, well-meaning doctors.

A cultural competence e-Learning course can be found on the e-Learning for Healthcare website (see Further reading).

Understanding global cosmetic dermatology practices

Being aware of global cosmetic skin, hair and nail practices, potential complications and their relationship to disease is a key skill for dermatologists wherever we work (Chapter 21). For example, we are all well aware of the increasing number of presentations of allergic contact dermatitis secondary to cosmetic acrylic nails in the UK. There are a number of cosmetic practices performed by certain ethnic and cultural groups that may be important in certain disease presentations to a dermatologist. Skin whitening will be discussed to illustrate this point, but there are multiple other cultural cosmetic practices relevant to a dermatologist, including cultural hair practices.

Skin lightening as a cosmetic procedure has been carried out for hundreds of years, and historians have attributed this to be linked with wealth, social class, limited outdoor labour, desirability and purity. This is opposed to the 'bronzed skin' appearance that is currently fashionable in the UK. Skin-whitening practices are very popular in Asia, but they also frequently occur in other communities, including in Africa. A study of skin-whitening products available in the European Union documented commonly found legal and illegal ingredients. Illegal cosmetic ingredients included corticosteroids, hydroquinone and mercury.

Corticosteroids could lead to skin atrophy, hydroquinone to cutaneous ochronosis and mercury to mercury poisoning, so these illegal products expose people to dangerous side-effects. These illegal cosmetics could also contain incorrectly labelled ingredients and packaging, and unregulated drug concentrations. Skin-whitening cosmetic practices raise some contentious social and ethical issues. Are these practices acceptable and down to personal choice, or do they perpetuate and reinforce negative and racist stereotypes and body images?

Future global health opportunities

The International Alliance for Global Health Dermatology (GLODERM) is a recently established international community of dermatologists. Its primary focus is on the advancement of skin health in resource-limited communities, but this is to be done locally and globally through sustainable and integrated approaches to clinical care, education, research, policy and advocacy. GLODERM aims to build connections between dermatologists, trainees and health professionals around the world to improve skin health.

The British Association of Dermatologists has provided support for global health dermatology by running an annual Global Health Day and offering specific funding and awards to support projects. Well-established programmes exist, such as with the Regional Dermatology Training Centre in Tanzania (Figure 9.2).

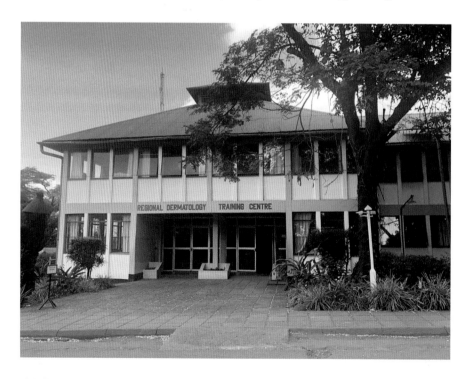

Figure 9.2 The Regional Dermatology Training Centre in Tanzania. © Professor C.E.M. Griffiths.

Plenty of opportunities may arise to get involved in this exciting and developing field, even after completion of training. The key theme is to engage with patients with an open mind, trying to understand their cultural point of view to increase patient satisfaction and improve the doctor–patient relationship. This will, in turn, increase adherence with treatment and reduce and help eliminate racial and ethnic healthcare disparities.

Pearls and pitfalls

- Global health dermatology seeks to improve the wellbeing of people in relation to skin disease throughout the world. Intervention transcends national borders and requires interdisciplinary collaboration, combining population-based health prevention with individual-level medical intervention.
- The World Health Organization has a list of 20 neglected tropical diseases, most of which have dermatological manifestations and are often subject to stigma and healthcare inequalities.
- The General Medical Council recommends 'wherever possible, to meet patients' language and communication needs'. It is not acceptable to just 'get by', when a professional interpreter could be used.
- Identify whether traditional medicine is relevant to your dermatology consultation. Manage any risks posed by traditional medications.
- Engage your patient to be adherent with evidence-based treatment, while allowing them to meet their health, socio-cultural, psychological and holistic healthcare needs, which may involve aspects of traditional medicine.
- Cultural competence will increase patient satisfaction and improve the doctor–patient relationship. This will improve adherence to treatment and help to eliminate racial and ethnic healthcare disparities.

SCE Questions. See questions 38–40.

FURTHER READING AND KEY RESOURCES

Ernst E. Adverse effects of herbal drugs in dermatology. *Br J Dermatol* 2000; **143**:923–9.

Flohr C, Hay R. Putting the burden of skin diseases on the global map. *Br J Dermatol* 2021; **184**:189–90.

Hay RJ, Augustin M, Griffiths CEM, Sterry W. The global challenge for skin health. *Br J Dermatol* 2015; **172**:1469–72.

Johnston GA, Bilbao RM, Graham-Brown RA. The use of complementary medicine in children with atopic dermatitis in secondary care in Leicester. *Br J Dermatol* 2003; **149**:566–71.

Juckett G, Unger K. Appropriate use of medical interpreters. *Am Fam Physician* 2014; **90**:476–80.

McKesey J, Berger TG, Lim HW *et al*. Cultural competence for the 21st century dermatologist practicing in the United States. *J Am Acad Dermatol* 2017; **77**:1159–69.

Nuwaha F, Okware J, Ndyomugyenyi R. Predictors of compliance with community-directed ivermectin treatment in Uganda: quantitative results. *Trop Med Int Health* 2005; **10**:659–67.

Williams HC, Langan SM, Flohr C. Public health in dermatology. In *Fitzpatrick's Dermatology in General Medicine* (Goldsmith LA, Katz S, Gilchrest BA, Paller AS, Leffell DJ, Wolff K, eds), 8th edn. New York: McGraw-Hill, 2017; Chapter 4.

Textbook

Babulal S, Kumar P, eds. *Essentials of Global Health*. Amsterdam: Elsevier, 2019.

Useful websites

British Association of Dermatologists. Fellowships and awards. Available at: https://www.bad.org.uk/healthcare-professionals/fellowships-and-awards.

Campus Connect. Fair Trade Learning. Available at: https://compact.org/ftl.

e-Learning for Healthcare. Cultural competence. Available at: https://www.e-lfh.org.uk/programmes/cultural-competence.

Fair Trade Learning. Advancing just global partnerships. Available at: https://docplayer.net/47431341-Fair-trade-learning-advancing-just-global-partnerships.html.

GLODERM. Available at: www.gloderm.org.

InfoNTD. Guides on stigma and mental wellbeing. Available at: https://www.infontd.org/toolkits/stigma-guides/stigmaguides.

International Alliance for the Control of Scabies. Available at: www.controlscabies.org.

Neglected Tropical Disease NGO Network. One Health for the WHO NTD road map. Available at: https://www.ntd-ngonetwork.org/one-health-for-the-who-ntd-road-map.

University of Minnesota. Tropical dermatology: a syndrome-based approach. Available at: https://learning.umn.edu/search/publicCourseSearchDetails.do?method=load&courseId=19315064.

World Health Organization. Ending the neglect to attain the sustainable development goals. Available at: https://www.who.int/neglected_diseases/Ending-the-neglect-to-attain-the-SDGs--NTD-Roadmap.pdf.

World Health Organization. Guidelines for the management of sexually transmitted infections. Available at: https://www.who.int/hiv/topics/vct/sw_toolkit/guidelines_management_sti.pdf.

World Health Organization. Traditional, complementary and integrative medicine. Available at: https://www.who.int/health-topics/traditional-complementary-and-integrative-medicine.

Section 3

General
dermatology

10

Medical dermatology

Victoria J. Lewis and Giles Dunnill

Introduction

The diagnosis and management of patients with inflammatory skin disease remain challenging but rewarding aspects of 'core' dermatology practice. Thorough history taking and examination, sometimes aided by histopathology, remain at the heart of good clinical care. Skills in the management of chronic disease need to be developed, underpinned by a good doctor–patient relationship. A thorough understanding of how the disease impacts the patient's life is key, and will facilitate assessment and communication of the risk–benefit ratio of various therapeutic strategies for shared decision making with the patient. This chapter is not meant to cover the entire breadth and depth of medical dermatological practice, but instead will provide those early in their dermatology career with sound fundamental knowledge on common conditions seen routinely in the outpatient clinic, along with practical management tips.

Skin inflammation results in a variety of colour changes primarily due to vasodilation, but also due to effects on melanocytes. Simply asking the patient if they have noticed a change in their skin colour may be useful. In white skin, inflammation mainly causes redness but can lead to other colour changes. In skin of colour, inflammation may cause violaceous, grey, brown–dark brown or even black colour changes, as well as redness. As such changes can be subtle in darker skin, it can be helpful to look for other signs of inflammation such as pain, heat, swelling, peeling, texture or contour changes, or prominent skin papules and pores. Using good lighting or a dark contrasting background can also aid in the detection of inflammation in skin of colour.

Dermatologists should become familiar with current national guidelines in the UK, published by the British Association of Dermatologists. New topical and systemic therapies are being developed for a number of skin conditions, ranging from inflammatory dermatoses such as psoriasis to skin cancer. Remember to take an appropriate, cautious approach to new therapies. Over the last 30 years several new drugs have been introduced with much optimism and marketed extensively, only to be withdrawn because of poor effectiveness or adverse events. You must take a long-term view for your patients who have long-term disease.

Psoriasis

Epidemiology

Overall, 2% of the population worldwide has psoriasis vulgaris. Countries further from the equator have higher prevalence rates (Northern Europe and North America up to 3%; Africa and Asia

Dermatology Training: The Essentials. Edited by Mahbub M.U. Chowdhury, Tamara W. Griffiths and Andrew Y. Finlay.
© 2022 The British Association of Dermatologists. Published 2022 by John Wiley & Sons Ltd.
Companion website: www.wiley.com/go/chowdhury/dermatologytraining

< 1%). Psoriasis can first appear from infancy up to the eighth decade. There is a bimodal peak in the age of onset seen in the late teens and early 20s (often more severe, and with a positive family history) and at 50–60 years. Psoriasis affects males and females equally, but onset is often earlier in females.

Aetiology

Psoriasis is thought to arise from an environmental trigger, in addition to a genetic susceptibility.

Genetic susceptibility

In psoriasis, the genetics are complex and polygenic. Evidence for genetic factors comes from family and twin studies, showing increased concordance in both dizygotic and monozygotic twins. Research has been extensive on human leucocyte antigen (HLA) linkage and genetic loci.

The most important identified so far are:

- HLA C*06:02: strongest association with severe disease of early onset, and with guttate psoriasis.
- *CARD14* gene region (previously named *PSORS2*; chromosome 17q25.3).

Environmental triggers and exacerbating factors

Psoriasis is known to be triggered or exacerbated by several factors:

- **Trauma.** The occurrence of psoriasis in an area of trauma or a scar is known as the Koebner phenomenon (Figure 10.1) The Koebner phenomenon also occurs in lichen planus and vitiligo and with viral warts.
- **Infection.** Streptococcal throat infection has a strong association with acute guttate psoriasis (Figure 10.1) and is also linked with flares of chronic plaque psoriasis.
- **HIV.** Psoriasis can occur for the first time following HIV seroconversion and may be the initial clinical sign of HIV infection. HIV can also make existing psoriasis worse. It is therefore important to check HIV serology in severe new adult presentations of psoriasis.
- **Drugs.** Some drugs can precipitate or worsen psoriasis. These include lithium, beta blockers, non-steroidal anti-inflammatory drugs, antimalarials and angiotensin-converting enzyme inhibitors, and the withdrawal of corticosteroids.
- **Sunlight.** Most patients' psoriasis improves in the sun but in about 10% it gets worse.
- **Metabolic.** Pregnancy generally improves psoriasis but it can worsen post-partum.
- **Generalised pustular psoriasis.** This can be triggered post-partum or exacerbated by hypocalcaemia.
- **Obesity.** Linked with psoriasis; weight loss can improve psoriasis in patients with obesity.
- **Stress.** There is strong evidence that stress can exacerbate psoriasis. Patients with high levels of worry respond less well to therapy.

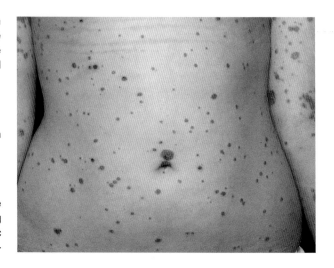

Figure 10.1 Guttate psoriasis. Note the small, widespread scaly plaques on arms and torso. Also note the Koebner phenomenon, a plaque of psoriasis just above the umbilicus, due to the trauma of piercing. © Medical Illustration Cardiff and Vale UHB.

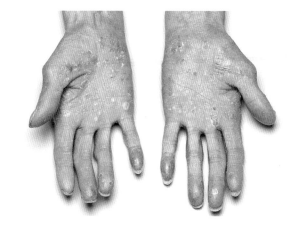

Figure 10.2 Palmoplantar pustulosis. Note the different colours of the pustules, indicating different maturity of the lesions. © Medical Illustration Cardiff and Vale UHB.

- **Alcohol.** Heavy consumption can worsen existing disease.
- **Smoking.** There is a strong link between smoking and palmoplantar pustulosis (Figure 10.2), particularly in women.

Pathogenesis

The three main features are:

- Epidermal proliferation and loss of differentiation, clinically causing scaling and thickening.
- Dilatation and proliferation of dermal blood vessels, clinically causing redness.
- Accumulation of inflammatory cells, mainly neutrophils and T lymphocytes.

The T lymphocyte

Psoriasis is a T-cell-mediated disease. T helper 1 (Th1) cells predominate and are activated by interleukin (IL)-12 and IL-23 to secrete IL-17, tumour necrosis factor-α and interferon-γ. This occurs via the signalling pathway involving the Janus kinase (JAK) protein and tyrosine kinase 2 enzyme. All of these mediators are now targets of various biologic therapies for psoriasis.

Psoriasis and cardiovascular disease

Adults with severe psoriasis are at an increased risk of cardiovascular disease and the condition should be considered more as a systemic disease. Assessing cardiovascular risk in this group can allow appropriate intervention of other, modifiable risk factors. It is appropriate to ask the patient's general practitioner (GP) to do this. Some biologic clinics will measure fasting lipids, weight and body mass index, and feed back to the GP for further management.

Clinical features of chronic plaque psoriasis

Sharply demarcated, papulosquamous plaques occur (Figure 10.3), often on the extensor surfaces (Figure 10.4). They can vary in size from < 1 mm to > 20 cm, and are covered in silvery-white scale, which when scratched off may cause pinpoint bleeding. This is known as the 'Auspitz sign' (not recommended to be used diagnostically). When covered with emollient the scale is more transparent and so the underlying plaque colour is more visible. In skin of colour, plaques tend to appear red/brown to violaceous with grey scale but, in white skin, plaques are a reddish colour. Post-inflammatory hypo- or hyperpigmentation may occur. Inflamed skin at the edge of a plaque indicates active psoriasis and is useful to assess response to therapy.

Diagnosis

The diagnosis of psoriasis is usually straightforward but confusion can arise in flexural psoriasis, scalp psoriasis and palmoplantar pustulosis.

Flexural psoriasis

There are some patients who present with indistinct inflammatory lesions in the flexural areas and who have inflamed skin at some typical psoriatic sites (always check for psoriasis at the umbilicus in this case), but who also have involvement at sites typical of seborrhoeic dermatitis. The groin area, vulva, axilla, submammary cleft and gluteal cleft can be affected, again with minimal scale to cause some diagnostic confusion with intertrigo (intertrigo and psoriasis can also coexist). This 'sebopsoriasis' may need to be treated initially with a combination of topical antifungals and moderately potent topical steroids. Do not worry if this presentation at first leaves you feeling unsure of the diagnosis – it can be very difficult. A biopsy is usually not helpful, as mixed

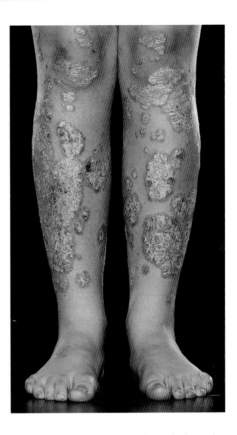

Figure 10.3 Typical plaques of psoriasis on the lower legs, with redness, scaling and slight excoriation. © Medical Illustration Cardiff and Vale UHB.

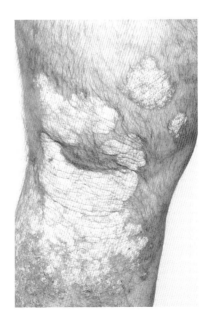

Figure 10.4 Chronic plaque psoriasis. Note the thick scaly plaque on the knee. © Medical Illustration Cardiff and Vale UHB.

inflammatory features are seen, but one is occasionally needed to exclude other flexural dermatoses.

Scalp psoriasis

Scalp psoriasis is usually easy to diagnose: there are typical lesions elsewhere and the lesions are very clearly defined. Plaques on the scalp can develop severe adherent scaling, termed pityriasis amiantacea. Hair growth is generally normal unless the scalp is severely affected. Topical coal tar, calcipotriol and/or corticosteroid preparations are useful treatments.

Occasionally you will see patients misdiagnosed as having scalp psoriasis, even though they have the typical diffuse changes of seborrhoeic dermatitis and no evidence of psoriasis elsewhere. Remember the value of topical antifungals in this setting.

Palmoplantar pustulosis (Figure 10.2)

Psoriasis of the palms or soles can sometimes be difficult to differentiate from chronic eczema. Look carefully for vesicles, as these clear sago-like small blebs are diagnostic of eczema (and usually very itchy). A mixture of large fresh yellow and older brown pustules is typical of palmoplantar pustulosis. However, in eczema, vesicles can sometimes get infected, also producing pustules, but no typical burnt-out older brown areas. This is a difficult condition to treat, and potent topical corticosteroids (with or without occlusion), localised psoralen plus ultraviolet A, ciclosporin or oral retinoids are standard treatments.

Assessment of disease severity

The reality of most consultations with patients with psoriasis is that severity is based on both the patient's and clinician's overall view as to whether the disease is getting better or worse. However, you should know about some basic methods of psoriasis severity assessment. These include body surface area estimation, the Psoriasis Area and Severity Index (PASI) scoring system and methods to measure the impact of psoriasis on quality of life, for example the Dermatology Life Quality Index (DLQI) (Chapter 8). It is suggested that current severe psoriasis can be defined by the Rule of Tens: body surface area > 10% *or* PASI > 10 *or* DLQI > 10.

Variants of psoriasis

Overall, 10% of people with psoriasis have a variant of the condition.

Generalised pustular psoriasis

Sheets of small, sterile pustules appear in areas of inflamed skin. When these are generalised, the patient can be systemically unwell, and this is a dermatological emergency. It may occur post-partum, as a rebound to withdrawal of topical or systemic steroids, or following infection. Emollients and

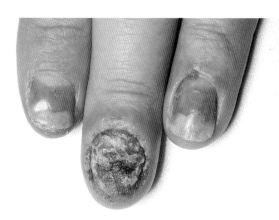

Figure 10.5 Psoriasis of the nails. Note the onycholysis and nail pitting. © Medical Illustration Cardiff and Vale UHB.

moderately potent topical steroids are used and, in addition to these, oral methotrexate or biologic drugs are often the first-line treatment options.

Nail psoriasis

About 25–50% of people with psoriasis have nail changes (Figure 10.5). These include pitting, ridging and discoloration of the nail, subungual hyperkeratosis, onycholysis and a circular 'oil spot' appearance (due to hyperkeratosis of the nail bed).

Acrodermatitis continua of Hallopeau

There are painful pustules on the tips of the fingers and under the nail bed, often with shedding of the nail plate. This can be a relentless condition, resistant to treatment.

Psoriatic arthritis

Arthritis occurs in 5–30% of patients with psoriasis. This can be:

- Mono/asymmetrical arthritis.
- Distal interphalangeal joint involvement, associated with nail involvement.
- Rheumatoid arthritis-like pattern.
- Arthritis mutilans.
- Spondylitis/sacroiliitis, increased in HLA B27 haplotypes.

It is important to assess for arthritis at the first presentation using the Psoriasis Epidemiology Screening Tool: patients scoring ≥ 3 should be referred to a rheumatologist for further assessment.

Management of chronic plaque psoriasis

Dermatology textbooks list the various options for treating psoriasis but few address the reality of the decision-making process. This is a complicated matter involving patient education and negotiation of shared decision making. It is heavily influenced by the individual patient's previous experience of different therapies, their attitudes towards risk, the practicalities of using topical therapy and the current impact that the disease is having on the patient's work–life balance.

Table 10.1 gives the main topical and systemic treatments used for psoriasis. More details are given in Chapters 17 and 18. The Psoriasis Association is a useful point of contact and information for patients.

Eczema

Eczema, or dermatitis (used as interchangeable terms), is an inflammatory skin condition featuring itching, redness, scaling and clustered papulovesicles. Eczema can be endogenous (from within the body) or exogenous (from an external trigger) (Table 10.2). Eczema is common in all skin types but may have varied appearances across different skin types (Figures 10.6 and 10.7).

Table 10.2 Types of exogenous and endogenous eczema

Types and causes of exogenous eczema

- Irritant contact dermatitis
- Allergic contact dermatitis
- Photoallergic or photoaggravated dermatitis
- Infective (secondary to bacterial, viral or fungal infection)
- Post-traumatic (rare, and *not* Koebner phenomenon)

Types of endogenous eczema

- Atopic dermatitis
- Seborrhoeic dermatitis
- Asteatotic eczema
- Discoid eczema
- Hand eczema
- Gravitational or varicose eczema
- Eczematous drug eruptions
- Lichen simplex

Table 10.1 Management of psoriasis

Therapy	Key points
Bath additives, soap substitutes, emollients	Emollients essential (Table 10.4). Paraffin-based emollients are flammable (please warn the patient)
Topical vitamin D analogues	First-line treatment. Can use in combination with topical steroids for limited periods. Some preparations can irritate sensitive areas of skin
Topical corticosteroids	Often first choice for sensitive areas of skin. Potent steroid use or withdrawal can lead to a rebound flare of psoriasis, or transformation to generalised pustular psoriasis
Topical coal tar	Some preparations are messy and smelly. Particularly good for small plaque or guttate psoriasis (apply to all of skin) or scalp
Topical dithranol (anthralin)	Works well on thin plaques. Start at a low concentration and build up. Apply to plaques only. Can irritate and stain surrounding skin
Narrowband ultraviolet B (TL-01)	Main complications are burning and skin cancer risk. Patient consent required and skin lesion/mole check should be considered in some patients before commencing. Starting dose determined by minimal erythemal dose. Stop once skin is clear or improvement plateaus. See Chapter 25
Psoralen plus ultraviolet A (UVA)	Psoralen drug can be oral or topical (bath, gel, paint). If taking oral preparation, the eyes must be protected from UV light for 24 hours (UVA opaque glasses). See Chapter 25
Systemic treatments	See Chapter 18. Acitretin, ciclosporin, methotrexate, mycophenolate mofetil
Biologic drugs	See Chapter 18. Antibodies, fusion proteins or receptor blockers to tumour necrosis factor-α, interleukin (IL)-12, IL-23, IL-17, Janus kinase, tyrosine kinase 2. Most require subcutaneous or intravenous administration. The main problems are increased risk of infections, particularly reactivation of tuberculosis. All are expensive

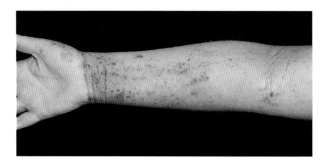

Figure 10.6 Atopic eczema. Note the flexural redness, lichenification and secondary infection of the skin. © Medical Illustration Cardiff and Vale UHB.

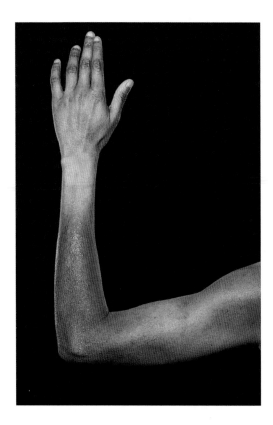

Figure 10.7 Eczema of the arm, showing hyperpigmentation and papular thickening. © Medical Illustration Cardiff and Vale UHB.

Atopic dermatitis

Epidemiology

Atopic dermatitis (AD) has a prevalence of 10–20%, the highest prevalence being in the most-developed 'Westernised' countries. Overall, 90% of cases begin before the age of 5 years. In England, eczema is more prevalent in children and adults of Black, Asian

Table 10.3 UK Working Party diagnostic criteria for diagnosis of atopic dermatitis
The person must have an itchy skin condition (or parental report of scratching or rubbing in a child), plus three or more of the following:
Onset below age of 2 years (not used if child is aged under 4 years)
History of skin crease involvement (including cheeks in children under 10 years)
History of generally dry skin
Personal history of other atopic disease (or history of any atopic disease in a first-degree relative in children under 4 years)
Visible flexural dermatitis (or dermatitis of cheeks or forehead and outer limbs in children under 4 years)

and mixed backgrounds than in those of White ethnic background. The prevalence of atopic diseases in general, and AD in particular, has been increasing over the last four decades.

Diagnosis

This is made according to the UK Working Party's validated refinement of Hanifin and Rajka's diagnostic criteria for AD (Table 10.3).

Aetiology

AD is thought to arise from an interaction of genetic and environmental factors.

Genetic and other factors

Parental (particularly maternal) history of atopy is one of the strongest risk factors for the development of atopy. Filaggrin null mutations, female sex, having asthma and higher birthweight are all also associated with higher risk of AD.

Environmental factors

- **Pollution**. Both indoor (e.g. cigarette smoke) and outdoor (e.g. industrial) pollutants may increase the prevalence of AD.
- **The hygiene hypothesis**. Children from large families, and those living in the developing world, have lower prevalence of AD. This may be due to early exposure to microbes, particularly those causing faeco-oral infection, thus driving the immune system to a protective response.
- **The home environment**. In moderate-to-severe eczema, some small studies show that reduction of house dust mite levels in the home may be of modest benefit, mainly in childhood AD. Measures that can be tried include:
  - Frequent vacuuming of carpets or avoidance of carpets.
  - Frequent dusting and ventilation of the bedroom.

o Covering bedding with dust-tight mattress and pillow covers.

o Frequent washing of soft toys, or putting them in the freezer for 24 hours.

Other points of advice for the home are:

o Avoidance of animal dander.

o Wearing cotton clothes rather than wool.

o Washing clothes in non-fragranced, non-biological detergents, at high temperatures (> 50 °C).

- **Food**. Food allergy can potentially aggravate AD in children less than one year old. After this age, its role is much less clear and more unlikely. The best advice, if parents insist on following a dietary route, is to eliminate a certain food from the diet singly, for six weeks only, to determine the effect of its avoidance (in the case of milk avoidance ensure other sources of calcium are given). The involvement of a dietician may be helpful to advise on safe and appropriate dietary manipulation. Specific IgE blood tests are available to diagnose food allergy, but the relationship between these antibodies in the blood and the effect on the skin is not predictable, thus these tests are not a reliable basis for practical advice and are best avoided.

Immunology

Patients with eczema have dry skin, with disruption of the epidermal barrier, increased transepidermal water loss and increased entry of environmental allergens, so inducing the Th2-dominant immune response.

T helper cells, in their development, differentiate into Th1 cells (secreting cytokines IL-2 and interferon-α) or Th2 cells (secreting cytokines IL-4, IL-5 and IL-13). Which helper cell they become depends on what signals they receive externally. In eczema, Th2 cells are predominant, secreting IL-4 and IL-5, which stimulates B cells to produce more IgE, the main immunoglobulin involved in the pathogenesis of atopic disease.

Skin and gut microbiome

There is increasing evidence that patients with AD lack microbial diversity on their skin and in their gut (early antibiotic use may be a factor in this). The gut microbiome is responsible for the production of short-chain fatty acids from the breakdown of complex carbohydrates. These fatty acids have a role in determining the microbial composition of the skin, resulting in protective effects against inflammation and allergic response. Microbiome correction is currently a topic of great interest as a possible therapeutic option for AD, acne and a wide variety of other inflammatory skin conditions.

Clinical features

These include:

- Itching.
- Dry skin.
- Macules, papules or papulovesicles.

- Brown, dark brown or grey lesions in skin of colour (Figures 10.7 and 10.8) and reddish lesions in white skin (Figure 10.6).
- Follicular papules.
- Discoid plaques.
- Dyspigmentation (Figure 10.9).
- Crusting.
- Excoriation and lichenification.
- Secondary bacterial or viral infections.

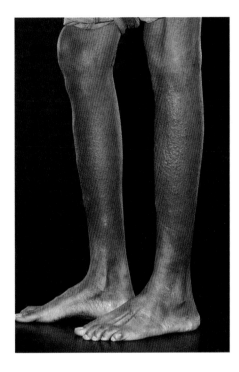

Figure 10.8 Eczema of the lower legs, showing hyperpigmentation and papular thickening, giving a 'cobblestone' appearance. © Medical Illustration Cardiff and Vale UHB.

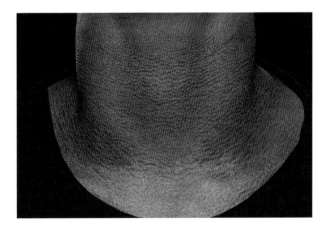

Figure 10.9 Linear hyperpigmentation of the neck in atopic dermatitis. © Medical Illustration Cardiff and Vale UHB.

Distribution

Distribution of AD varies with age:

- **Infants**. Usually most severe on the face (especially if excessive drooling is present). When crawling, extensor surfaces can become rubbed and affected by eczema.
- **Children**. Mainly affects elbow and knee flexures, neck, wrists and ankles. The neck can show fine pigmentation, a 'dirty neck'. Discoid, follicular and extensor distribution of eczema is often seen in children of African and South Asian origin.
- **Adults**. Eczema has a similar distribution to that in children, often with lichenified areas.

Natural history of atopic dermatitis

In 90% of affected children, the eczema starts before the age of five years. It tends to run a course of remissions and exacerbations. Four different trajectories of the condition in children have been described: severe-frequent, moderate-frequent, moderate-declining and mild-intermittent. Generally, there is a tendency towards spontaneous improvement throughout childhood. Clearance occurs in around 60% by teenage years. Severe persistent adult AD is seen but it is much less common than childhood eczema.

Complications

- **Bacterial infection** is secondary, and is often streptococcal or staphylococcal, mainly with *Staphylococcus aureus*.
- **Viral infection**. Secondary infection with herpes simplex virus can cause eczema herpeticum (Figures 10.10 and 10.11). This is a dermatological emergency (Chapters 12 and 16). There is sudden onset of numerous painful, small fluid-filled vesicles. These can become secondarily impetiginised, can cause systemic upset and can also affect the conjunctivae. Systemic antivirals are indicated (oral is usually adequate) and topical corticosteroids or immunosuppressants should be stopped. Viral warts and molluscum contagiosum have a tendency to spread on eczematous skin. However, varicella zoster virus affects people with eczema in the same way as it would those with normal skin.
- **Ocular abnormalities** include conjunctival irritation, the rare condition keratoconus (a conical cornea leading to marked visual disturbance) and cataract (mainly if severe facial eczema or with use of strong topical or systemic corticosteroids).

Measurement of severity of eczema

This can be measured physically, for example by the Eczema Assessment and Severity Index (EASI) or Scoring Atopic Dermatitis (SCORAD) (see Chapter 8). It is also important to ask about the effect of eczema on quality of life, either with specific measures, such as the DLQI or Children's Dermatology Life Quality Index, or by general enquiry about itch, sleep loss and

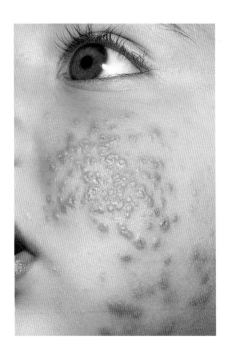

Figure 10.10 Eczema herpeticum (early). Note the numerous tiny fluid-filled vesicles on the cheek. © Medical Illustration Cardiff and Vale UHB.

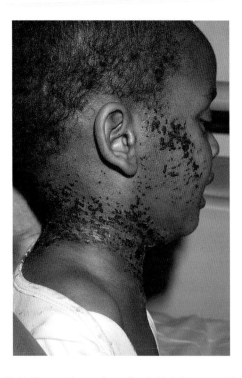

Figure 10.11 Eczema herpeticum (late). No blisters remain, but there are tiny discrete erosions and secondary bacterial infection and crusting on the cheek and neck. © Medical Illustration Cardiff and Vale UHB.

loss of time at work. Children's growth and progress at school should be particularly noted. All of these factors should influence shared decision making regarding management.

Treatment

As with any chronic inflammatory condition of the skin, time should be taken to develop a good relationship between the dermatologist and the patient, particularly in increasing understanding about the nature and course of the disease. Management should be based on a specific overall regimen, including bath additives, soap substitutes, emollients and either topical steroids or topical immunosuppressants (Chapter 17).

This maintenance regimen should be written down for the patient. A second regimen specifically for flare-ups should also be written down for them, specifying in addition when they can go back to their usual treatments. The quantity of topical treatments required should be discussed and, if possible, demonstrated during the consultation. Treatment concordance is the biggest problem to tackle and any reluctance to use the prescribed medication should be discussed (e.g. treatments that sting, fear about side-effects of topical steroids, reluctance to ask GP for repeat prescriptions). This all takes time but is well worth it in the long term. Always inform the patient or parents about the National Eczema Society, which is an excellent source of information.

For very severe and persisting AD, systemic therapy may be indicated. A summary of specific treatments is given in Table 10.4.

'What if my patient is not improving with conventional eczema treatment?'

If eczema fails to improve with correct treatment, or worsens, the following should be considered:

- Is the diagnosis correct? Other differential diagnoses include
  o Scabies: always look for scabies burrows, particularly on the finger webs, abdomen and genital area.
  o Seborrhoeic dermatitis: this mainly affects the scalp, eyebrows and creases on the face. Greasy scales are clinically visible.
  o Patch-stage mycosis fungoides: patches are static and are not always itchy.
  o Pre-bullous pemphigoid: before the blistering stage, this condition can resemble eczema that is resistant to conventional treatment.
- Is there an element of irritant contact dermatitis?
  o Patients with AD are more prone to this, particularly on the hands.

Table 10.4 Management of atopic dermatitis

Therapy	Key points
Bath and shower additives or soap substitutes	All patients should be advised to avoid soaps, bubble bath and shower gels. Some bath additives and soap substitutes contain antiseptic, which is important if the patient has recurrent infections. Care must be taken, as some products make the bath or shower very slippery
Emollients	These are essential and should be applied liberally. They vary in consistency. Stick with one that the patient likes and tolerates, and is willing to use, as they will then actually put it on! Paraffin-based emollients are *flammable* (please warn the patient)
Topical corticosteroids	These come in a range of potencies and a 'step-up' and 'step-down' regimen can be used according to the severity of eczema. More potent corticosteroids should be used for palms and soles, and less potent drugs for the face and neck. Some contain antibiotics and/or antifungals, which are useful in flexural areas, but antibiotic resistance can develop. See Chapter 17
Topical immunomodulators: tacrolimus, pimecrolimus	These are steroid sparing, so useful particularly on the face and neck, or where the patient requires potent topical steroids for long periods. These should be applied intermittently, beginning at the first signs of a new flare. They may cause a 'burning' sensation for the first few days of application but this often improves. Ensure sun protection to reduce potential skin cancer risk. See Chapter 17
Narrowband ultraviolet B (TL-01)	As for Table 10.1, but may need a tapering regimen once clearance is achieved
Systemic treatments	See Chapter 18. Azathioprine, ciclosporin, methotrexate and mycophenolate mofetil
Biologic drugs	Dupilumab (interleukin-4 and interleukin-13 inhibitor), baricitinib (Janus kinase inhibitor)

○ Eczema in localised sites (e.g. the face or hands) or eczema that is unresponsive or worsening, may indicate an allergic contact dermatitis. Patients with AD are more prone to contact allergy. They are also more likely to become sensitised to fragrances, topical steroids or preservatives in their treatments. Patch testing is indicated if this is suspected (Chapter 23).

Acne

Acne is a chronic inflammatory disorder of the pilosebaceous units. A pilosebaceous unit consists of a hair follicle, erector pili muscle, sebaceous gland and associated apocrine and eccrine sweat glands.

Epidemiology

Acne usually starts in adolescence and mainly resolves by the mid-20s, although 10–20% of cases persist into adulthood, particularly in women. Almost 95% of male and female adolescents develop acne to varying degrees, 10% of whom have severe acne. The peak prevalence is 14–16 years for females and 16–19 years in males, reflecting earlier onset of puberty in females.

'Is it my hormones, doctor?'

Androgen excess, for example in adrenal hyperplasia, polycystic ovarian syndrome (PCOS) or adrenal or ovarian tumours, can trigger acne. You must consider this, particularly if there is a history of:

- Irregular menstruation.
- Hirsutism: excessive hair growth in a male pattern.
- Virilisation: increased body hair, deepening of the voice, increase in muscle bulk.

Blood tests for DHEA-5 (dehydroepiandrosterone), total testosterone and free testosterone should be checked. Anti-androgenic drugs, such as the combined oral contraceptive pill Dianette™, may be of most help if PCOS is causing the acne. Spironolactone has proved helpful in many cases, if the combined oral contraceptive pill is contraindicated or in patients older than 45 years.

Acne can have some additional external causes, which should be considered and enquired about in patients with atypical or refractory acne:

- **Premenstrual flaring of acne.** This type of acne responds best to hormonal therapy (Table 10.5).
- **Occupation.** Patients dealing with heavy-duty oils and crude tars in their work are more susceptible. Those working with chlorinated hydrocarbons, if they are accidentally released, may develop chloracne, which is relatively resistant to treatment and may take several years to resolve.
- **Physical factors.** Certain cosmetics, particularly those with an oily base, are comedogenic. Oils and pomades used on Afro-textured hair also have a comedogenic effect.
- **Drugs.** The commonest acne-inducing drugs are anabolic steroids, corticosteroids, phenytoin, lithium, isoniazid and iodides. It is important to ask about prescription and non-prescription drugs.

Pathogenesis

The following contribute to causing acne:

- **Increased sebum production**. This is mainly dependent on androgenic sex hormones of gonadal or adrenal origin.
- **Genetically inherited distribution of sebaceous glands**. Increased numbers and size of glands appear to have a strong familial tendency, particularly in severe acne. The genetic influences for the development of acne are complex and not fully delineated.
- **Hypercornification of the pilosebaceous duct forming micro-comedones**. Comedones are due to abnormalities in proliferation and differentiation of ductal keratinocytes. Several factors are involved in this, including sebaceous lipid composition, bacteria, local cytokine production and androgens.
- **Abnormality of microbial flora**, especially *Cutibacterium acnes* (formerly *Propionibacterium acnes*): patients with acne have more *C. acnes* on their skin but levels do not correspond to clinical severity. The bacteria may induce inflammation.
- **Production of inflammation**. This is partly due to duct rupture, bacterial colonisation and hormonal factors.

Clinical features (Figures 10.12–10.14)

The main features are:

- Seborrhoea.
- Open and closed comedones: 'blackheads' and 'whiteheads'.
- Papules.
- Hyperpigmentation (post-inflammatory).
- Nodules (Figure 10.14).
- Deep pustules.
- Pseudocysts.
- Scarring.

'Is this "just" severe acne?'

Severe acne can cause systemic symptoms or may be part of a wider disorder. Keep these variants in mind when you see a patient with severe acne:

- **Acne conglobata**. Multiple inflamed nodules and scarring.
- **Acne fulminans**. Sudden-onset severe acne conglobata with systemic symptoms such as fever and joint pains.
- **SAPHO syndrome**. Synovitis, acne, pustulosis, hyperostosis, osteitis.
- **PAPA syndrome**. Pyogenic arthritis, pyoderma gangrenosum, acne.
- **Gram-negative folliculitis**. This presents as 'worsening' of existing acne already treated with prolonged courses of topical or oral antibiotics. Examination shows monomorphic pustules. It is caused by Gram-negative bacteria, seen on swab and culture.

Table 10.5 Management of acne

Therapy	Key points
Topical benzoyl peroxide and topical azelaic acid	Antimicrobial. All topical treatments for acne can irritate or dry the skin. Benzoyl peroxide can bleach clothes or bedclothes
Topical retinoids	Anti-comedonal. For oily skin, gels are often better to dry the skin. Topical retinoids are contraindicated in pregnancy
Topical antibiotics in combination with benzoyl peroxide or zinc	Some preparations can glow under ultraviolet strobe lights. Antibiotic resistance can occur
Oral antibiotics	At least three months of treatment should be given
Tetracyclines (e.g. lymecycline and doxycycline)	Contraindicated in pregnancy and children who do not have all their adult teeth yet (causes staining of teeth)
Erythromycin	Low dose 250 mg twice daily. Best choice for 'spot pickers'
Trimethoprim	High (unlicenced) dose 300 mg twice daily
Hormonal treatments	
Cyproterone acetate	Anti-androgen, thus suppresses sebum production
Spironolactone	Particularly useful for premenstrual flare of acne, or for acne related to polycystic ovarian syndrome. Useful in older females or where combined oral contraceptive pill is contraindicated. Contraindicated in pregnancy
Isotretinoin	Most common side-effects are dryness of lips and mucous membranes (dose related). Hair thinning, nosebleeds, muscle and joint pains, skin fragility (no hair waxing!) and reduced night vision can be problematic. Isotretinoin is teratogenic and the pregnancy prevention plan must be followed if there is any risk of pregnancy. Erectile dysfunction is a rare complication but needs to be mentioned. It is extremely important to monitor for depression and suicide risk and the patient should be assessed throughout treatment for this
Blue light, red light	Mixed trial results show equivalence to moderate acne treatments such as oral antibiotics
Laser and NLite	These have moderate effects, are not available in the UK NHS, and are contraindicated if taking isotretinoin
Physical treatments	
Intralesional triamcinolone	This can be helpful for early acne nodules or hypertrophic or keloid scars
Electrocautery	Closed comedones can respond to this

Treatments for acne scarring	These are not usually available in the UK NHS. They consist of:
	
	    Excision or subcision of scars
	    Dermabrasion
	    Laser resurfacing
	    Fractionated CO_2 laser (Fraxel®)
	    Microneedling
	    Chemical peels

How to assess the severity of acne

Acne should be assessed both in physical terms and in terms of its effect on the individual, in order to decide on the best management options for the patient. A measure of physical severity frequently used for research purposes is the Leeds Acne Grading System. However, this scale was developed before the introduction of isotretinoin and is biased towards extremely severe acne. It is useful to have a descriptive record of areas involved and presence or absence of cysts, scars, pustules and papules.

The psychological and social effects of acne should not be underestimated. Often acne starts in adolescence, a time where embarrassment and lack of confidence are already highest. Social contact may become limited, bullying may occur at

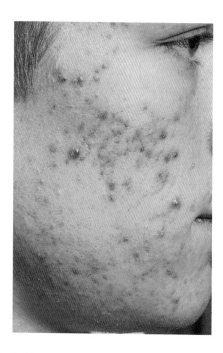

Figure 10.12 Moderate-to-severe acne. Note the papules, pustules, comedones and mild scarring on the cheek. © Medical Illustration Cardiff and Vale UHB.

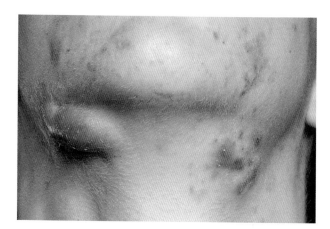

Figure 10.14 Severe nodulocystic acne. Note the open and closed comedones, cysts and keloid scarring under the chin (this should not be surgically excised). © Medical Illustration Cardiff and Vale UHB.

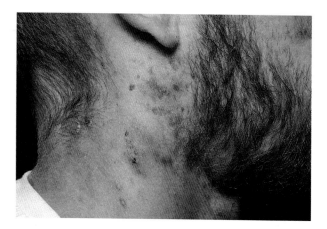

Figure 10.13 Acne on the right side of the face and neck, showing papules, pustules and signs of inflammation. © Medical Illustration Cardiff and Vale UHB.

school, and it may even affect employment prospects. More formal measures of quality of life can be used such as the DLQI, or an acne-specific measure such as the Cardiff Acne Disability Index or the Acne Quality of Life Scale.

Differential diagnosis

The main alternative diagnoses to consider are:

- **Rosacea**. Typically, there are no comedones in rosacea.
- **Perioral dermatitis**. There is often a history of topical steroid use to the perioral area. This is considered a form of rosacea (steroid-provoked rosacea) and is a misnomer as it is not a 'dermatitis'.
- **Folliculitis**. Gram-negative organisms such as *Malassezia* (previously 'pityrosporum') and demodex mite can cause a folliculitis, which may present as acne refractory to treatment. A trial of topical antibiotic, anti-yeast preparation or permethrin can help to differentiate between these conditions.

Management (Table 10.5)

When managing a patient with acne, it is important to address any misconceptions about what has caused it, for example:

- **Diet**. Many patients believe that eating fats or chocolate can cause acne. However, there is no convincing evidence to suggest that this is the case, but dairy products may play a part in the development of acne due to stimulating insulin swings, and this increases testosterone production.
- **Lack of hygiene**. Some patients believe that 'blackheads' are due to dirt and use abrasive or irritating preparations to cleanse their skin excessively. It is important to explain that the 'black' in a 'blackhead' is pigment, not dirt, and that excessive cleansing of the skin can make acne worse, as well as irritating the skin, causing dryness and soreness. A bland, non-irritating preparation or just water should be used to wash the skin.
- **Make-up**. There is some truth that greasy make-up can cause acne. It is important to recommend a non-comedogenic formulation of make-up and also to advise that it is completely removed before going to sleep at night. It is unrealistic to expect adolescent girls to go without make-up, so a compromise should be reached on this.
- **Emotional stress**. Raised cortisol levels can cause excess sebum production, thereby exacerbating existing acne.

How to treat a patient safely with isotretinoin

Isotretinoin is a very effective drug for severe, scarring or non-responsive acne. However, it also has many side-effects, some of which are serious and the benefits and risks of this treatment should be carefully weighed up before starting the course. The following section describes the current guidelines for the use of isotretinoin, but always consult the British Association of Dermatologists' website for the most up-to-date guidelines.

At first consultation, a Medicines and Healthcare products Regulatory Agency (MHRA)-approved written patient information booklet should be given to the patient, and the main side-effects (particularly the possible link with depression and suicide), indications and course of treatment discussed. It is useful to record any personal or family history of depression at this stage. Isotretinoin is teratogenic and any female patient considered for treatment with this drug should be assessed for their potential risk of pregnancy. A contraception information booklet should be given, if required. There is no impact on future fertility or teratogenic effects beyond one month. Baseline screening blood tests (including full blood count, liver function tests and fasting lipids) should also be performed.

At a second consultation, provided the patient would like to go ahead with treatment and all baseline blood tests are normal, a male patient can commence therapy with follow-up every 2–3 months. All other topical acne treatments and systemic antibiotics should be stopped. Any female patient considered at risk of pregnancy should be entered into the pregnancy prevention programme.

Pregnancy prevention plan

The prescriber, pharmacist and patients must follow these rules:

- Pregnancy test just before starting therapy. Pregnancy tests can be of blood or urine but they must be medically supervised. Isotretinoin should be started on the second day of the next period.
- One reliable and preferably two forms of contraception are to be used from at least one month before until at least one month after the completion of the course of isotretinoin.
- Monthly pregnancy tests throughout therapy.
- Pregnancy test five weeks after stopping the course of therapy.
- Isotretinoin prescriptions should be for only one month of therapy at a time. Prescriptions are valid for seven days only.
- Complete the *checklist for prescribing to female patients* at each stage, i.e. before treatment, at monthly visits during treatment and at the post-treatment visit.

If the patient is not regarded as at risk of pregnancy, for example they have had a hysterectomy or are sterilised, and does not enter the pregnancy prevention plan, the reason for this should be recorded in the notes.

'What if my patient becomes pregnant while on isotretinoin?'

If pregnancy occurs or is suspected in any female patient during treatment or in the five weeks after therapy:

- The patient should stop isotretinoin immediately.
- The patient should receive advice from a physician specialised or experienced in birth defects.
- The patient should inform the primary prescriber of the isotretinoin treatment and their GP. The supplier and the MHRA should be informed if pregnancy is confirmed.

'How much isotretinoin can I give?'

The standard dose of isotretinoin in the UK is up to 1 mg/kg/day for 16 weeks and a single treatment course is sufficient for the majority of patients. A further improvement of acne can be observed up to eight weeks after discontinuation of treatment, so a further course should not be considered until this time has elapsed. Patients are able to have longer courses of treatment (up to 24 weeks) or a repeat course as necessary but there is no substantial additional benefit beyond a cumulative treatment dose of 120–150 mg/kg.

'What if my patient has a flare of their acne when starting isotretinoin?'

All patients should be warned that this may happen in the first few weeks of their treatment. In very severe acne, this can be minimised by starting on a half-standard dose (0.5 mg/kg/day) or by the use of topical or oral corticosteroids to manage a severe flare should it occur.

'What if my patient is slow to respond or fails to respond to isotretinoin?'

Check if your patient is taking the tablets! If so, ensure that the patient is on the full dose according to weight. Some patients will be slower to respond and a prolonged course (up to 24 weeks) can be given, provided side-effects are tolerable. Note that acne cysts and large nodules will often require physical treatments to improve their appearance. Treating these by physical means such as cautery before starting a course of isotretinoin can be beneficial.

'What about isotretinoin and mood changes?'

This is a very important complication to become familiar with. It can happen to anyone, at any dose, at any time during treatment and the risk remains for up to a year after stopping treatment. Vigilance is key. Ask your patient to let friends and relatives know they are on the drug – they often spot mood changes when the patient does not.

Your patient's mood must be assessed at each follow-up visit and if there are any concerns a more formal assessment must be made, such as using the Hospital Anxiety and Depression Scale (HADS) to screen for depression, or the Patient Health Questionnaire (PHQ-9) to measure depression. It is important that your patient's consultant is aware of any problems and oversees reducing the dose or stopping the drug, as required. Remember that they, as well as you, carry ultimate responsibility if anything goes wrong.

Hidradenitis suppurativa

Hidradenitis suppurativa (HS) is a chronic painful condition consisting of recurrent flares of inflammatory nodules, with 'rope-like' scarring. It occurs mainly in the axillae (Figure 10.15), groin, buttocks and submammary areas. The key features are inflammatory nodules or abscesses, comedones and skin tunnels (sinus tracts).

HS usually starts in adolescence or young adulthood and can persist for decades. People with HS experience a major impact on their quality of life, because of pain that limits movement, odour and pus from the lesions, the need for dressings and the appearance of the skin. The impact on personal relationships is often severe. Its prevalence is approximately 1% in the UK, with a female-to-male ratio of 3:1. HS is associated with Crohn's disease and with comorbidities including obesity, type 2 diabetes, hypertension and depression. Rates of cardiovascular mortality and risks of completed suicide are double those of the background population.

The cause of HS is still unclear. It is no longer considered to be a disease of sweat glands (as suggested by its name), though follicular occlusion of apocrine ducts is seen. Genetic,

environmental (smoking, obesity), bacterial and endocrine influences may all play a role. About 40% of patients report a family history of the condition.

'Hurley staging' is used to classify the baseline severity of HS in each skin region: these stages reflect the extent and distribution of lesions and the degree of scarring. However, for monitoring purposes, dynamic physical signs instruments such as the Hidradenitis Suppurativa Clinical Response (HiSCR) end point, lesion counts, a pain numerical rating scale score from 0 to 10 and quality-of-life instruments are used.

Management is very challenging: patients are often understandably extremely distressed by the condition and there are no easy solutions. Adequate pain relief, wound dressings and other symptomatic approaches are essential. Screening for mental health problems using validated questionnaires and management of cardiovascular disease risk factors are important for holistic care. Support for smoking cessation and weight management should be provided where relevant.

Oral tetracyclines or the combination of oral clindamycin and rifampicin may partially reduce the inflammation. Adalimumab is now a licensed treatment at a dose of 40 mg per week and may produce significant improvement in the inflammation. Infliximab may benefit some patients and there is optimism that further biologics may be helpful in the future. Medical treatment should be integrated with surgical approaches for optimal care. Wide surgical excision of affected areas, a procedure with high morbidity, is sometimes the only hope for permanent improvement.

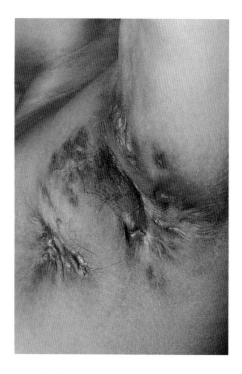

Figure 10.15 Hidradenitis suppurativa affecting the axilla.
© Medical Illustration Cardiff and Vale UHB.

Rosacea

Rosacea is a disorder characterised by frequent flushing, persistent redness or darker colour changes and telangiectasia, with episodes of inflammation, papules and pustules, but no comedones.

Epidemiology

Rosacea is very common: 10% of the population seek treatment for it. It is mainly seen in fair-skinned individuals who easily blush or have persistent background redness. It is more common in women in their third and fourth decades.

Aetiology and pathogenesis

These are unclear and rosacea is probably due to many factors, with the most likely being a vascular abnormality.

- **Vascular abnormality**. This has been proposed as possible vascular hyper-reactivity or long-standing vascular damage from solar radiation.
- **Demodex mite**. The demodex mite is present on everyone but some studies have found higher densities on the skin of patients with rosacea. Treatment directed at the mite has, in some cases, led to clinical improvement especially in HIV-infected patients.

- **Helicobacter pylori**. Many patients with peptic ulcers treated with antibiotics to eradicate *H. pylori* have incidental improvement in their rosacea. However, a role for *H. pylori* in rosacea is still unproven.

Clinical features (Figures 10.16 and 10.17)

The cheeks, nose, forehead and chin are the most commonly affected areas, with occasional involvement of scalp and torso.
Rosacea often progresses in a stepwise fashion:

- Transient redness.
- Persistent redness and telangiectasia.
- Papules and pustules.
- Chronic thickening and induration of skin.
- Rhinophyma (Figure 10.18).

Rosacea in skin of colour

Rosacea occurs in darker skin types, but its prevalence may be underestimated. The history is important. Patients often complain of burning and stinging of the face and are likely to describe a warm sensation of the face rather than 'flushing'. Affected skin becomes a reddish/brown–violet colour. Telangiectasia can be difficult to appreciate and so dermoscopy is useful.

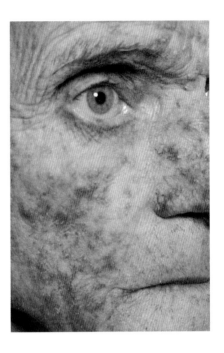

Figure 10.17 Rosacea on the right cheek. Chowdhury MMU *et al. Dermatology at a Glance*, 2nd edn. Chichester: Wiley, 2019.

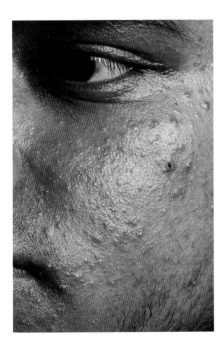

Figure 10.16 Rosacea on the left cheek, typically showing papules but no comedones. © Medical Illustration Cardiff and Vale UHB.

Table 10.6 Management of rosacea

Therapy	Key points
General management	Regular use of sunscreen. Avoiding alcohol, spicy foods and hot drinks may also reduce flushing
Topical azelaic acid	First line
Topical metronidazole	Can cause irritation
Topical ivermectin	Can be as effective as oral antibiotics
Oral antibiotics, tetracyclines, erythromycin	See Table 10.5 (acne)
Isotretinoin	See Table 10.5 and main text for acne
Pulsed-dye laser, KTP laser, intense pulsed light laser	Can treat facial thread veins and improve long-term control (Chapter 22)
Surgical excision and electrocautery	May be indicated for rhinophyma
Cosmetic camouflage	Green pigmentation conceals redness
Brimonidine gel, oxymetazoline 1% cream	Can be used for occasional control of flushing. Regular use can make rosacea worse

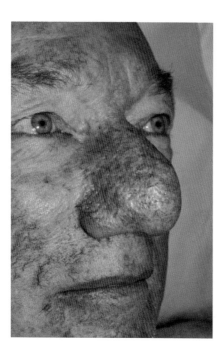

Figure 10.18 Rhinophyma with distortion of the shape of the nose. Chowdhury MMU *et al. Dermatology at a Glance*, 2nd edn. Chichester: Wiley, 2019.

Ocular rosacea

This occurs in 50% of patients causing irritation and redness of the conjunctiva, blepharitis, styes and occasionally keratitis. First-line treatment is with artificial tears and systemic tetracyclines (Table 10.5).

Rhinophyma

In rhinophyma there is distortion of the normal skin surface of the nose, leading to great cosmetic disfigurement (Figure 10.18). Once the active rosacea has been treated, surgical remodelling with electrosurgery, CO_2 or Nd:YAG laser can be performed (see Chapter 22).

Differential diagnosis

Consider the following conditions:

- **Acne vulgaris**. Comedones are also present.
- **Systemic or discoid lupus erythematosus**. No pustules occur. Scarring, scaling and follicular plugging are the prominent features of discoid lupus.
- **Seborrhoeic dermatitis**. The major feature is scaling on the scalp, eyebrows and external ear canals.

Management

The management of rosacea is summarised in Table 10.6. The cosmetic appearance of rosacea, and its effect on the patient, should be considered when deciding on management options.

Variants of rosacea

Steroid-induced rosacea

Prolonged facial application of potent topical steroids can induce rosacea. The steroid needs to be withdrawn (often with reducing steroid potency initially). Concomitant use of topical or systemic antibiotics or topical tacrolimus reduces the likelihood of the condition flaring on stopping topical steroids.

Rosacea fulminans ('pyoderma faciale')

This is a very severe variant of rosacea, mainly affecting adult female patients, with marked redness or darker colour changes, pustules and oedema. It can lead to severe scarring. It has been linked with use of the oral contraceptive pill and pregnancy, suggesting a hormonal trigger. Patients require treatment with systemic corticosteroids and isotretinoin (see 'Acne' section).

Perioral dermatitis

Small papules and pustules appear around the mouth, sparing the lip margins. There is also a peri-ocular variant (peri-ocular dermatitis). It is caused and exacerbated by topical steroid use. Management consists of stopping any topical steroids (an initial flare may occur) and starting topical or systemic antibiotics, as in standard rosacea treatment (Table 10.6).

Table 10.7 Common causes of lichenoid eruptions
Lichen planus
Drug eruption: gold, mepacrine, quinine, tetracyclines, thiazide diuretics, amlodipine
Graft-versus-host disease
Pityriasis lichenoides
Keratosis lichenoides chronica (Nekam's disease)
Lichen nitidus
Lichen striatus
Cutaneous T-cell lymphoma (mycosis fungoides)
Lichen aureus
Lichen simplex
Lichen planus pigmentosus

Lichen planus and lichenoid disorders

'Lichenoid' describes the clinical appearance of a flat-topped, shiny, papular rash. Confusingly, the word is also used to describe the histological appearance of a band-like inflammatory infiltrate in the superficial dermis, with liquefaction of the basal layer. This distinct histology usually makes a biopsy of such a rash helpful diagnostically. A lichenoid eruption can occur due to a number of causes (Table 10.7), and again histology can be helpful in distinguishing between the various causes. This section will focus on lichen planus only. Lichen planus is an idiopathic condition that occurs primarily in people aged 40–60 years. It can affect the skin, buccal mucosa and nails.

Epidemiology

Overall, 75% of patients with cutaneous lichen planus have oral involvement, so looking in the mouth is essential and helpful in diagnosing the condition. Around 10–20% of patients develop oral lichen planus first, and so often present to the dentist or oral surgeon (see Chapter 29).

Pathogenesis

Lichen planus is a T-cell-mediated autoimmune inflammatory condition. Its cause is unknown, although small studies have suggested a familial tendency, and also a possible association with hepatitis C, so check the serology.

Clinical features

Shiny, flat-topped violaceous papules occur on the skin, in a variety of configurations (Figures 10.19 and 10.20). These can

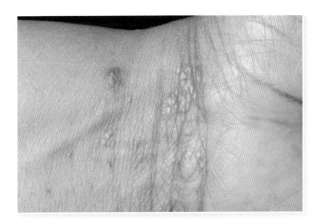

Figure 10.20 Typical lichen planus: shiny papules on the wrist. Chowdhury MMU *et al. Dermatology at a Glance*, 2nd edn. Chichester: Wiley, 2019.

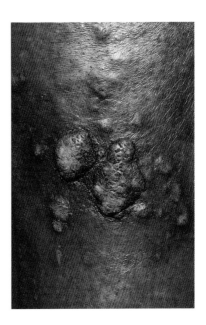

Figure 10.21 Hypertrophic lichen planus on the shin. © Medical Illustration Cardiff and Vale UHB.

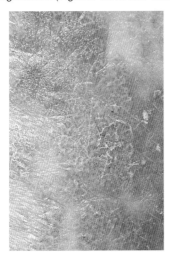

Figure 10.19 Lichen planus. A close-up view showing a violaceous plaque topped by Wickham's striae. © Medical Illustration Cardiff and Vale UHB.

be small papules or linear or annular lesions and may appear violaceous, grey, brown or even black in skin of colour. They are usually itchy. Lichen planus can also display the Koebner phenomenon, arising at a site of trauma. On the surface, a lace-like, white pattern is often seen – Wickham's striae (Figure 10.19). The papules can also become hyperpigmented, especially in skin of colour, and can become hypertrophic particularly on the ankles and shins (Figure 10.21). The condition is usually self-limiting, although it can take months to years to resolve completely. The course can be recalcitrant and chronic, particularly with oral disease.

Differential diagnosis

A skin biopsy is very helpful in confirming a lichenoid eruption, and also in identifying its cause. Other conditions that should be considered are plane warts, lichenified eczema, lichen simplex chronicus, lupus erythematosus, psoriasis and secondary syphilis.

Lichen planus of mucous membranes

- **Oral mucosa**. In the mouth, lichen planus has the appearance of white lace-like patches, often symmetrically distributed. If the patient has coexisting lichen planus of the skin, it is reasonable to treat the oral lesions in the first instance with topical corticosteroids. Amalgam fillings can cause adjacent lichenoid changes and are usually unilateral. A strong corticosteroid in a base designed for oral administration (e.g. triamcinolone in oral paste) is usually helpful. A patient with non-responding, atypical or asymmetrical lesions, particularly if they smoke, should be referred to the oral surgeons for consideration of biopsy. Remember that squamous cell carcinoma can occasionally arise in these lesions, so again atypical ulceration or new lumps in the mouth should be investigated (Chapter 29).
- **Genital area**. Lichen planus here can affect people regardless of sex, but it is more common on the vulva and can be difficult to treat. At worst, the lesions on the vulva can ulcerate causing painful scarring. A biopsy should be taken to differentiate it from lichen sclerosis, which can have a similar appearance (Chapter 28).

Other sites (Chapter 27)

- **Nails**. In 10% of cases there is nail involvement, particularly of the fingernails, with ridging and thinning of the nail plate. The nail can be completely lost or can form a 'pterygium' (severe narrowing of the nail resulting from partial destruction).
- **Scalp**. Lichen planus of the scalp can cause scarring alopecia and skin atrophy, which should be looked for (again a biopsy is very helpful) and treated early to try to avoid permanent scarring.

Treatment of lichen planus

The first-line treatment of localised areas of lichen planus is topical steroids with occlusion to increase absorption and also to reduce rubbing of the affected area. However, use of potent corticosteroids, especially under occlusion, carries the risk of skin atrophy and topical immunosuppressants may be a useful alternative. More widespread or non-responsive lesions require systemic treatment, with oral corticosteroids in the first instance (unless contraindicated), or with acitretin or narrowband ultraviolet B as second-line therapy.

Chronic spontaneous urticaria

Chronic urticaria/angio-oedema is defined as weals, angio-oedema or both, with daily or almost daily symptoms lasting for more than six weeks. In 50% of cases the cause is unknown (chronic spontaneous urticaria).

Presentation of urticaria

Urticaria occurs in 2–3% of individuals and is characterised by red, raised, itchy weals with a pale centre. The weals are a few millimetres to several centimetres in diameter (Figure 10.22). In very dark skin there may be no change in colour and no central pallor, but dilated follicular openings can be appreciated within weals. They usually appear and spread quickly and individual lesions last no more than 24 hours. The appearance is due to activation of mast cells in the papillary dermis of the skin, which release histamine causing vasodilation, increased blood flow and increased permeability of blood vessels.

Presentation of angio-oedema

Angio-oedema is caused by the same mechanism but with deeper tissue swelling, usually of the submucosa, deep reticular dermis and subcutaneous tissue (Chapter 16). It most commonly affects the face and oropharynx but can also affect the gastrointestinal tract or genitalia. The swelling is often painful and longer lasting than the weals on the skin.

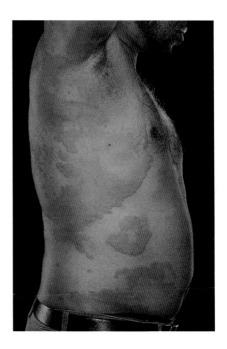

Figure 10.22 Widespread urticaria, showing a clear edge with faded areas centrally. © Medical Illustration Cardiff and Vale UHB.

Causes of urticaria (if not 'spontaneous')

A good history is very helpful in deciding what might be triggering the urticaria and therefore in directing what specific tests need to be done (Table 10.8 and Figure 10.23).

- **Food or other IgE-mediated allergy**. A good history or food diary can identify possible triggers, such as nut allergy or latex allergy. A blood test for specific IgE to individual allergens may confirm this. From the history you should try to narrow down possibilities so that only a small number of IgE tests are required. These tests should not be used indiscriminately to 'screen' for allergens, as there may be false positives that are not clinically relevant.
- **Drug induced**. Angiotensin-converting enzyme inhibitors can cause urticaria (angio-oedema only), sometimes after several years of use. This is more common in people of Afro-Caribbean

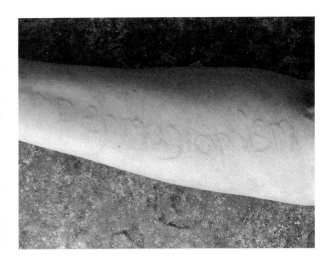

Figure 10.23 Dermographism in urticaria. Note the raised weals, a response to physical pressure. © V.J. Lewis.

origin. Non-steroidal anti-inflammatory drugs or opiates can provoke urticaria and should be changed or stopped, if possible.
- **C1 esterase inhibitor deficiency**. This can be inherited (hereditary angio-oedema) so ask about similar problems in the family. It can also be acquired, associated with paraproteinaemias.
- **Infection**. Complement activation can occur due to immune complex formation. Viral infections including Epstein–Barr virus and hepatitis B or C, or parasites such as threadworms can trigger this.
- **Vasculitis**. Often the weals will last for longer than 24 hours, may be tender rather than itchy, may display residual bruising and may make the patient feel generally unwell.
- **Physical stimuli**. Exercise, heat, cold, pressure, water (aquagenic urticaria), sun (solar urticaria) and vibration usually trigger immediate reactions, which fade within an hour. Delayed-pressure urticaria is an exception: it comes on more slowly after physical pressure, such as from waistbands or carrying bags. It can last for several hours to days.
- **Autoimmune**. This is associated with thyroid autoantibodies or antinuclear antibody positivity.

Treatment of chronic spontaneous urticaria

It is important to give the patient information about their condition, and explain that treatment only relieves symptoms rather than 'curing' the urticaria. Patients should understand that the condition can wax and wane and can often go away by itself and no real indication can be given as to how long it is likely to last.

Antihistamines form the mainstay of treatment for urticaria and all dermatologists need to have a good working knowledge (and usually have their own favourites) of both sedating and non-sedating antihistamines (Table 10.9). The algorithm in Figure 10.24

Table 10.8 Assessment of urticaria

History	Duration of weals (more or less than 24 hours)?
	Triggered by physical stimuli?
	Food or contact in the preceding 60 minutes?
	Drugs taken?
	Family history of similar symptoms?
	Recent viral illness?
Examination	Urticaria alone, urticaria plus angio-oedema or angio-oedema alone?
	If nothing to see today, does the patient have photos?
	Is dermographism present (a weal and flare response to physical pressure, Figure 10.23)?
	Is there residual bruising (indicating possible vasculitis)?
Basic blood tests	Full blood count: raised eosinophils could indicate parasitic infections
	C-reactive protein: if raised could indicate chronic infection or vasculitis
	Thyroid function test and thyroid autoantibodies
	Complement: C3/C4. If abnormal check C1q
Other tests	Antinuclear antibodies, iron, B_{12}, immunoglobulins or protein electrophoresis: if indicated from initial history, examination or blood tests
	Urinalysis or skin biopsy: perform if vasculitis suspected

Table 10.9 H1 antihistamines used in urticaria

Dose	Licensed daily dose	Other comments and side-effects
Acrivastine	8 mg three times daily	Second-generation antihistamine. Rapid onset of action, not long lasting, excreted unchanged in urine; non-sedating; 'on-demand' therapy
Bilastine	20 mg	Second-generation antihistamine
Cetirizine	10 mg	Second-generation antihistamine
Chlorphenamine	4 mg four times daily	First-generation antihistamine. Not for long-term use; injectable; short half-life; sedating
Desloratadine	5 mg	Second-generation antihistamine
Fexofenadine	120–180 mg	Second-generation antihistamine
Hydroxyzine	25 mg–100 mg	First-generation antihistamine. Not for long-term use; sedating
Levocetirizine	5 mg	Second-generation antihistamine
Loratadine	10 mg	Second-generation antihistamine
Mizolastine	10 mg	Second-generation antihistamine
Promethazine	10–20 mg three times daily	First-generation antihistamine. Not for long-term use; injectable; sedating
Rupatadine	10 mg	Second-generation antihistamine

Powell RJ et al. Clin Exp Allergy 2015; **45**:547–65.

covers the main stepwise treatment recommendations for urticaria. Note that off-licence use of antihistamines, such as levocetirizine and desloratadine, at higher dosages (up to four times normal daily doses) is recommended in most guidelines for urticaria. However, GPs will usually seek advice about this prior to commencing higher off-licence dosages. The exact dosages vary and should be checked in the *British National Formulary*.

Non-sedating antihistamines are used as first-choice therapy in urticaria and include levocetirizine, fexofenadine and desloratadine. For non-sedating antihistamines, side-effects include dry mouth, headache, nausea and drowsiness but these are much less common with second-generation tablets.

Sedating antihistamines are also used for general pruritus (usually at night) and include promethazine, hydroxyzine and chlorphenamine. The main side-effects of sedative antihistamines include drowsiness, impairment in using heavy machinery and driving, dry mouth, difficulty with micturition and blurred vision. Patients should specifically be warned about driving and potential interactions such as with anxiolytics and alcohol.

There is no strong evidence to suggest any antihistamine is more effective, but specific ones may be better tolerated by some patients and rotating antihistamines may be required to get the best effect if used for chronic urticaria. Many patients will of course be familiar with and be able to buy antihistamines over the counter for other conditions such as hay fever and not all will need to be prescribed.

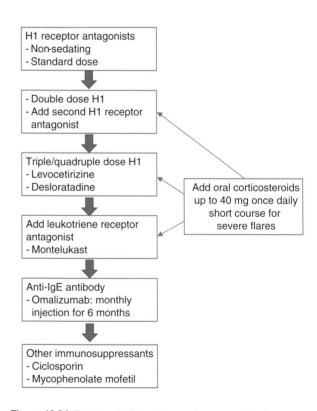

Figure 10.24 Treatment of chronic spontaneous urticaria.

Connective tissue diseases

Several connective tissue disorders present in the skin (Table 10.10). Lupus erythematosus (LE) will be discussed here.

LE can present with systemic manifestations of multiple organ systems being affected or only with cutaneous features. Around 80% of patients with systemic LE are affected by cutaneous LE. LE is more common in females and in patients of Afro-Caribbean origin. It is more prevalent in people who smoke.

Clinical presentation

- Malar or 'butterfly' rash of systemic LE.
- Subacute cutaneous LE: widespread inflamed patches and plaques on sun-exposed sites (Figure 10.25).
- Chronic discoid LE: scaly, scarring plaques, mainly on the face and scalp, causing a scarring alopecia (Figure 10.26).
- Bullous or chilblain-like lesions: uncommon.

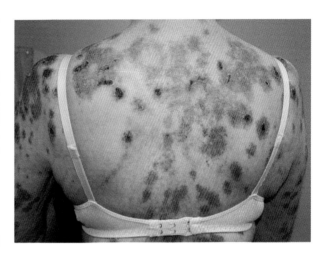

Figure 10.25 Subacute cutaneous lupus erythematosus. Marano AL *et al.* Subacute cutaneous lupus erythematosus and dermatomyositis associated with anti-programmed cell death 1 therapy. *Br J Dermatol* 2019; **181**:580–3.

Investigations

- Blood tests: full blood count may show a low lymphocyte count; complement C3 and C4 levels may also be low.
- Blood antibody tests: antinuclear antibodies are positive; anti-dsDNA is positive in systemic LE; anti-Ro (anti-SSA) and anti-La (anti-SSB) antibodies are positive in subacute cutaneous LE.

- Blood antiphospholipid antibodies are positive in associated antiphospholipid syndrome.
- Skin biopsy of discoid LE shows follicular plugging, atrophy and scarring, with an interface dermatitis. Direct immunofluorescence is positive in lesional skin.

Table 10.10 Connective tissue diseases (excluding lupus erythematosus)

Disease	Clinical presentation	Investigations	Important tips
Dermatomyositis	Red/purple patches on sun-exposed sites Purple 'heliotrope' rash on eyelids Purple plaque on bony prominences, especially knuckles (Gottron's papules) Prominent nailfold capillaries Proximal muscle weakness	Blood test: raised creatine kinase MRI scan of affected muscle, e.g. quadriceps (shows inflammation) Electromyography of muscles (shows atypical activity even at rest)	There is a strong association with malignancy: take a detailed history for 'red flag' symptoms
Systemic sclerosis	Widespread thickened, sclerotic skin	Blood test: anti-Scl70 antibody positive	Affects multiple organs, needs rheumatology care
Limited systemic sclerosis (formerly known as CREST syndrome)	Calcinosis, Raynaud's phenomenon, oesophageal dysmotility, sclerodactyly, telangiectasia	Blood test: anti-centromere antibodies	
Morphoea	Localised scleroderma (skin thickening) Plaque, nodular, linear patterns Can be dyspigmented	Blood test: negative anti-Scl70 antibody, negative anti-centromere antibodies Skin biopsy shows atrophic epidermis, thickened, hyalinised collagen	40% are associated with autoimmune disorders: particularly check for thyroid disease

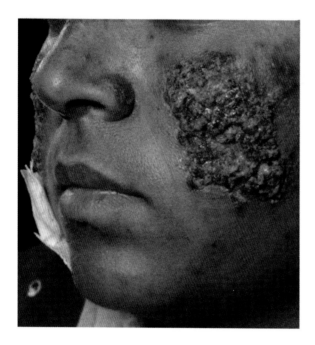

Figure 10.26 Thick plaque of discoid lupus erythematosus. This lady two years later developed systemic lupus erythematosus. Chowdhury MMU *et al. Dermatology at a Glance*, 2nd edn. Chichester: Wiley, 2019.

Conclusions

This chapter has given only a brief introduction to several conditions that make up the majority of cases seen in a general medical dermatology clinic. It is important in the early years of training in dermatology that trainees read extensively about these conditions and learn from the patients encountered. Get to grips with these core conditions and then extend your reading much more widely: you need to become familiar with a huge range of diseases. However, you have to start by becoming knowledgeable about the details of the most common ones.

In dermatology there are many conditions that can be cured or that are self-limiting. Obviously, these satisfactory outcomes lead to discharge from follow-up. However, this leaves a very large number of people who have chronic skin conditions and who need continuing review, and about whom difficult clinical decisions have to be taken spanning many years. Part of the art of becoming an expert dermatologist is developing skills to manage chronic diseases, skills that are generic to several fields of medicine. This includes, for example, learning how to develop a framework of care for individual patients and learning the techniques of appropriately discharging patients (Chapter 2).

There can be great satisfaction in getting to know patients with chronic disease, tailoring their treatment and wider management to put into practice the goal of delivering high-quality personalised medicine and skin care for dermatology patients.

Treatment

In discoid LE, very potent or potent topical steroids are required, along with sun protection. This can lead to skin atrophy on the face. Topical calcineurin inhibitors can be used as an alternative. If the condition fails to respond, oral hydroxychloroquine helps in approximately 80% of patients. LE is a spectrum of disease and localised discoid LE may still progress to systemic LE (in about 4% of cases). Therefore, it is important to check antinuclear antibodies approximately twice a year to ensure there is no progression.

Skin conditions associated with systemic diseases

Many systemic diseases may also involve the skin; a few are summarised in Table 10.11. One of the many satisfactions of being an expert in skin is the ability to diagnose or raise the possibility of a systemic disease, simply from examining the skin and from your detailed knowledge of the implications of specific skin signs. You should be encouraged to develop close links with your colleagues across other medical specialties in your hospital, as shared discussion of difficult cases is both helpful to patients and rewarding for you.

Pearls and pitfalls

- Sudden onset of numerous painful, small fluid-filled vesicles in a person with atopic dermatitis may be eczema herpeticum, a dermatological emergency.
- When managing a child or adult with atopic dermatitis, provide a written summary of the maintenance regimen to guide and enhance adherence.
- Always examine the oral mucosa if cutaneous lichen planus is suspected.
- When treating urticaria with antihistamines, high doses may be required but GPs will not routinely prescribe higher than standard dosages without authorisation first from dermatology secondary care.
- Although pyoderma gangrenosum has no clear diagnostic histopathology features, biopsy is still important to rule out other diagnoses such as malignancy.
- When treating a woman of childbearing age with isotretinoin, ensure that adequate contraception continues for at least four weeks after stopping therapy.

SCE Questions. See questions 11 and 12.

Table 10.11 Skin conditions associated with systemic diseases

Disease	Signs	Associated medical conditions	Important tips
Granuloma annulare	Annular, smooth plaques, particularly over knuckles Can present with a generalised rash	If widespread, may be associated with diabetes mellitus	Check blood sugar levels
Necrobiosis lipoidica (NL)	Shiny red, waxy plaques, usually on the shins Atrophy, prominent telangiectasia, fragility and ulceration can occur	Up to 65% of patients with NL can have diabetes One in 300 patients with diabetes have NL	Check blood sugar levels
Vasculitis	Presentation depends on the size of the vessel affected Palpable purpura and ulceration can occur Long-term haemosiderin deposition can occur	Can affect similarly sized blood vessels internally, such as in kidneys or bowel	Check blood pressure, urine dipstick Ask about abdominal pain, which may indicate bowel involvement
Neutrophilic disorders			
Pyoderma gangrenosum	Very painful nodule, which rapidly enlarges and ulcerates, usually on the lower legs	Inflammatory bowel disease: Crohn's disease and ulcerative colitis Rheumatoid arthritis Blood dyscrasias	Skin biopsy: not diagnostic but is used to exclude other causes such as skin cancer
Acute febrile neutrophilic dermatosis (Sweet's syndrome)	Tender papules, nodules or vesicles Can be large nodules or annular lesions	Rheumatoid arthritis Inflammatory bowel disease (Crohn's disease and ulcerative colitis) Blood dyscrasias	Associated with fever and general malaise Check full blood count for myelodysplasias and leukaemia

FURTHER READING AND KEY RESOURCES

Kroenke K, Spitzer RL, Williams JBW. The PHQ-9: validity of a brief depression severity measure. *J Intern Med* 2001; **16**:606–13.

de Lusignan S, Alexander H, Broderick C *et al*. The epidemiology of eczema in children and adults in England: a population-based study using primary care data. *Clin Exp Allergy* 2021; **51**:471–82.

Powell RJ, Leech SC, Till S *et al*. BSACI guideline for the management of chronic urticaria and angioedema. *Clin Exp Allergy* 2015; **45**:547–65.

Zaenglein AL, Pathy AL, Schlosser BJ *et al*. Guidelines of care for the management of acne vulgaris. *J Am Acad Dermatol* 2016; **74**:945–73.

Textbooks

Bolognia JL, Shaffer J, Cerroni L, eds. *Dermatology*, 4th edn. Amsterdam: Elsevier, 2017.

Griffiths CEM, Barker JN, Bleiker TO, Hussain W, Simpson RC, eds. *Rook's Textbook of Dermatology*, 10th edn. Oxford: Wiley-Blackwell, 2022; in press.

Lebwohl M, Heymann W, Coulson I, Murrell D. *Treatment of Skin Disease*, 6th edn. Amsterdam: Elsevier, 2021.

Useful websites

British Association of Dermatologists. Patient information leaflets. Available at: https://www.bad.org.uk/for-the-public/patient-information-leaflets.

Cardiff University School of Medicine. Quality of life question-naires. Available at: www.cardiff.ac.uk/medicine/resources/quality-of-life-questionnaires.

National Eczema Society. Available at: www.eczema.org.

National Institute for Health and Care Excellence. Quality statement 4: assessing cardiovascular risk. Available at: http://www.nice.org.uk/guidance/qs40/chapter/quality-statement-4-assessing-cardiovascular-risk.

Psoriasis Association. Available at: www.psoriasis-association.org.uk.

11

Paediatric dermatology

Lindsay Shaw

Introduction

Dermatology is the only medical specialty in which you have the pleasure, and challenge, of being responsible for the care of both adults and children. This can be a little daunting if you have had no specific paediatric training. Do not fear! With paediatric medical and nursing colleagues on the ward and in outpatients to guide you, you will soon start to develop an appreciation of the differences you need to consider when dealing with children and to develop some basic skills.

There is a wide range of conditions you will see in children that you need to learn about. The aim of this chapter is to explain the fundamentals of good paediatric care, including how treating children with skin conditions differs from treating adults, and to consider some clinical scenarios you will encounter in paediatric dermatology.

How children are different

The range of skin disease that you will see in paediatric dermatology is not the same as that in the general adult dermatology clinic. Presentations of common skin conditions may look different in children, and there are several specific entities unique to the paediatric population that you should be familiar with. These are covered in the paediatric dermatology curriculum.

The physiological response to skin disease may vary with age, so presentation of the same condition may change with time. For example, think about eczema and how its distribution and pattern tend to shift as the skin matures and is exposed to different environmental factors.

Children's understanding, experience and psychological reactions to skin problems also vary with age, and these affect how skin conditions are experienced and how they present. Think, for example, about the very different challenges toddlers and teenagers may have with topical treatments.

Skin conditions and their treatments can have an impact on children's growth and development. Growing up with a chronic skin condition can affect sleep, behaviour and the ability to concentrate and learn, and can even affect the development of personality traits and resilience. Having a chronic skin condition as a child may influence major life-changing decisions, such as which sports to concentrate on, which type of higher education to choose and what career to aim for.

Dermatology Training: The Essentials. Edited by Mahbub M.U. Chowdhury, Tamara W. Griffiths and Andrew Y. Finlay.
© 2022 The British Association of Dermatologists. Published 2022 by John Wiley & Sons Ltd.
Companion website: www.wiley.com/go/chowdhury/dermatologytraining

Changes occur quite quickly over time, so just when you think you have got to know a particular child, the next time you see them everything may be different!

When your patient is a child, formal clinical etiquette does not always apply. You may need to start your examination first before the history, looking at the bit that gets shown to you, before you even start talking. You may find yourself dealing with a child who will not speak to you at all or one who constantly interrupts your careful history taking with questions while turning the tap and the lights on and off.

You will almost always see your patient with other family members, whose different perspectives and worries need to be understood and balanced with the voice of the patient themselves. Usually this means you are working together with parents and carers, but occasionally your role may be to advocate what you think is in the child's best interest even if that conflicts with the wishes of parents.

The services available for children are different from those for adults, especially in the community, and it is helpful to familiarise yourself with the roles of other professionals who may be involved with your patient.

Younger children will soon get bored; there should be plenty of toys available for them to play with while the adults talk.

Older children will be able to contribute and should be encouraged to do so, but they may find it difficult to describe symptoms, and need their parents to chip in and explain what the problem has been. Sometimes older children and young people need privacy from their parents for aspects of the discussion and examination.

History taking in children differs slightly from that for adults. There are some specific questions that need to be covered:

- Birth history: were the pregnancy, labour and delivery normal?
- Birthweight.
- Feeding: bottle or breast? Has weaning started? Has the diet been manipulated in any way (e.g. change of formula milk, exclusion of cow's milk)?
- Immunisations.
- Hospitalisations.
- Development: for older children, which school do they attend? How are they getting on in school? For children under school age, ask if the parents have any concerns about the child's development.

The clinical nurse specialist

Spending some time with the clinical nurse specialist (CNS) at the beginning of your paediatric dermatology attachment is a good idea, to familiarise yourself with all aspects of topical treatment, including the appropriate strengths of topical steroids and the use of bandages. The CNS can play a vital role in patient and parent education, particularly for children with atopic eczema.

Often the reason for referral is poor compliance with treatment, nearly always because the parents have had inadequate guidance on how to use the treatments. Parents and children like to try out different emollients in the clinic, and they may leave the nurse consultation with several samples to try at home, thus encouraging better compliance. The CNS can also provide follow-up support in person and remotely.

Taking the history and examining the child (Figure 11.1)

When interviewing a child with a skin problem, it is best not to make assumptions at the start of the consultation. First introduce yourself, then politely ask the adults with the child what their relationship is to the child, as it could be a grandparent, older sibling or childminder. Find out by what name the child is usually known and use it when talking to the child and the family. Usually the carer who brings the child can give the history.

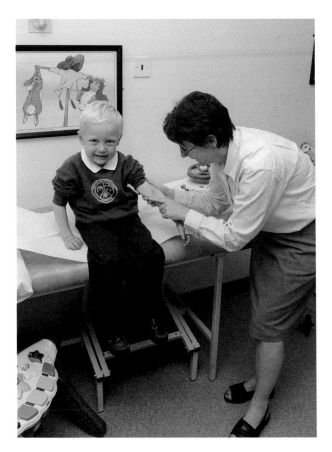

Figure 11.1 Examining a child. © Swansea Bay UHB.

- Family history: a brief enquiry into other family members' health can be very valuable, for example having other family members with an itchy rash suggests scabies, and knowing that a relative died of melanoma helps to explain why a simple naevus is causing so much anxiety. If an inherited disorder is suspected a more detailed family history should be taken.

It is useful to observe a young child playing, as it will guide your examination of the child later. If the child is confident to leave their parents to play on the floor, they will probably let you examine them even if you have to get down on the floor to do so. However, if the child remains clinging to mum's leg, you are unlikely to get much cooperation by prising them away, and it is better to limit the examination to what you can see while they sit on the parent's knee.

The way to take a history and examine a child or young person depends very much on their age. A toddler may well say no to any question asked directly! If you ask this child if you can examine them and they say no, then you are stuck in a tricky situation. If you are confident and gentle and let them see that their mum is comfortable with the plan, you are more likely to be successful. You should explain to them that you are going to look at their skin and start with a non-threatening area such as a hand or arm. Babies enjoy smiley eye contact and vocalisation; toddlers need encouragement and you may find yourself discussing and examining their toy or their parent first.

You will learn your own style of putting children at ease, but in general be open and clear and do not expect the same formula to work each time.

Growth monitoring

Assessment of a child's growth is an important part of paediatric examination. All children attending hospital should be weighed and measured as a routine. The appropriate weight and height charts (Figure 11.2), which are sex and age specific, should be available and be used in the clinic. For example, if the weight plots 'on the second centile', this means that only 2 out of every 100 children of this age weigh less. A single measurement is only a snapshot and what really matters is the trend over time.

Familiarise yourself with the 'Red Book', which is a parent-held record and should have information on previous weights. The weight gain should roughly follow centile lines, and when centile lines are crossed you should consider reasons for this such as dietary restriction, food allergies or underlying health problems. If you are concerned, make sure that the child will be seen again and monitored by the health visitor, who should check for weight change and flag up concerns as necessary.

Faltering growth may indicate the effect of severe illness, dietary restriction or treatments, all of which may be relevant in children with eczema and other skin conditions. It is important to look at a trend over time rather than a snapshot of a single measure.

Excessive height is usually familial, but a tall girl referred with early-onset acne may have precocious puberty or isolated adrenarche, thus measuring the child could prompt referral for endocrine investigations.

Obesity in childhood is increasingly common, and type 2 diabetes mellitus is seen in children and teenagers. There are several skin abnormalities associated with insulin resistance, such as acanthosis nigricans, so the first point of referral to secondary care could be the dermatology clinic.

Prescribing for children

Many topical and systemic drugs used to treat dermatology patients have not been specifically tested for paediatric use and so many are unlicensed for children, particularly those under two years of age. Nevertheless, these drugs are used: the *British National Formulary for Children* should be utilised as a reference guide. The diseases they are used for may be different in children and the formulations may have to be altered, for example tablets crushed or drugs in liquid form.

The epidermis in a full-term infant is well developed, but in pre-term children the stratum corneum is poorly developed and barrier function may be poor. This results in an increased rate of transepidermal water loss, causing problems with fluid control and increased absorption of topical therapies. Babies and young children also have a greater body-surface-to-weight ratio than adults and so are more likely to experience systemic side-effects from topical drugs. Other factors affecting drug penetration are given in Table 11.1. Some drugs that can cause toxicity in children after topical application are outlined in Table 11.2.

Genetics

Genetic influences impact on every aspect of human life and illness, and so separating out genetics as an individual topic in dermatology is somewhat arbitrary. It is important to be aware of the modes of inheritance of genetic conditions and the ever-improving tools used to identify genetic abnormalities, including single-gene sequencing, targeted panels, exome sequencing and genome sequencing. You should learn the diagnostic criteria for common neurocutaneous conditions, and for those that cause increased cancer susceptibility. It is important to understand how the embryology of skin development results in presentation in mosaic patterns and along Blaschko's lines, as well as how constellations of features arise in tissues with a common embryological origin.

You are not expected to recognise and immediately diagnose every rare genetic skin condition. However, you may be in a position to make a difference to the outcome for a neonate or older child with a range of skin presentations using the first principles of your dermatology expertise.

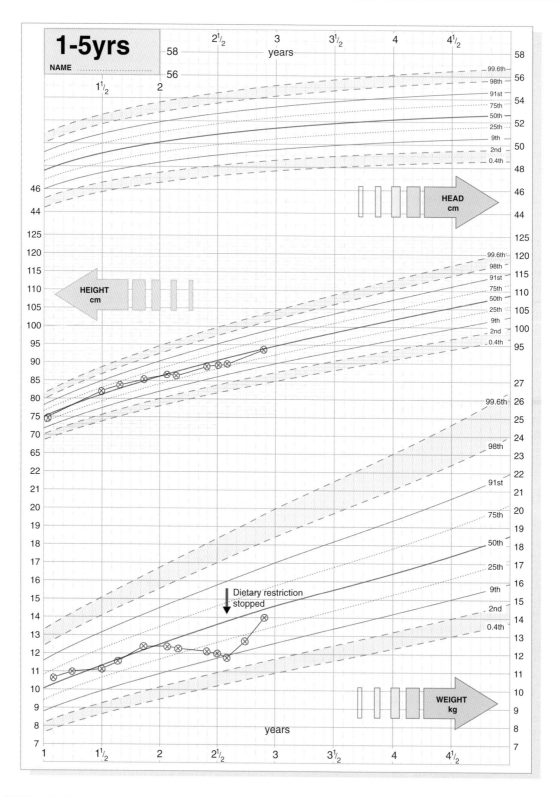

Figure 11.2 Standard height and weight growth chart. The 2-year-old had been on a restricted diet and his weight had fallen to the 9th percentile. He gained weight following topical therapy and a normal diet. © Child Growth Foundation.

Table 11.1 Factors influencing drug permeability through skin

Age

Site: eyelid > forearm > sole of foot: flexures greater than other sites

Damage to skin: lichenification reduces permeation, inflammation increases permeation

Drug type: pH, particle size, water or lipid solubility

Vehicle type: ointment, cream, gel or lotion

Application method: occlusion under plastic increases topical steroid absorption

Table 11.2 Drugs that can cause toxicity in children after topical application

Adrenaline (epinephrine): local application can cause local pallor and tachycardia

Corticosteroids: problems of undertreatment from underuse (steroid phobia) common. Side-effects are more likely if potent steroids are used, and if for prolonged periods:

  Local: striae and skin atrophy, infection, hirsutism and acne, hypopigmentation, rebound flare of inflammation after discontinuation

  Systemic (very rare): Cushing's syndrome, hypothalamic–pituitary axis suppression, glaucoma and cataracts; failure to thrive

Immunomodulators: tacrolimus ointment and pimecrolimus cream. A tingling or burning sensation is quite common on initial use, but often improves

Iodine: widely used as an antiseptic. If used in neonates or over large areas such as burns, may cause abnormal thyroid function

Neomycin: ototoxic if used widely topically

Salicylic acid: used as a keratolytic. Can cause salicylism – serious as metabolic acidosis may occur

Scabicides; lindane can cause central nervous system toxicity and aplastic anaemia in infants. Malathion in high concentration can cause toxicity and hyperglycaemia

Topical anaesthetics: EMLA (eutectic mixture of local anaesthetics) cream containing 2.5% lidocaine and 2.5% prilocaine is applied for 1–5 hours before injection of local anaesthetic for skin surgery. Local effects include redness or darker colour changes and dermatitis. Benzocaine gel can cause methaemoglobinaemia after application to skin or mucous membranes

When seeing a child with a skin condition that could be inherited, the first step is to take and record a detailed family history. You may need to involve the genetics team in assisting with diagnosis and with giving expert genetic counselling to the family. Here are some examples.

Naevoid basal cell carcinoma syndrome (Gorlin syndrome, Gorlin–Goltz syndrome) (Figure 11.3)

An autosomal dominant condition. The *PTCH* gene, a tumour suppressor gene located on chromosome 9q22.3-q31, is the site of the mutation. This results in numerous basal cell carcinomas at a young age. Other features include jaw cysts (first seen around puberty), palmar and plantar pits and skeletal abnormalities.

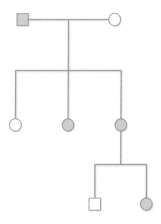

Figure 11.3 Naevoid basal cell carcinoma syndrome: family tree. Finlay AY, Chowdhury MMU. Specialist *Training in Dermatology.* © 2007 Mosby Elsevier.

Xeroderma pigmentosum (Figure 11.4)

This is an autosomal recessive condition. There are several different complementation groups, all with variable mutations at different chromosomal locations. Diagnosis is made by demonstrating abnormal DNA repair after ultraviolet radiation of cultured fibroblasts. The clinical picture is a child with photosensitivity, early onset of skin cancers, pigmentary changes with marked freckling, and conjunctivitis. Ataxia, deafness and mental decline occur in complementation group A and are progressive. Prenatal testing is possible.

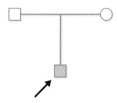

Figure 11.4 Xeroderma pigmentosum: family tree. Finlay AY, Chowdhury MMU. *Specialist Training in Dermatology.* © 2007 Mosby Elsevier.

X-linked ichthyosis (steroid sulfatase deficiency) (Figure 11.5)

An X-linked recessive disorder, so the condition is seen in males. Carrier females are unaffected or may have corneal opacities and mild skin changes. Brown scaly skin occurs, most noticeably in the flexures from about 6 months of age (Figure 11.6). The faulty gene on the X chromosome codes for the enzyme steroid sulfatase. Lack of this enzyme leads to accumulation of cholesterol sulfate, and high plasma levels are diagnostic. Low enzyme activity in the placenta leads to low levels of oestriol in maternal plasma and urine, with possible slow progression of labour when an affected male is being born.

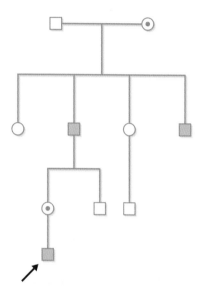

Figure 11.5 X-linked ichthyosis: family tree. Finlay AY, Chowdhury MMU. *Specialist Training in Dermatology.* © 2007 Mosby Elsevier.

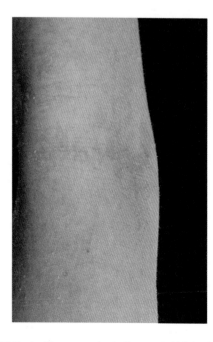

Figure 11.6 Typical brown scales in flexures in X-linked ichthyosis. © Medical Illustration Cardiff and Vale UHB.

Infected eczema

A two-year-old with extensive infected eczema has been unwell for a couple of days (Figure 11.7). She also has asthma. She has a pulse rate of 110 beats per min and a respiratory rate of 24 breaths per min. Should you be concerned?

This question highlights the point that physiological parameters vary with age and you should expect to look things like this up in readily accessible online sources. These parameters mentioned are within the normal range. You may be the first doctor to assess an acutely unwell child and should be aware of red flags in presentations that indicate acute life-threatening illness (see Further reading). Points to look out for include pale mottled skin, reduced level of consciousness, grunting respiration, tachypnoea, reduced skin turgor or just generally looking unwell.

Although you will be involved in the care of children with skin problems on the ward and in the emergency department, you should not be expected to make a full assessment of acutely unwell children and should always ask for help if unsure. Most of the specialty registrars seeing children will be paediatric trainees. Other healthcare professionals such as nurses may think of you as a paediatric trainee and ask, for example, if you think the child is well enough to go home. You have to leave such decisions to the acute paediatric team and you need to explain that clearly.

Food allergy in infancy

A 12-month-old child with atopic eczema comes to your clinic. He has been awake and scratching frequently at night for months. His mother is exhausted: she is concerned that this is caused by food allergy and wants him to be tested.

This is one of the commonest scenarios you will come across and it can be challenging. Parents may have had to be very persistent to get a referral for their child's problem and have waited a long time to finally come to the hospital and find out what is causing it. Sometimes the last thing they want is a discussion about yet more creams. The first appointment is the most important to make sure that the family feel all their concerns have been addressed. This may take some time, and where possible it is useful to involve the nurse specialist for at least some of the appointment.

Parents of young children with eczema experience a difficult combination of factors. They are often physically tired and emotionally exhausted, having been awake through the night trying to stop their child scratching. They are likely to have tried many different treatments as advised by their general practitioner, pharmacist, friends and even someone in the supermarket (as everyone has an opinion about eczema!) and have had a lot of conflicting and sometimes worrying information. This can lead to feelings of guilt about causing possible harm with treatments or just not having tried hard

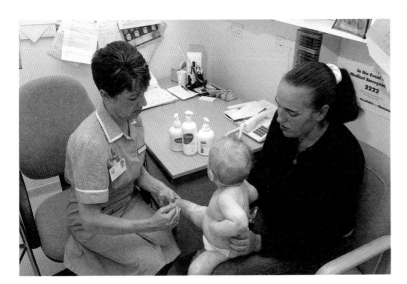

Figure 11.7 Child with extensive atopic eczema, with mother and nurse specialist. © Swansea Bay UHB.

enough. On top of this they may have dismissed the condition as 'only eczema' and not a serious illness, that there is 'not much anyone can do and it will clear up'. Family conflict and breakdown and the involvement of social services are understandably quite common for these families.

You will see children for whom maximal topical treatment is not working and you need to understand the indications for considering systemic treatments. In general, carers need to have the confidence to use enough of a sufficiently potent anti-inflammatory treatment to work and a clear plan about how to deliver this during the child's normal daily life.

Sometimes foods do make eczema worse, and foods that parents notice consistently cause a reaction with worsening of eczema should be avoided. However, eczema is not just an allergy to something. In this case of a 12-month-old child, foods that are commonly allergenic such as peanuts and dairy should not be avoided unless there is a clear history of a reaction, and weaning should not be delayed. Avoiding allergenic foods such as peanuts may reduce the development of oral tolerance and increase the risk of true allergy.

Food allergy testing is largely unhelpful in elucidating an underlying cause of eczema. Skin prick testing or specific IgE tests (radioallergosorbent test, RAST) only assess IgE-mediated reactions, whereas foods that drive eczema do so mostly by non-IgE mechanisms. Tests are generally only indicated in children who have immediate reactions to certain foods (for contact dermatitis and patch testing see Chapter 23).

During weaning, new foods should be introduced cautiously one at a time, because there is an increased risk of immediate food reactions in children with eczema. An immediate food reaction is IgE mediated, and most develop immediately or within 30–60 minutes of eating or touching a food. Your history should explore immediate food reactions. Children with immediate reactions who also have asthma are most at risk of severe reactions and should be referred to allergy services. There are a number of quite complex concepts to communicate, so observe a few of these conversations with your consultant and try to have a clear understanding of how this all fits together. Do not be pressured into performing random IgE tests unless justified.

The family should leave the consultation with a feeling of being heard and the confidence that they will be supported to use treatments that they previously may have worried were dangerous. It is helpful to give them a route to ask further questions and check that the plan is working, so it can be improved and changed as needed. A follow-up appointment with a nurse specialist a few weeks later is ideal.

Atopic eczema: treatment at school

A child with severe atopic eczema has not been able to have topical treatment put on at school. Who can help?

Schools are sometimes wary of topical treatments and may have their own regulations regarding supervision of medications. There may be all sorts of other issues that affect children with eczema in school. If you are lucky enough to have a dermatology nurse specialist as part of your hospital team, they should be the first person you ask to be involved. Each school will have a school nurse associated with them who can be contacted. For children whose health problems are having a significant effect on their schooling and function, you should consider also involving community paediatric services. The structures of these vary slightly between regions, but they are usually much more comprehensive than adult services and there will always be a local team responsible for supporting children with significant health needs in school. Look them up in your area.

Psoriasis

An eight-year-old girl attends your clinic with a recent onset of guttate psoriasis. How do you manage this?

Psoriasis is much less common than eczema in children. Its pattern may be atypical compared with adults and treatment options more limited, especially at delicate sites such as the face, flexures and nappy area, which are often affected in children.

A careful history including family history of psoriasis, arthritis and inflammatory bowel disease should be taken. Ask about eye and joint problems and examine the nails and areas such as axillae, umbilicus, groin/natal cleft and scalp.

Infection is a common trigger, especially streptococcal sore throat. Ask specifically about this in the history and consider a throat swab and a course of oral penicillin in the acute phase. Where recurrent infection causes recurrent flares, consider early treatment of any febrile episode with penicillin. Tonsillectomy may occasionally be indicated.

Treatment starts with soap avoidance and use of emollients, as in adults. A mild-potency topical steroid, such as hydrocortisone, or tacrolimus could be considered for the face and delicate flexural sites. More potent steroid–calcipotriol combinations can be used in older children on less delicate areas. Many children over the age of seven years will cope with phototherapy where necessary. Systemic treatments including methotrexate, and biologics can also be considered if the psoriasis is persistent and severe.

Differentials to think about are pityriasis rosea and pityriasis lichenoides. These have clues in the history and specific morphological signs. Any persistent scaly reddish rash in the nappy area should raise suspicion of Langerhans cell histiocytosis: look carefully for any petechial or purpuric lesions.

Haemangiomas

A 17-month-old boy with a haemangioma over the lower back (Figure 11.8) is pulling himself up to stand but not walking. Should you refer him to anyone?

There are red flag developmental milestones you should be aware of (which are easy enough to look up), but again you are not expected to do a full developmental and neurological examination. You should refer for paediatric assessment if a child is clearly failing to meet milestones. This developmental level is borderline and may well be normal for this child.

Segmental (big, flat, atypical) haemangiomas can be associated with underlying abnormalities and, in the lumbosacral and perineal area, early MRI is indicated to look for spinal problems. You should not wait and monitor, as neurosurgical intervention may be needed to prevent complications.

Other congenital abnormalities overlying the lumbosacral midline such as skin pits, sinuses and hair tufts can be associated with spinal abnormalities and should be investigated with spinal ultrasound in the first few weeks of life, before bony fusion makes ultrasound assessment difficult.

Segmental facial haemangiomas can also be associated with underlying abnormalities (PHACES syndrome), and children with these should have cerebrospinal MRI and echocardiogram.

Typical, small and well-circumscribed haemangiomas including in the nappy area do not cause the same concern, and the usual developmental monitoring by the health visitor, as for any other child, would then be indicated.

Haemangiomas at high risk of causing complications should be treated early with beta blockers. The UK guideline about this use of propranolol is given under 'Further reading'.

Consent in children

At what age can a child give consent for a procedure? And at what age can consent be refused?

Capacity to consent is presumed, as for adults, from the age of 16 years. Under 16 years of age, this is quite complex and involves case law. In general, if the doctor, carer and patient are in agreement about the best treatment option, there is no problem.

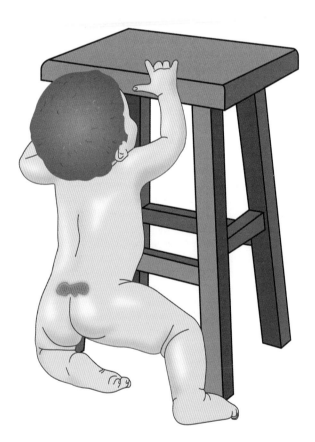

Figure 11.8 Haemangioma on the lower back.

Gillick (or Fraser) competency permits those under 16 years of age to consent to medical treatment 'if the child shows sufficient understanding and intelligence to enable them to understand fully what is proposed. This includes the purpose, nature of treatment, likely effects and risks, chances of success and the availability of other options.' It was established as a legal principle in 1985 in a House of Lords ruling about a case involving prescription of contraception to a girl under the age of 16 years without the permission, or even knowledge, of her parents. This means you have to consider these criteria for each individual child for each situation and, like assessment of capacity in adults, they depend on the complexity of the procedure.

You may judge, quite reasonably, that the same 13-year-old can give their consent for cryotherapy but not for a bone marrow transplant. You are the person judging competency to consent and not the parent. You should always seek to establish consensus where possible, but your focus is on the best interests of the child (as required in the Children Act) and the right of the child to be involved in medical decision making where possible.

Children and young people should feel safe in confiding in medical professionals and seeking treatment where it is needed, regardless of any views their parents might hold. This may mean you actively seeking a private conversation in some situations, for example when prescribing a potentially teratogenic drug and considering the need for contraception. The rules of confidentiality apply to people of all ages, and information can only be disclosed where not to do so risks significant harm.

The legal framework is slightly different concerning 16–18-year-olds who refuse consent to a treatment that both medical professionals and their parents feel is essential. That situation is rare and usually requires formal legal advice.

Problems during a procedure

You have injected local anaesthetic into a six-year-old's arm and she suddenly cries and says she wants to go home. You are planning to do a punch biopsy. What do you do next?

This is where clinical judgement and common sense come into play in the thorny issue of consent. Firstly, you should not get into a situation where you are doing something that is not medically important to a child who is too young to give informed consent themselves (e.g. cryotherapy or removal of asymptomatic lesions that the parent finds unsightly). If the biopsy makes a difference to management and is medically important, you are committed to facilitating that as painlessly and quickly as possible. This means preparation, such as consideration of doing the procedure under general anaesthetic in the first place, appropriate play therapy and ensuring nurse support and parental involvement in any necessary brief physical restraint. Your guiding principle is getting the best outcome and treatment for the child while minimising pain and distress. For this situation you should muster all the distraction and parental or nursing support at your disposal and get the procedure done as quickly as possible.

Non-accidental injury

Examining a four-year-old boy, you notice an odd-looking linear superficial erosion over the buttock. He also has an unusual-shaped bruise over the thigh. His mum thinks he may have scratched himself, but you are concerned about non-accidental injury. How do you proceed?

You should take a full history, including a history of the presentation of the visible marks you are concerned about, and examine the rest of the skin as part of your routine process. You should obtain consent to photograph the relevant areas, as well as the skin problem or lesion that was presented.

You should ask yourself the question: 'Does the explanation match the clinical findings?' A full description of the presenting features of child abuse is not possible here. Features in the history of an injury that raise suspicion of physical abuse are described in the Royal College of Paediatrics and Child Health *Child Protection Companion* (see Further reading and Table 11.3).

Protecting children and young people is the responsibility of all doctors. Where you have suspicions, you must share these concerns with your local safeguarding team and document that you are doing so. There will be a clearly established pathway for raising concerns in your hospital through the child safeguarding team ('named' doctor and nurse team), who are available to discuss the next steps. You should find out who they are and look up the local referral protocol in case you need it.

As a trainee, your first conversation should be with the consultant and, where relevant, the paediatric nurse or nurse specialist in clinic with you. It is good practice to explain to the carer that you are discussing these concerns, but if you feel unable to explain this to the carer you can still share your concerns with other professionals. If your concerns turn out to be unfounded, you will not be criticised as long as the concerns are honestly held and reasonable, and you take action through appropriate channels.

Neonatal skin abnormalities

You have been asked to see an inpatient on the neonatal unit who has some skin abnormalities. How do you approach this?

If there is skin blistering or loss, or suggestion of skin fragility:

- Consider staphylococcal scalded skin syndrome and treat for infection. Handle with care.
- Children with genetic skin fragility such as epidermolysis bullosa (EB) experience most of their skin damage in the early hours of life. Accurate up-to-date guidance about initial treatment is available from the national EB services. The general principles are to avoid shearing forces when handling, to dress in soft seamless (or seams on the outside) clothing and to avoid name tags or any adherent dressings or tape.

Table 11.3 Features in the history of an injury that raise suspicion of physical abuse

A significant injury where there is no explanation

An explanation that does not fit with the pattern of injury seen

An explanation that does not fit with the motor developmental stage of the child

Injuries in infants who are not independently mobile. This age group rarely has accidental injuries

An explanation that varies when described by the same or different parents or carers

Multiple explanations that are proposed but do not explain the injury seen

An inappropriate time delay in seeking appropriate medical assessment or treatment

Inappropriate parent or carer response (e.g. unconcerned or aggressive)

A history of inappropriate child response (e.g. did not cry, felt no pain)

Presence of multiple injuries

Child or family known to children's social care or subject to a child protection plan

Previous history of unusual injury or illness, e.g. unexplained apnoea

Repeated attendance with injuries that may be due to neglect or abuse

- A stitched umbilical line placed early can be very useful for any necessary blood samples.
- A biopsy and blood for genetics are usually needed. This should be done only once and only by someone specifically trained to do it, such as one of the nurse specialists from the EB service. Contact them as soon as possible.

If there is abnormally dry red or thickened skin or a collodion membrane:

- Think about transepidermal water and heat loss, and nutritional needs.
- Applying a bland, greasy emollient and nursing in an incubator are important first steps.
- A range of rare genetic and metabolic conditions can present in this way, so it is a good idea, with permission, to take and store blood for genetics. Children do not always survive beyond early life with some of these conditions and you do not want to miss an opportunity for possible future pregnancy planning.

- Severe immunodeficiency and storage disorders are also a possible cause, so arrange simple blood tests for full blood count, blood film and biochemistry, and store serum for further possible tests.
- A biopsy is rarely helpful in this clinical situation and does not need to be done urgently.

Conclusions

There is a vast amount for you to learn in paediatric dermatology: it can be even more challenging than adult dermatology, as few trainees have previous paediatric experience. When starting, do not be scared or daunted but work closely with your supervisor. As with adults, every patient needs to be handled differently and you also have to establish a good relationship with the parents or carer. You will learn your own style of putting children at ease, but be open and clear and do not expect the same formula to work each time. In urgent situations, always ask for help; this may be obvious, but it is especially important in paediatrics, where clinical situations can change fast.

The demand for paediatric dermatology services and shortage of dermatologists is leading to closer collaboration and support of paediatricians to be involved in paediatric dermatology. There is now a recognised training route for paediatricians with an interest in paediatric dermatology within paediatrics. Paediatric dermatologists have the opportunity to share their dermatology expertise with paediatric colleagues. There is a reciprocal benefit in sharing paediatric knowledge as part of a joined-up service to deliver the best possible care for children with skin problems.

Pearls and pitfalls

- When to ask for help early: if a child seems acutely unwell, if there are possible underlying systemic or developmental problems, or if there are concerns about possible abuse.
- Before your first clinic appointment for a child with eczema, observe your consultant to learn how to address common themes.
- The first appointment is critical to ensure that the family feel all their concerns have been addressed.
- Learn from your clinical nurse specialist about the practicalities of topical treatment.
- Infantile haemangiomas are usually harmless and self-resolving, but around the eye, lip or airway, consider early beta blockers.
- If haemangiomas are atypical, especially on the face or lumbosacral and perineal area, screen early for underlying abnormalities.

SCE Questions. See questions 58–62.

FURTHER READING AND KEY RESOURCES

Solman L, Glover M, Beattie PE *et al.* Oral propranolol in the treatment of proliferating infantile haemangiomas: British Society for Paediatric Dermatology consensus guidelines. *Br J Dermatol* 2018; **179**:582–9.

Textbooks

Hoeger P, Kinsler V, Yan A, eds. *Harper's Textbook of Pediatric Dermatology*, 4th edn. Chichester: Wiley-Blackwell, 2019.

Lewis-Jones MS, Murphy R, eds. *Oxford Specialist Handbook of Paediatric Dermatology*, 2nd edn. Oxford: Oxford University Press, 2020.

Websites

British Society for Paediatric Dermatology. For useful links to guidelines, publications, fellowships and recommended courses and meetings. Available at: www.bspd.org.

DEBRA. Epidermolysis bullosa support charity. Available at: www.debra.org.uk.

National Institute for Health and Care Excellence. Atopic eczema in under 12s: diagnosis and management. Available at: https://www.nice.org.uk/guidance/cg57/resources/atopic-eczema-in-under-12s-diagnosis-and-management-pdf-975512529349.

National Institute for Health and Care Excellence. Traffic light system for identifying risk of serious illness. https://www.nice.org.uk/guidance/ng143/resources/support-for-education-and-learning-educational-resource-traffic-light-table-pdf-6960664333.

Royal College of Paediatrics and Child Health. *Child Protection Companion*. Available at: https://childprotection.rcpch.ac.uk/child-protection-companion.

12

Infections and infestations

Cherng Jong and Roderick Hay

Introduction

General practitioners (GPs) see a large number of patients with skin infections and infestations; when these become difficult to manage, they may be referred to dermatology. Be mindful that if they are referred to secondary care, the presentation may be atypical. It is therefore important to maintain an index of suspicion for those presenting with papulosquamous or vesiculobullous disease.

Interdepartmental referral is also common, and sometimes clues to a diagnosis may be obtained by knowing the circumstance of the referral, for example cellulitis in a patient with a contaminated post-operative wound. Where infection or skin infestation is suspected, it is important to take a good history, including history of recent contact with a possible index case and a travel history. Most infections and skin infestations occur in short or recurrent bursts. This chapter briefly discusses some of the common conditions that dermatologists may encounter in their daily work.

As children may not be able to communicate clearly how they are unwell, it is important to obtain as much information as possible from their parents or carers. The majority of children seen in dermatology outpatient clinics are not acutely ill and many present with localised skin infections. Although this chapter describes common infections and infestations first in children, then in adults, many of the conditions described can occur at any age.

Be aware of varied presentations with infections in skin of colour. Skin inflammation results in a variety of colour changes

Dermatology Training: The Essentials. Edited by Mahbub M.U. Chowdhury, Tamara W. Griffiths and Andrew Y. Finlay.
© 2022 The British Association of Dermatologists. Published 2022 by John Wiley & Sons Ltd.
Companion website: www.wiley.com/go/chowdhury/dermatologytraining

primarily due to vasodilation, but also due to effects on melanocytes. In white skin, inflammation causes redness (erythema). In skin of colour, inflammation may cause violaceous, grey, brown–dark brown or even black colour changes, rather than redness. As such changes can be subtle in darker skin, it can be helpful to look for other signs of inflammation such as pain, heat, swelling, peeling, texture or contour changes, or prominent skin papules and pores. Using good lighting or a dark contrasting background can also aid in detection of inflammation in skin of colour, or simply ask the patient if they have noticed a change in their skin colour.

Basic microbiology

Skin infections and infestations require interaction between the host (human) and the invading organisms. Normally the skin microbiome contains an array of microorganisms that exist in equilibrium. For example, the forearms and back are mainly colonised by Gram-positive bacteria and *Malassezia* yeast, whereas in the more moist groin and axillae, organisms are more varied and numerous and include Gram-negative bacteria (Table 12.1). The microbiome can change as a result of many factors such as climate, underlying disease or alterations in the local skin environment following the use of topical or systemic antibiotics and corticosteroids.

The skin defends against microorganisms by maintaining epidermal integrity, by the presence of its normal flora and by innate and acquired immune pathways. Skin infection and signs of disease develop via three mechanisms: breach of intact skin, bloodborne infection and toxin-mediated damage (Figure 12.1).

It is useful to have an understanding of the basic microbiological investigation techniques to confirm a clinical diagnosis. These are shown in Table 12.2.

Table 12.1 The normal flora

Body sites	Organisms
All body sites	*Staphylococcus aureus*
	Staphylococcus epidermidis
	Micrococcus spp.
Intertriginous areas (axilla, groin, perineum, skin folds, digital webs)	*Corynebacterium spp.*
	Acinetobacter spp.
	Candida spp.
Skin rich in sebaceous glands and hair follicles (scalp, upper back)	*Cutibacterium spp.*
	Malassezia spp.

Skin infection and infestation in a well child

Warty lesions

Common viral warts (human papillomavirus, most commonly types 1, 2 and 4) usually present on children's fingers, and plantar warts on children's feet, but they can also occur on the face (Figure 12.2). These are areas exposed to repeated trauma and warts spread through contact. Warts may show areas of typical thrombosed capillaries (small dark dots in the lesion). Asymptomatic warts do not usually require treatment as they tend to resolve spontaneously; however, in secondary care settings, resistant and problematic warts may be seen. Finger biting and sharing of personal items, for example sandals, should be discouraged. Walking barefoot in a swimming pool may be a source of infection. When treatment is required in painful nail fold or plantar warts, over-the-counter salicylic acid-based wart preparations applied over several months can be used. Cryotherapy is painful and is not well tolerated by most children. For genital warts in children, the possibility of sexual abuse should be considered if there is other supporting evidence.

Umbilicated papular lesions

Firm, umbilicated and papular lesions, which appear in groups, are molluscum contagiosum caused by a poxvirus (Figure 12.3). They are usually distributed on the neck, trunk and axilla and are often asymptomatic. Molluscum contagiosum is more florid in children with atopic eczema due to localised immune dysregulation. Simple expression of lesions hastens their resolution. Parents can treat the lesions with 5% potassium hydroxide, which is available over the counter. Some clinicians treat them with cryotherapy or cantharidin, but cantharidin is not easily available. It is important to reassure the parents that the condition is self-limiting and unlikely to scar unless a severe inflammatory response or secondary infection occurs. Sharing of personal items such as towels should be discouraged.

Crusted lesions

Lesions with yellow or golden crusts on the face and around the nose and mouth suggest impetigo (caused by *Staphylococcus aureus* or group A streptococci), which is seen in general practice but seldom in secondary care (Figure 12.4). Children who present early may have intact pustules or sometimes blisters that are indicative of staphylococcal infection. Impetigo is highly infectious and children often self-inoculate themselves by scratching. A swab should be taken from the affected areas for bacterial culture and sensitivity if the infection recurs or is slow to resolve. Treatment is with topical fusidic acid or mupirocin. Eradication of nasal carriage with topical mupirocin is appropriate in recurrent cases. Oral flucloxacillin, erythromycin or cephalexin may be required to treat extensive infection.

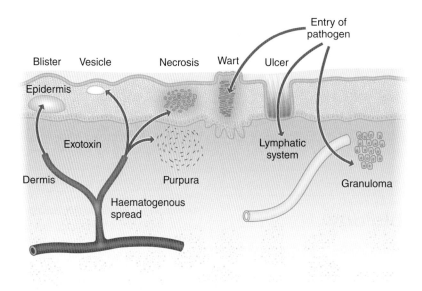

Figure 12.1 Mechanisms of mucocutaneous lesions. Invasion can occur directly via skin or be blood borne. Toxins and immune complexes also arrive via the blood. Finlay AY, Chowdhury MMU. Specialist Training in Dermatology. © 2007 Mosby Elsevier.

Table 12.2 Techniques of microbiological investigations

Techniques	Where they are indicated
Culture and sensitivity	
Skin swab	Bacterial infection
Blister fluid	Viral infection
Skin scraping	Fungal infection
Tissue biopsy	Mycobacterial infection
Staining	Bacterial infection (e.g. Gram stain)
	Mycobacterial infection (e.g. Ziehl–Neelsen for *Mycobacterium tuberculosis*)
	Fungal infection: periodic acid–Schiff (PAS) or methenamine silver
Serum for initial and convalescence serology	Suspected viral infection
Electron microscopy	Orf
Tissue for histology	Viral infection (e.g. vacuolation, inclusion body)
Polymerase chain reaction	Viral infection, mycobacterial infection, leishmaniasis

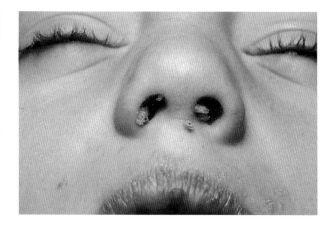

Figure 12.2 Common viral warts on a child's nose. © Medical Illustration Cardiff and Vale UHB.

Ecthyma is an ulcerated deeper infection covered with a haemorrhagic crust, caused by *Streptococcus pyogenes* or *Staphylococcus aureus*, and this can accompany insect bites.

Grouped vesicles and erosions

Painful and localised vesicles, pustules or erosions suggest herpes simplex (caused by human herpesvirus 1 or 2) (Figure 12.5). When the infection is localised, the child is usually asymptomatic.

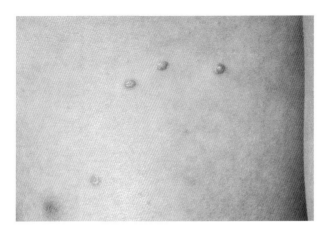

Figure 12.3 Molluscum contagiosum on a child's trunk. © Medical Illustration Cardiff and Vale UHB.

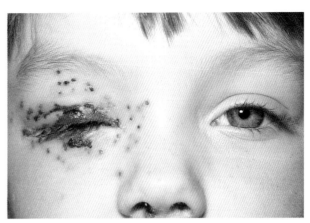

Figure 12.5 Herpes simplex affecting the periocular region. © Medical Illustration Cardiff and Vale UHB.

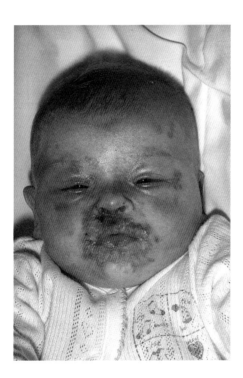

Figure 12.4 Staphylococcal impetigo affecting the face of a young child. © Medical Illustration Cardiff and Vale UHB.

However, the child may be ill with fever and have enlarged regional lymph nodes. The infection is typically localised (herpes gingivostomatitis, herpes keratoconjunctivitis and herpes labialis), but in neonates it may be truncal and extensive. Referral to other specialties may be required if there is ocular or genital involvement. For mild, localised and uncomplicated herpes simplex, topical aciclovir is adequate. For severe or recurrent eruptions, treatment with oral valaciclovir or aciclovir for short- or long-term therapy (400 mg twice daily for six months) should be considered. The differential diagnoses of herpes zoster, impetigo and non-infective dermatosis, for example dermatitis herpetiformis, should be considered.

Eczema herpeticum is widespread infection with herpes simplex in a patient with atopic eczema and may be misdiagnosed as bacterial infection or exacerbation of eczema. Multiple discrete crusted or vesicular lesions are seen, often affecting the face. It is frequently severe and can be life threatening, particularly in neonates or the immunocompromised, with potential to affect the eyes, brain, lung and liver. It must be treated aggressively with systemic antivirals such as aciclovir or valaciclovir (Chapter 16). Kaposi varicelliform eruption is a term often used to refer to herpes infection in patients without eczema, for example those with Darier's disease, Hailey–Hailey disease, pemphigus vulgaris or ichthyosis.

In hand, foot and mouth disease (caused by Coxsackie A and other enteroviruses) the vesicles are oval and are distributed in the mouth, hands and feet. The child may feel unwell and have a mild fever. The vesicles quickly break down to form ulcers that heal over a week. Viral samples taken from vesicular fluid can be detected using polymerase chain reaction (PCR). However, the diagnosis is usually clinical.

Blisters

Blisters may be caused by insect bites, trauma (friction or thermal burn) or infection (impetigo). The diagnosis can usually be made based on careful history and clinical appearance. When taking a history, consider whether the blisters come in crops and are recurrent, as they may coincide with insect bites or activity to suggest trauma. Blisters can also be caused by non-infectious and autoimmune conditions (Chapters 11 and 16).

Red scaly and annular lesions

Itchy, scaly, well-circumscribed and annular lesions (often unilateral) with central clearing are suggestive of dermatophyte fungal infection or tinea (usually species of *Microsporum* or *Trichophyton*). In inflamed lesions, pustules may occasionally be seen. Tinea can occur at any body site, and clinical descriptions depend on the sites involved. It is important for dermatologists to be aware of the correct nomenclature: tinea corporis means tinea of the trunk and limbs, tinea capitis the scalp (Figure 12.6), tinea faciei the face, tinea pedis the feet and tinea manuum the hand. It is important to take a history to find out about the child's contact with other cases or pets, as this may suggest a source of infection (e.g. *Microsporum canis* from dogs and cats; *Trichophyton mentagrophytes* from rodents) (Table 12.3). Kerion (Figure 12.7) is an inflamed, boggy and pustular scalp lesion often caused by animal ringworm; it may lead to scarring alopecia if treatment is delayed.

The differential diagnoses of a scaly and well-circumscribed lesion include erythrasma (scaly plaque with wrinkling), discoid eczema and psoriasis. Atypical and non-scaly tinea resulting from inappropriate topical steroid treatment is called tinea incognito. Non-scaly asymptomatic annular lesions suggest granuloma annulare, which is also common in childhood.

Hair examination under a filtered ultraviolet A (Wood's) lamp is useful only in ectothrix dermatophyte scalp hair infection (e.g. hair will fluoresce bright green in *Microsporum canis* infection).

Skin scrapings should be taken from the edge of lesions for potassium hydroxide examination and culture or PCR prior to the start of treatment. However, it may be necessary to start treatment on clinical grounds before the result is available, because culture results may take up to four weeks. In tinea

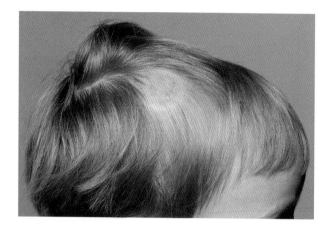

Figure 12.6 Tinea capitis on a child's scalp. © Medical Illustration Cardiff and Vale UHB.

Table 12.3 Dermatophytes and their sources

Source	Fungi
Anthropophilic: human	*Microsporum audouinii* (West Africa)
	Trichophyton mentagrophytes
	Trichophyton interdigitale
	Trichophyton rubrum
	Trichophyton tonsurans (endemic in the UK)
	Trichophyton violaceum (North Africa, India, Middle East)
	Trichophyton schoenleinii
	Epidermophyton floccosum
Zoophilic: animal	*Microsporum canis* (cats, dogs)
	Trichophyton verrucosum (cattle)
	Trichophyton equinum (horse)
	Trichophyton mentagrophytes (also in rodents)
	Trichophyton erinacei (hedgehogs; Europe)
	Microsporum gallinae (fowl)
Geophilic: soil	*Nannizzia gypsea* (previously *Microsporum gypseum*)

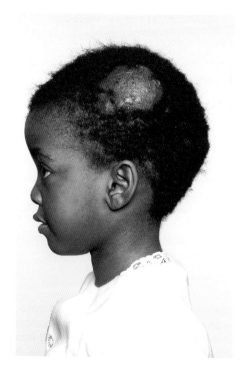

Figure 12.7 Kerion on a child's scalp. © Medical Illustration Cardiff and Vale UHB.

capitis and kerion, hair should be plucked to include the roots (not usually painful as the hair comes away easily) for potassium hydroxide examination. Kerion should be treated aggressively in order to minimise scarring alopecia due to a robust inflammatory response. A short course of oral steroids may be required in conjunction with systemic antifungal agents.

Localised tinea corporis, tinea cruris, tinea manuum and tinea pedis can be treated with topical terbinafine for 1–4 weeks, whereas tinea capitis should be treated with oral griseofulvin for 8–10 weeks or terbinafine (unlicensed in children) for 4 weeks or more. Published guidelines on the management of tinea capitis are updated regularly.

If tinea corporis is suspected in an adult, be sure to check the feet and groin, as these are also likely to be positive. Tinea manuum in an adult often presents as 'one hand, two foot disease' and may have been treated inappropriately as hand dermatitis with topical steroids to transform to tinea incognito.

Beefy-red rash with satellite pustules in the nappy (diaper) area

This description is suggestive of a cutaneous *Candida* infection. The differential diagnoses are irritant contact dermatitis and flexural eczema. Topical imidazole-based (clotrimazole) preparations or topical polyenes (nystatin) with each nappy change for about five days are effective. Where the diagnosis is in doubt, a skin swab for microscopy and culture should be performed.

In young children referred with painful perianal 'dermatitis', swabs should be taken to rule out streptococcal infection. In older children, flexural psoriasis needs to be considered.

Very itchy papules on the fingers and feet in an irritable child

The infant or toddler may be crying and miserable and there may be a history of contact with persons who have been treated recently for scabies. There are itchy papules on the interdigital webs of the fingers and flexural aspects of the wrists, elbows, axillae, feet and genitalia. The papules may become excoriated in older children, as a result of intense scratching. There may be short, wavy burrows at the sites mentioned above. The GP may have tried topical steroids without any benefit. The history and clinical features are very suggestive of scabies (infestation by the mite *Sarcoptes scabiei*). Direct contact is required to transmit scabies. The differential diagnosis is eczema.

In crusted scabies, there is scaling of the affected areas. In doubtful cases, skin scraping taken from a burrow should be examined in a drop of potassium hydroxide or mineral oil, to look for an eight-legged mite; dermoscopy will also show the mite present in the burrow (see Figure 7.34). Treatment is by applying 5% permethrin cream from scalp to toe. The treatment is left on for 12 hours and then washed off. Emphasise to the parents or carers that the treatment needs to be applied thoroughly to the total body surface area. This process is repeated seven days later to ensure maximum efficacy, as this will eliminate newly hatched mites during the interim period. All persons in the same household and any other close contacts should be treated at the same time, and all bedding and clothes used within the previous week should be laundered and dried with high heat.

Head lice

In a child with head lice, the scalp may be itchy and there may be scratch marks and excoriations (Figure 12.8). Head lice are equal-opportunity parasites and they do not respect socioeconomic boundaries. Infestation does not imply a lack of hygiene in their host. Head lice can be treated by using two applications of malathion, permethrin or phenothrin (leave on for 12 hours before washing off) a week apart so that all the lice that hatch within the treatment week are also targeted. Encourage your patients or their carers to comb their hair with a fine-toothed or nit comb on a daily basis, but not to share the comb. All affected members of the household should also be treated at the same time, and pillowcases and sheets should be washed and dried with high heat.

Skin infection and infestation in an unwell child

When reviewing an unwell child, if there is doubt in the outpatient clinic or emergency department about a diagnosis or the

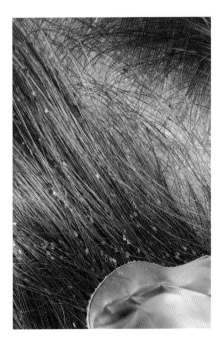

Figure 12.8 Head-louse eggs on hair shafts. © Medical Illustration Cardiff and Vale UHB.

significance of skin signs, the child should be admitted for observation and the management shared between the dermatology and paediatric teams. This is especially needed when there is an extensive skin area involved and if other systemic symptoms are present. Dermatologists also may be called to see unwell children with skin signs on the ward.

Multiple pustules

Numerous and widespread vesicles and pustules that appear in successive crops over a few days suggest a diagnosis of chickenpox caused by varicella zoster virus. The child may have a low-grade fever and appear slightly unwell. The incubation period is 2–3 weeks, and a secondary bacterial infection of the skin lesions may occur. The diagnosis is chiefly clinical and the differential diagnoses of herpes simplex and herpes zoster should be considered in patients with a more localised vesicular pustular eruption. In doubtful cases, tests can be performed after discussion with your local microbiologist (swab and culture, acute and convalescent serology, viral DNA PCR of samples taken from scraping of the base of or fluid from a vesicle). Children with mild symptoms require only symptomatic treatment, whereas in immunocompromised children oral or intravenous aciclovir is indicated. Ideally children with varicella should be isolated from other healthy individuals until all lesions have crusted over.

Secondary bacterial infection of lesions confirmed by culture should be treated with oral antibiotics. If vesicles are localised to the hands, feet and mouth, then hand, foot and mouth disease (caused by Coxsackie A and sometimes enteroviruses) should be considered.

Macular rash

The child with macular rash may have very mild symptoms or may present with prodromal fever, malaise and upper respiratory symptoms (Table 12.4). In rubella, the incubation period is around 2–3 weeks. The child develops a macular rash that starts from the head and spreads to the feet over 24 hours. This rash is accompanied by occipital lymph node enlargement. The rash takes three days to clear. Non-immune mothers who become

Table 12.4 Causes of a macular rash

Rubella
Measles
Erythema infectiosum
COVID-19
Roseola
Infectious mononucleosis
Scarlet fever
Drug eruption

exposed in the first trimester are most at risk of having an affected foetus.

Measles causes a similar but more maculopapular rash and it spreads from the face to involve other parts of the body more slowly, over 2–3 days. The prodromal symptoms in patients with measles are very similar to those that occur in rubella, but in measles the incubation period is slightly longer and symptoms more severe. Preauricular lymph nodes may be enlarged, and white (Koplik's) spots may be found on the buccal mucosa. Measles may be complicated by otitis media, pneumonia and encephalitis.

Acute and convalescence serology can be performed to detect these infections. Acute IgM and a fourfold rise in IgG confirm their presence.

Although childhood preventative immunisation is recommended for both conditions, there are increasing numbers of children who are not immunised. Normal human immunoglobulin is indicated for active measles in immunocompromised children, non-immune pregnant women and infants aged under nine months who have been exposed to measles.

Erythema infectiosum presents as a macular rash and is caused by a human parvovirus B19 infection. This usually starts with intense redness of the cheek (slapped-cheek appearance) and later the child develops a more widespread lacy pink or dull-red macular rash involving the trunk, arms and legs. The incubation period is between one and two weeks and the disease is transmitted via respiratory droplets or blood products. If the child appears anaemic, the full blood count should be checked, as aplastic crisis can be a rare complication. In pregnant women infected during the first and second trimesters, foetal monitoring may be indicated. Specific IgM can be measured to detect an acute infection. Uncomplicated infection requires only symptomatic treatment.

In roseola (caused by human herpesvirus 6), the child usually has a high fever and, when the fever subsides, a rose pink papular eruption appears on the trunk and neck. The incubation period is about two weeks. The disease is transmitted by saliva or respiratory droplets. The child is usually under three years of age. The infection may be complicated by febrile convulsions because of the high fever. Uncomplicated infection requires only symptomatic treatment.

If infectious mononucleosis, seen in older children or adolescents, is inappropriately treated with a beta lactam penicillin antibiotic such as amoxicillin, a widespread rash can occur. However, most other patients with infectious mononucleosis do not develop a rash. The incubation period of infectious mononucleosis, caused by Epstein–Barr virus, is 1–2 months. Patients usually have a fever, lymphadenopathy and a sore throat that may have been treated recently with penicillin. Hepatosplenomegaly sometimes occurs. Splenic rupture, thrombocytopenia, haemolytic anaemia and cardiac involvement are rare but can occur. Therefore it is important to examine thoroughly all children and adults with rashes.

When infectious mononucleosis is suspected it is important to perform a full blood count, and the diagnosis should be supported by a Paul–Bunnell test or Monospot screening test. Both of these tests detect a heterophile antibody (IgM) that agglutinates mammalian red cells. Serology to detect specific IgM and a rising IgG should also be performed. Anti-streptolysin O titre should be checked to exclude scarlet fever.

Scarlet fever (caused by *Streptococcus pyogenes*) is characterised by a rapid onset of headache, fever, anorexia, tonsillitis and lymphadenopathy. A red macular rash spreads from the neck downwards over the trunk to the extremities. A white or red strawberry tongue, circumoral pallor and linear petechiae (along skin folds) may be found. A throat swab for culture and blood test for anti-streptolysin O titre should be performed to confirm the diagnosis. The disease should be treated with penicillin for 10 days. Possible complications from this disease are myocarditis, rheumatic fever, arthritis, osteomyelitis and meningitis.

Purpuric rash

In an unwell child this raises the concern of meningococcaemia and the patient should be managed as an emergency by a paediatric team. Initial blind therapy using intravenous ceftriaxone (child aged 1 month to 11 years: 80–100 mg/kg once daily; 12 years to adult: 2–4 g daily) should be given urgently, with circulatory support to combat shock; benzylpenicillin or ampicillin is an alternative. There is a rapid PCR-based test that can be performed on blood or, where appropriate, on cerebrospinal fluid.

Inflamed skin and desquamation

There are several differential diagnoses to consider: staphylococcal scalded skin syndrome (SSSS), toxic shock syndrome (TSS) and toxic epidermal necrolysis (TEN). In SSSS, the child, usually under the age of five years, may have a focus of infection (e.g. skin, respiratory tract), which is followed by a fever and a widespread red, inflamed skin eruption and blister formation. The skin becomes tender to touch, and gentle rubbing on the skin results in epidermal separation, leaving a shiny, moist and red surface (i.e. positive Nikolsky sign). Periorbital and perioral crusting may be evident.

TSS, on the other hand, can occur at any age, but is seen typically in adolescents and young adults. A focus of skin infection may be evident. All patients have a fever and hypotension. They may have evidence of renal failure. Patients may develop diffuse skin inflammation, redness and oedema or a scarlatiniform rash, which is followed a week or two later by desquamation of the skin on the palms and soles.

TSS may be caused by *Staphylococcus aureus* or group A *Streptococcus* and both TSS and SSSS are mediated by an exotoxin. Blood should be taken for culture and sensitivity. TEN may be confused with SSSS and in both cases the Nikolsky sign is positive. In TEN, the dusky red skin is necrotic and it comes off in large sheets. Skin biopsy shows a subepidermal split in TEN, and a subcorneal split in SSSS.

The choice of antibiotics in SSSS and TSS should be discussed with the local microbiologists, for example beta-lactamase-resistant antibiotics or flucloxacillin to cover staphylococci, and co-amoxiclav to cover streptococci.

Skin infection and infestation in an adult

Some infections have been described in the children's section, but can also occur in adults.

Viral warts

Most patients with viral warts seen in the outpatients department are immunocompetent. However, viral warts are more likely to develop, become more numerous and be more resistant to treatment in patients who are immunosuppressed. This includes patients on long-term immunosuppressive drugs (e.g. tacrolimus, azathioprine or ciclosporin) and those with HIV infection. Patients have usually tried topical preparations containing salicylic acid. Salicylic acid should be avoided for warts on the face as it can cause severe irritation at that site. Adults are tolerant of physical destructive treatment, such as cryotherapy or curettage, in combination with salicylic acid preparations. Plantar warts are generally harder to treat, presumably because of poor drug penetration as a result of the thicker cornified layer. Laser and surgical excision are not usually recommended due to risk of recurrence, but intralesional bleomycin can be considered for debilitating recalcitrant warts.

Genital warts can be effectively treated with cryotherapy or with 5% topical imiquimod cream, three times a week for 16 weeks. Alternatively, purified podophyllotoxin 0.5% solution, which is applied twice daily for three consecutive days, can be used under the direct supervision of a genitourinary medicine physician. This treatment may need to be repeated to produce clinical clearance.

Molluscum contagiosum

In adults this is more commonly seen in association with atopic eczema or with immunosuppression due to HIV infection or immunosuppressant drugs. The papules can be treated by expression of their content, with 5% potassium hydroxide, with cryotherapy, or by applying 5% imiquimod cream three times a week for four weeks.

Discrete inflamed pustules and tender red nodules

Lesions arising as a result of exogenous infection are usually confined to hair-bearing areas. The presentations of pus-containing lesions depend on the depth of the lesions and range from a pustule (in folliculitis) to a tender red nodule (a furuncle or boil). The predisposing factors include occlusive bandaging in the treatment of eczema (seen on dermatology wards), obesity, depilation, long-term antibiotics and corticosteroid use. These are usually caused by *Staphylococcus aureus* infection. Hot tub usage is associated with *Pseudomonas* folliculitis. A skin swab should be taken for culture and sensitivity.

Flucloxacillin or a macrolide is the treatment of choice. However, if patients do not respond, consider infection with staphylococcal strains carrying the Panton–Valentine leucocidin (PVL) virulence factor and liaise with your microbiology department. Pustules on the beard area may be due to a foreign-body reaction 'pseudofolliculitis barbae'. In recurrent cases this is treated with long-term tetracycline and patients should be advised to reduce the frequency of shaving. Folliculitis, which is usually itchy, on the back may be due to *Malassezia furfur*; this is treated with itraconazole 200 mg daily for 10 days.

Inflammatory forms of tinea corporis, and those mistakenly treated with potent topical corticosteroids, characterised by papulopustules (often on the buttocks), can be confused with bacterial folliculitis, but the treatment is with oral antifungal agents rather than antibiotics.

Large red and hot area on a limb

This is usually either cellulitis or a deep vein thrombosis or both. In cellulitis (affecting the dermis and subcutaneous tissue), the skin is red and inflamed with a spreading edge and sometimes has tracking proximal red streaks due to lymphangitis. Regional lymph nodes may be enlarged and there may be signs of the source of infection (e.g. fungal infection between the toes, fissured eczema or a thorn injury). The affected limb is swollen and painful and the patient may be pyrexial. Skin swabs and blood culture are rarely positive, although an anti-streptolysin O test may become positive after 7–10 days; the decision to treat is made on clinical grounds. Erythema nodosum can appear very similar to cellulitis, but in erythema nodosum there are usually several diffusely red large raised tender nodules. Cellulitis is treated with flucloxacillin (for staphylococci) and benzylpenicillin (for streptococci) or a macrolide such as erythromycin if the patient is allergic to penicillin, for 14 days. Dermatologists are often asked to see patients who have had several courses of antibiotics for cellulitis associated with a chronic leg ulcer. In such cases, one should always make sure that the 'cellulitis' is not contact dermatitis, deep vein thrombosis or redness due to haemosiderin deposition, or lipodermatosclerosis (Chapter 26).

Erysipelas (Figure 12.9) is usually more clearly demarcated (affecting the dermis) than cellulitis and is less swollen. It may occur on the face, legs and feet.

If there has been a rapid deterioration of an area of cellulitis such as the skin turning blue-grey, increasing pain, bulla formation, a malodorous discharge or crepitation, the diagnosis of necrotising fasciitis should be considered. The patient is usually ill with fever, diarrhoea, nausea and vomiting, which can be associated with a high mortality rate. At first, pain may be out of proportion to the initial limited clinical findings. There may be a history of recent surgery, ulcer formation or penetrating trauma affecting the lower limbs, abdomen or perineum. Surgeons should be consulted urgently for surgical debridement of necrotic skin. Depending on the site affected and suspected organisms, a broad-spectrum antibiotic with Gram-positive and Gram-negative cover (e.g. penicillin G for group A *Streptococcus* and

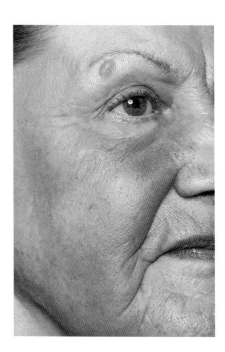

Figure 12.9 Erysipelas affecting a woman's cheek. © Medical Illustration Cardiff and Vale UHB.

Clostridium spp.), metronidazole (for anaerobes) and gentamicin or piperacillin/tazobactam (for *Pseudomonas* infection) may be required. Appropriate samples (skin, blood, urine, faeces) should be sent for culture and sensitivity.

Grouped vesicles and erosions

Herpes simplex also occurs in adults. It usually affects the perioral region and less commonly the fingers (herpetic whitlow). Severe and recurrent cases of herpes simplex, and especially when these are accompanied by erythema multiforme, should be treated with short- or long-term aciclovir, respectively (400 mg aciclovir for six months).

As in children, eczema herpeticum (or Kaposi varicelliform eruption) can occur in patients with atopic dermatitis and other dermatoses, such as Darier's disease or Hailey–Hailey disease (benign familial pemphigus). When one or several dermatomes are involved (e.g. trigeminal or thoracic), then shingles or herpes zoster should be considered. Ophthalmology advice is required in ophthalmic zoster because this can be accompanied by zoster keratitis, and blindness if untreated. Presentation may be subtle, but if a vesicle on the nasal tip is evident (Hutchinson's sign) this indicates ocular involvement via the nasociliary nerve. Herpes zoster should be treated urgently, to limit disease progression and to reduce the risk of post-herpetic neuralgia (Chapter 16). High-dose oral aciclovir or oral valaciclovir (better oral absorption than aciclovir) is indicated. The staff caring for inpatients with herpes zoster should be aware that the patient will require careful infection control procedures until the blisters have dried up.

An ill adult with numerous pustules

Chickenpox occurs less frequently in adults than in children, but adults tend to experience more severe systemic symptoms. There is also a higher chance of developing complications such as pneumonia or hepatitis.

A farmer who has a reddish blue swelling on a finger

In orf, the lesion usually starts as a small papule, which develops into a haemorrhagic nodule or pustule (Figure 12.10). Often there is a central crust. The patient may have regional lymph node enlargement and fever. The parapoxvirus is acquired from handling live sheep or goats, meat, or a contaminated barn door or feeding trough. The disease is usually diagnosed clinically, but it can be confirmed histologically and with PCR. The differential diagnosis includes herpetic whitlow. Patients may also develop erythema multiforme.

A keeper of tropical fish with a non-healing plaque on the hand

The nodules, sometimes in a sporotrichoid distribution along the line of lymphatic vessels, are suggestive of fish tank granuloma (Figure 12.11) caused by *Mycobacterium marinum* infection. This is acquired from handling fish or cleaning out a fish tank. A tissue biopsy should be obtained for histopathology culture, but these may be false negative and the history of exposure to tropical

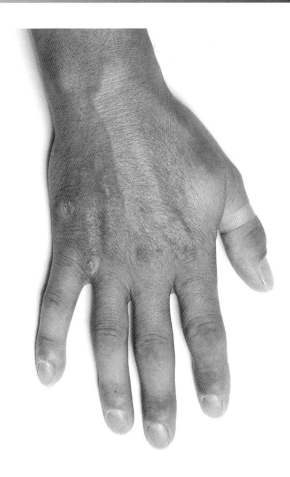

Figure 12.11 Purple-red nodules of *Mycobacterium marinum* infection. © Kings College London NHS Trust.

fish may provide the only clue. This is sometimes because the culture needs to be grown at lower temperatures, hence it is good to warn the microbiologists of the clinical suspicion when the biopsy sample is sent. The infection is treated with either rifampicin or co-trimoxazole, combined with clarithromycin for three months.

Other atypical mycobacteria, such as *Mycobacterium chelonae*, can cause non-sporotrichoid infection, which is rarely seen but can occur in immunosuppressed individuals, in contaminated tattoos (Figure 12.12) or after cosmetic procedures. It is prudent to inform and discuss treatment with a local microbiologist, public health and a specialist in infectious diseases.

Thick and crumbly nails

Dermatophyte infection due to *Trichophyton rubrum* is the most common cause of nail infections (Figure 12.13), and scaling on the soles or between the toe web spaces provides an additional clue. Nail clippings and scrapings should be sent for microscopy and culture for mycology. Dermatophyte infection is treated with terbinafine for 6 weeks for fingernail infection and 12 weeks for toenail infection. Candida onychomycosis is treated with

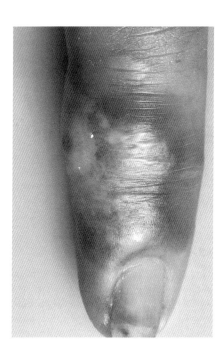

Figure 12.10 Orf on a finger. © Medical Illustration Cardiff and Vale UHB.

(a)

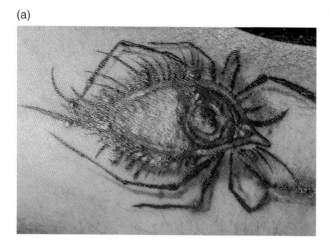

(b)

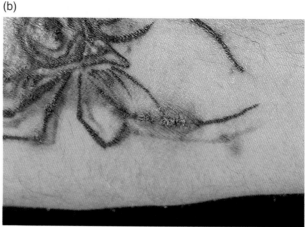

Figure 12.12 Mycobacterium chelonae infection within a tattoo. © Medical Illustration Cardiff and Vale UHB.

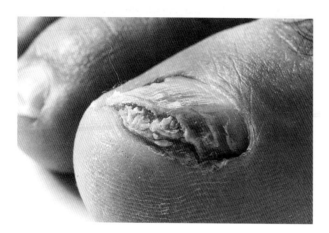

Figure 12.13 Onychomycosis. © Medical Illustration Cardiff and Vale UHB.

2–4 pulses of itraconazole (one week per month). Published guidelines on the treatment of onychomycosis are updated regularly.

Green discoloration of the nail is a sign of *Pseudomonas aeruginosa* infection and can be treated with gentamicin–ciprofloxacin drops applied under the nail.

Numerous itchy papules and crusted eczema-like areas in an elderly patient

The scenario is usually of an elderly person who has been admitted from a nursing or a long-stay ward (e.g. elderly care or rehabilitation ward). This history is suggestive of scabies. The patient may have several itchy red papules on the fingers. If these are also present on the scrotum or penis, this is highly suggestive of scabies. Less commonly, an immunosuppressed patient may have crusted eczema-like areas suggesting crusted scabies. The treatment is the same as in children, but patients need to be isolated as the infestation is highly contagious in hospital settings. Oral ivermectin is indicated for crusted scabies.

Multiple white or brown-pink patches with fine scaling on the trunk and upper arms

Asymptomatic multiple fine-scaled hyperpigmented (in pale-skinned individuals) or hypopigmented (in dark-skinned individuals) patches on the trunk, axillae and limbs are suggestive of pityriasis versicolor caused by the yeast *Malassezia furfur*. GPs or other physicians may have erroneously diagnosed vitiligo and alarmed the patient. The other differential diagnosis is pityriasis alba, which is seen (usually on the face) in atopic individuals and is more common in patients with skin of colour, including children. Where diagnosis is difficult, Wood's lamp examination (yellow fluorescence in pityriasis versicolor) and skin scraping and potassium hydroxide examination (looking for hyphae and spores) are useful. The treatment options include selenium sulfide or ketoconazole shampoo (to wash with), ketoconazole cream daily for 10 days, or oral itraconazole [child age 1 month to 12 years: 3–5 mg/kg (maximum 200 mg) once daily for a week; age 12 years to adult: 200 mg once daily for a week].

Multiple coppery red papules and plaques

The differential diagnoses to be considered here are pityriasis rosea, lichen planus and syphilis. In syphilis the palms are usually affected and there may be associated signs of fever, weight loss and generalised lymphadenopathy, which are not seen in pityriasis rosea. Diagnosis is by non-specific screening tests using rapid plasma reagin and Venereal Disease Research Laboratory tests, and by specific tests (e.g. treponemal enzyme immunoassay or chemiluminescent assay, or fluorescent treponemal antibody absorption test). Syphilis is treated with benzathine penicillin G, 2.4 million units intramuscularly (IM) as a single dose or procaine benzylpenicillin IM for 14 days.

Skin infection or infestation in a returned traveller

It is essential to enquire where the patient has travelled from and the activities that they have carried out while overseas, including where they have visited, slept or swum.

A returned traveller from Central Africa may present with a burning or itchy round papule with central black punctum, called tungiasis. The condition is caused by a burrowing sand flea, *Tunga penetrans* (jigger), due to walking barefoot. Although the condition is self-limiting, most dermatologists advise removing the flea surgically.

An intensely itchy, creeping, raised, red serpiginous tract suggests cutaneous larva migrans (Figure 12.14). The organisms responsible for this condition are *Ancylostoma caninum*, *Ancylostoma braziliense* and *Uncinaria stenocephala*, which are acquired by walking barefoot. These organisms are distributed sparsely in Europe and are mainly acquired in tropical areas including the Caribbean, Africa and Latin America. Eggs and larvae may be found in the faeces in systemic infection. Although most infections usually resolve spontaneously within six weeks without treatment, localised disease is generally treated with a single dose of ivermectin or albendazole.

A persistent brown plaque on a patient originating from a tropical country should alert a dermatologist to the diagnosis of an infectious granuloma such as lupus vulgaris or deep fungal infection. The differential diagnosis includes sarcoidosis, and a biopsy sample should be taken for Ziehl–Neelsen staining and culture or PCR to detect mycobacterial DNA. A chest X-ray should be taken to exclude pulmonary tuberculosis. Lupus vulgaris is treated with isoniazid, rifampicin, pyrazinamide and ethambutol for the first two months and isoniazid and rifampicin for a further four months.

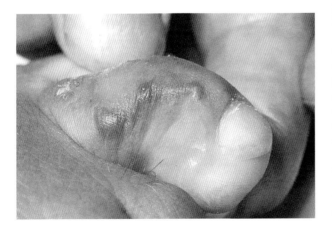

Figure 12.14 Cutaneous larva migrans affecting a patient's toe. © Medical Illustration Cardiff and Vale UHB.

A hypopigmented patch, an anaesthetic plaque with red, raised edges or numerous hypopigmented or red macules in a patient from the Indian subcontinent, Asia, Africa or South America may suggest leprosy. Peripheral nerves may also be enlarged. A skin scraping, skin biopsy or slit-skin smear should be taken for staining with Ziehl–Neelsen to look for *Mycobacterium leprae*. Patients should be referred to a specialist leprosy centre.

A large and expanding inflamed plaque on the leg after returning from a camping trip in the UK, Europe or North America could indicate erythema chronicum migrans caused by *Borrelia burgdorferi* (Lyme disease). The patient may not recall a tick bite. Localised skin disease is treated by doxycycline 100 mg twice a day for three weeks. Systemic infection, where there is lymphadenopathy, and complicated cases, where there may be arthritis, myocarditis, neuropathies, meningoencephalitis or hepatitis, should be referred to a specialist in infectious disease. The infection can be confirmed by the detection of an antibody to *Borrelia burgdorferi*, which should be confirmed in a reference laboratory. The positive predictive value of these serology tests depends on the local prevalence of Lyme disease and therefore, if any doubt, the opinion of a microbiologist should be sought at an early stage.

A nodule or a non-healing ulcer that has developed over several months on the arm or nasal mucosa in a traveller from the Mediterranean basin, Northern Africa, India or South America suggests the lesion may be cutaneous leishmaniasis. A slit-skin smear or a tissue biopsy should be obtained, stained and examined to look for parasites. Tissue histology may show granulomas. DNA detection using PCR is available in some hospitals. The treatment of different species of *Leishmania* should be discussed with a microbiologist or infectious diseases specialist and may need referral to a specialist centre.

Skin manifestations of COVID-19

In 2019, the world saw the emergence of COVID-19, which led to a pandemic. This coronavirus infection affects patients of all ages. Individuals who are elderly and have underlying health issues are particularly adversely affected by the virus, including having a higher risk of death.

The virus is transmitted by respiratory droplets generated by coughing and sneezing and through contact with contaminated surfaces. This occurs during pre-symptomatic and symptomatic periods. The incubation period is up to 14 days with a median of 5 days. The main symptoms of the infection include fever, dry cough, shortness of breath and loss (or altered) sense of smell or taste. A significant number of infected individuals are asymptomatic.

Dermatologists can assist in diagnosing COVID-19, especially prior to a positive test result. A significant proportion of patients may present with cutaneous signs prior to other symptoms. Be aware that clinical presentations may vary in skin of colour and knowledge in this area is rapidly evolving.

Observational studies in different populations have highlighted multiple cutaneous presentations of COVID-19, as follows.

(a)

(b)

(c)

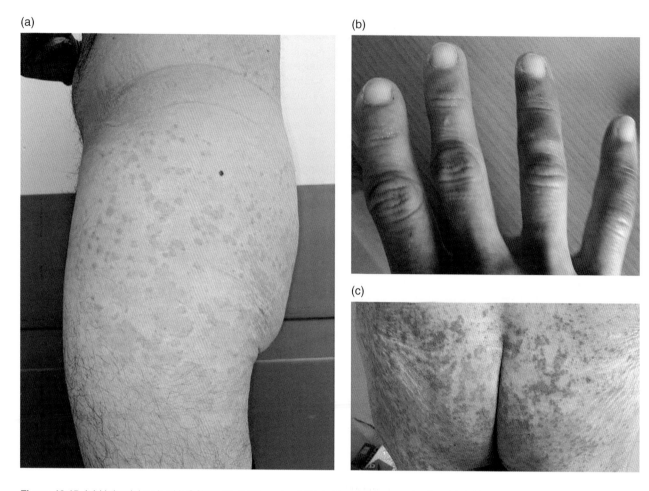

Figure 12.15 (a) Urticarial rash with COVID-19. (b) Pseudo-chilblain-like changes on the fingers. (c) Livedoid eruption on the buttocks. *Galván Casas et al. Br J Dermatol* 2020; **183**:71–7.

- **Urticarial pattern**. This is similar to other forms of urticaria, but can be more resistant to treatment with antihistamines and require oral corticosteroids. This pattern may be seen early in the course of the infection (Figure 12.15a).
- **Red papules and vesicles.** These may occur and can be very itchy and scaly. This pattern presents during or after COVID-19 (sometimes weeks later) and may be relapsing and last for weeks.
- **Pseudo-chilblain/acral erythema pattern**. This presents with red, painful, oedematous plaques or blisters, usually in an asymmetrical distribution (Figure 12.15b). This pattern has been mainly observed in younger patients and less severe cases. This pattern resembles chilblains and typically appears later in the evolution of COVID-19.
- **Livedo/vasculitic pattern**. This can present with reticular ('net-like') cyanotic discoloration of the skin, which can lead to vasculitic lesions usually seen on the limbs (Figure 12.15c). This pattern is mostly observed in older and hospitalised

patients and has been linked with a mortality rate of 10%. Early hospitalisation and intervention are recommended, including checking for clotting abnormalities, and multisystem organ involvement can occur.
- **In children**. Skin manifestations of COVID-19 may be similar to those in adults, but there may be other less common presentations such as oral mucosal findings (tongue swelling), erythema multiforme and Kawasaki disease-like inflammatory syndrome (paediatric inflammatory multisystem syndrome; PIMS).

Conclusions

There are a wide number of skin infections and infestations to be aware of as a practising dermatologist. Some of these you may only see intermittently in your career, as they are rare in the UK or present more often to primary care physicians. The diagnosis is frequently based on clinical features, with appropriate testing for confirmation. However, this may not be obvious due to the stage at which the disease presents, previous treatments used and other confounding factors such as immunosuppression and skin colour. It is important to be vigilant and not miss the possibility of infection or infestation in patients who do not respond to treatment as expected. Always keep an open mind and, if in doubt, discuss the case with a consultant colleague, a consultant microbiologist or an infectious diseases consultant. Most skin infections and infestations can be cured, and hence treating these conditions is a very rewarding task with grateful patients who improve with the correct management.

Pearls and pitfalls

- Consider staphylococcal scalded skin syndrome in young children who are irritable and who may have been referred for suspected eczema flare or toxic epidermal necrolysis. TEN is usually drug induced and is rare in children.
- Eczema herpeticum is often misdiagnosed as an eczema flare. The appearance of monomorphic punched-out erosions with haemorrhagic crusts is characteristic.
- Consider tinea corporis in patients with asymmetrical 'eczema' affecting one limb (usually the leg). On the other hand, consider eczema in patients who may have been misdiagnosed with chronic bilateral cellulitis.
- Consider Panton–Valentine leucocidin *Staphylococcus aureus* or MRSA infection in patients with recurrent purulent infection, often where pain, redness and inflammation are out of proportion to the severity of skin sepsis. A positive contact is a clue to the diagnosis.

SCE Questions. See questions 63–65.

FURTHER READING AND KEY RESOURCES

Ameen M, Lear JT, Madan V *et al*. British Association of Dermatologists' guidelines for the management of onychomycosis 2014. *Br J Dermatol* 2014; **171**:937–58.

Andina D, Belloni-Fortina A, Bodemer C *et al*. Skin manifestations of COVID-19 in children: parts 1–3. *Clin Exp Dermatol* 2021; **46**:444–50; 451–61; 462–72.

Fuller LC, Barton RC, Mohd Mustapa MF *et al*. British Association of Dermatologists' guidelines for the management of tinea capitis 2014. *Br J Dermatol* 2014; **171**:454–63.

Galván Casas C, Català A, Carretero Hernández G *et al*. Classification of the cutaneous manifestations of COVID-19: a rapid prospective nationwide consensus study in Spain with 375 cases. *Br J Dermatol* 2020; **183**:71–7.

Sterling JC, Gibbs S, Haque Hussain SS *et al*. British Association of Dermatologists' guidelines for the management of cutaneous warts 2014. *Br J Dermatol* 2014; **171**:696–712.

Useful websites

British Association of Dermatologists (BAD). Covid-19 skin patterns. Available at: https://covidskinsigns.com.

BAD. Patient information leaflets. Available at: https://www.bad.org.uk/for-the-public/patient-information-leaflets.

DermNet NZ. Available at: www.dermnetnz.org.

13

Skin cancer

Alla M. Altayeb and Richard J. Motley

Introduction

Due to the combination of sun exposure and the ageing population, skin cancers have now formed a major part of a dermatologist's workload. Familiarity with the diagnosis and management of common skin tumours is therefore essential.

Much of clinical dermatology care consists of suppressing or alleviating chronic disease. In contrast, treatment of skin cancer in the vast majority of cases results in complete cure. This makes the care of these patients very satisfying, usually with the outcome of a happy and grateful patient. However, there are many potential pitfalls in this complex area to understand and avoid. There are also several aspects of therapy, especially surgical techniques, that can greatly influence the prognosis and cosmetic outcome. Although reaching a high level of skill is challenging, the huge skin cancer workload will allow you to develop rapidly. During this process it is essential to work with and learn from experts in dermatological surgery.

Malignant melanoma

Malignant melanoma (MM) is a type of cancer arising from melanocytes. It is one of the most dangerous and unpredictable skin cancers, with prognosis closely related to the thickness of the lesion. Early recognition and excision of melanomas give the greatest opportunity for cure. MM occurs in adults of all ages; it metastasises easily and can develop anywhere in the body (not just sun-exposed areas, e.g. in skin of colour).

The incidence of melanoma varies from 3–5 per 100,000 per annum in Mediterranean countries to 50 per 100,000 in Australia and New Zealand. In the UK the incidence has quadrupled over the last 40 years and is now around 16 per 100,000 per annum.

MM is described as *in situ* (if a tumour is confined to the epidermis), invasive (if a tumour has spread into the dermis) or metastatic (if a tumour has spread to other tissues).

Types of melanomas

Four major histological types have been described:

- Superficial spreading melanoma (most common) (Figure 13.1).
- Nodular melanoma.
- Lentigo maligna melanoma.
- Acral lentiginous melanoma (Figure 13.2; and Chapter 14).

Aetiological factors

MM occurs mainly due to extensive sun exposure, but some individuals are more susceptible due to genetic factors. Some of the risks of developing MM are shown in Table 13.1.

Dermatology Training: The Essentials. Edited by Mahbub M.U. Chowdhury, Tamara W. Griffiths and Andrew Y. Finlay.
© 2022 The British Association of Dermatologists. Published 2022 by John Wiley & Sons Ltd.
Companion website: www.wiley.com/go/chowdhury/dermatologytraining

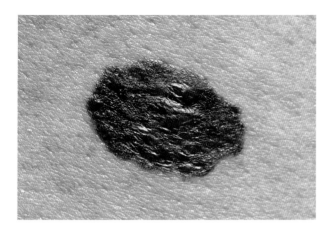

Figure 13.1 Superficial malignant melanoma. © Medical Illustration Cardiff and Vale UHB.

Table 13.1 Risk factors for melanoma skin cancer

Ultraviolet light exposure is the major risk factor
Fair skin, red hair and freckles
Increasing age (however, it is the most common cancer in people < 30 years old)
History of melanoma (especially for age < 40 years) or any other skin cancer
History of at least eight moles greater than 6 mm diameter
History of a changing mole
Some hereditary conditions: dysplastic naevus syndrome and xeroderma pigmentosum
Family history of melanoma
Large congenital naevus (> 15 cm)
Immunosuppression

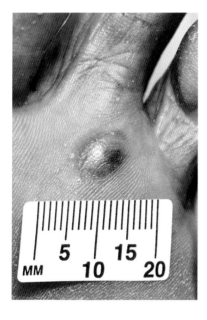

Figure 13.2 Acral malignant melanoma in skin of colour. © Medical Illustration Cardiff and Vale UHB.

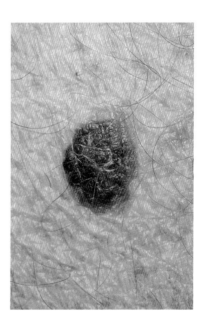

Figure 13.3 Asymmetry in colour, shape and edge of a malignant melanoma. © Medical Illustration Cardiff and Vale UHB.

Some gene mutations have been linked with the risk of developing MM. Knowledge of the exact genetic mutation can be helpful in providing targeted therapy and for selection of patients for clinical trials:

- *BRAF*, *CDKN2A*, *NRAS* and *TP53* gene mutations in cutaneous melanoma.
- *BRAF*, *NRAS*, *NF1* and *KIT* gene mutations in acral melanoma.
- *SF3B1* gene mutation in mucosal melanoma.

Initial assessment and diagnosis

The key feature suggesting a diagnosis of MM is asymmetry. There may be irregularity in colour (light to dark brown, black

and red colours) and irregularity in the shape, surface or edge of the lesion (Figure 13.3). Bleeding is a late sign in advanced melanoma, but there may be a history of irritation, changing colour or recent growth. These changes have been abbreviated within aide-mémoires such as the seven-point checklist (Table 13.2) and the ABCD(E) rules (Table 13.3).

Any patient with a suspicious pigmented lesion should have a full skin examination, including careful examination for lymphadenopathy and hepatomegaly. The site and size of the pigmented lesion should be documented, and a record should be made of

Table 13.2 Glasgow seven-point checklist

Major features

    Change in size

    Irregular shape

    Irregular colour

Minor features

    Largest diameter 7 mm or more

    Inflammation

    Oozing

    Change in sensation

Lesions with any major feature or three minor features are suspicious of melanoma

Table 13.3 American ABCD(E) system for diagnosing melanoma

Asymmetry

Border irregularity

Colour variation: three or more colours

Diameter more than 6 mm

Evolution of the lesion (change in size, shape or colour)

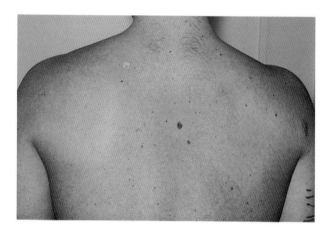

Figure 13.4 The ugly duckling sign. © Medical Illustration Cardiff and Vale UHB.

Table 13.4 Dermoscopic features of malignant melanoma (Chapter 7)

Peripherally situated black or brown dots or globules (indicating active growth)

Blue-white veil appearance over the lesion

Irregular pseudopods of pigment

Radial streaming (asymmetric parallel linear extensions of pigment at the radial margins)

Regression (white scarring)

other pigmented lesions. Clinical photographs and mole mapping may be helpful.

Melanomas may arise *de novo*, or in an acquired or congenital melanocytic naevus. Giant naevi frequently give rise to MM during the teenage years. Prospective studies have failed to identify an increased risk of malignancy in small congenital naevi, but dermatologists commonly see melanoma that has arisen in small congenital moles; this association suggests there may be an increased risk. For this reason, removal of small congenital naevi may be advocated to prevent future malignancy.

The 'ugly duckling sign' is useful in highlighting moles that stand out as being irregular compared to other moles; these should be treated with a high degree of suspicion (Figure 13.4).

Dermoscopy allows a closer examination of pigmented lesions, and in the hands of an experienced physician it enhances the diagnostic accuracy (Table 13.4).

Biopsy of suspected melanoma

Any suspected MM should be removed in its entirety with a 2–3-mm margin of normal skin. For small lesions, the biopsy wound is usually closed primarily. If the lesion is of a significant size, the wound may be left open with planned regular dressings until the histological diagnosis is confirmed.

Shave and punch biopsies are not recommended. Incisional biopsy is occasionally acceptable when suspecting a lentigo maligna on the face or acral melanoma.

Histology

The most essential pathological feature is the maximum depth, usually described by Breslow thickness or Clark level. This normally determines the type of treatment and prognosis. The histology report should describe the presence of ulceration, vascular invasion, atypical mitoses, the extent of regression and clearance of surgical margins.

Breslow thickness

This Breslow thickness is the distance in millimetres from the overlying epidermal granular layer to the deepest point of tumour invasion, and it is the strongest predictor of prognosis. Tumours less than 1 mm thick are considered low risk; those 1–2 mm are intermediate risk; 2–4 mm are high risk and > 4 mm are very high risk. It is important to assess the Breslow thickness accurately, therefore a shave biopsy is not appropriate.

Clark level

Another method of assessing melanomas is via the Clark level. It describes the melanoma according to the layers of skin involved using a scale of I–V (Table 13.5). As skin thickness varies considerably throughout the body (e.g. eyelid skin versus heel skin), the level of invasion is more qualitative than quantitative. Most often both descriptors are used to define a melanoma (e.g. Clark level III, 1.5 mm Breslow depth).

Management of melanoma

Once histology confirms a diagnosis of MM, a multidisciplinary team should be involved. Dermatologists follow the 2018 American Joint Committee on Cancer (AJCC) TNM (tumour–nodes–metastasis) staging system (see Further reading) and treatment is planned accordingly.

Investigations

- No investigations are necessary for patients with stage 0–IA melanoma (i.e. non-ulcerated tumours of < 0.8-mm Breslow thickness).
- For tumours of > 0.8-mm Breslow thickness, the first step is to offer sentinel lymph node biopsy (SLNB), followed by wide local excision with a 1–2-cm margin depending on the Breslow thickness (Table 13.6). If patients test positive on SLNB the melanoma is classed as stage III or higher, depending on the presence of any distal metastasis, and they may qualify for adjuvant immunotherapy.
- Complete lymph node dissection is not routinely recommended for sentinel node-positive patients due to the associated morbidity, but it is recommended for patients with clinically detectable (macroscopic) lymph node metastasis.
- Patients with melanoma of stage IIC and above should have:
  - Computed tomography (CT) scan with contrast of head, neck, chest, abdomen and pelvis. Patients should be advised they will have six-monthly surveillance CT scans for three years, followed by annual CT scans for a further two years.
  - Bloods to check the liver function, lactate dehydrogenase level and full blood count.
  - *BRAF* gene mutation testing, which can be done on a tumour sample or on blood.

Adjuvant therapy (Chapter 18)

Patients with stage III or higher melanomas should be evaluated for adjuvant immunotherapy agents such as ipilimumab (human anti-cytotoxic T-lymphocyte-associated protein 4), nivolumab or pembrolizumab (anti-programmed death 1) and trametinib (anti-mitogen-activated protein kinase monoclonal antibody).

Targeted therapies such as vemurafenib or dabrafenib against the mutated *BRAF* gene (occurring in 50% of MMs) have also been used in addition to the above immunotherapies for patients who are BRAF positive. They inhibit the mutated BRAF protein, hence preventing further growth of the MM.

Adjuvant radiotherapy may be considered for cases of inadequate resection margins or after resection of bulky disease.

Radiotherapy to the primary tumour is only considered in rare palliative cases when excision is not possible, either due to the patient's comorbidities or when morbidity of the excision is too great. Radiotherapy in these situations is not curative.

Informing patients of the diagnosis of melanoma

Breaking the news of a diagnosis of MM requires sensitivity and careful timing. A face-to-face follow-up appointment should be arranged, and the patient advised to bring a relative or friend to the appointment. Patients should also be assigned to a skin cancer specialist nurse. It is usual practice to plan follow-up two weeks after the excision, and pathologists are informed of the date to ensure report availability.

Prognosis

Prognosis is estimated using prognostic indicator tables (Table 13.7). It is good practice to do this before discussing the diagnosis with the patient. However, prognosis may improve in the future due to the continuous advances in targeted immunotherapies.

Patient education

All patients should be taught self-examination due to the high risk of recurrence. Vitamin D levels should also be checked and supplemented if needed. Some educational points for patients with MM are listed in Table 13.8.

Table 13.5 Clark levels of melanoma

Clark level I: melanoma confined to the epidermis (*in situ*)

Clark level II: melanoma spread to the upper dermis

Clark level III: melanoma involves most of the upper dermis

Clark level IV: melanoma spread to the lower dermis

Clark level V: melanoma invaded the subcutaneous tissue

Table 13.6 Recommended surgical excision margins for malignant melanoma

Breslow thickness	Excision margins to achieve complete histological excision
In situ	0.5 cm
< 1 mm	1 cm
> 1 mm	2 cm

Table 13.7 Breslow thickness and 5-year survival for malignant melanoma

Breslow thickness	5-year survival
In situ	90–100%
< 1 mm	80–90%
1–2 mm	70–80%
2–4 mm	60–70%
> 4 mm	50%

Table 13.9 Risk factors for non-melanoma skin cancers

Sun exposure is a major risk factor
Skin type, especially Fitzpatrick types I and II
Elderly age
Immunosuppression, e.g. organ transplant patients
Multiple previous skin cancers, solar keratoses or Bowen's disease
Inherited syndromes, e.g. Gorlin syndrome and xeroderma pigmentosum

Table 13.8 Education points for patients with malignant melanoma

Sun protection advice (sun-protective clothing and sunscreens)
Lifelong self-examination of the skin and peripheral lymph nodes
Possible recurrence within the melanoma scar
Patient must be aware that family members have an increased risk of developing melanomas
Vitamin D levels should be measured, and supplements given if needed

Follow-up

Patients with *in situ* melanomas do not require follow-up. Patients with stage IA require six-monthly follow-up for one year. Melanomas of stage IB and above require three-monthly follow-up for three years, then every six months for two years; however, there remains no global consensus on the optimal follow-up schedule.

Basal cell carcinoma

Basal cell carcinoma (BCC) is the most common skin cancer; in fact, it is the most common malignancy in humans. It is a slow-growing skin cancer usually seen on sun-exposed areas (head and neck) in elderly White individuals. However, with increasing sun exposure, these tumours are now seen in adults in the fourth decade or younger. Risk factors are shown in Table 13.9.

BCC is a locally destructive tumour that almost never metastasises; however, it will inevitably destroy surrounding tissue if left untreated. The typical BCC appears as a skin-coloured pearly nodule, often with prominent overlying telangiectasia.

Clinical assessment

When assessing a possible BCC, it is very helpful to wet the surface of the tumour with an alcohol wipe followed by oblique illumination using a light source. This will highlight

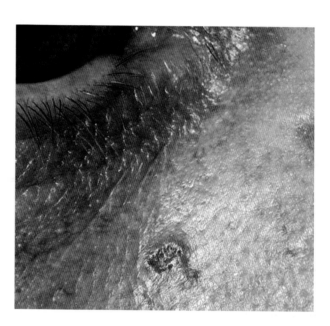

Figure 13.5 Rodent ulcer. © Medical Illustration Cardiff and Vale UHB.

surface changes, such as the characteristic rolled edges and telangiectasia. For assessment in skin of colour see Chapter 14.

Any slight changes to the skin surface surrounding the tumour should be viewed with suspicion and considered as extension of the tumour until proven otherwise.

BCCs are usually soft in consistency and easily damaged by minimal trauma, such as shaving or washing. Once damaged the surface will often remain ulcerated, giving rise to the term 'rodent ulcer' (Figure 13.5). If the lesion is crusted, it is usually necessary to remove the crust before the characteristic features can be seen. Magnification via dermoscopy improves diagnostic accuracy by highlighting some of the lesion's common dermoscopic features (Table 13.10). Be aware that elderly patients may have multiple BCCs and therefore a thorough examination of sun-exposed areas is advisable.

Table 13.10 Dermoscopic features of basal cell carcinoma (Chapter 7)

Arborising vessels and redness
Leaf-like areas
Blue-grey nests or globules
Erosions and ulcerations
Spoke wheel pigmentation

Points to note:

- Secondary bacterial infection (usually *Staphylococcus aureus*) can occur in ulcerated BCCs leading to increased risk of infection after surgery.
- Prophylactic antibiotics (e.g. flucloxacillin 250 mg four times daily) are given for 5–7 days starting on the day of surgery.

Types of basal cell carcinoma

There are several morphological variants of BCC, and these can only be determined by histological examination. However, the clinician may suspect an infiltrative tumour if the margins of the lesion are not clearly visible.

Nodular basal cell carcinoma

This is the commonest subtype and accounts for more than 60% of cases (Figure 13.6). It presents as a pearly or translucent papule or nodule with overlying telangiectatic vessels. Nodular BCCs exhibit a very definite 'footprint' on the skin surface with clear tumour margins. They may ulcerate and the patient may give a history of bleeding and crusting.

Some nodular BCCs (especially in skin of colour or easily tanned skin) show brown or black pigmentation, known as 'pigmented BCC', which may be sometimes confused with a melanoma. Others have soft fluctuant centres and may mimic a cyst. Therefore, it is important to send all samples for histology.

Superficial basal cell carcinoma

These are the second most common subtype, accounting for 15% of all BCCs. The lesions commonly affect the torso. They present as scaly pink to red patches or plaques, often with central clearing and a characteristic thin pearly border, more easily seen on stretching the skin (Figure 13.7). They are slowly progressive, do not usually ulcerate and may be confused with psoriasis or eczema.

Morphoeic basal cell carcinoma

These appear as a sclerotic (scar-like), waxy or red plaque or papule (Figure 13.8). The border is ill defined, and the tumour often extends well beyond the clinical margins. Ulceration, bleeding and crusting are uncommon. These account for 3% of

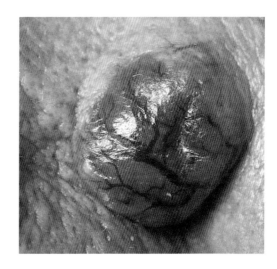

Figure 13.6 Nodular basal cell carcinoma. © Medical Illustration Cardiff and Vale UHB.

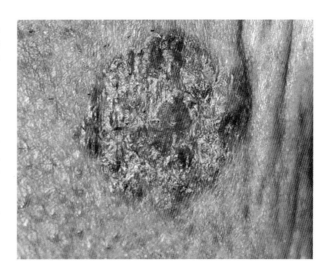

Figure 13.7 Superficial basal cell carcinoma. © Medical Illustration Cardiff and Vale UHB.

BCCs and occur almost exclusively on the face; treatment is with Mohs surgery (Chapter 19).

Infiltrative basal cell carcinomas

These comprise 5% of all BCCs and are characterised clinically by an ill-defined margin. This subtype requires histological confirmation, where infiltrative strands and islands of tumour are seen.

Basosquamous basal cell carcinoma

These are mixed basal and squamous cell carcinomas; histologically they have features of both. They are infiltrative and potentially more aggressive than other forms of BCC.

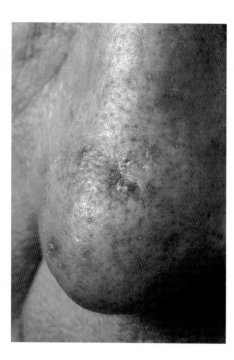

Figure 13.8 Morphoeic basal cell carcinoma. © Medical Illustration Cardiff and Vale UHB.

Fibroepithelioma of Pinkus

This is a rare variant that presents as a pink, dome-shaped, pedunculated papule or nodule on the torso or extremities.

Diagnosis

In most cases, diagnosis of BCC tends to be based on clinical appearance. However, where doubt exists, a biopsy is recommended. This should consist of a small sample from the upper part of the tumour, usually by a 'shave' or 'curettage' biopsy. Punch biopsies carry the risk of displacing the tumour beneath the natural base of the lesion.

Histology

The common histological findings are nests of neoplastic basaloid cells, which are organised as lobules, islands or chords, with tumour cells aligning more densely at the periphery (Chapter 5). In the dermis, intense inflammatory infiltrate is common. Cleft formation (known as retraction artefact) occurs between BCC nests and stroma due to shrinkage of mucin during tissue fixation and staining. Specific histological subtypes are recognised by the architectural pattern of tumour cell aggregates and the accompanying stromal reaction.

It is important to note the following:

- Be clear whether the intention is to take a biopsy – in which case a *small* superficial sample of the tumour should be taken – or to fully excise the lesion.

- An over-generous biopsy could eliminate the tumour trace, without adequate margins of excision. This is problematic especially if further surgery is required, in addition to increasing the risk of recurrence.

Treatment

Treatment of BCC depends on its type, size and location. The number of lesions to be treated and patient factors (e.g. patient's choice and comorbidities) should also be considered. Most are treated surgically.

Surgical excision

Excision is the appropriate treatment for the majority of BCCs; it can be usefully combined with curettage, which better delineates the extent of the tumour, before excising with a 3-mm margin of normal skin around the curetted defect. In the absence of curettage, a 4–5-mm margin may be appropriate. If these large margins will have an adverse impact on the surgical and cosmetic outcomes, consider Mohs surgery instead. The excised tissue should be examined histologically to confirm the diagnosis and to assess the adequacy of the excision. Excision adequacy should never be compromised due to concerns regarding wound repair. Most wounds are closed primarily as a simple elliptical closure into a straight line, but dermatologists with interest in cutaneous surgery should become familiar with second-intention wounds, skin grafts and skin flaps (Chapter 19).

Curettage and cautery/electrodesiccation

The soft consistency of BCCs allows them to be scooped away easily from the skin using a curette. Disposable curettes have a scalpel-like razor-sharp edge, which should be used with light pressure, and a blunt edge that can be applied more firmly for curettage. After curettage, the base of the wound is heated with cautery or electrodessication to secure haemostasis. This technique is effective for simple nodular BCCs, but cannot be expected to remove infiltrative tumour strands. The adequacy of this treatment cannot be assessed histologically, and the wound usually heals with an unsightly depressed scar. For these reasons, curettage and cautery or curettage and electrodesiccation should be reserved for tumours in non-cosmetic locations and situations where recurrence of the tumour is of less concern (e.g. trunk and limbs).

Mohs micrographic surgery (Figure 19.11)

Micrographic surgery, pioneered by Dr Frederic Mohs, is a technique in which the entire surgical margin of the excised tissue is examined histologically on the day of surgery; more tissue is removed repeatedly if necessary until the margins are clear. It achieves the highest cure rates for BCCs and is indicated for tumours with ill-defined margins (e.g. morphoeic BCCs), aggressive tumours (e.g. those with perineural or perivascular involvement), recurrent tumours and those arising at critical anatomical sites where preservation of normal tissue is paramount (e.g. eyelids, nose).

Other treatment modalities

Treatment options include radiotherapy, cryotherapy, phototherapy, photodynamic therapy and topical treatments such as 5-fluorouracil (Efudix®, Mylan, Hatfield, UK) and imiquimod (Aldara®, Meda Pharmaceuticals, Bishop's Stortford, UK). They all lack histological confirmation of treatment adequacy and therefore should be used with caution in sites where recurrence may become a problem.

- **Radiotherapy** is particularly valuable for large tumours in elderly patients. The tumour is irradiated over 1–2 weeks and subsequently crusts over and heals in 4–6 weeks. Several visits are required. The initial result may be cosmetically excellent, but over a few years the skin becomes atrophic and telangiectatic.
- In skilled hands, **cryotherapy** using liquid nitrogen spray gives cure rates comparable with those of other treatments for small, well-defined BCCs. Cryotherapy causes a pale, atrophic scar and moderate-to-severe discomfort. The wound (a localised 'frostbite') is often weepy and oedematous and takes several weeks to heal. Cryotherapy works because the tumour cells are less able to withstand low-temperature injury than the normal surrounding dermal fibroblasts.
- In **photodynamic therapy** a topical photosensitising cream (methyl aminolaevulinic acid) is applied to the skin tumour for several hours and then an appropriate light source is shone onto the tumour (Chapter 25). The light activates the photosensitiser cream, causing destruction of the tumour cells. This treatment can be inconvenient due to the long duration of cream application and can be painful (although there is no reason to withhold local anaesthesia). The treated skin usually heals well with excellent cosmetic results, but long-term cure rates are disappointing and lower than with other treatments.
- **Topical chemotherapy** is best reserved for small superficial lesions, especially when multiple lesions exist on extensive areas of photodamaged skin. Imiquimod 5% cream (Aldara) is the preferred choice of topical treatments for superficial BCCs. It is applied nightly or five times per week for six weeks; 5-fluorouracil cream (Efudix) can also be used. The inflammatory response to these agents can be uncomfortable, but can indicate good response for tumour destruction.
- **Non-treatment of BCCs** is an option as not all BCCs require treatment. Aggressive treatment might be inappropriate for patients of advanced age or poor general health, especially for asymptomatic low-risk lesions that are unlikely to cause significant morbidity. Some elderly or frail patients with symptomatic or high-risk tumours might prefer less aggressive treatments designed to palliate rather than cure. Local availability of specialised services and the experience of the dermatologist managing the case are factors that will influence the choice of therapy.

Follow-up

After the post-operative review, patients with completely excised BCCs do not require long-term follow-up. Patient education is important prior to discharge, as a significant proportion will develop more BCCs.

Squamous cell carcinoma

Squamous cell carcinoma (SCC) is the second most common skin cancer. It is a malignant tumour arising from the keratinocytes of the epidermis or its appendages.

Unlike in BCC, with SCCs there is a risk of metastasis, especially in immunosuppressed patients (e.g. those on long-term immunosuppressive drugs for organ transplant, those with latent leukaemia, or the very elderly). It is the commonest skin cancer in this cohort of patients. Patients with a past history of psoralen–ultraviolet A (PUVA) therapy may be at increased risk of SCC, which may be exacerbated if they subsequently receive immunosuppressants. The risk of metastasis is associated with the size of the tumour and the degree of invasion at the time of removal.

Clinical features and diagnosis

SCCs arise mainly on sun-exposed skin. They present as indurated, crusted, nodular or ulcerated lesions that are often tender on palpation (Figure 13.9). Compared to BCCs, they are more frequently seen on the ears, lips and dorsa of the hands. SCCs can grow rapidly and are usually tender, a symptom that can be useful in distinguishing SCCs from other warty lesions in transplant patients. For SCCs in skin of colour see Chapter 14.

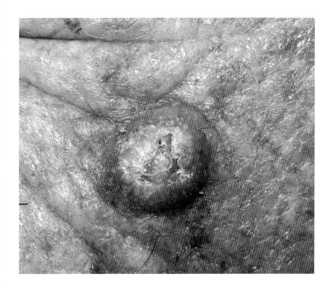

Figure 13.9 Squamous cell carcinoma. © Medical Illustration Cardiff and Vale UHB.

The induration typically extends beyond the visible margins. On the lips or genitalia, SCC generally presents as a fissure or non-healing ulcer. Regional lymph nodes may be enlarged due to infection of the ulcerated lesion or metastases (hard, irregular nodes). Haematogenous spread is uncommon.

The diagnosis of SCC is established histologically, but in addition to clinical features certain dermoscopic features may aid in the diagnosis (Table 13.11; also Chapter 7).

Histology

Irregular masses or nests of varying proportions of normal and anaplastic squamous cells are seen. Well-differentiated tumours are marked by the presence of horn pearls and are lower risk than moderately or poorly differentiated lesions.

Treatment

The goal of treatment is complete removal of the primary tumour. Treatment choice depends on the size, location and level of risk for that particular SCC (Table 13.12).

Surgical excision

Excision is the treatment of choice for most SCCs. The recommended surgical margins depend on the risk of the tumour, and complete excision is defined by at least 1-mm histological clearance of all margins.

Recommended excision margins are:

- 4 mm for a low-risk SCC.
- 6 mm for a high-risk SCC.
- 10 mm for a very high-risk SCC.

Mohs micrographic surgery

Consider Mohs surgery for ill-defined and high-risk lesions, particularly in sites where tissue conservation is important for function. Once the margins are cleared, the wound is closed if possible or left to heal by second intention. If Mohs surgery is not available, the wound should be left open until histological confirmation of excision adequacy is achieved.

Other treatment modalities

- Curettage and cautery may be used for small, low-risk lesions. Histology of the curetted lesion should be reviewed to ensure there are no high-risk features.
- Various modalities such as radiotherapy, cryotherapy, laser and intralesional cytotoxic therapy have been used for localised disease. Chemotherapy can be used for more widespread disease when surgery is likely to result in an unacceptable functional or aesthetic outcome.
- Primary radiotherapy can be offered if surgery is not feasible or treatment is mainly symptomatic.
- Adjuvant radiotherapy may be offered after surgery for high-risk SCCs.
- Immunotherapy may be considered for metastatic SCCs or inoperable locally advanced SCCs that are not amenable to radical radiotherapy.
- Chemotherapy may be offered to patients with metastatic SCCs who have contraindications to immunotherapy. It can also be considered in the palliative setting.

Table 13.11 Dermoscopic features of squamous cell carcinoma (Chapter 7)

Central yellow keratinous plug
Arborising vessels centrally
Hairpin vessels peripherally

Table 13.12 Squamous cell carcinoma risk classification

	Low risk	High risk	Very high risk
Size and depth	Tumour diameter ≤ 20 mm	Diameter > 20–40 mm	Diameter > 40 mm
	Tumour thickness ≤ 4 mm	Thickness > 4–6 mm	Thickness > 6 mm
Invasion	Invasion into dermis No perineural invasion No lymphovascular invasion	Invasion into subcutaneous fat Perineural invasion present in the dermis only Lymphovascular invasion	Invasion beyond subcutaneous fat. Any bone invasion Perineural invasion present beyond the dermis
Histology	Well-differentiated or moderately differentiated histology	Poorly differentiated histology	High-grade histological subtype: adenosquamous, desmoplastic, spindle/sarcomatoid/metaplastic
Site		Tumour site: ear or lip	In transit metastasis
		Tumour arising within a scar or area of chronic inflammation	

Follow-up

The recommended frequency and duration of follow-up depend on the SCC risk. All patients should be encouraged to self-examine, with particular attention to the possibility of recurrence at the original site and in the draining lymph nodes. Elderly patients might find it difficult to adequately self-examine, and therefore a dermatologist or specialist nurse may undertake regular follow-up.

For low-risk SCCs a single post-operative follow-up is offered to conduct skin surveillance and facilitate patient education. For high-risk SCCs, patients are followed up every four months for one year, then every six months for a further year. For very high-risk SCCs, follow-up should be every four months for two years, then six-monthly for a further year.

Prevention of excessive sun exposure (sunscreens and protective clothing) reduces the incidence of future SCCs.

Prognosis

Most patients with primary cutaneous SCC have a very good prognosis, with < 5% mortality. Conversely, those with distal metastasis have a five-year survival rate of 20–40%. Up to 95% of metastases and local recurrences are detected within the first five years, with 70–90% occurring within the first two years.

Keratoacanthoma

Keratoacanthoma (KA) is a rapidly growing epithelial tumour of hair follicle origin. It can strongly resemble an SCC both clinically and histologically. It usually presents as a solitary lesion, but multiple lesions are described as part of Ferguson–Smith and Muir–Torre syndromes.

Clinical features and diagnosis

KA presents as a rapidly growing nodule with a central crater containing a keratin plug (Figure 13.10). It often reaches 2 cm or more in diameter within 4–6 weeks, after which it begins to involute and heals spontaneously, leaving a depressed scar (Figure 13.11).

KA arises commonly in hair-bearing sun-exposed skin in elderly patients. The face, neck and dorsa of the upper extremities are common sites; truncal lesions are rare. KAs have also been observed in subungual and mucosal areas, indicating non-follicular origin in some cases.

History of rapid growth to a relatively large size, spontaneous resolution and typical clinical features of a regular crateriform keratotic plug with undamaged surrounding skin all suggest the diagnosis of KA.

Histology

KAs are composed of well-differentiated squamous epithelium with a mild degree of pleomorphism and masses of keratin that constitute the central core of the KA. However, it can be very difficult histologically to differentiate KA from SCC.

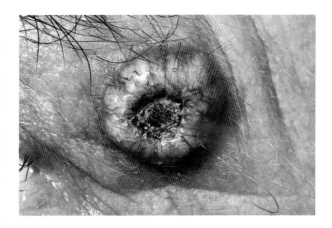

Figure 13.10 Keratoacanthoma. © Medical Illustration Cardiff and Vale UHB.

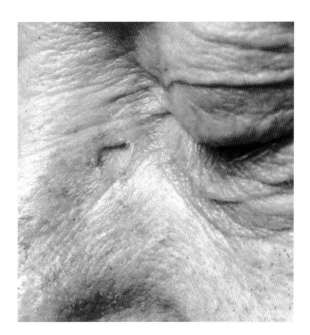

Figure 13.11 Moon-crater scar seen in a healed keratoacanthoma. Eghlileb AM, Finlay AY. Healed keratoacanthoma: the 'moon-crater' sign. *J Eur Acad Dermatol Venereol* 2008; **22**:521–2.

Treatment

Due to the strong clinical resemblance of KA to an SCC, excision is recommended to confirm the diagnosis by histological examination, and to minimise the tissue damage that will occur if the lesion is allowed to pursue its natural course. It is not uncommon for the histology to be suggestive of an SCC, and so the diagnosis is heavily dependent on the correlation of the histopathology with the clinical history and appearance.

Actinic keratosis

Actinic keratosis (AK) is the commonest sun-related skin growth. Affected individuals are usually elderly fair-skinned patients who burn easily and tan poorly. Along with excessive sun exposure, ionising radiation and exposure to products of coal distillation are important causative agents.

The presence of multiple AKs is a risk factor for SCC, with an estimated risk of < 1% per annum with a latent period of 10 years. Solitary lesions rarely evolve into SCCs.

Clinical features and diagnosis

AKs commonly present as pink-to-red scaly papules or plaques on sun-exposed areas. The face, ears, scalp and the dorsa of the hands are the commonest sites (Figure 13.12).

Diagnosis is usually clinical, but for suspicious, tender or indurated lesions, biopsy is indicated to rule out malignant change.

Histology

Acanthosis and dyskeratosis with mitotic figures in the epidermis are common features. Usually, marked hyperkeratosis and areas of parakeratosis with loss of the granular layer are present. The basement membrane is intact and dyskeratotic changes rarely extend into adnexal structures.

Treatment

Spontaneous resolution often occurs. Common treatment modalities are curettage and cautery, cryotherapy and topical 5-fluorouracil, imiquimod or diclofenac, especially when treating multiple smaller lesions. Larger, tender and indurated lesions should be excised for histological diagnosis. Daylight phototherapy may be effective.

Bowen's disease

Bowen's disease is a form of *in situ* SCC. It has the potential to progress to an invasive SCC, seen in 3% of patients, but spontaneous partial regression may also occur. Chronic solar damage, arsenic exposure, immunodeficiencies, viral infections (human papillomavirus), therapeutic radiation and other ionising radiations have all been linked to the aetiology of Bowen's disease.

Clinical features and diagnosis

Bowen's disease appears as a gradually enlarging well-demarcated pink to red scaly macule or plaque (Figure 13.13). It can appear anywhere, but it usually occurs on the lower limbs in elderly patients. Lesions are generally asymptomatic in the absence of ulceration and can mimic an inflammatory dermatosis, though their fixed and static location may aid in diagnosis. The palms and soles can sometimes be affected, but this is rare.

Diagnosis is primarily on the basis of typical clinical features, but if suspicion exists, a skin biopsy is required to rule out an invasive malignancy. Differential diagnosis includes scaly macules of eczema, psoriasis, AK or superficial spreading BCC.

Key facts about Bowen's disease:

- Rare before 30 years of age.
- Peak incidence in the seventh decade.
- Multiple lesions in up to 20% of people.
- Predominantly occurs in women.
- 75% of patients have lesions on lower legs.

Histology

The epidermis is replaced with abnormal keratinocytes with disordered maturation and loss of polarity. Atypical mitotic figures

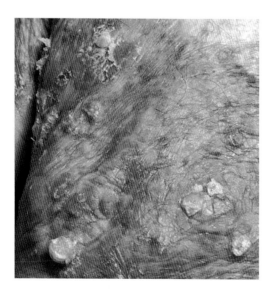

Figure 13.12 Actinic keratosis. © Medical Illustration Cardiff and Vale UHB.

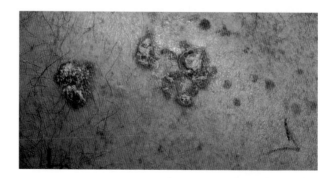

Figure 13.13 Bowen's disease. © Medical Illustration Cardiff and Vale UHB.

are characteristic. Similar changes extend deep into the pilose-baceous unit. A loss of granular layer with parakeratosis is typical. The basement membrane is intact.

Treatment

Commonly used treatment modalities are topical 5-fluorouracil or imiquimod cream, cryotherapy and curettage. Surgical excision and photodynamic therapy are other second-line therapies. In elderly patients with slowly progressive lesions, especially in areas of poor healing (e.g. lower limbs), observation rather than intervention may be appropriate.

Merkel cell carcinoma

Merkel cell carcinoma (MCC) is a rare, highly aggressive skin cancer with an incidence of 0.3–1.5 per 100,000 population, with higher rates in Australia. About one-third of patients die of the disease, thus it has a higher fatality rate than MM.

MCC was previously thought to be derived from Merkel cells (pressure receptors), but current theories include a possible derivation from a precursor of B-cell lymphocytes. Polyomavirus-causing gene mutations have been detected in 80% of patients with MCC. People at risk include elderly patients, the immuno-suppressed (e.g. organ transplant patients on long-term ciclosporin or azathioprine, or patients with haematological malignancies) and those with a history of other skin cancers. Virus-negative tumours have been associated with chronic UV radiation exposure.

Clinical features and diagnosis

MCC presents as a solitary red-to-violet papule or nodule on sun-exposed sites (head and neck). It is similar to BCC in appearance, but has more rapid growth (Figure 13.14). Lesions rarely ulcerate. Local (in transit metastasis) and regional lymph node involvement is present in 30% of patients at presentation. This has the potential for distal metastasis, and most recurrences happen within the first two years after diagnosis.

It is difficult to make a clinical diagnosis of MCC as the lesions are usually mistaken for BCC, amelanotic melanoma or metastatic cancer deposits. Strong suspicion is required, especially if the lesion is non-tender or expands rapidly, and in at-risk patients (Table 13.13). A biopsy is essential for diagnosis; immunochemistry can be helpful, as cytokeratin-20 is positive in 95% of MCCs.

Histology

Nodular or diffuse patterns of aggregated, deep-blue-stained, small basaloid cells in the dermis are seen, usually arranged in a trabeculated pattern. Membrane-bound neurosecretory granules and perinuclear whorls of intermediate filaments are structural hallmarks of MCC.

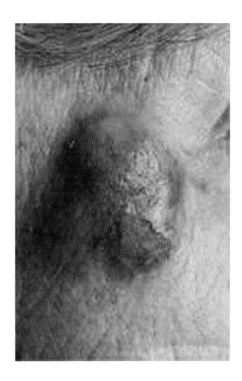

Figure 13.14 Merkel cell carcinoma. Chowdhury MMU *et al. Dermatology at a Glance*, 2nd edn. Chichester: Wiley, 2019.

Table 13.13 The acronym AEIOU is used to aid in diagnosis of Merkel cell carcinoma

Asymptomatic lesion
Expanding rapidly
Immunosuppressed patients
Over 50 years old
Ultraviolet exposed

Treatment

Once diagnosed, multidisciplinary input is required. Aggressive management may not always be possible, especially in frail patients.

- Wide local excision (1–2-cm margin) is usually indicated, with possible post-operative radiotherapy for large tumours > 1 cm, those with limited surgical margins and those located on the head and neck.
- MCCs are radiosensitive tumours and adjuvant radiotherapy has shown promising results in disease-free survival, especially in early-stage tumours.
- Despite the general agreement that patients without clinical nodal involvement may still harbour subclinical nodal metastases, the role of SLNB remains unclear.

- Staging CT is recommended, especially for patients with palpable lymphadenopathy or those with positive SLNB.
- Prophylactic lymph node dissection or irradiation is advocated for patients with positive SLNB and for patients with high risk of regional metastasis (e.g. due to previous recurrence), regardless of the SLNB status.
- For metastatic disease, the prognosis is usually poor and treatment is focused on improving quality of life. Radiotherapy and/or chemotherapy may be administered. Up to 50% response rates have been reported in patients on immunotherapy, for example pembrolizumab, avelumab and nivolumab (anti-programmed death 1 monoclonal antibodies). The five-year survival rates are 30–60% depending on the stage at diagnosis.

Follow-up

As most recurrences occur within the first two years, patients are usually seen every 3–6 months for two years, and then the frequency of follow-up is subsequently reduced. No further follow-up is required if the patient remains disease free at five years.

Primary cutaneous lymphoma

Primary cutaneous lymphomas can be broadly divided into two categories: cutaneous T-cell lymphomas (CTCLs) and cutaneous B-cell lymphomas (CBCLs).

Cutaneous T-cell lymphoma

CTCL is a group of diseases characterised by malignant monoclonal proliferation of T-cell lymphocytes in the skin, and it accounts for 65% of all lymphomas. There are several types of T-cell lymphomas (Table 13.14), with mycosis fungoides (MF) and Sézary syndrome (SS) being the most common variants, compromising around 50% of all CTCLs. Diagnosis can

be challenging, as often they mimic other common benign skin conditions such as eczema and psoriasis, and early histological changes may be subtle. It can take up to 10 years with multiple skin biopsies required to confirm the diagnosis in some patients.

The aetiology of CTCLs remains unclear, but the current hypothesis includes genetic, environmental and infectious causes.

Mycosis fungoides

The peak incidence of MF occurs in the fifth and sixth decades; it is more common in men than in women. MF has an indolent clinical course and usually presents with a red/brown scaly patch in non-sun-exposed areas. Patches may be atrophic, and patients may or may not complain of itch. These patches then slowly develop into discrete, well-demarcated plaques or tumours with an asymmetrical distribution (Figure 13.15).

Folliculotropic MF (affecting hair-bearing skin), pagetoid reticulosis (affecting the distal extremities) and granulomatous slack skin (affecting the intertriginous regions) are well-recognised subtypes of MF.

Sézary syndrome

SS is characterised by erythroderma, lymphadenopathy and Sézary cells (malignant T lymphocytes) in the blood and lymph nodes. SS may present *de novo* or arise from pre-existing MF. An absence of Sézary cells in the blood helps differentiate erythrodermic MF from SS. It tends to affect elderly White men more than other demographic groups. Patients present with a generalised, intensely red and pruritic exfoliative rash (Figure 13.16). The prognosis of SS is generally poor, with a median survival between 2 and 4 years.

Diagnosis

A clinically suspected diagnosis of CTCL should be confirmed by biopsy. Histological confirmation may require serial skin

---

Table 13.14 Types of cutaneous T-cell lymphoma (World Health Organization 2008 classification)

Indolent (slow growing/low grade) clinical behaviour	Aggressive clinical behaviour

- Mycosis fungoides (MF) and subtypes
  o Folliculotropic MF
  o Pagetoid reticulosis
  o Granulomatous slack skin
- CD30⁺ lymphoproliferative disorders
  o Primary cutaneous anaplastic large cell lymphoma
  o Lymphomatoid papulosis
- Subcutaneous panniculitis-like T-cell lymphoma (histiocytic cytophagic panniculitis)
- Primary cutaneous CD4⁺ small/medium pleomorphic T-cell lymphoma
	- Sézary syndrome
	- Adult T-cell leukaemia/lymphoma
	- Extranodal natural killer/T-cell lymphoma, nasal type; this is associated with Epstein–Barr virus
	- Primary cutaneous peripheral T-cell lymphoma, unspecified
	  o Primary cutaneous aggressive CD8⁺ T-cell lymphoma
	  o Cutaneous γ/δ T-cell lymphoma

(a) (b)

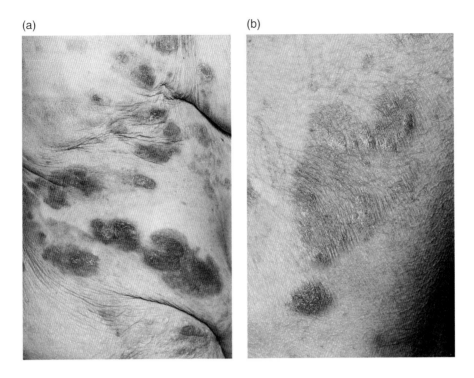

Figure 13.15 Mycosis fungoides. © Medical Illustration Cardiff and Vale UHB.

(a) (b)

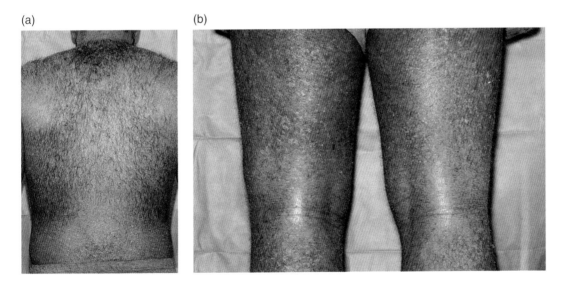

Figure 13.16 Sézary syndrome. © Medical Illustration Cardiff and Vale UHB.

biopsies, as early CTCL can be difficult to differentiate from other skin conditions, particularly eczema.

In challenging cases, immunohistochemistry and T-cell gene rearrangement studies can be helpful. MF immunohistochemistry usually shows a predominance of CD4+ T cells with fewer CD8+ cells. T-cell gene rearrangement studies demonstrate a clonal population of T cells in most cases, but often repeated investigations in individual patients may be needed to isolate or prove this.

Enlarged lymph nodes can be biopsied and blood films examined for Sézary cells.

Patients with advanced CTCL may need CT or magnetic resonance imaging scans to determine the extent of the spread.

Histology

In MF, the histopathology is characterised by infiltrates of malignant T cells, with irregular cerebriform nuclei. The clinical stages (patch, plaque, tumour) correlate with the progressive density of the malignant T cells.

In patch-stage MF there is a superficial lichenoid infiltrate, mainly lymphocytes and histiocytes and a few atypical cells infiltrating the epidermis without significant spongiosis. This stage may be very subtle and mimic other dermatoses such as eczema or lichenoid dermatoses.

Plaque and tumour-stage MF show a denser dermal infiltrate, and there may be intraepidermal collections of atypical cells (Pautrier micro-abscesses).

Treatment

This depends on the stage of the disease. For early-stage MF, general emollient therapy and topical steroids with or without phototherapy (ultraviolet B, PUVA) are usually enough to control the disease. However, MF runs a chronic course and may remit and relapse, so regular follow-up is essential.

For later stages, radiotherapy, immunotherapy, oral retinoids and chemotherapy could be considered. Extracorporeal photopheresis may be used for patients with SS and erythrodermic MF.

Cutaneous B-cell lymphoma

CBCL is a group of diseases characterised by the malignant proliferation of B-cell lymphocytes and accounts for 20% of all skin lymphomas. It generally affects patients in their sixth decade, but can affect children and young adults. It is rarely associated with *Borrelia* infection.

CBCLs are divided into:

- **Follicle centre lymphoma**: a solitary nodule or a cluster of lesions, usually on the scalp, forehead and back.
- **Marginal zone lymphoma**: a red/brown plaque, usually on the extremities or trunk.

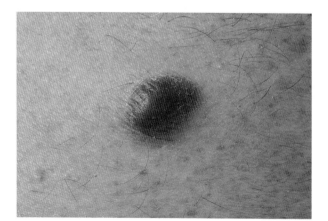

Figure 13.17 Diffuse large B-cell lymphoma. © Medical Illustration Cardiff and Vale UHB.

- **Diffuse large B-cell lymphoma**: usually on the lower legs of elderly women and often ulcerated (Figure 13.17).

There are other very rare types that do not fit into any of the above subtypes.

Diagnosis

As with any other lymphoma, the clinical suspicion should be confirmed by biopsy. Blood investigations including a blood film and T-cell rearrangement studies could be useful in detecting clonal B-cell proliferation. Histologically, CBCL shows a diffuse monotonous population of centroblasts and immunoblasts, but immunohistochemical tests are required to classify the exact type of CBCL.

Treatment

Patients with confirmed CBCL on biopsy should be referred to the haematologists for full assessment. Solitary nodules and localised disease can be treated with radiotherapy or surgery. For patients with more aggressive disease (e.g. diffuse B-cell lymphoma), treatment with chemotherapy or rituximab may be required.

Conclusions

Within just a few decades, skin cancer has become a major part of every dermatologist's workload. It is vital that all dermatologists are able to provide basic care for skin cancer and to recognise high-risk lesions. In addition, a significant proportion of the dermatology workforce needs to become specialists in this particular field, with skills in surgery and other advanced techniques and therapies.

Our goal should be early identification and treatment of all skin tumours, as well as leading efforts to prevent skin cancer. For patients with advanced and metastatic disease there have been great advances in targeted therapies for melanoma, BCC and SCC. Dermatologists will increasingly work with oncologists to deliver these new treatments, which may lead to a significant improvement in disease prognosis especially for patients with advanced skin cancer.

Pearls and pitfalls

- Be aware that early amelanotic melanoma can appear as a featureless pink macule or plaque; if the diagnosis is in doubt, always biopsy.
- Patients with *in situ* melanomas should be reassured once excision is complete, and they do not require regular follow-up.

- When assessing a possible BCC, it is very helpful to wet the surface of the tumour with an alcohol wipe and to use oblique lighting to highlight the pearly edges of the lesion.
- Ulcerated tumours carry a high risk of wound infection; use pre-operative antibiotics for 5–7 days starting on the day of surgery.
- Take care when taking a biopsy for a possible BCC at a critical site; do not remove the entire lesion, as subsequent treatment will be difficult if no residual tumour is visible after the biopsy.
- SCCs grow rapidly and are usually tender compared to other benign warty lesions, especially in transplant or immunosuppressed patients.
- MF can be very challenging to diagnose; multiple skin biopsies may be necessary and the diagnosis should be suspected in patients with chronic skin complaints, such as eczema or psoriasis, that appear unresponsive to conventional therapy.
- In patients with erythroderma unresponsive to conventional therapies, look for Sézary cells in the blood.

SCE Questions. See questions 18–20.

FURTHER READING AND KEY RESOURCES

Garcia-Carbonero R, Marquez-Rodas I, de la Cruz-Merino L et al. Recent therapeutic advances and change in treatment paradigm of patients with Merkel cell carcinoma. *Oncologist* 2019; **24**:1375–83.

Karunaratne YG, Gunaratne DA, Veness MJ. Systematic review of sentinel lymph node biopsy in Merkel cell carcinoma of the head and neck. *Head Neck* 2018; **40**:2704–13.

Keohane SG, Botting J, Budny PG et al. British Association of Dermatologists guidelines for the management of people with cutaneous squamous cell carcinoma 2020. *Br J Dermatol* 2021; **184**:401–14.

Keohane SG, Proby CM, Newlands C et al. The new 8th edition of TNM staging and its implications for skin cancer: a review by the British Association of Dermatologists and the Royal College of Pathologists, U.K. *Br J Dermatol* 2018; **179**:824–8.

Keung EZ, Gershenwald JE. The eighth edition American Joint Committee on Cancer (AJCC) melanoma staging system: implications for melanoma treatment and care. *Expert Rev Anticancer Ther* 2018; **18**:775–84.

Michielin O, van Akkooi ACJ, Ascierto PA et al. Cutaneous melanoma: ESMO Clinical Practice Guidelines for diagnosis, treatment and follow-up. *Ann Oncol* 2019; **30**:1884–901.

Nasr I, McGrath EJ, Harwood CA et al. British Association of Dermatologists guidelines for the management of adults with basal cell carcinoma 2021. *Br J Dermatol* 2021; in press; doi: 10.1111/bjd.20524.

Radu O, Pantanowitz L. Kaposi sarcoma. *Arch Pathol Lab Med* 2013; **137**:289–94.

Rubin AI, Chen EH, Ratner D. Basal-cell carcinoma. *N Engl J Med* 2005; **353**:2262–9.

Textbook

Creamer D, Baker J, Kerdel FA, eds. *Acute Adult Dermatology: Diagnosis and Management*. Boca Raton, FL: CRC Press, 2011.

14

Dermatology for skin of colour

Sharon A. Belmo

Introduction

Skin of colour describes individuals with darker skin tones than White Europeans and includes those of African, Asian, Middle Eastern or Hispanic/Latin descent. In addition, inter-racial mixing should be taken into account.

Biological differences in the structure and function of the skin exist among racial groups. There are also conditions that are unique, more prevalent or clinically variable in darker skin. Additionally, there are cultural beliefs and habits among certain ethnic groups that may impact the skin and hair, for example hair grooming practices, hair coverings, traditional Chinese medicine, homeopathy and Ayurvedic medicine.

The demographics of the UK are rapidly diversifying. It is therefore important that dermatologists become confident and competent in diagnosing and managing dermatological conditions in skin of colour. In this chapter, several aspects of dermatology pertaining to skin of colour will be discussed.

Structure and function of skin of colour

Skin colour is determined mainly by the presence of melanin, a photoprotective pigment, produced by melanocytes and packaged into melanosomes. There are two types of melanin in the skin: eumelanin, a brown-black colour, and phaeomelanin, a

Dermatology Training: The Essentials. Edited by Mahbub M.U. Chowdhury, Tamara W. Griffiths and Andrew Y. Finlay.
© 2022 The British Association of Dermatologists. Published 2022 by John Wiley & Sons Ltd.
Companion website: www.wiley.com/go/chowdhury/dermatologytraining

yellow-red pigment. Darker skin possesses more eumelanin than phaeomelanin, whereas the reverse is true for those with lighter skin. The number of melanocytes is equal among all races; however, melanin production, as determined by melanocyte activity, is higher in darker skin. The characteristics of melanosomes vary with skin tone. Broadly speaking, melanosomes in light-skinned individuals are small, clustered and confined to the stratum basale and are broken down more quickly in the stratum spinosum. Melanosomes in darker-skinned individuals tend to be larger and non-aggregated, present throughout the epidermis and broken down more slowly. They also remain in the stratum corneum for longer. Variations are observed among intermediate skin tones within different racial groups.

The thickness of the stratum corneum has been shown to be similar in black and white skin, but it is more compact and cohesive in black skin. Ceramide levels are lower in black skin than in Asian and white skin, both of which exhibit similar levels. This has implications for dry skin in black or richly pigmented skin tones.

Racial differences in the dermis have also been demonstrated. In comparison to white skin, the dermis in black skin is thicker and more compact, displays less elastosis and has higher quantities of fibroblasts that are also larger and multinucleated or binucleated. Furthermore, collagen fibre bundles have been shown to be smaller and more closely packed than in white skin.

The aforementioned biological and structural differences observed in skin of colour are likely to be linked with reduced rates of skin cancer and slower ageing. Paradoxically, they may contribute to increased susceptibility to keloids and pigmentary disorders.

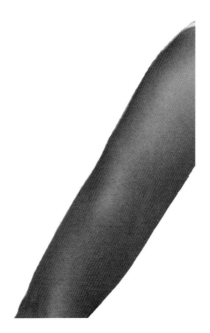

Figure 14.1 Futcher's line on the arm. © Dr Sharon Belmo.

Normal variants in skin of colour

Pigmentary demarcation lines

Pigmentary demarcation lines represent abrupt areas of transition between light and dark pigmentation of the skin. They are thought to be due to mosaicism. They are most commonly reported in Black and Japanese individuals, with a female sex predilection. Six variants of pigmentary demarcation lines have been described, corresponding to different parts of the body. Type A, Futcher's lines (also known as Voigt's lines), are the most common and represent abrupt linear demarcations on the flexor surface of the upper arm (Figure 14.1). In Black children, hairlines occurring in a similar pattern as Futcher's lines may be observed in the pre-auricular region (Figure 14.2).

Palmoplantar hyperpigmentation

It is not uncommon to find hyperpigmented macules on the palms and soles of Black adults, particularly those with darker skin tones (Figure 14.3).

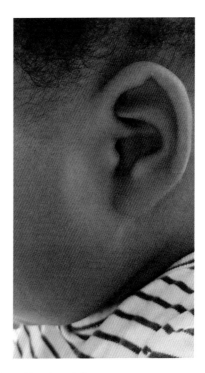

Figure 14.2 Hairline in an infant. © Dr Sharon Belmo.

Mucous membrane hyperpigmentation

Mucous membrane pigmentation is common in skin of colour and may affect the lips, gums, buccal mucosa and conjunctiva. People of colour are also prone to developing post-inflammatory hyperpigmentation (PIH) of the oral cavity.

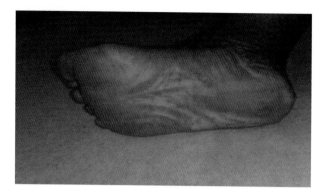

Figure 14.3 Hyperpigmentation of the sole. © Dr Sharon Belmo.

Longitudinal melanonychia

Longitudinal melanonychia is a very common pattern of pigmented bands on the nails in people of colour, particularly Black and Japanese. The incidence increases with age; nearly all Black people over the age of 50 years will have this. It typically presents on the central or lateral aspects of the nail (Figure 14.4). There may be several bands on one nail and they tend to be darker in those with darker skin.

Idiopathic guttate hypomelanosis

Idiopathic guttate hypomelanosis is a common benign acquired disorder seen in all races. It is characterised by small, sharply defined white asymptomatic macules on the arms and legs and so is more striking in skin of colour (Figure 14.5). It may therefore be of cosmetic concern. It is frequently seen in the elderly

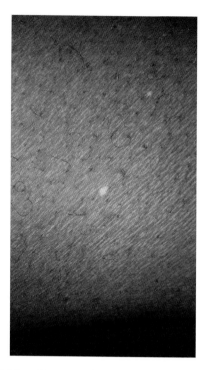

Figure 14.5 Idiopathic guttate hypomelanosis. © Dr Sharon Belmo.

and has no relation to vitiligo or other pigmentary disorders. The cause is unclear, but factors such as skin ageing, ultraviolet radiation, trauma and genetic predisposition have been proposed. No treatment is required and reassurance is key.

Presentation of common dermatoses in skin of colour

Common dermatological disorders may vary in appearance in skin of colour for a number of reasons (Table 14.1). Due to background pigmentation, redness associated with inflammation may be less visible. Alternatively, inflammation may present as shades of purple, red-brown, grey, brown or very dark brown-black. It is important to retrain the eye to assess redness in darker skin. Comparing involved skin to uninvolved skin can be helpful, as can additional clues such as oedema, itching or tenderness.

Lability of melanin during or after inflammatory processes can result in marked pigmentary changes. Additionally, there is a predisposition to develop distinctive cutaneous reaction patterns to common dermatoses, in comparison to white skin. These include the following patterns:

- Follicular
- Annular
- Papular
- Granulomatous
- Keloidal
- Ulcerative

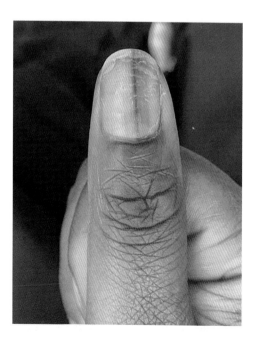

Figure 14.4 Longitudinal melanonychia. © Dr Sharon Belmo.

Table 14.1 Comparison of common dermatological conditions

Condition	White skin	Skin of colour
Inflammation	Pink, red	No colour change, pink, red, purple, grey, brown, dark brown or black
Eczema	Mainly flexural in children	Commonly extensor in children
		Discoid, papular and follicular patterns common
		Lichenification common
		Post-inflammatory hypo- and hyperpigmentation common
Psoriasis	Salmon-pink plaques with silvery scale	Pink, violaceous, hypopigmented or hyperpigmented plaques
		Post-inflammatory hypo- and hyperpigmentation common
Lichen planus	Violaceous papules and plaques	Violaceous, grey, dark brown or black papules or plaques
		Post-inflammatory hyperpigmentation very common
		Hypertrophic plaques common
		Variants such as lichen planus pigmentosus more common
Acne	Post-inflammatory redness common	Post-inflammatory hyperpigmentation common
	Cystic acne more common	Keloid scarring more common
		Pomade acne more common
Seborrhoeic dermatitis	Salmon-pink scaly patches	Pink or hypopigmented scaly patches
		Petaloid variant more common
		Hypopigmentation more common

Eczema

Higher incidences of eczema have been reported in Black and Asian ethnic groups in comparison to their White counterparts. Children of African heritage are also twice as likely to experience severe disease than children of European heritage.

The distribution of eczema in skin of colour may differ from that seen in white skin. For example, eczema affecting the extensor surfaces is observed in children of colour. This is rarely seen in White children, who tend to present with flexural eczema. Discoid, papular and follicular patterns are common in skin of colour. Follicular eczema (1–3-mm papules in eczema-prone sites) may present in the absence of more typical signs of eczema (Figure 14.6a–c). It is important to be aware of these clinical variants to avoid unnecessary biopsies and delays in treatment. Lichenification and nodular prurigo are more common in individuals of African descent. Individuals of East Asian descent may be more prone to having psoriasiform eczema (Figure 14.6d, e).

Post-inflammatory hypo- and hyperpigmentation are common sequelae and may persist for several months. This can cause significant distress, and in some individuals it may be more concerning than the active eczema. It is important that this too is acknowledged and treated where possible.

Psoriasis

Psoriasis affects all races. However, it is less prevalent in skin of colour (Black 1.9%, Hispanic 1.6%, others 1.4%) in comparison to white skin (3.6%). Psoriasis is reported to be more severe with a greater psychosocial impact in African Americans than in White individuals. However, epidemiological data for non-White populations is limited.

Psoriasis may present differently in darker skin. The 'classic' salmon-pink plaques with overlying silver scale might rather appear violaceous, grey, hypopigmented or hyperpigmented (Figure 14.7). Plaques may also be more hypertrophic. Post-inflammatory hyper- or hypopigmentation can be problematic and cause marked psychosocial burden. The earlier that psoriasis is diagnosed and treated, the lower the extent of dyspigmentation that will follow. Irrespective of skin type, psoriasis has the same pattern of presentation. This should aid diagnosis in skin of colour. Treatment is the same for all skin types. Phototherapy is safe and effective in skin of colour.

For scalp psoriasis, be mindful when prescribing treatments in women with afro-textured hair, who, due to the dry and fragile nature of the hair, should wash their hair weekly rather than daily. Some women may have specific preferences for vehicle of treatment; for example, those with

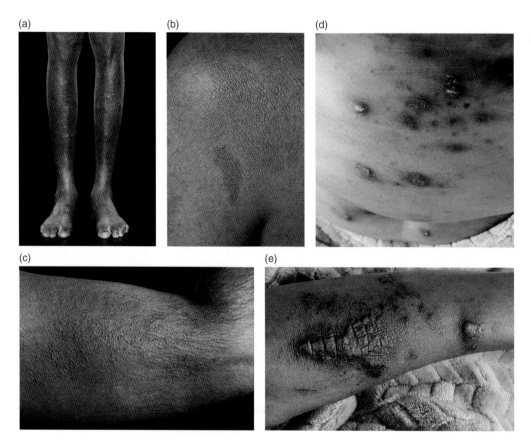

Figure 14.6 (a) Acute severe eczema on the legs. (b) Papular eczema on the shoulder. (c) Papular eczema on the arm. © Medical Illustration Cardiff and Vale UHB. (d) Nodular prurigo on the abdomen. (e) Lichenification on the arm. © Croydon University Hospital.

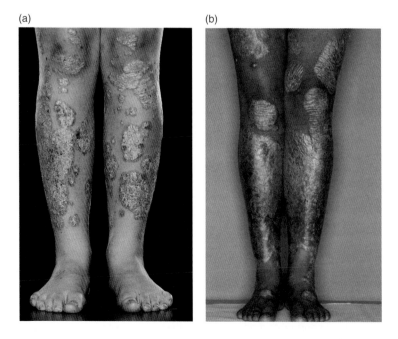

Figure 14.7 Psoriasis on the lower legs. (a) © Medical Illustration Cardiff and Vale UHB. (b) Griffiths CEM *et al.* Psoriasis. *Lancet* 2021; **397**:1301–15.

chemically straightened hair are not likely to want to use water-based scalp treatments.

Ointments and pomades are more likely to be welcomed in those with afro-textured hair than in those with straight hair. Open discussions and clear instructions prior to prescribing treatments might result in better adherence.

Seborrhoeic dermatitis

Seborrhoeic dermatitis is prevalent in Black women and may even be considered normal by some patients. There may be an increased incidence. Inappropriate use of oils and pomades on the scalp and infrequent hair washing may contribute. In skin of colour, particularly in those with darker skin, hypopigmentation is prominent, with hypopigmented (rather than pink to red) scaly patches occurring at the typical sites (Figure 14.8). A subtype known as petaloid seborrhoeic dermatitis may also been seen in individuals of colour. This is characterised by pink or hypopigmented petal-shaped patches on the face and hairline. Children with skin of colour may not present with cradle cap as seen in White children, and more often present with flaking, hypopigmentation and/or redness.

Treatment of seborrhoeic dermatitis is the same for all skin types but, as for scalp psoriasis, particular attention and care must be taken where afro-textured hair is concerned. Ketoconazole and other anti-dandruff shampoos are extremely drying to afro-textured hair and should preferably not be used more than once weekly. Such patients must also be advised against applying oils and pomades directly to the scalp, as this can result in product build-up and further scalp irritation.

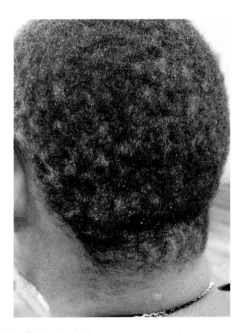

Figure 14.8 Seborrhoeic dermatitis on the scalp. © Dr Sharon Belmo.

Vitiligo

Vitiligo is a chronic acquired depigmenting disorder of the skin. It occurs in all racial groups, but is more striking in appearance in skin of colour. As a result, it is often associated with cultural stigmatism, profound psychosocial distress and low self-esteem. The exact prevalence is unknown, but it is in the range of 0–2.2%, with one-third to one-half of cases presenting in childhood. The highest incidence rates have been reported in India, but worldwide incidence reporting is variable. Vitiligo is likely to affect males and females equally, although some studies have reported a slight preponderance in younger females.

The cause of vitiligo is poorly understood, but it is felt to be a multifactorial autoimmune disorder that presents in genetically susceptible people. It is particularly associated with autoimmune thyroid disease, as well as other autoimmune diseases such as pernicious anaemia, Addison's disease, systemic lupus erythematosus, inflammatory bowel disease, rheumatoid arthritis and type 1 diabetes mellitus.

Clinical features

Vitiligo presents as distinct patches of complete pigment loss. It commonly affects the face, neck and eyelids (Figure 14.9), flexures, fingertips, lips and genitalia. The hair and eyes might also be affected. Vitiligo displays the Koebner phenomenon, whereby areas of depigmentation appear in areas of trauma. It may also occasionally start as multiple halo naevi. It runs a very unpredictable course that varies from person to person. Vitiligo has been classified into four main groups (Table 14.2).

Management

Treatment of vitiligo is largely unsatisfactory, with high rates of recurrence. It is important that cultural implications are taken into consideration, patient expectations are managed and psychological support is offered where possible.

The following treatment options may be used with varying levels of success:

- Cosmetic camouflage
- Photoprotection
- Topical steroids
- Topical calcineurin inhibitors
- Topical vitamin D analogues
- Phototherapy
- Depigmentation (of normal skin)
- Surgical therapies

Lichen planus

Lichen planus does not have any racial predilection. The characteristic papules and plaques are classically described as purple or violaceous. In skin of colour, the lesions may appear purple, but can also appear grey, brown, dark brown or black. PIH is common and often more troublesome. Hypertrophic lichen planus is considered to be more common (Figure 14.10a).

(a)

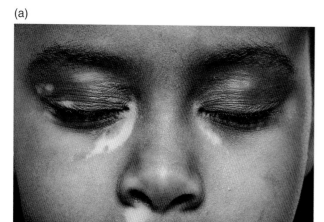

(b)

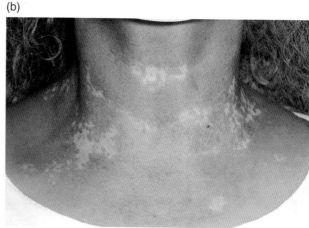

Figure 14.9 Vitiligo on (a) the face and (b) the neck. © Medical Illustration Cardiff and Vale UHB.

Table 14.2 Classification of vitiligo

Classification	Subtype
Non-segmental vitiligo	Focal, mucosal, acrofacial, generalised, universal
Segmental vitiligo	Focal, mucosal, unisegmental, bi- or multisegmental
Mixed vitiligo	Non-segmental and segmental vitiligo
Unclassified vitiligo	Focal at onset, multifocal, asymmetrical non-segmental, unifocal mucosal

Wickham's striae of the buccal mucosa are usually more striking in those with darker skin.

Lichen planus actinicus is a variant of lichen planus that is more common in those of Middle Eastern, African and Asian descent. It is characterised by a photodistributed lichenoid eruption. Unlike in classic lichen planus, pruritus, nail involvement and Koebnerisation are uncommon.

Lichen planus pigmentosus is a pigmented variant of lichen planus that is also more common in skin of colour (Figure 14.10b). It is characterised by greyish to dark brown/black patches on sun-exposed sites or flexures.

Treatment of lichen planus is the same for all skin types.

Acne

Acne is common in all skin types. However, there are unique presentations and treatment needs in patients of colour. Rates of nodulocystic acne are reportedly lower in Black patients than in those of other races.

Pomade acne, presenting as widespread comedones on the forehead and temples, is observed in some Black people as a result of the use of comedogenic skin and hair products (Figure 14.11). Keloids are long-term sequelae of acne in skin of colour.

Hyperpigmentation may be the only obvious presenting feature of acne in skin of colour. You are likely to have a dissatisfied patient if this is dismissed as PIH with no treatment. Palpation of the skin will often reveal underlying papules. In skin of colour, subclinical inflammation has been observed histologically in simple comedones and perilesional skin. This is likely to contribute to both peri- and post-inflammatory hyperpigmentation. Studies have shown that for non-White women, clearance of PIH is more important than actual lesion clearance.

The treatment of acne is the same for all skin types, but particular attention must be paid to hyperpigmentation in skin of colour. This should ideally be managed concurrently with active acne with products that are effective at treating both, such as topical retinoids and azelaic acid. Persistent PIH may warrant hydroquinone preparations. Care must be taken to avoid iatrogenic dyspigmentation as a result of irritating topicals. Slowly building up use of the products mentioned previously while buffering with a non-comedogenic moisturiser may improve tolerance, minimise irritation and prevent further hyperpigmentation. Patients should also be advised to use sunscreen.

Rosacea

Although the prevalence of rosacea in skin of colour is lower than in those with lighter skin, it does occur, and is most probably underdiagnosed. The granulomatous variant has been predominantly reported in Black individuals. The masking of redness and telangiectasia by epidermal melanin poses a challenge in diagnosing rosacea (Figure 14.12). Other features such as papules, pustules or oedema should be sought. Examining in good lighting or using a dark contrasting background can also be helpful. Cultural sensitivity should be demonstrated when counselling patients of colour with respect to sunscreen use,

(a)

(b)

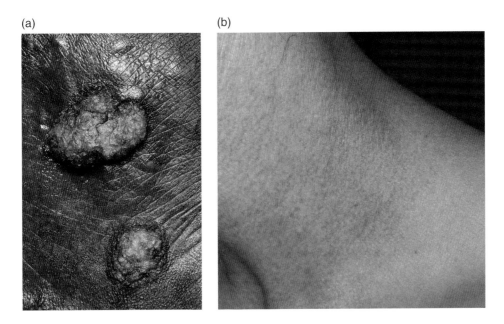

Figure 14.10 (a) Hypertrophic lichen planus on the leg. © Medical Illustration Cardiff and Vale UHB. (b) Lichen planus pigmentosus on the neck. Vashi NA, Kundu RV. Facial hyperpigmentation: causes and treatment. *Br J Dermatol* 2013; **169**:41–56.

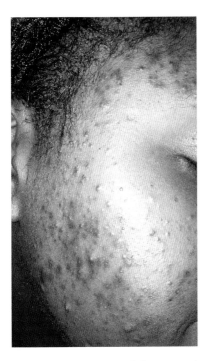

Figure 14.11 Acne with peri- and post-inflammatory hyperpigmentation. © Dr Sharon Belmo.

spicy food intake and use of potentially irritating skin-lightening creams. Treatment is the same for all skin types; however, caution should be exercised if laser is to be used due to the very high risk of dyspigmentation.

Skin cancer and skin of colour

The annual incidence in the USA of melanoma and non-melanoma skin cancer is approximately 5 per 100,000 in Hispanic and 2 per 100,000 in Asian and African American individuals, compared to an incidence of 31 per 100,000 in White populations. There is a paucity of data for the UK. Despite the lower incidence, mortality among Black patients is disproportionately high. Reasons for the poorer prognosis are likely to include delays in diagnosis, more advanced disease at presentation, lack of diversity in skin cancer public health campaigns, and misconceptions among both patients and clinicians about the occurrence of skin cancer in skin of colour. Delayed diagnoses may occur as a result of unfamiliarity with variation in presentation of skin cancer in skin of colour.

Squamous cell carcinoma

Squamous cell carcinoma (SCC) is the most common skin cancer in Black and Indian populations and the second most common skin cancer in White, East Asian and Hispanic groups. The majority of SCCs in skin of colour develop on sun-protected sites, as opposed to sun-exposed sites in white skin. They typically present as pink to red patches, plaques or nodules, but may vary in appearance. SCCs tend to develop in the setting of chronic inflammation, chronic scarring, burns, leg ulcers, chronic discoid lupus erythematosus, albinism and human papillomavirus. Common sites include the lower legs and anogenital region. SCCs in Black patients are potentially more aggressive with a poorer prognosis. It is therefore important that they are diagnosed and treated early.

(a) (b)

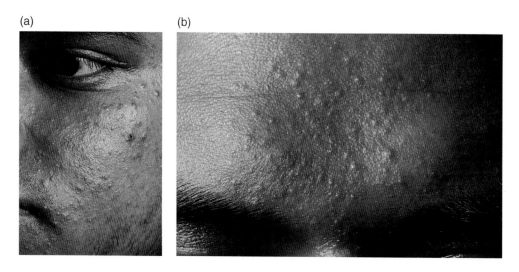

Figure 14.12 Rosacea on (a) the cheek and (b) the forehead. © Medical Illustration Cardiff and Vale UHB.

(a) (b)

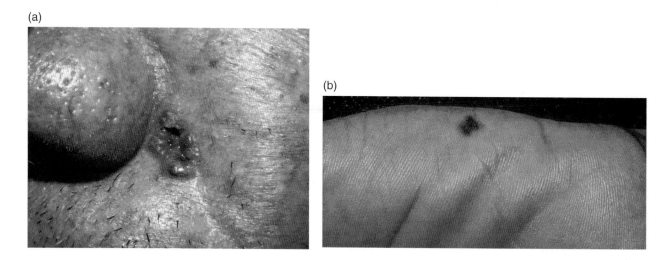

Figure 14.13 (a) Pigmented basal cell carcinoma. © Waikato District Health Board. (b) Acral melanoma. Gohara M. Skin cancer: an African perspective. *Br J Dermatol* 2015; **173**:17–21.

Basal cell carcinoma

Basal cell carcinoma (BCC) is the second most common skin cancer in Black individuals and those from the Indian subcontinent, and the most common skin cancer in White, Hispanic, Chinese vand Japanese populations. Unlike for SCC and melanoma, ultraviolet radiation plays a significant role in the development of BCC in skin of colour. The head and neck region is the most common site in all racial groups. BCCs can also occur in unusual or sun-protected sites. BCCs in skin of colour are often pigmented and have been described as having a 'black pearly' appearance in East Asian skin (Figure 14.13a). Telangiectasiae and the pearly rolled border can be difficult to discern in dark skin. As a result, they are often misdiagnosed as seborrhoeic keratoses or even melanoma.

In contrast to SCC, BCC is not associated with an increased morbidity in Black people.

Melanoma

In comparison to White patients, people of colour with melanoma are more likely to die. The five-year survival rate among Black patients is the lowest at 72.2%, in comparison to 80.2% in Asian and 89.9% in White patients. Melanoma in skin of colour more commonly presents on non-sun-exposed sites such as the palms, soles, mucous membranes and subungual region. Acral lentiginous melanoma is the most common subtype in Black and Asian patients (Figure 14.13b and Figure 13.2). There is a lack of evidence to confirm that ultraviolet radiation is a risk factor for melanoma in skin of colour.

Conditions more common in skin of colour

Traction alopecia

Traction alopecia (TA) is hair loss and thinning due to repetitive or prolonged tension to the hair (Figure 14.14). It is an important and common cause of alopecia in women and girls of African descent due to hair grooming practices and the inherent fragility of afro-textured hair. It can also occur in other ethnic groups. History taking is very important when TA is suspected, and women should be specifically asked about their hair grooming practices. Patients may give a history of having sore papules or pustules on their scalp directly after having certain hairstyles installed such as braids or weaves.

Clinical features

Marginal TA is the most common type and is seen on the fronto-temporal hairline. There is often a strip of retained hairs along the hairline known as the fringe sign. Non-marginal or patchy TA can also occur, where the hair loss is observed in different areas on the scalp, for example due to hair clips. TA is initially non-scarring, but if the traction forces are chronic, the hair loss progresses and becomes scarring.

Differential diagnoses of TA include frontal fibrosing alopecia (FFA), ophiasis (involving the occipital and lateral scalp), alopecia areata, androgenetic alopecia and telogen effluvium. FFA is likely to be underdiagnosed in women of colour and may be diagnosed mistakenly as TA. Of course, bear in mind that these diagnoses may coexist.

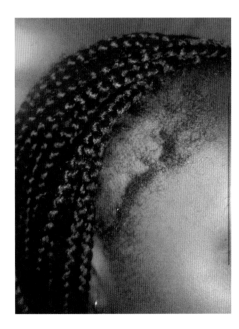

Figure 14.14 Traction alopecia. © Dr Sharon Belmo.

Management

Preventing TA is worthwhile as it is reversible at early stages of progression. Hairstyling advice should be given; for example, keeping hairstyles loose, avoiding tight or painful braids or weaves, and being careful with religious hair coverings that may rub on the hairline.

Treatment is aimed at suppressing the inflammation seen at early stages and may consist of topical or intralesional steroids at the periphery of the hair loss, topical or oral antibiotics, and topical minoxidil. In the case of scarring disease, hair transplantation is an option.

Central centrifugal cicatricial alopecia

Central centrifugal cicatricial alopecia (CCCA), previously known as hot comb alopecia, is a lymphocytic primary cicatricial alopecia that most commonly affects women of African descent (Figure 14.15). It is the most common cause of scarring alopecia in Black women, but has also been reported in men.

The aetiology of CCCA is likely to be multifactorial. It is very clear that it is not caused by the hot comb, although modern hairstyling practices may be implicated. An autosomal pattern of inheritance has been reported in families affected by CCCA in South Africa. *PADI3* gene mutations have recently been identified in CCCA-affected scalp biopsies. Critical genes implicated in fibroproliferative disorders such as fibroids and keloids have been shown to be upregulated in CCCA-affected scalp tissue. It is clear that ongoing research is required.

Clinical features

CCCA presents with scarring hair loss of the crown, with peripheral spread, usually sparing the lateral and posterior scalp. Patchy cases have also been reported. It may be associated with burning, itching and soreness, but can be asymptomatic or present with

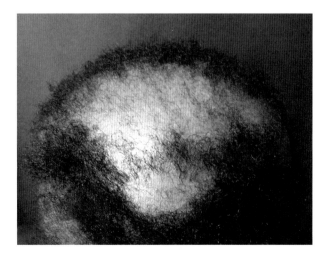

Figure 14.15 Central cicatricial centrifugal alopecia. Source: DermNet New Zealand Trust.

broken hairs on the crown. Differential diagnoses include female pattern hair loss and lichen planopilaris (Chapter 27).

Management

As with most scarring alopecias, early diagnosis of CCCA is crucial. Treatment is aimed at suppressing inflammation and stopping the scarring process, thus preventing further hair loss. Treatment usually involves a combination of daily topical steroids or calcineurin inhibitors, and 4–6-weekly intralesional steroids, applied to the periphery of hair loss. Doxycycline may also be used for its anti-inflammatory action. In more refractory cases, systemics such as hydroxychloroquine, mycophenolate mofetil or ciclosporin may be required to halt the inflammation. Minoxidil can also be helpful in some cases.

Pseudofolliculitis barbae

Pseudofolliculitis barbae, also known as 'razor bumps', is a chronic inflammatory disorder affecting the beard area. It is caused by a foreign-body reaction to ingrown shaved hairs, resulting in follicular and perifollicular inflammation. Due to the curly nature of afro-textured hair, it is most common in Black men (or women), but can occur in other races. Pseudofolliculitis barbae can also develop in other sites bearing curly hair where skin is regularly shaved, such as the axillae or pubic region.

Clinical features

Pseudofolliculitis barbae is characterised by the presence of inflammatory papules and pustules in shaved parts of the beard area (Figure 14.16). They tend to occur a few days after close shaving. PIH and hypertrophic and keloid scarring may occur. The condition can cause significant psychosocial burden among those affected. They may look to self-treat by purchasing over-the-counter products, which often contain salicylic acid.

Management

Cessation of shaving will abate symptoms after approximately three months, but for various reasons this may not be acceptable. Shaving practice recommendations can be helpful in this condition (Table 14.3).

Medical treatments include topical steroids, antibiotics and benzoyl peroxide as monotherapy or in combination. These aim to reduce inflammation, colonisation and secondary infection. For severe disease, or in the presence of pustules, oral antibiotics such as tetracyclines should be used. Intralesional steroids may be used to treat both inflammation and keloids. Hypopigmentation is a risk in darker skin. Topical retinoids, glycolic acid or salicylic acid peels can be used to reduce hyperkeratosis. PIH can be concerning and should also be managed (see page 194).

Alternative methods of hair removal include chemical depilatories and electrolysis. Chemical depilatories have the potential to cause irritant dermatitis and are therefore not widely used. Electrolysis is expensive, painful and often unsuccessful. For those who fail more conservative treatment, the only definitive cure for

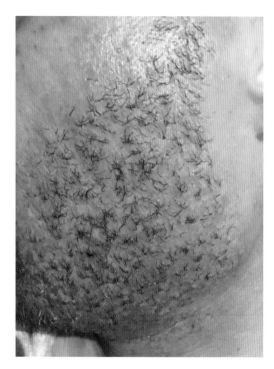

Figure 14.16 Pseudofolliculitis barbae. © Dr Sharon Belmo.

Table 14.3 Shaving recommendations for pseudofolliculitis barbae

Wash beard area with warm water prior to shaving
Release ingrown hairs using a sterile needle before shaving (optional)
Avoid shaving with a razor, particularly blunt razors
Shave with an electric clipper leaving 1 mm of hair behind
Avoid pulling or stretching skin when shaving
Avoid dry shaving
Shave in the direction of hair growth
Apply a therapeutic agent as aftershave, e.g. topical retinoid or antibiotic

pseudofolliculitis barbae is laser hair removal. Care must be taken when utilising lasers in skin of colour. The long-pulsed 1064 nm Nd:YAG has been shown to have the lowest incidence of adverse effects associated with laser hair removal in darker skin.

Folliculitis keloidalis

Folliculitis keloidalis (synonymous with acne keloidalis nuchae and folliculitis keloidalis nuchae) is a chronic and progressive folliculitis that leads to a scarring alopecia. The term acne keloidalis nuchae is misleading, as there is no acne, the lesions formed are not true keloids and the condition can affect more than the nuchal region.

Folliculitis keloidalis most commonly affects Black men after puberty, although it can be seen in White individuals. There is a male-to-female preponderance of 20:1. The exact cause remains unknown. Suggested risk factors include mechanical irritation from shirt collars, low-grade folliculitis, having afro-textured hair, and associated hair cutting practices. It has been postulated that folliculitis keloidalis occurs as a result of an aberrant immune reaction that results in scarring hair loss.

Clinical features

Folliculitis keloidalis is characterised by firm follicular and perifollicular papules on the occiput or posterior neck that coalesce to form keloidal plaques (Figure 14.17a, b). Keloidal plaques can grow to up to 10 cm in diameter and can be very disfiguring (Figure 14.17c). Alopecia, polytrichia (tufted hairs) and pruritus are common associations. Comedones are not present.

Complications such as secondary infections, abscesses and sinus formation may occur.

Management

Preventative measures are imperative. Patients should be advised to avoid mechanical irritation (very close or bald haircuts, tight-fitting collared shirts, razors or electric clippers at the posterior hairline). They can also wash with antimicrobial soaps to prevent secondary infection.

There is no single cure for folliculitis keloidalis. A combination of treatments is more likely to be effective, such as topical and/or intralesional steroids and topical retinoids. Topical antibiotics may be used in the presence of pustules or infection. If there is no improvement, swabs should be taken and appropriate oral antibiotics should be given according to sensitivities. A combination of oral antibiotics and steroids may be required for abscesses or draining sinuses.

For extensive or end-stage disease, lesions can be surgically excised and closed primarily. The base of the excision should

(a)

(b)

(c)

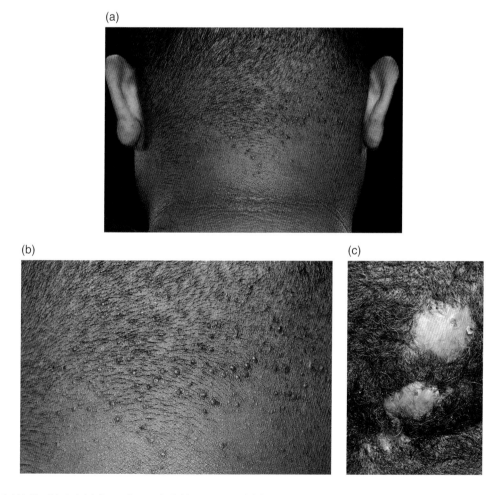

Figure 14.17 (a) Folliculitis keloidalis on the neck; (b) in close-up. (c) Folliculitis keloidalis with large plaques on the scalp. © Medical Illustration Cardiff and Vale UHB.

extend below the hair follicles. Larger lesions should be excised in multiple stages and can be left to heal by second intention. Other treatment options include lasers (CO_2, Nd:YAG 1064 nm, long-pulse diode) and cryotherapy.

Keloids

Keloid scars develop due to an exuberant or exaggerated wound healing response, commonly seen as a consequence of trauma or cutaneous inflammation such as acne. The trauma preceding the keloid may be negligible, giving the impression that the scars have occurred spontaneously. They may appear weeks to months after the original insult. Keloids can occur in all races, but individuals with darker skin are more susceptible. Prevalence rates of up to 16% have been reported in those of African, Asian and Hispanic descent. The risk is highest among Black populations, with incidences 5–16 times higher than in White people. Keloids are seen more commonly in adolescents and young adults and can be associated with significant disfigurement and psychosocial burden.

The pathogenesis of keloid scarring remains unclear. Several factors are implicated, including genetics, and fibroblast and keratinocyte activity. It is felt that melanocytes may have an effect on keloid formation, as suggested by the higher prevalence in darker skin and absence in melanocyte-poor sites such as palms and soles.

Clinical features

Keloids are characterised by smooth, firm, red, skin-coloured or hyperpigmented papules, plaques or nodules (Figure 14.18). In contrast to hypertrophic scars, keloids extend beyond the wound margin, do not regress spontaneously and may become more indurated and hypopigmented with time. Patients often complain of pain and itch. They most commonly present on the head, neck, ears, upper chest and arms, but can present anywhere. Differential diagnoses in skin of colour include hypertrophic scars, dermatofibroma, sarcoidosis and dermatofibrosarcoma protuberans.

Keloid scars versus hypertrophic scars

Hypertrophic scars vary from raised red to hyperpigmented scars that arise after trauma. They occur in all skin types and may be hard to distinguish from keloid scars. Taking a good history is helpful. Table 14.4 outlines the differences between these two types of scars.

Table 14.4 Comparison of keloid and hypertrophic scars

Keloid scar	Hypertrophic scar
Associated with darker skin	Associated with all skin types
Strong familial tendency	Not commonly familial
Preceding injury not always obvious	Always results from injury
Delayed onset (up to one year or more)	Immediate onset (less than three months)
Extends beyond wound margin	Confined to wound margin
Very rarely resolves spontaneously	Usually spontaneously resolves
Poor response to treatment	Good response to treatment
Painful, itchy	Usually asymptomatic

(a)

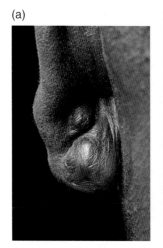

(b)

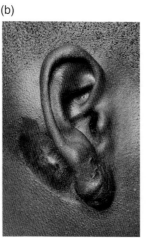

(c)

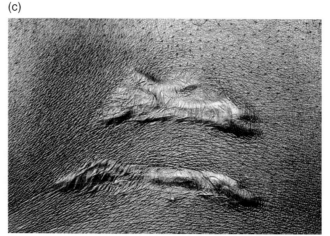

Figure 14.18 (a, b) Keloid on the ear. (c) Keloids on the chest. © Medical Illustration Cardiff and Vale UHB.

Table 14.5 Keloid preventative measures

Avoid tattoos, ear piercing or elective cosmetic surgery if there is a history of keloids

Close surgical wounds with minimal tension

Follow skin creases when making incisions

Avoid mid-chest incisions

Limit skin stretching during healing

Fixable garments, bandages, tape, silicone gel sheets post-operatively

Intralesional triamcinolone immediately post-operatively

Radiotherapy immediately post-operatively

Management

Keloid scars are chronic and difficult to treat. They may be recalcitrant to treatment and the recurrence rate is high. Preventative measures are advisable (Table 14.5).

A combination of two or more of the treatment strategies listed here is more effective at delaying recurrence than monotherapy:

- Silicone gel or dressings.
- Compression therapy.
- Topical steroid under occlusive dressings or corticosteroid tape.
- Intralesional steroid injections repeated every few weeks.
- Cryotherapy.
- Intralesional interferon α2b.
- Surgical excision.
- Radiotherapy (post-operative).
- Laser therapy.
- Imiquimod (post-operative).
- Intralesional 5-fluorouacil.
- Intralesional bleomycin.

Melasma

Melasma (synonymous with chloasma and mask of pregnancy) is a common acquired disorder of hyperpigmentation, mainly affecting sun-exposed areas of the body, particularly the face. It can affect all races and is commonly seen in women of reproductive age, particularly affecting areas of intense ultraviolet radiation. It is particularly common and may be more obvious in skin of colour. It has also been reported in men. Given the predilection for the face, melasma can cause significant psychosocial and emotional distress. This can be disproportionate to the clinical appearance and should be taken into consideration when treatment decisions are being made.

The exact cause of melasma remains unclear. Known risk factors for developing melasma include ultraviolet radiation, exogenous hormones (oral contraceptive pill, hormone replacement therapy), genetic predisposition, anti-epileptic and phototoxic drugs, and thyroid disease. Melasma is triggered by pregnancy or oral contraceptive use in up to 50% of cases, but it can occur in men or nulliparous women. In lighter-skinned women, pigmentation may resolve completely within one year of delivery; however, it may persist in darker skin. Recurrences are common in subsequent pregnancies. Ultraviolet radiation and visible light are strongly implicated in the development of melasma.

Clinical features

Melasma presents with irregular brown to grey-brown patches, mainly on the face (Figure 14.19). It may also occur on the chest and forearms and has been observed on the nipples and external genitalia. Three patterns of facial melasma have been described:

- Centrofacial: forehead, cheeks, nose, upper lips (sparing the philtrum) and chin.
- Malar: cheeks and nose.
- Mandibular: jawline.

The centrofacial pattern is the most common, but combinations of patterns may occur. Using Wood's lamp, melasma can be further classified into epidermal, dermal or mixed variants. Epidermal melasma responds better to treatment; however, many patients have a mixed pattern of melasma.

The differential diagnosis of melasma is wide ranging (Table 14.6). Thorough history and examination are useful, but a biopsy may still be required in cases of diagnostic uncertainty.

Management

Treatment of melasma is challenging. A multifaceted approach is required. It is important to communicate the chronicity and high recurrence rates of the disorder to patients, thus managing expectations appropriately.

First line. Preventative measures include stringent use of broad-spectrum sunscreen with a sun protective factor of at least 30 and high ultraviolet A protection with physical blockers. Remember that ultraviolet A can penetrate window glass, such as when driving in a car. Use of tinted formulations containing titanium oxide, zinc oxide or iron oxide should be advised to provide protection against visible light. Additional preventative measures include behavioural sun avoidance and stopping the oral contraceptive pill or hormone replacement therapy, if possible. Given the inherent risk of vitamin D deficiency in those with darker skin, sun protection advice should be accompanied by vitamin D supplementation and recommendations for intake of vitamin D-rich food.

Hydroquinone is the 'gold standard' of melasma treatment, either as monotherapy or as combination therapy with a retinoid and fluorinated steroid. It is a tyrosinase inhibitor and is commonly used at concentrations of 2–4%, although higher strengths can be prescribed. Irritant reactions can occur, particularly when it is combined with retinoids.

Triple-combination preparations are more efficacious than hydroquinone monotherapy. Pigmanorm® (hydroquinone 5%, tretinoin 0.1%, hydrocortisone 1%; Widmer, Lorsch, Germany)

(a)　　　　　　(b)　　　　　　(c)

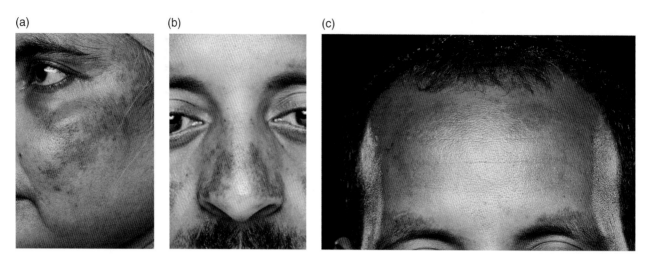

Figure 14.19 Melasma on (a) the cheek, (b) the nose and (c) the forehead. © Medical Illustration Cardiff and Vale UHB.

Table 14.6 Differential diagnosis of melasma

Post-inflammatory hyperpigmentation

Drug-induced hyperpigmentation, e.g. minocycline

Lichen planus pigmentosus

Exogenous ochronosis

Riehl melanosis (pigmented contact dermatitis)

Erythema dyschromicum perstans (ashy dermatosis)

Bilateral naevus of Ota

Hori's naevus

Solar lentigines

is available in the UK as a British Association of Dermatologists 'Special' (Chapter 17), although not all health boards will fund it. It can be used for up to six months. Exogenous ochronosis is a paradoxical blue-black discoloration of the skin that can occur after prolonged use of hydroquinone, especially when it is formulated with resorcinol (Figure 14.20). To avoid exogenous ochronosis, it is advisable to switch to a non-hydroquinone-based lightening agent as soon as possible.

Azelaic acid 20% is an alternative tyrosinase inhibitor that is readily available and can be prescribed by general practitioners. Used twice daily, it can have similar efficacy to hydroquinone 4%. Associated side-effects include redness, itching and scaling.

Other skin-lightening agents that may be useful include kojic acid, arbutin (plant extract), niacinamide, cysteamine, liquorice root extract and ascorbic acid.

Second line. Oral tranexamic acid 250 mg twice daily has been shown to be effective in the management of melasma. It is a plasmin inhibitor that can competitively inhibit tyrosinase, reduce inflammation and downregulate vascularisation occurring in melasma.

Chemical peels can be useful adjuncts to melasma treatment. Superficial peels such as salicylic acid 20–30% and glycolic acid 20–70% can be used effectively in darker skin. Trichloroacetic acid peels should be avoided due to the risk of scarring and PIH.

Third line. Lasers and light therapy may be considered for refractory melasma, but should be used with extreme caution in patients with darker skin due to the high incidence of post-inflammatory hyperpigmentation.

Post-inflammatory hyperpigmentation

PIH is an acquired hypermelanosis that occurs in response to cutaneous inflammation or injury. It can occur in all skin types, but is more common in skin of colour, with the pigment intensity often being greater in those with darker complexions.

The exact pathogenesis of PIH is not fully understood; however, it is felt to be due to stimulation of melanocyte activity by inflammatory mediators. Melanin deposition may occur in the epidermis, dermis or both. Dermal hyperpigmentation can be persistent. The causes of PIH are wide ranging (Table 14.7). Common associated conditions include acne, eczema, lichen planus and drug reactions.

Clinical features

PIH presents as pigmented macules or patches distributed at the sites of the original injury or inflammation (Figure 14.11). Epidermal pigmentation appears tan or brown to dark brown, whereas dermal pigmentation appears blue-grey in appearance. The pigment may take months or years to fade without treatment. It may even be permanent, particularly in the case of dermal pigment. Ultraviolet radiation or repeated inflammation or injury will exacerbate PIH or delay the course of resolution.

(a)

(b)

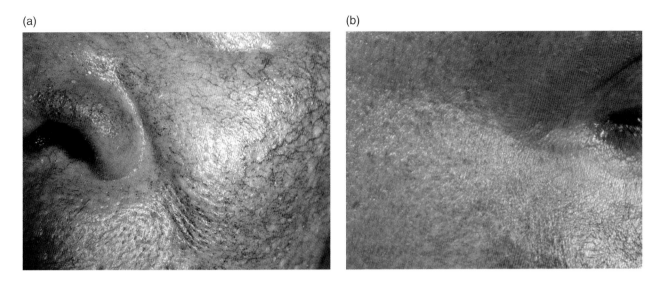

Figure 14.20 Exogenous ochronosis. (a) © Waikato District Health Board. (b) Vashi NA, Kundu RV. Facial hyperpigmentation: causes and treatment. *Br J Dermatol* 2013; **169**:41–56.

Table 14.7 Common causes of post-inflammatory hyperpigmentation

Dermatological disorders	Acne
	Eczema
	Psoriasis
	Lichenoid disorders, e.g. lichen planus
	Infections, e.g. impetigo
	Vesiculobullous disorders, e.g. pemphigus, pemphigoid
Dermatological treatments	Drug eruptions
	Topical agents, e.g. retinoids
Cosmetic procedures	Chemical peels
	Microdermabrasion
	Cryotherapy
	Laser therapy
	Dermal fillers
Trauma	Burns
	Cutaneous injury
	Friction

Management

The most important step in the management of PIH is to treat the underlying cause. Efforts to treat the pigmentation will be futile if this is not addressed. Treatment is otherwise very similar to that of melasma. Caution must be exercised when using irritating topicals as they can potentially further exacerbate post-inflammatory pigmentation. Many of the products listed below can be purchased over the counter. Patients may have already tried a variety of cosmeceuticals and/or illegal skin-lightening products before seeking treatment.

Suggested methods of management are:

- Photoprotection.
- Hydroquinone monotherapy or combination therapy.
- Topical retinoids, e.g. tretinoin or adapalene.
- Azelaic acid.
- Cysteamine.
- Kojic acid.
- Arbutin.
- Niacinamide.
- Ascorbic acid.
- Chemical peels.
- Laser.

Conclusions

Dermatology for skin of colour focuses on skin and hair disorders in non-white skin. Given the variability in presentation of dermatological conditions and prevalence of conditions unique to specific ethnic groups, it is imperative that skin of colour is incorporated into dermatology teaching and training. This chapter provides an overview of common conditions pertaining to skin of colour. It is now essential that exposure to a number of patients with varying skin tones is sought throughout training. This clinical experience, in combination with further reading, will provide you with the knowledge as a dermatologist to treat people with all skin types appropriately and with confidence.

Pearls and pitfalls

- Higher incidence of eczema has been reported in Black and Asian ethnic groups in comparison to their White counterparts, with follicular patterns being more common.
- Be aware of specific issues relating to afro-textured hair and hair care practices when treating scalp psoriasis or seborrhoeic dermatitis.
- Hyperpigmentation may be the only obvious presenting feature of active acne in skin of colour.
- Melanoma in skin of colour has a poorer prognosis than in White patients, and is more common in sun-protected sites such as the palms, soles, mucous membranes and subungual regions.
- Early diagnosis and treatment of traction alopecia and central centrifugal cicatricial alopecia are crucial to prevent permanent hair loss.
- The importance of broad-spectrum sun protection should not be underestimated in the management of melasma and post-inflammatory hyperpigmentation.

SCE Questions. See questions 51 and 52.

FURTHER READING AND KEY RESOURCES

Alexis AF. Lasers and light-based therapies in ethnic skin: treatment options and recommendations for Fitzpatrick skin types V and VI. *Br J Dermatol* 2013; **169** (Suppl. 3):91–7.

Davis EC, Callender VD. A review of acne in ethnic skin: pathogenesis, clinical manifestations, and management strategies. *J Clin Aesthet Dermatol* 2010; **3**:24–38.

Gloster HM Jr, Neal K. Skin cancer in skin of color. *J Am Acad Dermatol* 2006; **55**:741–60.

Rajanala S, Maymone MBC, Vashi NA. Melasma pathogenesis: a review of the latest research, pathological findings, and investigational therapies. *Dermatol Online J* 2019; **25**:13030/qt47b7r28c.

Salam A, Aryiku S, Dadzie OE. Hair and scalp disorders in women of African descent: an overview. *Br J Dermatol* 2013; **169** (Suppl. 3):19–32.

Textbooks

Dadzie OE, Petit A, Alexis AF. *Ethnic Dermatology: Principles and Practice*. Hoboken, NJ: Wiley-Blackwell, 2013.

Kelly AP, Taylor SC, Lim HC, Serrano AMA. *Taylor and Kelly's Dermatology for Skin of Color*, 2nd edn. New York: McGraw-Hill Medical, 2015.

Useful websites

British Association of Dermatologists. Describing erythema in skin of colour. Available at: https://www.bad.org.uk/healthcare-professionals/inclusivity-and-representation/erythema-in-skin-of-colour.

British Association of Dermatologists. Educational resources for clinicians on skin of colour. Available at: https//www.bad.org.uk/healthcare-professionals/education/skin-of-colour-resources.

British Association of Dermatologists. Improving descriptors in dermatology. Available at: https://www.bad.org.uk/healthcare-professionals/inclusivity-and-representation/descriptors-in-dermatology.

Centre of Evidence Based Dermatology. Skin of colour resource. Available at: https://www.nottingham.ac.uk/research/groups/cebd/resources/skin-of-colour/index.aspx.

MIMS Learning. Dermatology for skin of colour learning plan. Available at: https://www.mimslearning.co.uk/pages/mims-learning-dermatology.

15

Psychodermatology

Anthony Bewley

Introduction

Psychodermatology is an increasingly recognised and important branch of dermatology, and is the interface between dermatology and psychiatry/psychology (thus 'psychocutaneous medicine' or 'psychodermatology'). It encompasses disease that involves the complex interaction between the brain, the cutaneous nerves, the cutaneous immune system and the skin. Patients with psychocutaneous disease are often variably managed, as dermatologists struggle, in general dermatology clinics, to meet the complex needs of these patients. Most patients with psychocutaneous disease are reluctant to attend purely psychiatric clinics. For these reasons, over the last few decades, the subspecialty of psychodermatology has emerged to address the clinical needs of this group of patients, and to support an academic focus in developing this specialty.

Patients with psychocutaneous disease are common. They fall into four categories (Table 15.1), with the first two categories being the bulk of the workload: patients with primarily psychiatric disease who present to dermatology healthcare professionals (HCPs), for example delusional infestation and body dysmorphic disorder; and patients with skin disease (e.g. psoriasis, atopic eczema, vitiligo and acne) for whom there are large psychosocial comorbidities such as anxiety, depression and even suicidal ideation. Management of patients with psychodermatological disease requires a multidisciplinary team (MDT) approach (Table 15.2). Such clinics are relatively rare and there is a growing body of evidence that management of patients with psychodermatological disease in MDT clinics is cost-effective and also produces the best clinical outcome for patients (Table 15.3). There are various ways in which psychodermatology can be delivered (Table 15.4), which may rely on the availability of local expertise. However, in order to

Dermatology Training: The Essentials. Edited by Mahbub M.U. Chowdhury, Tamara W. Griffiths and Andrew Y. Finlay.
© 2022 The British Association of Dermatologists. Published 2022 by John Wiley & Sons Ltd.
Companion website: www.wiley.com/go/chowdhury/dermatologytraining

Table 15.1 Psychodermatological disease categories

1. Primary skin disease with psychosocial comorbidities (e.g. psoriasis and anxiety or depression)

2. Primary psychiatric disease presenting to dermatology healthcare professionals (e.g. delusional infestation and body dysmorphic disorder)

3. Skin disease as a consequence of psychotropic medication (e.g. psoriasis as a result of lithium for bipolar depression) and psychiatric disease as a result of dermatological medication (e.g. isotretinoin and depression)

4. Comorbidity of skin disease with another psychiatric disorder (e.g. alcoholism)

Table 15.2 The psychodermatology multidisciplinary team

Dermatologists

Psychiatrists

Psychologists

Dermatology nurses

Child and adolescent mental health specialists (CaMHS)

Paediatricians

Geriatricians and older-age psychiatrists

Social workers

Table 15.3 Organisations that lead clinical–academic excellence in psychodermatology

All Party Parliamentary Group on Skin; Skin Disease and Mental Health (2020) Report: https://www.appgs.co.uk/mental-health-and-skin-disease-report-2020

Psychodermatology UK: www.psychodermatology.co.uk

European Society for Dermatology and Psychiatry: www.psychodermatology.net

British Association of Dermatologists, Skin Support: www.skinsupport.org.uk

Table 15.4 Models of provision of psychodermatology services

A dermatologist who refers to a clinically adjacent psychiatrist or psychologist (i.e. a colleague who is running a separate clinic nearby)

A dermatologist who refers to a psychiatrist or psychologist who is in a remote clinic (who will be able to support and supervise decisions taken by a dermatologist)

A dermatologist who has a psychiatrist sitting in clinic at the same time. Patients are seen by both specialists concurrently

A dermatologist who has a clinically adjacent psychologist (psychologists rarely sit in on clinics with dermatologists or psychiatrists)

deliver comprehensive psychodermatology services, a dermatologist and psychiatrist seeing patients together in the same room (for at least some of the time) is probably the best model.

Primary dermatological disease with psychological comorbidities

Skin disease commonly has psychosocial comorbidities. These include depression, anxiety, changes in self-esteem and body image, other affective disorders, obsessive and compulsive spectrum disease, suicidal ideation, substance abuse and psychosis.

Anxiety, depression and suicidal ideation are potential comorbidities for patients living with atopic eczema, acne, alopecia or psoriasis. Depression is particularly significant and may be independently related to pro-inflammatory brain patho-aetiology. Many patients indicate that stress has triggered the onset of the skin disease, but the latent period between a significant life stress and the onset or exacerbation of skin disease has been difficult to assess. Also, patients with skin disease may feel stigmatised and have a very altered sense of self-perception. Stigmatisation describes the situation where an individual believes that they are disqualified from full social acceptance, and patients with skin disease may believe that this is because of their appearance or their disease, or both.

Assessment and management of psychosocial comorbidities in patients with dermatological disease

Assessment of psychosocial comorbidities and health-related quality of life

Psychosocial comorbidities (e.g. depression and anxiety) are a different concept from health-related quality of life (HRQoL) issues. Listening to and engaging patients in a clinical consultation is of immense importance, and HCPs can obtain excellent assessments of affective disease and HRQoL by asking simple Socratic open questions (e.g. 'how are you feeling?'). However, there are well-validated tools to screen and grade psychosocial comorbidities and HRQoL, which may be general medical, dermatology, disease, age, patient or family specific (Table 15.5).

Managing the psychosocial comorbidities of dermatological disease

In managing the psychosocial comorbidities of primary skin disease, it is important to remember the 'golden rules' of

Table 15.5 Well-validated questionnaires and tools to assess psychosocial comorbidities in patients with dermatological disease

Dermatology Life Quality Index (DLQI)

Skindex-16 and Skindex-29

Cardiff Acne Disability Index

Hospital Anxiety and Depression Score (HADS)

Generalised Anxiety Disorder (GAD, GAD-7)

Patient Health Questionnaire 9 (PHQ-9)

Measurements of the impact of skin disease on carers and younger patients

Children's Dermatology Life Quality Index (CDLQI)

Family Dermatology Life Quality Index (FDLQI)

Table 15.6 Coping strategies and simple signposting for patient support

Healthy eating

Do not suffer in silence

Connecting with other people (family and friends)

Talk to professionals, e.g. general practitioners

Signposting to patient advocacy groups

Signposting to general support

Maintaining healthy sleeping patterns

Maintaining healthy exercise patterns

Take time out for reflection (e.g. meditation or mindfulness)

Avoid non-helpful coping strategies (e.g. alcohol)

Be self-compassionate

Table 15.7 Coping strategies suggested by Changing Faces

3-2-1 Go! Prepares a patient with a visible difference with the following coping strategies:

- Three things to do if someone stares at you:
  o Look back and smile
  o Look back, smile and say, *'I'm sorry, do we know one another?'*
  o Ask them not to stare
- Two things to say if someone asks you what happened:
  o *'I have a skin condition but I'd rather not talk about it'*
  o *'I've had psoriasis for a few years but it's not contagious'*
- One thing to think if someone appears to turn away:
  o *'It's OK, they didn't mean any harm'*

Modified from Tools to help you cope with each other people's reaction, coping with people's reactions, Changing Faces.

Table 15.8 The Changing Faces REACHOUT mnemonic to assist coping with living with different facial appearance

- R – Reassurance: putting someone at ease
- E – Energy: creating an interest in what they say
- A – Assertiveness: taking the initiative
- C – Courage: being strong and taking control
- H – Humour: introducing fun or a joke
- O – Over there! Distracting away from the skin condition
- U – Understanding: being aware that seeing a skin condition can be difficult
- T – Tenacity: try again, use a different strategy if the first does not work

psychodermatology: 'In managing patients with psychocutaneous disease always (i) exclude organic disease, and (ii) appropriately assess and treat the dermatological disease at the same time as appropriately assessing and treating the psychological disease.'

It is also important to guide patients into developing coping strategies in taking control of their psychosocial comorbidities. Simple advice about appropriate coping strategies (Table 15.6) can be of significant benefit. Changing Faces, a support group for people with altered appearance, has also developed some helpful coping strategy tools (Table 15.7) and has suggested a REACHOUT mnemonic to remember key social strategies (Table 15.8).

There are two broad categories in managing psychosocial comorbidities of primary dermatological disease: talking therapies and pharmacological therapies. For general dermatology clinics, a simple knowledge of the basic talk therapies and how to refer or signpost patients to access these therapies is sufficient. For pharmacological management of affective disease, a basic knowledge of the medications and how to use them is essential. Basic affirmative cognitive behavioural therapy (active listening and non-judgemental support) of patients is necessary, and some dermatology trainees may choose to formally develop further skills in psychotherapy.

For trainees in general and psychodermatology clinics, under the supervision of senior or psychodermatology team colleagues, the initiation, maintenance and monitoring of patients on psychotropic medication are appropriate, where such skills have been developed. If trainees are uncertain about the use of psychotropic medication, then referral to primary care, psychiatry or psychodermatology services may be necessary.

There is good evidence that patients with affective disease will respond to either talking therapies or psychotropic medication, and that the combination of both concurrently leads to fewer recurrences of the affective disease.

Psychological therapies

The use of psychotherapies in disorders is common and is usually talking based. The relationship between the HCP and the patient has a potentially powerful therapeutic (or sometimes counter-therapeutic) effect, even before formal psychological techniques are considered. The effect of an empathic approach can be very powerful. Although psychological treatments are effective and common, some patients may have a preconceived bias or feel stigmatised regarding the use of talking therapies. The opportunity to express their anxieties and fears may provide significant relief. The effect of actively listening within a therapeutic relationship (Rogerian cognitive behavioural therapy) allows patients to address their own problems and is the basis of client-centred counselling.

Cognitive behavioural therapy

Increasingly, cognitive behavioural therapy (CBT) has become the first-line psychological therapy in depression and anxiety disorders. CBT explores the interaction between thoughts, feelings and behaviour. The theory of CBT is that the patient automatically responds to certain situations and stimuli with ingrained negative thoughts. These thoughts in turn lead to negative emotions such as fear or depression, and behavioural consequences such as avoidance or rituals. Treatment in CBT is based around the process of sympathetically, through the development of a treatment alliance, challenging these negative automatic thoughts and exploring alternative responses that may not lead to behavioural and emotional pathology. Often, adjunctive relaxation and anxiety management techniques are an integral part of the therapy. There is a range of CBT techniques, such as:

- Patient-centric CBT.
- Acceptance and commitment therapy.
- Bibliotherapy.
- Group therapy.
- Family therapy.

Choosing the best CBT for a patient may involve the assessment of a psychologist or other HCP working together with the patient (the patient is always at the centre of decision making). In the UK, provision of psychological therapies has been enhanced through the Improving Access to Psychological Therapies (IAPT) programme. However, other longer-term psychotherapy programmes also have a place in a patient's management.

Dynamic psychotherapies and psychoanalysis

Psychodynamic and psychoanalysis therapies are longer-term, more exploratory techniques that can closely examine the relationship, causes and analysis of approaching an individual's behaviour and responses to situational stimuli. Psychodynamic concepts such as transference, counter-transference, projection and identification can help explore the relationship between physical or psychological distress, or both. Short-term forms of dynamic therapies (defined as fewer than 40 sessions) have been shown to have efficacy in a wide range of common mental health disorders. Many forms of dynamic therapies and psychoanalytic therapy are long lasting and intensive. Access to such therapies is often via psychiatry.

Drug treatments

Antidepressants and anti-anxiety medication

Antidepressants are widely used, not only in depression but also for anxiety and panic disorder, obsessive–compulsive disorder and body dysmorphic disorder, post-traumatic stress disorder, and bulimia nervosa and pain (Table 15.9). Before starting an antidepressant, it is important to ensure that the patient understands the rationale for their use and has information about what to expect. Emphasise to the patient that depression is an illness that is treatable. Explain that antidepressants work by increasing the levels of certain brain chemicals, and that this takes a while so the therapeutic effect is not immediate. An effect from antidepressants can be evident at one week, and by 2–3 weeks an effect is often seen if the antidepressant is taken at a therapeutic dose. If there is minimal effect, consider increasing the dose after 3–4 weeks, but if there is no response at all after 3–4 weeks consider changing to another agent. However, side-effects can be more immediate, for example the sedative and appetite-increasing side-effect of mirtazapine. Explain what side-effects to expect and whether these will settle.

Patients are often concerned that antidepressants are addictive. Explain that they are not, but that they can cause a discontinuation syndrome in which if the antidepressant is stopped suddenly the patient may experience flu-like symptoms and odd electric shock sensations. These symptoms disappear on restarting the antidepressant, which should then be withdrawn gradually. Antidepressants with a shorter half-life, for example paroxetine, are particularly prone to have a discontinuation syndrome, whereas fluoxetine with its long half-life is much less likely to manifest this problem. After starting an antidepressant, the patient should be monitored carefully for the possible side-effect of suicidal ideation; this is especially important for patients under the age of 25 years, in whom the risk of this effect is greater. A review after one week may be important for those felt to be at high risk of self-harm, or those under 25 years of age, while a review after 2–6 weeks is suitable for others. Antidepressants should be continued for 6–9 months past the remission of symptoms, as this helps reduce the risk of relapse. The Maudsley prescribing guidelines can be accessed for more information.

Selective serotonin reuptake inhibitors (SSRIs; e.g. fluoxetine, citalopram) are now recommended as first choice for use in depression, obsessive–compulsive disorder (including body dysmorphic disorder) and anxiety disorders. This is due to their relatively low side-effect profile, good tolerance and lower toxicity

Table 15.9 Antidepressants used in psychodermatology

Name	Dose (adult under 65 years)	Indications	Type of antidepressant
Fluoxetine	20–60 mg/day	Depression	Selective serotonin reuptake inhibitors
Sertraline	50–200 mg/day	Obsessive–compulsive disorder	
Citalopram	20–40 mg/day		
		Body dysmorphic disorder	
		Bulimia nervosa	
		Panic disorder	
		Post-traumatic stress disorder	
		Social anxiety disorder	
		Generalised anxiety disorder	
Venlafaxine	37.5–225 mg daily	Depression, generalised anxiety disorder	Serotonin and norepinephrine reuptake inhibitors. Used often by pain clinics as some evidence helpful in neuropathic pain
Duloxetine	30–120 mg daily		
Mirtazapine	15–45 mg	Depression	NaSRI (noradrenergic–serotonergic reuptake inhibitor)
			Side-effects include weight gain, sleepiness and sexual dysfunction
Amitriptyline	10–150 mg	Depression, anxiety, neuropathic pain	Tricyclics. Can be used in very low doses (though not as an antidepressant) for pain relief. Can be used for pruritus and dysaesthesias
Doxepin	25–50 mg, usually at night		Potentially cardiotoxic

in overdosage compared with the older tricyclic antidepressants. The most common side-effects are nausea, dyspepsia and gastrointestinal upset, headache, agitation and anxiety, sweating and different drug-related rashes, insomnia and sexual dysfunction. Rarely, SSRIs may lead initially to an exacerbation of anxiety, and, in patients under the age of 18 years, the association with agitation leading to increased suicidal behaviour and hostility has led to the recommendation that SSRIs are only prescribed by child and adolescent mental health specialists (CaMHS). Hyponatraemia and increased risk of bleeding due to an effect on platelets can rarely occur. The SSRIs are generally regarded as having low cardiotoxicity, but recent studies have indicated that citalopram and escitalopram can prolong the QT interval, thus increasing the risk of fatal arrythmias. Citalopram should now not be used in doses above 40 mg. Caution should be exercised and the prescriber should avoid combination with other drugs known to cause a prolonged QT interval.

Serotonin and norepinephrine reuptake inhibitors, for example venlafaxine and duloxetine, act on both serotonin and norepinephrine and are used as second-line agents. Generally they are less well tolerated than SSRIs, but are better tolerated than the old tricyclic agents. They have similar side-effects to the SSRIs in terms of gastrointestinal side-effects and increased anxiety, but

they generally have fewer sexual side-effects (such as decreased libido). SSRIs can heighten alertness, which may worsen insomnia. Mirtazapine belongs to the class called noradrenergic and specific serotonergic antidepressants (NaSSA). It has minimal sexual side-effects, but is sedative and causes increased appetite and weight gain. These side-effects can be helpful in patients with insomnia and loss of appetite, but it is important to warn patients of the risk of gaining weight and they are best avoided in overweight patients.

Tricyclic antidepressants are no longer recommended for first-line use in depression. They are still useful when sedation is required, as this can provide some immediate relief from the insomnia of depressive states, and aid in concordance. In lower doses tricyclics are commonly used by dermatologists for pruritus and urticaria (as patients may find both the anti-pruritic and sedative effects useful), and for dysaesthesias and atypical pain syndromes (e.g. burning mouth syndrome). Side-effects include dry mouth, blurred vision, constipation, sedation, urinary retention, open-angle glaucoma and postural hypotension. Cardiotoxicity, including heart block, is recognised if they are taken in larger doses or in overdoses. Prolongation of QT interval is caused by most tricyclics; amitriptyline in particular can cause marked QT prolongation, so caution needs to be exercised in use of high doses or if there is a potential combination with other drugs that prolong QT interval. Do not prescribe in patients with a risk of overdose as this will likely be lethal with these drugs. Reduction of the seizure threshold is greater than with the SSRIs, so tricyclics should be avoided in epilepsy.

Alternative therapies

There has been a long tradition of the use of complementary therapies in dermatology, but especially for those diseases where there is a psychological component. Most reports of therapy are anecdotal. Acupuncture, biofeedback and hypnosis have been used in skin disease. Hypnotherapy has been the most frequently studied and has an associated medical literature. Alternative herbal medications may be used both topically and systemically.

Suicide in dermatological patients

The mistake often made by non-dermatology HCPs is assuming that skin disease does not carry a mortality risk. 'Suicide' refers to a range of self-destructive behaviours ranging from non-lethal acts, which have been called suicidal gestures, attempted suicide, parasuicide and more recently self-injury, to a lethal action in which a patient dies, defined as a completed suicide. The rates of completed suicide in the UK are 8–10 per 100,000 people. In 2019, the England and Wales male suicide rate of 16.9 deaths per 100,000 was the highest since 2000; for females, the rate was 5.3 deaths per 100,000 and the highest since 2004. The rate is rising, particularly in young men. Suicide is an essential feature of depressive disease and 15% of patients with major depression kill themselves. It is therefore one of the 10 most common causes of death in the UK in younger men and women. Psychiatric disorders are the main risk factors, but numerous studies have also identified physical illness as an important contributory factor (Table 15.10).

Unfortunately, some dermatology patients become so unhappy that they succeed in committing suicide. Dermatologists must explore suicidal thoughts. Simple assessments to consider should include:

- Has the patient attempted suicide before?
- Are there any risk factors for suicide (Table 15.10)?
- What are the supports for the patient (family or others)?
- Has the patient prepared for suicide (e.g. written a note)?
- Does the patient have immediate plans?
- Is the patient safe right now?

If a dermatology HCP is satisfied that the patient is currently safe, then it is important to ensure that the patient has access to support if a suicidal impulse arises (e.g. friends, family, access to websites such as the Samaritans). If an HCP is sufficiently worried, then an immediate referral to the local acute mental health team is crucial.

Table 15.10 Risk factors for suicide

Male gender
Substance abuse
Isolation
Long-standing physical disease
Psychiatric disease, especially:
• Depression
• Body dysmorphic disease
Unemployment
Skin diseases with known suicidal risk include:
• Acne
• Psoriasis
• Pruritus associated with any skin disease

Primary psychiatric disease presenting to dermatologists

Delusional infestation

A primary delusion is a false, unshakeable belief that is not amenable to logic and is out of keeping with the person's educational and cultural background. Primary delusions can be an isolated phenomenon (a monosymptomatic hypochondriacal psychosis such as delusional infestation, DI) or part of a broader psychosis (e.g. schizophrenia). A secondary delusion more commonly occurs with affective disorder and the delusion is secondary to the mood (e.g. with nihilistic delusions in severe depression, the patient may believe that their skin is rotting away). The intensity with which a delusional belief is held may be variable. DI, for example, may arise as an overvalued idea or may be a very intensely held belief.

DI is an uncommon but very disabling condition, where the patient is convinced that they are infested with mites, parasites, bacteria, worms, viruses or inanimate fibres or other material. The patient will go to huge efforts to demonstrate the infestation, known as a positive 'specimen sign' (Figure 15.1). Patients with DI usually present to dermatology HCPs and struggle to engage with psychiatric services. Such patients have often seen a large number of HCPs without accepting any treatment. DI may be primary, where no underlying cause is found, or secondary to concomitant organic or psychiatric disease. Over two-thirds of patients presenting with DI have secondary DI, where they have an underlying psychiatric or organic disease, and the commonest cause of secondary DI is recreational drug usage (Table 15.11).

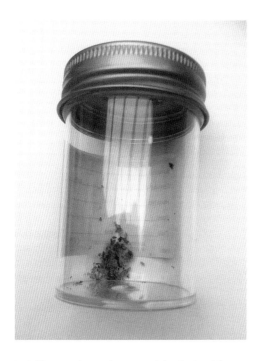

Figure 15.1 The specimen sign: material submitted from a patient with delusional infestation. © A. Bewley.

Shared delusions are common among family and friends of patients with DI:

- DI as a shared delusion (*folie à deux*): family members, carers and friends may commonly believe that they too are infested, or delusionally share the belief of the individual who is presenting with DI.
- DI by proxy: patients complain that their child, pet or friend is infested despite all evidence to the contrary.

The diagnosis of DI is usually made with the clinical history alone. However, it is crucial that HCPs carefully examine the skin of patients with suspected DI to check for a genuine infestation, to assess differential diagnoses and causes of DI and to engage with the patient. On examination, patients may have localised or generalised excoriations, erosions and sometimes ulceration. Some patients go to great lengths to eradicate the perceived infestation by using tools such as tweezers. Occasionally there are no physical signs, but the patient will still maintain that the infestation is present and the itching, biting or stinging sensations are there. Patients with DI are usually keen to prove their infestation. Many will demonstrate the 'specimen sign' by bringing along specimens of the organisms that they believe are infesting them. It is imperative that these specimens are taken seriously and carefully reviewed by clinicians. Skin debris and specimen material may be analysed for human

Table 15.11 Causes of delusional infestation (DI)

Primary DI	DI secondary to organic disease	DI secondary to psychiatric disease
No underlying disease	Substance abuse	Schizophrenia
	Alcohol	Bipolar depression with psychotic symptoms
	Recreational drugs	Borderline personality disorder
	Prescribed medications, e.g. anti-parkinsonian medication, such as ropinirole	Anxiety disorder
	Tuberculosis	
	HIV	
	Thyroid disease	
	Solid tumours	
	Haematological cancer	
	Liver disease	
	Renal failure	
	Metabolic disease	
	Vitamin B_{12} deficiency	
	Systemic lupus erythematosus	
	Multiple sclerosis	
	Cerebrovascular disease	
	Parkinson's disease	

pathogens by microscopy in the local microbiology laboratory. A catalogue of normal results will assist the patient in understanding that the clinician has insight into the patient's experience and continues to seek and exclude a genuine infestation. Assessment of coexistent affective disease, suicidality, and recreational drug and alcohol usage is important.

To engage the patient fully, HCPs must develop a sympathetic, understanding approach. It is usually futile to try to dissuade patients of the validity of their infestation. Instead, it is better to let the patient know that you understand the difficulties that they are experiencing, and that you have successfully looked after patients with similar disease. Recognition of your clinical experience with this condition often helps to engage the patient with appropriate treatments.

As always in psychodermatology, it is important to treat the skin appropriately in conjunction with the psychiatric disease.

Treatments

The aim is to manage the skin, the delusion and the risk to the patient simultaneously. Several strategies may be used:

- Antipsychotics are first line (choose according to the lifestyle of the patient). Treat with very low doses. Monitor for potential side-effects such as extrapyramidal parkinsonism symptoms. Be explicit about the use of the antipsychotic medication such as risperidone (0.5–4 mg), olanzapine (2.5–10 mg), amisulpride (50–400 mg), quetiapine (25–100 mg) or aripiprazole (5–15 mg).
- Emollients that contain antiseptics.
- Assessment of risk, suicidality and affective disease.
- Referral to a substance abuse unit if appropriate (and advise cessation of recreational drugs and excess alcohol)
- Treat the people who share the delusion with appropriate skin management. As the patient with DI improves, those who share the delusion will improve too.
- Refer any vulnerable adults or children to appropriate services.

The prognosis is usually good once patients are engaged. The longer a patient is left untreated, the less likely any antipsychotic treatment is likely to be beneficial. Confronting patients with the diagnosis is often futile. Writing to primary care physicians with the diagnosis is also unlikely to be helpful, as the patient will not agree with the diagnosis of DI. Instead, describing the clinical scenario to primary care colleagues (i.e. 'patient experiences sensations of a skin infestation' or 'patient believes that they have an infestation of the skin') is a preferred and less confrontational approach. Some centres will use prolactin levels as an objective measure of adherence as some antipsychotics, for example risperidone, may cause elevated prolactin levels. As patients improve, they will indicate that the infestation has 'gone' or 'stopped'. It is usually best to continue with medication for 3–6 months after the symptoms of DI have cleared. A small number of patients will clear with no treatment at all, though these are usually patients with overstated ideation of infestation rather than an intensely held delusional belief of infestation.

Olfactory delusions

Olfactory reference syndrome (ORS) describes the rare syndrome when a patient believes that their skin is emitting an unpleasant odour. Once fish odour syndrome has been excluded (by urinalysis for tryptophan), ORS is likely to be the cause of the patient's symptoms. It is usually a primary hypochondriacal psychosis, but rarely patients with nihilistic symptoms of depression can believe that they 'smell bad'.

Differential diagnoses include:

- A genuine body odour.
- Trimethylaminuria or 'fish odour syndrome': the patient has a genetic amino acid metabolic syndrome caused by abnormalities of the production or function of the enzyme flavin-containing monooxygenase 3, which leads to the build-up of trimethylamine (TMA) in body fluids. The ability to smell TMA objectively is genetic and variable. Urine analysis for TMA (usually compared to TMA oxide) is helpful to establish the diagnosis.
- Temporal lobe epilepsy or olfactory hallucinations, which are common.
- Other organic brain disease, Parkinson's disease or brain tumour.

Treatment

Once organic disease has been excluded, engagement of the patient is essential, with management of the skin and the ORS at the same time. Usually, the patient's skin is treated with antibacterial emollients and the ORS with antidepressants (typically SSRIs, see above) or low doses of antipsychotics (as for DI above).

Obsessive and compulsive behaviour

Obsessive–compulsive behaviour (OCD) is present in up to 25% of dermatology outpatients. OCD dermatological disorders include body dysmorphic disorder (BDD), lichen simplex chronicus, skin picking disorder, acne excoriée, trichotillosis (trichotillomania), onychophagia and onychotillomania (nail biting and chewing), nodular prurigo (Figure 15.2) and health anxieties.

Body dysmorphic disorder

BDD is characterised by a preoccupation with a real or an imagined defect in physical appearance. If there is a slight physical anomaly, then the concern is out of proportion to the anomaly. The defect that the patient experiences may seem trivial, but for the patient it is a major focus. BDD is common (1–2% in the general population), especially in those seeking aesthetic surgery. It is more common in younger individuals, and especially younger women. There is a high degree of comorbidity with mood disorders, OCD and social phobia.

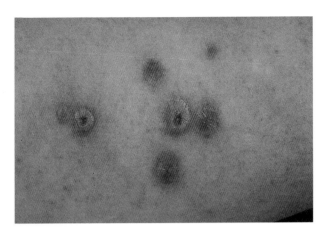

Figure 15.2 Nodular prurigo. Note nodules with overlying excoriation and others with healing and hyperpigmentation. © Barts Health NHS Trust.

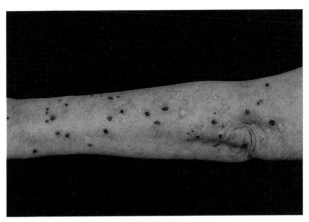

Figure 15.3 Skin picking syndrome. Note erosions and ulcers with serosanguinous crust from constant picking, and some areas of healing with hypopigmentation. © Barts Health NHS Trust.

Patients with BDD may present with a variety of perceived defects such as acne scarring, pigmentation, hair disorders or some (often real but objectively minor) visible difference about which they are extremely concerned. Patients will spend large amounts of time checking their skin, may have social avoidance (agoraphobia) and will frequently have persistent ruminant thoughts about the perceived defect. Often others will have told the patient that it appears a minor 'defect' or that it is imperceivable.

When assessing BDD:

- Assess for potential suicide risk and refer where necessary.
- Assess for any underlying abuse (vulnerable adult or child for both physical and mental abuse).
- Assess for underlying psychiatric disease (depression or anxiety, or both).
- Acknowledge genuine skin disease (e.g. hair loss or skin pigmentation changes).
- Investigate skin changes appropriately: this may mean no investigations at all or it may mean appropriately investigating a differential diagnosis.
- Ask about substance abuse.
- Investigate any underlying psychiatric disease.

Skin picking disorder and acne excoriée

Synonyms for these conditions include psychogenic excoriations, neurotic excoriations, compulsive skin picking, dermatillomania and psychogenic skin picking.

Skin picking is common. The lesions differ from artefactual disorders, as patients admit to picking their skin or acne. There may be an initial reluctance to own up to the self-damage, but patients are usually willing to discuss the picking as a 'response to stress'. Any area may be affected (the face and chest in acne excoriée), and the lesions may range from shallow erosions, excoriations and linear tears to deep, wide ulcers. Commonly there are ulcers and erosions at different stages of the healing or scarring process (Figure 15.3).

The aetiology may include traumatic life events or pre-existing skin disease (e.g. atopic eczema or acne); psychosocial comorbidities are very common, such as depression and/or anxiety. It is important to exclude excoriations caused by underlying pruritus with organic aetiology, autoimmune bullous disorders and inflammatory dermatoses.

Trichotillomania and trichotillosis

Hair pulling is common, but extensive and disfiguring trichotillomania is rarer. There appear to be two populations: those who present in childhood, mainly aged 5–12 years, and adults, usually women aged 30–45 years. Diagnostic criteria include:

- Pulling out one's own hair, resulting in hair loss.
- An increasing sense of tension immediately before pulling out the hair or when attempting to resist the behaviour.
- Pleasure, gratification or relief when pulling out the hair.
- The disturbance is not better accounted for by another mental disorder.
- The disturbance provokes clinically marked distress or impairment in occupational, social or other areas of functioning, or all of these activities.

Hair pulling and plucking are commonest from the scalp, but hair from any body area may be pulled and it is common for more than one site to be affected. Patients usually describe an irresistible drive to pull the hair, followed by a sense of relief and then guilt. The aetiologies are similar to those of BDD, as are the common comorbidities. On examination, there are often areas of hair loss together with areas of hair regrowth (stubble and longer hairs). Hair loss may be localised or more generalised. The differential diagnosis is that of hair loss, but the patient will usually admit to the habit of hair pulling if asked empathically. The complications of trichotillomania include permanent hair loss, folliculitis, scarring and trichobezoar (hair balls in the gastrointestinal tract).

Onychotillomania and onychophagia

The compulsive habits of nail picking and nail biting are common in children and adolescents. Damage to cuticles and nails causes paronychia, nail dystrophy and longitudinal nail scarring. In chronic cases, there is an association with trichotillomania.

Management (Table 15.12)

Several options are available for the management of obsessive and compulsive behaviour.

- **Skin treatment**. Patients with psychodermatological disease need to have their skin *and* their psychological disease treated concurrently. *Appropriate* treatment of the patient's skin will facilitate engagement of the patient. One difficulty is that such treatment may not satisfy the expectations of the patient, who may then go on to seek more extreme options such as inappropriate surgery. From the outset it is important to treat the psychological disease while also addressing the perceived skin disease. Often there are some skin changes (however minimal), and acknowledging these changes rather than dismissing them will facilitate patient engagement.
- **Education** for patients and their friends and family (see Further reading).
- **Psychopharmacological treatments**. SSRIs are the treatments of choice, along with CBT. Where possible, make a referral for CBT (see below) at the same time as considering SSRIs (Table 15.9) in higher doses. The use of CBT and SSRIs is probably more effective than either treatment in isolation, although the patient always remains at the centre of any treatment decisions.
- **Talking therapies**. There are various CBT techniques that can be used in the management of BDD. Clinicians may make a referral via the primary care physician or directly to community mental health teams. The range and choice of CBT involve the patient, may involve an assessment from a psychologist and may depend on local availability.
- **If the patient is still not improving**, it is usually an adherence issue. However, there are a group of patients with BDD who are either delusional (i.e. there really is nothing to see; or they are referring to a delusional 'defect', e.g. 'my eyebrows are moving higher up my forehead') or may have a personality disorder. These patients, and those not responding to other treatment plans, need to be referred to specialist psychodermatology units.

Dermatitis artefacta and factitious skin disease

Factitious skin disease refers to a spectrum of illness that depends on the level of intention to deceive at the time of the act, and the motivation for the induced illness. Factitious behaviour is defined in Table 15.13. Apart from dermatitis artefacta, there is a range of other factitious skin diseases, including dermatitis simulate, dermatological pathomimicry, dermatitis passivate, malingering, Munchausen's syndrome and Munchausen's syndrome by proxy.

Table 15.12 Treatment of dermatological obsessive–compulsive disorders (OCDs): general principles

1. Simple, empathetic supportive approaches from healthcare professionals are essential

2. Treat the skin appropriately (topical steroids, emollients)

3. Treat the OCD component with:
   i. Talk therapies (see body dysmorphic disorder, BDD). Psychotherapy can produce significant improvement. Cognitive behavioural therapy alone has improved some patients, although the management of underlying personality difficulties may require the specific skills of a psychotherapist
   ii. Pharmacological therapies (see BDD): selective serotonin reuptake inhibitors can be helpful. Usually, patients need to be encouraged to start treatment, with explanations that benefit will only start after 4–6 weeks. Higher doses may be necessary, but maximal recommended doses must not be exceeded. Clomipramine and doxepin may also be effective

4. Assess for comorbidities (e.g. suicidal ideation, substance abuse)

5. Try to find out why the patient has the 'habit'

6. Never attempt to tell the patient that it is 'all in their head' or that they 'need to snap out of it'

7. Habit reversal therapy may be useful. Details can be accessed online or via self-help publications (e.g. www.atopicskindisease.com)

8. The A-B-C model of habit disorders – **A**ffect regulation, **B**ehavioural regulation and **C**ognitive control – makes use of all modalities to help patients conceptualise and manage skin picking behaviours

9. A psychodermatology multidisciplinary team can be very helpful in management of complex disease

10. Second- and third-line treatments can be planned at a psychodermatology multidisciplinary team meeting or accessed through appropriate specialists

Table 15.13 Factitious skin disease criteria

A Falsification of physical or psychological signs or symptoms, or induction of injury or disease, associated with identified deception

B The individual presents himself or herself to others as ill, impaired, or injured

C The deceptive behaviour is evident even in the absence of obvious external rewards

D The behaviour is not better explained by another mental disorder, such as delusional disorder or another psychotic disorder

Adapted from American Psychiatric Association, *Diagnostic and Statistical Manual of Mental Disorders* (DSM-5®), 5th edition, American Psychiatric Publishing, 2013.

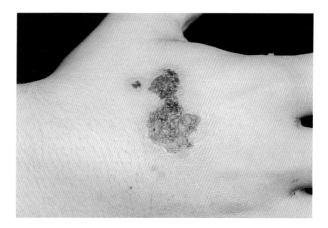

Figure 15.4 Dermatitis artefacta. Odd-shaped erosion over the dorsum of the hand. © Medical Illustration Cardiff and Vale UHB.

Dermatitis artefacta

Dermatitis artefacta (DA) is a mixture of different presentations of skin changes in which patients make changes to their skin in order to seek medical attention. It is usually very different from OCD-related dermatological disease, in that the patient makes some effort to conceal that they are manipulating their skin, and the changes in the skin are not consistent with one of the OCD-related dermatoses. Very frequently patients hide the responsibility for their actions from their HCPs. Very occasionally, patients may make changes to their skin in a fugue or dissociative state. Women are affected more often than men. Children may present with dermatitis artefacta from the age of 8 years and over, and in adolescence. For all age groups the commonest site of involvement is the face, but any part of the body may be affected.

Cutaneous lesions can include any physical skin signs such as excoriations, ulcers (Figures 15.4 and 15.5), scars, blisters, bruises, linear tears, pigmentation and petechiae. However, a key feature is that the lesions are unusual, linear, asymmetrical and sharp edged, and do not usually conform to a pattern of known cutaneous disease. In addition, often the patient describes the sudden appearance of complete lesions with little or no prodrome, there is no complete description of the genesis of individual skin lesions, and the lesions appear or are 'discovered', often on waking. Patients may show a *'belle indifférence'* to their skin disease and are often unable to give a clear account of how the lesions start, develop and clear (the hollow history). 'How' the patient is changing the skin is much less important than 'why' the patient is making the changes to the skin.

There are a range of different ways for 'how' the patient may generate DA on the skin, including picking, scratching, tape stripping, burning, freezing, crushing, bruising and using implements to make changes on the skin. Patients' motivations are variable. If there is an element of secondary gain (financial or other rewards) then the patient could be malingering. The reasons 'why' a patient generates DA range from bullying and difficult life events through to physical, social and sexual abuse. Patients will

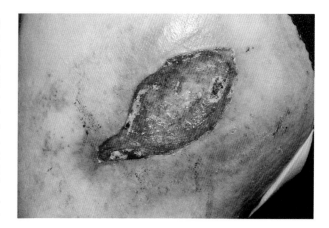

Figure 15.5 Dermatitis artefacta. Oval-shaped ulcer with surrounding bruising on the buttock. © Medical Illustration Cardiff and Vale UHB.

usually only discuss their underlying psychosocial disease when they feel engaged with the HCP and can trust that individual. It is always crucial that genuine organic disease is excluded before a safe diagnosis of DA can be made. The medical literature is studded with case reports of patients who have been misdiagnosed as having DA, only to later confirm that a genuine organic disease exists. However, similarly it is important to consider DA as a diagnosis if indicated by the clinical picture.

Management

The management of DA and other factitious skin diseases should be sympathetic and facilitative rather than confrontational:

● It is very unlikely that confronting the patient with the possibility that they are generating the skin lesions themselves will lead to a helpful consultation. It is usually best to indicate that the disease pattern does not conform to a known dermatological condition, and that often skin disease may be initiated or facilitated by stress. Taking time to allow the patient to engage with the HCP is likely to lead to a more helpful consultation.

- It is important to treat the skin appropriately.
- It is important to address *why* the patient is presenting with DA. Usually a cause for the DA will be revealed as soon as the patient feels safe with the clinician and the environment. This can be very quickly after presentation or it may take a very long time.
- Once a therapeutic relationship has been established between the patient and the clinician, the appropriate action can be initiated. This may mean tackling bullying at school, referral to social services or a range of different psychosocial measures.
- It may be necessary to refer the patient to a vulnerable adult service, or to psychiatry services if there are safeguarding issues or psychiatric comorbidities.
- It may be important to distance the patient from adopting a sick role (e.g. encouraging the patient to avoid opioid pain relief and suggesting other pain relief techniques).

The prognosis relates to that of the primary psychological disorder. Acute stress reaction can be addressed in a series of short consultations at the same time as when the dressings are changed. Approximately one-third to one-half of patients will continue to develop chronic lesions.

Dermatitis simulate

Apparent skin disease can be represented by patients who are ingenious enough to use external disguise to simulate disease. These patients do not significantly damage their skin. Make-up, glue, paint and other materials have been used to simulate skin disease or a birthmark. As expected, this is most common in children.

Dermatological pathomimicry

Some patients may intentionally aggravate or mimic an existing dermatosis using the explanation of its genesis given by their dermatologist, for example developing a rash that exactly mimics a known dermatological condition (e.g. lupus). Another example would be a non-healing ulcer following surgery that mimics infection or pyoderma gangrenosum; in this situation it is very important to make sure that there is no genuine, organic cause. Similarly, it is important to consider pathomimicry if the exacerbations appear at times of stress or just before contact with HCPs. In this situation, there is usually also a family member or friend who has the mimicked condition.

Dermatitis passivate (terra firma forme)

The cessation of normal skin cleansing results in an accumulation of keratin. The patient may describe symptoms related to the keratin build-up (pain, discomfort, fear of ulceration), and the lesions may appear anywhere on the body. Simple cleansing may remove the keratin, but a discussion about why the patient has developed the lesions is also important. In the elderly, or in patients with severe depression, there may be dementia or neglect, and this is different from true passivate, in that such patients simply forget or neglect to wash and so keratin builds up, as opposed to a determined conscious effort not to wash in order to generate a skin change.

Malingering

The essential feature of malingering is the intentional production of false or grossly exaggerated physical or psychological symptoms, motivated by external incentives such as avoiding work, seeking financial compensation, evading criminal prosecution or obtaining drugs.

Munchausen's syndrome

Munchausen's syndrome usually refers to patients who attend emergency or other medical departments with simulated disease (e.g. abdominal pain simulating appendicitis) to gain access to medical care, and to adopt a sick role with all the consequences. While dermatological complaints are uncommon in Munchausen's syndrome, simulated porphyria and connective tissue disease, for example, may present to the dermatologist. The internet is a rich resource of ideas for some patients with Munchausen's syndrome, who may present with textbook factitious reproductions of the diseases they have read about online. Cases have been reported showing the facility with which such individuals can attract attention, mobilise sympathy and control others.

Fabricated and induced illness or Munchausen's syndrome by proxy

Munchausen's syndrome by proxy (or fabricated and induced illness, FII) describes when someone causes a simulated disease on another individual (often a child or a vulnerable adult), for example by creating erosions or blisters on another individual to simulate autoimmune bullous disease.

The history is 'hollow' with a lack of detail. By contrast, most parents and carers can give a clear account of a skin disease if it is genuine. Risk factors for FII include being a single parent or young parent, previous abuse, frequent visits to general practitioner or accident and emergency departments, poverty and overcrowding. The victims have a persistent or recurrent illness that cannot be readily explained. The diagnosis of FII remains one that is made clinically. Symptoms with which the patient presents often do not respond to the treatment and laboratory tests are incongruous. If suspected, a referral to child or adult safeguarding is essential.

Deliberate self-harm (self-mutilation)

Self-mutilation of the skin, sometimes termed self-injury or self-harm, may present with a wide range of lesions. It is common, particularly in young women. Cutting and scratching are frequent, but other methods, such as grazing, burning with fire or chemicals, or insertion of foreign bodies under the skin, are also seen.

Deliberate self-harm is different from DA in that the patient admits that they are creating the skin manifestation themselves, though they will usually explain that they have an urge to 'cut' and a sense of 'control' and 'relief' afterwards. Working with families, schools and if necessary mental health services can be helpful.

Mental health legislation

The law in this area in the UK has been covered by the Mental Health Act 1983 and its amendments. A replacement Mental Health Bill is being considered in 2021 and so legislation is likely to change.

Sometimes dermatologists may believe that a patient is at risk of harm to themselves or to others, and that managing the patient as an inpatient is imperative. This is rare in dermatology. For the most part, psychiatrists will attempt to persuade patients whom they believe are at risk of harm to themselves or others to agree to a voluntary admission. Where dermatology HCPs believe that a patient may be at risk of harming themselves or others, the correct course of action is to contact the patient's primary care doctor and the local liaison psychiatry team. Primary care and/or the local crisis team will then be able to assess and set in motion all the necessary steps when a patient in these circumstances is not persuaded to agree to an inpatient admission (this usually involves a mixture of social workers and clinicians).

Conclusions

Managing patients with primary psychodermatological disease is usually best done via an MDT approach. Growing research indicates that dedicated comprehensive psychodermatology clinics are both clinically and cost-effective. Dermatology trainees and HCPs can manage patients with primary skin disease and psychosocial comorbidities in general skin clinics. Psychosocial comorbidities of dermatological disease occur very commonly. Psychodermatological disease can be severe and extensive, and patients prefer to be managed in dermatology units by an MDT.

Pearls and pitfalls

- In psychodermatology treat the physical disease and the psychosocial disease at the same time.
- Before establishing the diagnosis of dermatitis artefacta, always exclude organic disease. But do not be afraid to consider the diagnosis if the clinical picture suggests dermatitis artefacta in the differential.
- When managing a person with dermatitis artefacta, 'why' is usually much more important than 'how'.
- When caring for a patient with delusional infestation, engaging the patient is crucial. Negotiation about the validity of the patient's experience (e.g. 'Have you considered that the problem you are experiencing is all in your mind?') is likely to be unhelpful.

- Do not be afraid to ask about suicidal ideation in dermatology patients. To ask reduces the risk of patients acting on suicidal ideation, and provides an opportunity for signposting patients to helpful support.
- In patients with body dysmorphia, do not dismiss the 'defect' about which the patient is concerned. Instead, try to acknowledge the difference between how the patient perceives it and how others perceive it.

SCE Questions. See questions 49 and 50.

FURTHER READING AND KEY RESOURCES

Bewley A, Affleck A, Bundy C *et al.* Psychodermatology services guidance: the report of the British Association of Dermatologists' Psychodermatology Working Party. *Br J Dermatol* 2013; **168**:1149–50.

Textbooks

Bewley A, Taylor RE, Reichenberg J, Magid M, eds. *Practical Psychodermatology*. Chichester: Wiley, 2014.

Taylor DM, Barnes TRE, Young AH. *The Maudley Prescribing Guidelines in Psychiatry*. Hoboken, NJ: Wiley-Blackwell, 2018.

Taylor DM, Gaughran F, Pillinger T. *Practice Guidelines for Physical Health Conditions in Psychiatry*. Hoboken, NJ: Wiley-Blackwell, 2020.

Useful websites

Adult Improving Access to Psychological Therapies programme. Available at: https://www.england.nhs.uk/mental-health/adults/iapt.

All Party Parliamentary Group on Skin. Mental health and skin disease. Available at: https://www.appgs.co.uk/mental-health-and-skin-disease-report-2020.

Body Dysmorphic Disorder Foundation. Available at: https://www.bddfoundation.org/support-groups.

British Association of Therapeutic Hypnotists. Available at: www.bathh.co.uk.

British Hypnotherapy Association. Available at: www.hypnotherapy-association.org.

Changing Faces. Support group for people with different appearance. Available at: www.changingfaces.org.uk.

MIND. Mental health information and support charity. Available at: www.mind.org.uk.

National Health Service. Body dysmorphic disorder. Available at: https://www.nhs.uk/conditions/body-dysmorphia.

OCD-UK. Obsessive–compulsive disorder information and support charity. Available at: www.ocduk.org.

Skin Support. Emotional support for people with skin disease. Available at: www.skinsupport.org.uk.

16

Emergency dermatology

Ruwani P. Katugampola

Introduction

Being called to see a dermatological emergency when you are on call at the start of your dermatology training can be daunting. Non-dermatologists will look to you to make the correct diagnosis, initiate the appropriate treatment and 'sort out' the patient, who may be visibly distressed and covered in an itchy and/or painful red, scaly, blistering rash. There are some general tips in dealing with dermatological emergencies.

Ensure the patient is alert and vital functions are intact by checking **A**irway, **B**reathing and **C**irculation (ABC). This would usually have been assessed by the referring physician by the time you arrive on the scene. Stay calm and go back to the basics of good history taking, thorough clinical examination of the skin, and general examination, including palpation for lymph nodes. Good knowledge of the normal anatomy and physiological function of the skin is essential in these situations. Be aware that dermatological emergencies presenting in individuals with skin of colour may look different from what you are familiar with seeing in those with lighter skin colour and/or typical textbook images.

Complications of dermatological emergencies occur due to skin failure and loss of normal skin function. Restoring the physiological function of the diseased skin applies to the initial management of most dermatological emergencies, regardless of the diagnosis (Table 16.1). Undertake skin biopsy and relevant blood investigations based on your differential diagnosis to help guide further management of the patient, including the extracutaneous manifestations where appropriate. Once a definite diagnosis has been made, it is helpful to know where to find up-to-date guidelines on disease management, such as from the British Association of Dermatologists.

Erythroderma

Erythroderma is characterised by widespread redness, scaling and exfoliation of the skin affecting at least 90% of the body surface area (Figure 16.1). Be alert to these features when assessing individuals with skin of colour, as redness will not be so evident as in those with paler skin colour. The possible causes of erythroderma are summarised in Table 16.2. The age of the patient, in addition to a detailed clinical history and examination, will help with the differential diagnosis of erythroderma. However, about 20–30% of cases with erythroderma can be idiopathic, with no known underlying cause.

Management

- Provide supportive care.
- Manage the patient in a warm environment, ideally in a single cubicle.

Dermatology Training: The Essentials. Edited by Mahbub M.U. Chowdhury, Tamara W. Griffiths and Andrew Y. Finlay.
© 2022 The British Association of Dermatologists. Published 2022 by John Wiley & Sons Ltd.
Companion website: www.wiley.com/go/chowdhury/dermatologytraining

- Treat or prevent potential complications of erythroderma, as summarised in Table 16.1.
- Diagnose (e.g. by skin biopsy) and treat the underlying cause, withdraw the potential cause e.g. the suspect drug.
- Sedating antihistamines can provide symptomatic relief, if a patient is itchy.
- Consider oral prednisolone for drug-induced erythroderma.

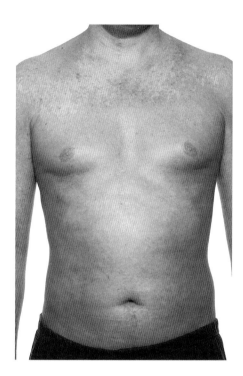

Figure 16.1 Erythroderma. © Medical Illustration Cardiff and Vale UHB.

Erythema multiforme

The typical presentation of erythema multiforme (EM) is multiple target-like skin lesions, often in an acral distribution (Figure 16.2). However, EM, as its name implies, can appear as pink to red lesions of many different shapes and forms. EM with only skin involvement is classified as EM minor; if mucosal surfaces are also involved this is classified as EM major.

In up to 50% of cases, the cause of EM is unknown. Known causes of EM include:

- **Infections**: mycoplasma, herpes simplex virus (HSV) or Epstein–Barr virus.
- **Drugs**: antibiotics (for example sulfonamides, penicillin) or non-steroidal anti-inflammatories.

Investigations

Where the clinical features of EM are atypical or involve the mucosal surfaces, a skin biopsy should be undertaken to exclude other differential diagnoses, including Stevens–Johnson syndrome (SJS) and other immunobullous diseases such as pemphigus vulgaris. Further investigations, such as routine bloods, septic screen or chest X-ray, will be dictated by the possible underlying cause.

Management

EM is usually self-limiting but can recur. In the acute phase, management includes identifying and withdrawing the potential causative medication or treating the underlying infective cause, and symptomatic treatment with regular emollients, antihistamines and mild-to-moderate-potency topical corticosteroids. Recurrent episodes of EM may require a course of long-term aciclovir, if reactivation of dormant HSV is thought to be the cause.

Table 16.1 Management of potential complications due to loss of skin function in dermatological emergencies

Loss of skin function	Complications	Management
Loss of skin barrier function	Skin infection, septicaemia	Monitor for evidence of infection, perform septic screen, commence systemic antibiotics if evidence of infection (guided by microbiological sensitivities)
Loss of thermoregulation	Hypothermia	Monitor core body temperature, manage patient in a warm environment, ideally in a single cubicle
Loss of regulation of transepidermal water loss	Dehydration Tachycardia and high-output cardiac failure Renal failure	Monitor blood pressure, pulse, fluid balance and renal function to guide oral or intravenous fluid and electrolyte replacement
Exfoliation with loss of albumin and protein	Peripheral oedema	Frequent application of emollients, monitor serum albumin, nutritional support

Table 16.2 Likely causes of erythroderma based on the age of the patient

	Neonate or infant	Child	Adult
Inflammatory skin diseases	Atopic dermatitis	Atopic dermatitis Psoriasis	Atopic dermatitis Allergic contact dermatitis Psoriasis Pityriasis rubra pilaris
Drug reactions	Antibiotics	Antibiotics Anticonvulsants	Antibiotics Anticonvulsants Allopurinol
Bullous skin disease			Bullous pemphigoid Pemphigus foliaceus
Malignancies			Cutaneous T-cell lymphoma Lymphoproliferative malignancies Sézary syndrome
Infection	Staphylococcal scalded skin syndrome Candidiasis	Staphylococcal scalded skin syndrome	
Immune deficiency	Severe combined immune deficiency		
Genetic	Ichthyosis (e.g. Netherton's syndrome, bullous ichthyosiform erythroderma)	Ichthyosis (e.g. Netherton's syndrome)	

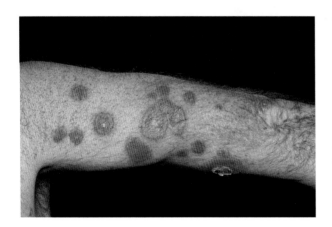

Figure 16.2 Erythema multiforme. Note the target-like skin lesions. © Medical Illustration Cardiff and Vale UHB.

Individuals with EM major require analgesia, supportive care and input from oral medicine and ophthalmology teams to manage the affected mucosal surfaces. A short course of oral prednisolone may need to be considered. These individuals require close monitoring as the differential diagnosis includes SJS.

Stevens–Johnson syndrome and toxic epidermal necrolysis

SJS (Figure 16.3) and toxic epidermal necrolysis (TEN, Figure 16.4) are both rare and comprise a potentially life-threatening disease spectrum of mucocutaneous exfoliation, which can affect any age group. They are often drug induced, but rarely they can occur due to infective causes (Table 16.3).

Clinical presentation of Stevens–Johnson syndrome and toxic epidermal necrolysis

SJS and TEN are defined by the area of skin detachment, measured by the affected body surface area (BSA):

- SJS: < 10% BSA
- SJS/TEN overlap: 10–30% BSA
- TEN: > 30% BSA

Skin pain is a diagnostic feature of TEN. Patients can present with feeling unwell, malaise, a dusky maculopapular rash, targetoid lesions, erosions and skin pain, progressing to detachment of the epidermis spontaneously or with minimal pressure (Nikolsky sign), leading to large areas of skin loss resembling burns. Mucosal exfoliation results in the extracutaneous manifestations of SJS and TEN, as summarised in Table 16.4.

Management of Stevens–Johnson syndrome and toxic epidermal necrolysis

A skin biopsy of the affected skin for routine histology, and perilesional biopsy for direct immunofluorescence (IMF) (Chapter 5), can be helpful in the initial stages of suspected TEN/SJS to distinguish it from other differential diagnoses such as staphylococcal scaled skin syndrome, pemphigus and epidermolysis bullosa acquisita. The typical histological feature of TEN is full-thickness necrosis of the epidermis.

The severity of illness score in TEN (SCORTEN) is a scoring system calculated within the first 24 hours of presentation that helps predict mortality (Table 16.4). Each factor scores one point, and mortality increases with increasing total score (score 0–1 = 3.2%, score ≥ 5 = 90% mortality).

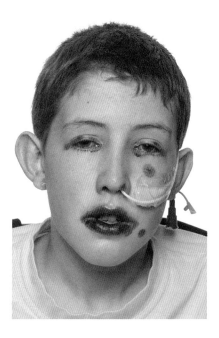

Figure 16.3 Stevens–Johnson syndrome. Note the stomatitis and conjunctival redness and erosions. © Medical Illustration Cardiff and Vale UHB.

(a)

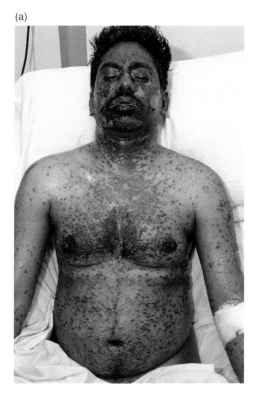

(b)

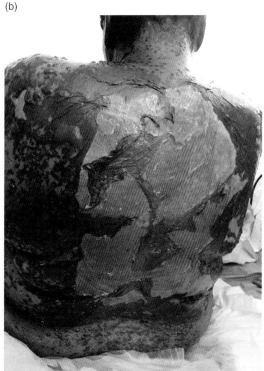

Figure 16.4 Toxic epidermal necrolysis. (a) Note the dusky maculopapular rash, targetoid lesions on the trunk and limbs, stomatitis and erosions on the face. © Salford Royal NHS Foundation Trust. (b) Note the detachment of the epidermis leading to large areas of skin loss resembling burns. Creamer D *et al. Br J Dermatol* 2016; **174**:1194–227.

Table 16.3 Causes of Stevens–Johnson syndrome and toxic epidermal necrolysis

Medication	Antibiotics, e.g. penicillin, sulfonamides
	Anticonvulsants, e.g. carbamazepine, phenytoin, lamotrigine
	Allopurinol
	Antiretroviral medication, e.g. abacavir
	Non-steroidal anti-inflammatory drugs
	Targeted anticancer therapy and immunotherapy, e.g. imatinib, rituximab
Infections	Epstein–Barr virus
	Herpes simplex virus
	Mycoplasma

Table 16.4 Factors used to calculate the severity of illness score in toxic epidermal necrolysis (SCORTEN)

Age > 40 years
Epidermal detachment of > 10% body surface area
Presence of malignancy
Pulse > 120 beats per minute
Serum glucose > 14 mmol/L
Serum urea > 10 mmol/L
Serum bicarbonate < 20 mmol/L

Management of the skin in SJS and TEN is similar to that in erythroderma, including stopping the suspect drug or treating the causative infection, and supportive care with regular analgesia, non-adherent dressing on the denuded skin and supportive care (Table 16.1). There are extensive areas of skin loss and potential life-threatening complications due to multisystem mucosal exfoliation in TEN (Table 16.5). Therefore, these patients are best managed in a high-dependency unit (HDU) or burns unit with input from a multidisciplinary team, including ophthalmology, oral medicine, respiratory medicine, gastroenterology, urology and dietetics, as well as dermatology. The use of systemic therapy for SJS and TEN is controversial. However, treatments such as systemic steroids, intravenous immunoglobulin (IVIg), oral ciclosporin and tumour necrosis factor-α inhibitors (such as infliximab) initiated early at the onset of the disease process have been reported to improve the prognosis of SJS and TEN.

Table 16.5 Extracutaneous manifestations of Stevens–Johnson syndrome and toxic epidermal necrolysis

Mucosal involvement	Manifestations
Lips and oral mucosa	Stomatitis
Conjunctiva and cornea	Conjunctivitis, erosions, scarring
Respiratory tract	Respiratory failure
Gastrointestinal tract	Oesophagitis, diarrhoea
Urinary tract	Dysuria, urinary retention

For detailed guidelines, care pathways, a discharge letter template and patient information leaflets for children, young people and adults with SJS and TEN, refer to the British Association of Dermatologists' guidelines.

Angio-oedema and anaphylaxis

Angio-oedema is characterised by painless oedema of the lips, tongue and eyelids, or more widespread oedema involving the hands and feet, gastrointestinal tract and laryngeal mucosa (Figure 16.5). Angio-oedema may last for up to a week and may be associated with urticaria in about 50% of cases. Angio-oedema may be idiopathic or caused by factors broadly divided into two categories: histamine-mediated and bradykinin-mediated angio-oedema (Table 16.6). It responds to different modes of treatment. The final common pathway is the release of vasodilatory substances and increased vascular permeability, resulting in swelling of the deep dermis and subcutaneous tissue and leading to the clinical manifestations. Anaphylaxis is a life-threatening emergency and is within the spectrum of histamine-mediated angio-oedema. It presents with rapid onset of oedema of the upper airway leading to difficulty in breathing and swallowing, with potential loss of consciousness, and requires emergency treatment.

Management

Anaphylaxis is potentially life-threatening and requires *immediate intervention* as follows:

- Assessment of **A**irway, **B**reathing and **C**irculation (ABC).
- Maintaining these vital functions with intubation or tracheostomy as required.
- Administration of high-flow oxygen.

- Intravenous fluid.
- Intramuscular adrenaline 500 μg for an adult (0.5 mL of 1:1000 adrenaline) to be repeated after 5 minutes if no improvement.
- Intramuscular or slow intravenous hydrocortisone 200 mg for an adult.
- Intramuscular or slow intravenous chlorphenamine 10 mg for an adult.

Once the patient is stable, the potential cause of the anaphylaxis should be investigated and a detailed history should be taken. The patient should be advised to wear a MedicAlert® bracelet (MedicAlert Foundation, Turlock, VA, USA) and be prescribed and shown how to use an EpiPen® (Mylan, Potters Bar, UK) in the event of further anaphylaxis.

Management of idiopathic and histamine-mediated angio-oedema consists of H1 antihistamines, a short course of oral steroids, EpiPen in the acute setting and IVIg. Consider ciclosporin for long-term management of recurrent disease. Management of hereditary angio-oedema consists of the anti-androgen danazol (not suitable for women of childbearing age or children, due to androgenic effects), infusion of C1 esterase inhibitor concentrate (in C1 esterase inhibitor deficiency) and fresh frozen plasma.

The most up-to-date management details and algorithm for anaphylaxis can be found on the UK Resuscitation Council website (see Further reading).

(a)

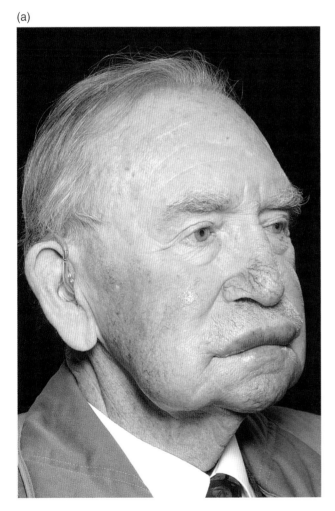

(b)

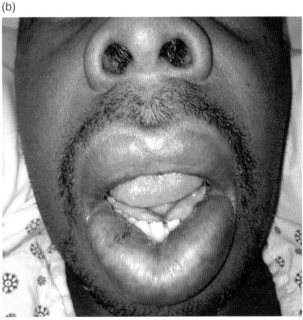

Figure 16.5 Angio-oedema. Note the swelling of the lips in individuals with (a) lighter skin and (b) skin of colour. (a) © Medical Illustration Cardiff and Vale UHB (b) Jung M *et al*. Angioedema in patients treated with sirolimus and ACE inhibitor post hematopoietic stem cell transplant. *Bone Marrow Transplant* 2014; **49**:1448–9.

Table 16.6 Causes of angio-oedema

Category	Causes	Pathogenesis
Idiopathic	Unknown	Unknown
Histamine mediated	Food, e.g. nuts, shellfish, strawberries Latex Contrast medium used in radiological procedures Bee or wasp sting Physical induced, e.g. cold exposure, pressure, physical activity (cholinergic)	IgE-mediated degranulation of mast cells and basophils leading to release of histamine (type 1 hypersensitivity reaction) Onset within minutes, lasts 12–24 hours May be associated with urticaria Bronchospasm, hypotension common
Bradykinin mediated	Hereditary C1 esterase inhibitor deficiency and defective function Acquired, e.g. medication (angiotensin-converting enzyme inhibitors, especially in patients of Afro-Caribbean origin; tacrolimus; sirolimus)	Production or inhibition of breakdown of bradykinin leads to activation of endothelial cells Onset within hours, lasts 48–72 hours Urticaria uncommon Bronchospasm, hypotension uncommon Gastrointestinal symptoms common

Investigations

A detailed history will help identify the likely cause of the angio-oedema and/or anaphylaxis and dictate the choice of further investigations and management. When IgE-mediated type 1 hypersensitivity reaction is suspected to a specific agent, such as latex or a particular type of nuts, this can be investigated by serum IgE and by the allergen-specific radioallergosorbent test (RAST). If specific IgE is negative, prick test to the suspect allergen could be considered with availability of full resuscitation facilities. Where C1 esterase inhibitor deficiency is suspected, serum C1 esterase inhibitor (including functional levels), complement C3 and C4 should be measured.

Blistering skin rashes

There are many causes of blistering rashes; a detailed clinical history and examination, including the distribution and morphology of the blisters, will assist to narrow down the differential diagnosis. Here are some tips to help you:

- **Age of the patient** (Table 16.7). In neonates and infants, the differential diagnosis should include inherited and acquired causes of bullous diseases.
- **Extent and distribution of the rash**. For example, localised painful and/or itchy urticated plaques and blisters in a linear streaky distribution appearing within 24 hours at the site of contact with plants containing photosensitising psoralen (e.g. celery, giant hogweed) and sunlight exposure cause phyto-photodermatitis. This is due to a phototoxic reaction within the skin. Blisters confined to sun-exposed skin and sparing the

Table 16.7 Differential diagnosis of blistering rashes based on the age of the patient

Neonate and infants
- Inherited: epidermolysis bullosa, bullous ichthyosiform erythroderma, incontinentia pigmenti
- Acquired: bullous impetigo, staphylococcal scalded skin syndrome, herpes simplex infection, eczema herpeticum, varicella zoster

Children
- Immunobullous: linear IgA disease
- Infectious causes mentioned above
- Other: insect bites, phytophotodermatitis, severe sunburn, dermatitis artefacta, Stevens–Johnson syndrome (SJS) and toxic epidermal necrolysis (TEN)

Adults and elderly
- Immunobullous: bullous pemphigoid, pemphigus, dermatitis herpetiformis
- Infectious causes: eczema herpeticum, herpes zoster
- Inflammatory: phytophotodermatitis, pompholyx eczema
- Drug reactions: SJS/TEN, fixed drug eruptions
- Other: insect bites, phytophotodermatitis, severe sunburn, dermatitis artefacta, bullous cutaneous porphyrias, pseudoporphyria

unexposed skin suggest the likelihood of photodermatoses, such as bullous cutaneous porphyrias.
- **Morphology of the blisters**. For example, blisters in an arc pattern ('string of pearls' distribution) in a child are characteristic

of linear IgA disease. Blisters in a linear blaschkoid distribution in a female neonate are highly suggestive of incontinentia pigmenti, an X-linked dominant disease. If the detachment is intraepidermal, there may be no clinically evident blisters, but merely erosions.

Most blistering skin diseases need to be biopsied to confirm the clinical diagnosis. A biopsy from the lesional skin should be taken for haematoxylin and eosin (H&E) staining and perilesional biopsy for direct IMF (Chapter 5). Blood investigations should include serum antibodies to the target antigen and for indirect IMF. When infective causes are considered in the differential diagnosis, a swab of the blister fluid should be sent for virology or microbiology, based on the clinical suspicion.

Some blistering skin diseases that may present as a dermatological emergency are described in further detail below.

Bullous pemphigoid

Bullous pemphigoid (BP) is an immunobullous disease that presents most commonly in elderly patients. BP occurs due to IgG autoantibodies directed against the basement membrane antigen BP180 (type XVII collagen) or BP230, resulting in cleavage of the dermoepidermal junction in the skin leading to subepidermal blisters. Medications can be associated with triggering or exacerbating BP (Table 16.8).

The onset of the blisters is often preceded by intense itching of the skin or by itchy urticated plaques. The tense skin blisters may be either localised or widespread, and occasionally also develop on mucosal surfaces, including the oral and genital mucosa. The skin blisters burst, leading to superficial erosions that heal without scarring (Figure 16.6). Cicatricial pemphigoid, on the other hand, presents with blisters mainly affecting the mucous membranes, including the oral, oesophageal and/or ocular mucosa, and heal with scarring leading to complications such as visual impairment and dysphagia.

Investigations

Investigation of BP is as described above, checking serum pemphigoid antibodies and lesional and perilesional skin biopsies for H&E and direct IMF, respectively. The characteristic histological features of BP are a subepidermal blister on H&E and linear deposition of IgG at the basement membrane on direct IMF.

Management

Management of BP depends on the extent of the disease, the patient's other comorbidities, potential triggers and exacerbating factors. The decision to discontinue a medication suspected of triggering or exacerbating BP, and choice of an alternative medication, should be made in consultation with the patient and

Table 16.8 Medications associated with bullous pemphigoid

Antibiotics
Angiotensin-converting enzyme (ACE) inhibitors
Anti-tumour necrosis factor-α
Beta blockers
Calcium channel blockers
Diuretics
Dipeptidyl peptidase 4 inhibitors, e.g. sitagliptin
Immune checkpoint inhibitors, e.g. pembrolizumab
Non-steroidal anti-inflammatories
Salicylates

(a)

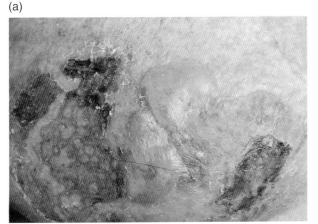

(b)

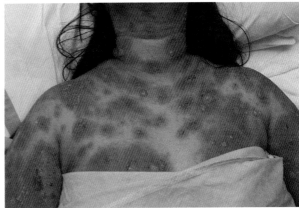

Figure 16.6 Bullous pemphigoid. (a) Note the tense blisters, some of which have burst, leaving superficial erosions in an individual with lighter skin colour. © Medical Illustration Cardiff and Vale UHB. (b) Note the dusky redness at the base of the blisters in an individual with skin of colour. © Salford Royal NHS Foundation Trust.

other healthcare professionals involved in their care. Localised BP can be treated with topical superpotent corticosteroids (e.g. 0.05% clobetasol propionate). More widespread disease requires a reducing course of oral prednisolone starting at 0.5 mg/kg/day, in combination with an oral immunosuppressant such as mycophenolate mofetil or azathioprine. Oral doxycycline 200 mg per day is an alternative option for those patients who are not suitable for oral immunosuppressant therapy. BP may relapse and remit, but it usually resolves within 3–5 years.

Cicatricial pemphigoid requires early intervention to prevent complications related to scarring. This includes the use of oral steroids with immunosuppressants such as mycophenolate mofetil, intravenous cyclophosphamide and the chimeric anti-CD20 monoclonal antibody rituximab.

Pemphigus

Pemphigus is a group of rare, potentially life-threatening immunobullous diseases that usually affect middle-aged individuals. It occurs due to IgG autoantibodies directed against the epidermal cell-surface proteins desmoglein 1 and 3, leading to loss of cell-to-cell adhesion and the characteristic acantholysis seen on histology. Acantholysis occurs at different levels within the epidermis, resulting in varying clinical presentations including flaccid, fragile blisters and/or superficial scaly erosions of the skin, with or without involvement of the mucosal surfaces (Figure 16.7).

Based on these features, there are three main types of pemphigus (Table 16.9). Paraneoplastic pemphigus is seen in association with lymphoproliferative diseases such as non-Hodgkin's lymphoma, chronic lymphocytic leukaemia, thymoma and Castleman's disease.

Investigations

Investigation of pemphigus includes lesional and perilesional skin biopsies for H&E and direct IMF, respectively (Chapter 5), serum indirect IMF, and enzyme-linked immunoassay for anti-

bodies to desmoglein 1 and 3. Patients with paraneoplastic pemphigus should be investigated for an underlying malignancy with routine blood tests, including a full blood count and blood film, lactate dehydrogenase and chest X-ray. Consider a full-body CT scan and further tests guided by the initial investigation results and the patient's clinical history and general examination findings.

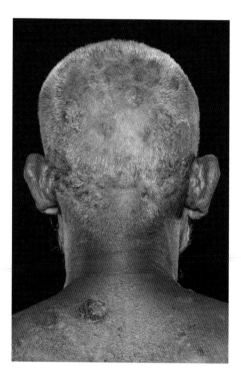

Figure 16.7 Pemphigus vulgaris. Note the superficial erosions and crusting, which are often seen rather than the fragile blisters. © Medical Illustration Cardiff and Vale UHB.

Table 16.9 Features of three main types of pemphigus

Type of pemphigus	Pemphigus vulgaris	Pemphigus foliaceous	Paraneoplastic pemphigus
Skin manifestation	Fragile, flaccid blisters	Superficial scaly erosions	Polymorphous lesions, including erosions, lichenoid lesions, targetoid lesions similar to erythema multiforme
Mucosal involvement	Often involved	Spared	Severely involved
Presence of serum autoantibodies	Desmogleins 1 and 3	Desmoglein 1	Desmogleins 1 and 3, epithelial plakin proteins (e.g. desmoplakin)
H&E histology	Suprabasal acantholysis	Subcorneal acantholysis	Suprabasal acantholysis
Direct IMF	Net-like pattern of cell-surface bound IgG in the epidermis	Net-like pattern of cell-surface-bound IgG in the epidermis	Net-like pattern of cell-surface-bound IgG in the epidermis

H&E, haematoxylin and eosin; IMF, immunofluorescence.

Management

Supportive care of the skin including use of non-adherent dressings applies to the management of all forms of pemphigus (Table 16.1). For pemphigus vulgaris and pemphigus foliaceous, a high-dose weaning course of oral prednisolone (up to 1 mg/kg/day) is needed in combination with an oral immunosuppressant such as azathioprine or mycophenolate mofetil. Other treatment options are IVIg, cyclophosphamide and rituximab. Due to the mucosal involvement in pemphigus vulgaris and paraneoplastic pemphigus, input from ophthalmology, oral medicine and other relevant specialties is essential to prevent complications due to ulceration and scarring. For paraneoplastic pemphigus, in addition to the treatments mentioned, the aim is to treat the underlying neoplasm, which needs a multidisciplinary management approach.

Table 16.10 Causative medications of acute generalised exanthematous pustulosis

Antibiotics
Angiotensin-converting enzyme (ACE) inhibitors
Anticonvulsants
Antimalarials
Antivirals
Allopurinol
Calcium channel blockers
Diuretics
Infections, including mycoplasma, parvovirus B19, cytomegalovirus and *Escherichia coli*
Psoralen and ultraviolet A (PUVA)

Drug reactions

You may see a range of different drug-induced rashes as a dermatological emergency. Some of these were described earlier in this chapter, and a few more will be described below. A detailed drug history (prescribed and over-the-counter medications, timing between the use of a medication and onset of the rash) is paramount in making a diagnosis of a drug reaction. In general, excluding immediate type 1 reactions, there is up to a three-month time interval between commencement of a new medication and the onset of a drug reaction. Initial management of any drug reaction is to withdraw the suspect medication and commence supportive care, as described earlier. The acute potentially life-threatening drug reactions require rapid intervention, as described in the individual sections.

Acute generalised exanthematous pustulosis

Acute generalised exanthematous pustulosis (AGEP) presents with an acute onset of widespread small, sterile pustules on a red background in a febrile individual. The rash often starts in the skin folds such as axillae, groin and/or submammary regions, prior to becoming more generalised. AGEP develops usually within 24–48 hours of ingestion of a causative medication and therefore a detailed drug history is important to make the diagnosis. The list of causative medications is extensive (Table 16.10).

The diagnosis of AGEP can be made clinically in most cases, based on the history and clinical features. The main differential diagnoses are acute generalised pustular psoriasis and subcorneal pustular dermatosis.

Investigations

A full blood count will show a neutrophilia, and the C-reactive protein will be elevated. A skin biopsy will help if the diagnosis is uncertain: it will show intraepidermal pustules, focal necrosis of keratinocytes and eosinophils within the pustules and/or dermis. If infectious causes are suspected, swab a pustule for microscopy, culture and staining, and undertake a septic screen based on clinical suspicion.

Management

Management of AGEP includes withdrawal of the suspect medication and supportive care as for erythroderma. The rash usually resolves within 1–2 weeks of stopping the causative medication.

Drug reaction with eosinophilia and systemic symptoms

Drug reaction with eosinophilia and systemic symptoms (DRESS) is a multisystem, potentially life-threatening condition associated with a mortality of up to 10%. In contrast to AGEP, DRESS tends to present 2–8 weeks after ingestion of the causative medication. The causative medications associated with DRESS include antibiotics, anticonvulsants and allopurinol.

The skin manifestations of DRESS can vary from a mild, itchy red maculopapular rash, AGEP-like presentation or blistering rash to exfoliative erythroderma. Mucosal surfaces are generally spared, a distinguishing feature from SJS and TEN. The extracutaneous complications of DRESS include pericarditis, pneumonitis, hepatitis and interstitial nephritis. The severity of the skin manifestations does not always correspond to the extra-cutaneous organ involvement, and therefore patients with suspected DRESS should be monitored closely for multiorgan involvement.

Investigations

Initial blood tests include a full blood count (leucocytosis with atypical lymphocytes and eosinophilia), renal and liver function (elevated liver enzymes) and C-reactive protein. A skin biopsy may be considered, to exclude other severe drug reactions such as SJS and TEN. The skin histological features of DRESS are not diagnostic, but include interface dermatitis with apoptotic keratinocytes. Further extracutaneous investigations including chest X-ray, echocardiogram or creatinine clearance will be dictated by the multidisciplinary team.

Management

DRESS may take several months to resolve following withdrawal of the medication. These individuals are best managed by a multidisciplinary team to ensure monitoring and prevention of multiorgan complications. Management of the skin includes supportive care as for erythroderma and a weaning course of oral prednisolone, in consultation with the multidisciplinary team, to prevent and/or treat multiorgan disease.

Vasculitis

Vasculitis is a very broad subject beyond the full scope of this chapter. However, this section will cover the basics of cutaneous vasculitis to guide you to manage these patients in the acute setting. Vasculitis develops secondarily to inflammation of blood vessel walls due to various causes and results in narrowing or obstruction of the vessel lumina. This leads to extravasation of blood to the extravascular tissue and ischaemia, and end-organ damage of the distal tissues. Therefore, vasculitis needs to be diagnosed and treated without delay to prevent end-organ damage. Vasculitis can be categorised based on the size of the affected vessels (Table 16.11).

Cutaneous manifestations are rare in large vessel vasculitis. In the other forms of vasculitis, the cutaneous features include urticaria, livedo reticularis, erythema multiforme, palpable purpura and ulceration, often on dependent body sites such as lower legs (Figure 16.8). Individuals with cutaneous features of vasculitis need to be assessed systematically to exclude or identify systemic involvement, such as of the renal, respiratory, ocular and/or central nervous system, and referred to the appropriate specialties for prompt treatment and to prevent complications.

The potential causes of vasculitis are summarised in Table 16.12. However, in about 60% of cases the underlying cause may not be identified.

Table 16.11 Classification of vasculitis based on the size of the affected vessels

Size of affected vessels	Examples
Large vessel vasculitis	Giant cell arteritis
	Takayasu's arteritis
Medium vessel vasculitis	Kawasaki disease
	Polyarteritis nodosa
Medium to small vessel vasculitis	Granulomatosis with polyangiitis (Wegener's granulomatosis)
	Eosinophilic granulomatous angiitis (Churg–Strauss syndrome)
Small vessel vasculitis	Henoch–Schönlein purpura
	Cutaneous small vessel vasculitis (leucocytoclastic vasculitis)
	Cryoglobulinaemia

(a)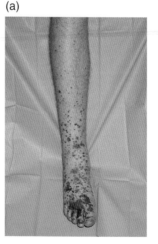
(b)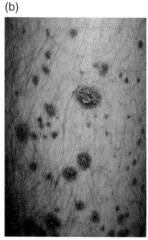

Figure 16.8 (a) Cutaneous small vessel vasculitis. (b) Note the purpura, which is palpable. © Medical Illustration Cardiff and Vale UHB.

Investigations

Patients need to be investigated to identify the cause of the vasculitis and the potential complications. The initial blood investigations include a full blood count, C-reactive protein, renal and liver function, autoantibody screen including antinuclear antibodies, double-stranded DNA, antineutrophilic cytoplasmic antibodies, cryoglobulins, antistreptolysin O titres and virology screen based on clinical suspicion. Other investigations

Table 16.12 The causes of vasculitis

Infections
Bacterial: streptococcal group A
Viral: hepatitis B and C, herpes simplex, HIV
Medication: antibiotics, thiazide diuretics
Autoantibodies: systemic lupus erythematosus, granulomatosis with polyangiitis, eosinophilic granulomatous angiitis
Malignancy: renal cancer, lung cancer, multiple myeloma

include a skin biopsy for H&E and direct IMF, urinalysis and blood pressure. Additional investigations such as chest X-ray, echocardiography and renal biopsy will be dictated by the other organs involved and the relevant specialties.

Management

Management of vasculitis involves identifying then withdrawing or treating the underlying cause, and treatment of affected organs. Small vessel vasculitis confined to the skin is often self-limiting and can be managed with rest and leg elevation, emollients, antihistamines and/or analgesia (non-steroidal anti-inflammatories if no contraindications), depending on symptoms. If the skin lesions are extensive, at risk of ulceration with signs of other organ involvement, a weaning course of oral prednisolone (0.5–1 mg/kg/day) should be considered in liaison with the other specialties. Other treatment options, as a single agent or in combination with oral steroids, include dapsone, colchicine, ciclosporin, methotrexate, azathioprine, IVIg and rituximab, based on the underlying cause and other organ involvement.

Skin infections

Skin infections such as eczema herpeticum, staphylococcal scalded skin syndrome and necrotising fasciitis may present acutely as a dermatological emergency. Be vigilant for the skin manifestations in association with COVID-19 infection. Refer to Chapter 12 for further details.

Conclusions

Dermatological emergencies are not common, but when presenting acutely, either during or out of hours, they need urgent input from dermatologists. Very often multidisciplinary care with admitting teams such as general physicians and possibly intensive care or regional burns units will be required. Drug reactions can present on any ward and also directly from general practitioners. Take every opportunity to see acutely ill patients urgently, with colleagues if needed, and be aware of and always consult the latest national guidelines and management recommendations, which are updated regularly. Experience gained under supervision is essential to progress in training. If in doubt regarding diagnosis or management, always ask your senior colleagues for advice.

Pearls and pitfalls

- The age of the patient can help you narrow down the likely differential diagnoses.
- When you are referred a patient with an acute-onset rash, ensure you see the patient as soon as possible, as the non-dermatological referral may not always use the correct dermatological terminology and may not appreciate the severity of the disease.
- Always consider multisystem involvement and/or complications in individuals presenting with dermatological emergencies. Do not be misled by the initial rash affecting a small body surface area.
- Be alert to history of skin pain: this can be a distinguishing feature of toxic epidermal necrolysis.
- Involve other relevant specialties from the outset for multidisciplinary management of mucocutaneous and vasculitic diseases to prevent long-term systemic complications.
- Patients commenced on long-term high-dose systemic steroids require osteoporosis prophylaxis and monitoring for steroid-induced complications such as gastrointestinal symptoms, diabetes and hypertension.
- For urgent acutely ill patients with a rash, if in doubt with either diagnosis or management, always ask for senior help.

SCE Questions. See questions 3 and 4.

FURTHER READING AND KEY RESOURCES

Creamer D, Walsh SA, Dziewulski P et al. UK guidelines for the management of Stevens–Johnson syndrome/toxic epidermal necrolysis in adults 2016. Br J Dermatol 2016; **174**:1194–227.

McPherson T, Exton LS, Biswas S et al. British Association of Dermatologists guidelines for the management of Stevens–Johnson syndrome/toxic epidermal necrolysis in children and young people, 2018. Br J Dermatol 2019; **181**:37–54.

Moro F, Fania L, Sinagra JLM et al. Bullous pemphigoid: trigger and predisposing factors. Biomolecules 2020; **10**:1432.

Watanabe H. Recent advances in drug-induced hypersensitivity syndrome/drug reaction with eosinophilia and systemic symptoms. J Immunol Res 2018; **2018**:5163129.

Useful website

Resuscitation Council UK. Emergency treatment of anaphylactic reactions: Guidelines for healthcare providers. Available at: https://www.resus.org.uk/library/additional-guidance/guidance-anaphylaxis/emergency-treatment.

Section 4

Therapeutics and procedural dermatology

Topical therapy

Maulina Sharma

Introduction

Topical therapy is usually the first-line treatment for skin diseases, including skin infections, infestations and inflammatory dermatoses. Topical treatments can also act as adjuncts to systemic therapies and to phototherapy for moderate-to-severe skin disease. While it is easy for us to prescribe a whole array of creams, lotions and potions, our patients may find these time consuming and tedious to apply, messy to use and difficult to apply to hard-to-reach areas (e.g. the back). The cost implications of topical therapy also need to be considered. As general medical training emphasises systemic therapy, dermatologists early in training may feel more confident in using systemic treatments for skin disease, but topical therapy should be the preferred choice wherever possible, and this requires knowledge and experience. Engaging and empowering patients with topical treatment plans, managing patient expectations and clear communication help patients and carers have a realistic approach in managing their skin disease. For example, the carer of a child with atopic eczema would benefit from a demonstration on how to apply topical emollients and corticosteroids on affected sites. This would help reassure the carer, build rapport, engage both the carer and the patient in their therapy plan and allay fears or doubts regarding use of topical therapy, especially corticosteroids.

Why is topical therapy for dermatology patients important?

Topical therapy has the advantage of reaching its target organ directly at an optimum concentration and providing local treatment. Percutaneous absorption of the active drug is enhanced by dissolving or suspending it in a vehicle base. Drugs that can be delivered topically include antibiotics, antifungals, antivirals, corticosteroids and retinoids. The drug diffuses through the horny layer, and then through the rest of the epidermis into the

Dermatology Training: The Essentials. Edited by Mahbub M.U. Chowdhury, Tamara W. Griffiths and Andrew Y. Finlay.
© 2022 The British Association of Dermatologists. Published 2022 by John Wiley & Sons Ltd.
Companion website: www.wiley.com/go/chowdhury/dermatologytraining

papillary dermis. How well the drug penetrates through the skin depends on factors related to the formulation of the product (e.g. molecular weight, concentration, vehicle base) and the properties of the involved skin (e.g. thickness and hydration of horny layer or temperature). Hydrated warm skin favours penetration (e.g. axillae), while thick palmar skin impedes permeability. As there is usually very little systemic absorption of topically applied drugs, side-effects on the bone marrow, liver and kidneys are minimised. However, it is important to be aware of the risk of systemic side-effects if a topical drug is applied frequently over extensive areas of inflamed skin.

For example, enough potent topical steroids may be absorbed to cause systemic steroid side-effects. Similarly, widespread application of salicylic acid, a keratolytic used to treat scaly, thickened skin conditions, may cause salicylism. Salicylism, or salicylic acid toxicity, occurs if the blood salicylate levels are above 35 mg/dL and could be acute or chronic. Patients may experience nausea, vomiting, tinnitus, dizziness and confusion. Hence care should be taken when prescribing topical salicylic acid in children and for treating conditions like psoriasis or ichthyosis with large body surface area involvement.

Vehicle bases for topical therapies

It is important to think about the vehicle bases you choose for the topical preparations for your patient. These can range from powders, lotions, creams, ointments and pastes, to sprays, gels or mousses. For example, dusting powders could help reduce friction in skin folds, while lotions help dry up weeping skin and evaporate quickly to help cooling of the skin. Creams are effective moisturisers and can be water-in-oil or oil-in-water emulsions, usually in a 50:50 ratio. Gels, being less greasy than creams, can be cosmetically more acceptable for patients, especially if used on the face and scalp. However, patients can develop an allergic contact dermatitis or contact urticaria to ingredients within topical medicaments and sunscreens. These ingredients include lanolin, fragrances or preservatives used in lotions, creams and gels [e.g. *para*-hydroxybenzoic acid esters (parabens), chlorocresol, sorbic acid and propylene glycol]. Ointments, which are water-in-oil (20:80 ratio) emulsions, need no preservatives and can provide an excellent safe alternative, especially for dry skin conditions.

Emollients

The useful role of emollients on itchy dry skin conditions such as eczema or psoriasis is often underestimated by patients and carers. Emollients or moisturisers help to soften the skin, act as artificial protective barriers to dysfunctional skin, help with symptom relief, for example by cooling the skin, and can reduce moisture loss. Although there is no reliable evidence that one emollient is better than another, patients may prefer urea-based products due to their keratolytic properties. The aim with moisturisers is to rehydrate the outer layer of the skin (stratum corneum), and they have been shown to prolong the time between eczema flares and reduce their frequency. Moisturisers also have a steroid-sparing effect, with less topical steroid required to gain control with concomitant use. When they are used alone or in combination with barrier creams (which act as physical barriers between skin and contaminants or irritants), there is a clinically important protective effect in the primary prevention of occupational irritant hand dermatitis. Emollient bath and shower products provide no clinical benefit when added to standard eczema care in children (BATHE Study). However, for other severe skin diseases, standard emollients may be useful as soap substitutes (Tables 17.1 and 17.2).

Before prescribing emollients consider:

- History and examination findings.
- Degree of 'dryness' noted in the skin condition or disease.
- Patient's lifestyle, age and acceptability of product on their skin (e.g. less greasy products better for the face).
- Ability and frequency of when they can be applied and suitability of dispenser (e.g. pump dispenser for elderly or those with arthritis, who may find opening and closing tubs difficult, and to avoid contamination).
- Previous use of emollients and their acceptability and effectiveness.
- Previous allergies or irritation to skin products.
- Availability of product in the local pharmacy, on prescription or over the counter.

How best to apply emollients

Patients and carers are often confused about how best to apply their topical treatments. Some simple 'to do' rules can come in handy:

- Keep readily accessible topical instruction sheets with written instructions on the amount and frequency of use as a reminder for patients at home. Always try to demonstrate how to apply the recommended emollient. There is a helpful video with a stepwise approach on how to apply topical emollients from the British Association of Dermatologists (see Further reading).
- Recommend applying after a shower or a wash.
- If prescribing a tub or a pot, instruct patients to use a clean spoon or spatula.
- Some recommend that the emollient be applied in the direction of hair growth to avoid folliculitis.
- Leave at least half an hour before or after use of emollients for any other topical product (e.g. steroid ointment or cream), except when using under occlusive bandaging, when only one active treatment should be used.
- Ointments contain fewer preservatives than cream formulations and can avoid potential allergies.
- Patients who are patch test positive to lanolin, fragrances or other preservatives should avoid products containing them.

Table 17.1 Some examples of emollients

Mild dry skin	Moderate dry skin		Severe dry skin
Less greasy			More greasy
Gels, lotions, creams	Creams, ointments		Ointments
Cetraben® emollient: 1050 g or 500 g pump dispenser, 50 g tube	Aveeno® cream: 100 mL tube (e.g. for facial eczema over age 2 years)	Doublebase®: 500 g pump dispenser	Hydromol® ointment: 500 g tube or pot, 125 g pot
Dermol® 500 lotion: 500 mL pump dispenser	Aquadrate® (10% cream): 100 g tube	Unguentum M®: 200 mL dispenser	Emulsifying ointment: 500 g pot
Diprobase® cream: 500 g pump dispenser	Dermol® cream (contains antimicrobial): 500 g pump dispenser		50% liquid paraffin in 50% white soft paraffin (also called 50:50 LP with WSP): 500 g pot
Eucerin® lotion (10% urea): 250 mL bottle	Epimax® ExCetra cream: 500 g easy squeeze dispenser		Emollin® spray: as alternative to WSP if difficult to apply, e.g. perianal area
E45 cream: 500 g pump dispenser	Zeroderm® cream: 500 g pump dispenser		Zeroderm® ointment: 500 g pot

Table 17.2 Soap substitutes

Aqueous cream BP: 30 g pot, 100 g tube, 500 g pot (Do *not* use as 'leave-on emollient', to avoid skin reactions)
Cetraben® emollient: 1050 g or 500 g pump dispenser, 50 g tube
Dermol® 500 lotion (contains antimicrobial), 500 mL pump dispenser
Dermol® cream, 500 g pump dispenser (contains antimicrobial)
Diprobase® cream, 500 g pump dispenser
Hydromol® ointment, 500 g tube or pot, 125 g pot
Oilatum Plus® (antibacterial), 500 mL bottle

- Prescribe enough (e.g. to cover the whole skin, 500 g weekly for an adult or 250 g weekly for a child).
- In difficult areas such as perianal areas and around stoma sites, consider white soft paraffin with liquid paraffin (50:50), or emollient spray as an alternative.

Adherence

The most important hallmark of effective topical therapy is patient adherence to the agreed treatment plan. Patients may over-optimistically anticipate a quick response to a therapy that they only partially adhere to. Unfortunately, it does take effort to put creams on day in, day out for a length of time and it can be easy to give up ('it doesn't work, doctor'). With skin disease, particularly a chronic condition such as eczema or psoriasis, perseverance definitely pays off!

You cannot stress enough to the patient the importance of maintaining a topical regimen and building the topical application into the patient's daily routine. This will not only help patients to be managed well on topical therapy, but it may also avoid or delay unnecessary progression to more toxic systemic treatment options. For example, you could suggest applying the cream, ointment, lotion or gel after a shower (and use soap substitute in the shower) in the morning, once again at lunch time and then before going to bed (i.e. application at least three times daily). Similarly, if suggesting a tapering course of therapy, keep it simple (e.g. weekend applications), with a helpful phone calendar or written reminders. Do check how much of the treatment in their tubes or pots the patient uses in a week. Treatments may simply be stocked up and not used. Ensure patients have a repeat prescription via their general practitioner (GP) and are not struggling to get their topical treatments when needed. It is helpful to copy to the patient the clinic letter and prescription instructions sent to the GP.

It is useful to consider the following to improve adherence (or 'concordance'):

- A trial of an emollient pack: a sample of products in small tubes or pots with varying levels of greasiness. The patient can try them out and decide which ones they prefer before you prescribe larger quantities. This may improve acceptability of treatment and thus adherence.

- Once it is sure which product the patient prefers, do not be stingy with the amounts prescribed! (Table 17.3)
- Use topical treatment instruction sheets for patients and carers to avoid confusion.

Specialist nurses in day case units can further educate patients about their treatments and provide support to those patients struggling with their topical applications.

For topical therapy for inpatients consider the following. (i) Always prescribe topical treatments on ward prescriptions with defined timed intervals, for example once, twice or three or four times daily, *not* 'as required (PRN)'. 'As required' risks the patient never having any treatment applied! (ii) Give topical treatment instructions (verbal and written) to a specific nurse, doctor, pharmacist and patient or carer if possible. Use topical treatment instruction sheets for patients and carers to refer to after discharge from hospital care.

Topical corticosteroids

Topical corticosteroids are the mainstay of treatment for inflammatory dermatoses. This is particularly true for eczema, both endogenous and exogenous. For example, for seborrhoeic der-

matitis of the face and scalp in both adolescents and adults, topical steroids work well and no difference in effectiveness has been found between mild (e.g. hydrocortisone) and potent (e.g. betamethasone) topical corticosteroids in the short term (up to four weeks). Corticosteroids and calcineurin inhibitors are equally effective, but corticosteroids have fewer short-term side-effects.

Topical corticosteroids are good therapeutic options in auto-immune dermatoses. Bullous pemphigoid (BP) is a common autoimmune blistering disease affecting elderly people. Very potent topical corticosteroids are effective and safe for treatment of BP, with lower-potency corticosteroids effective and safe for moderate BP. Of course, in the presence of extensive skin involvement, there may be limitations regarding side-effects and practicalities (such as needing help to apply to difficult-to-reach sites).

How to apply topical corticosteroids

Education of patients and carers of children and the elderly is paramount for the appropriate use of topical corticosteroids. There is a helpful video on how to apply topical corticosteroids from the British Association of Dermatologists (see Further reading). Underuse from the tendency to apply 'very sparingly' is counterproductive, with sub-therapeutic applications resulting in poor response to treatment. Patients may be misinformed about corticosteroid side-effects, including by various healthcare professionals.

Topical corticosteroids can be classified according to their potency. Think about the corticosteroid ladder: what appropriate strength of topical corticosteroid to use depends on the **p**otency, **a**ge of the patient, **s**ites where applied and the **s**everity of condition you are treating. The acronym PASS (**P**otency, **A**ge, **S**ites and **S**everity) can guide you (Table 17.4). As an example, the palms and soles of an adult have a thick stratum corneum, which allows much less penetration than on the face. Thus, a reasonable approach would be to use a potent or superpotent topical corticosteroid to treat hand dermatitis and reserve mild strengths for facial eczema. Proactive use of topical corticosteroids for two days per week between flares helps to prevent

Table 17.3 How much emollient cream to prescribe: minimum requirement if applied twice daily for a week

Age	Quantity for whole body
6 months	60 g
4 years	80 g
8 years	130 g
12 years	250 g (larger quantities may be needed for extensive skin involvement)
Adult (70 kg)	500 g (larger quantities for extensive skin involvement)

Table 17.4 Corticosteroid ladder in eczema (PASS: Potency, Age, Site, Severity)

Potency	Age	Site	Severity
Mild, e.g. hydrocortisone	Children and adults	All areas including face and flexures	Mild eczema, e.g. facial or flexural sites
Moderate, e.g. clobetasone/ Eumovate®, Synalar® 1:4 dilution, Betnovate RD®	Children (in special circumstances) and adults	All areas including face and flexures	Moderate eczema, e.g. facial or flexural sites
Potent, e.g. Elocon®, Betnovate, Locoid®, Mometasone®, Synalar	Adults	Avoid face and flexures, except with great caution	Severe eczema, e.g. areas of lichenification and palms and soles
Superpotent, e.g. clobetasol/ Dermovate®	Adults	Avoid face and flexures except with great caution	Severe eczema, e.g. areas of lichenification and palms and soles

eczema flares and therefore reduces the need for more intense periods of topical corticosteroid use, which may be associated with an increase in adverse events. Applying topical corticosteroids to wet skin after bathing, or use of wet wraps, may improve penetration and delivery of the cream or ointment into the upper layers, thus increasing the efficacy of the topical corticosteroid. However, there is also a risk of systemic absorption, particularly with a potent topical corticosteroid applied over a large body surface area.

The vehicle chosen for the corticosteroid prescribed (e.g. lotion, foam, ointment, cream, tape) will depend on the site and condition you are treating. Ointments usually work better on dry skin conditions and contain fewer preservatives, hence reducing the likelihood of allergic contact dermatitis.

A Cochrane review found no association between maternal use of topical corticosteroids of any potency and any increase in adverse pregnancy outcomes, including mode of delivery, congenital abnormality, pre-term delivery, foetal death or low Apgar score.

Once-a-day application of topical corticosteroid improves adherence compared to twice daily, and is usually enough to give benefit.

Avoid giving more than 200 g of mildly potent, 50 g of moderately potent or 30 g of potent corticosteroid per week for more than a month in an adult patient.

What is a fingertip unit (FTU)?

A fingertip unit is the amount of cream or ointment squeezed out of a tube (with a 5-mm nozzle) onto the tip of the index finger, reaching from the crease of the finger (distal interphalangeal joint) to the end of the finger: 1 FTU = ½ g or 2 handprint areas. A handprint is approximately 1% of the body surface area.

Give clear instructions to patients, with the help of written topical sheets and a body chart, describing how to use the FTU when at home (Figure 17.1).

Side-effects and cautions

High-potency topical corticosteroids, if used inappropriately on delicate skin sites and over a prolonged time, can cause both local and systemic side-effects.

Local side-effects include:

- Telangiectasia and skin colour change (redder, or darker or lighter).
- Skin atrophy.
- Easy bruising and fragility of skin.
- Striae.
- Folliculitis.
- Rosacea, acne, perioral dermatitis.
- Hirsutism.

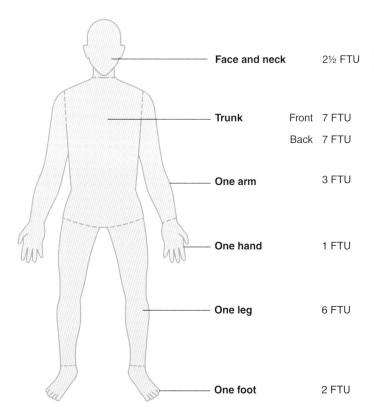

Face and neck		2½ FTU
Trunk	Front	7 FTU
	Back	7 FTU
One arm		3 FTU
One hand		1 FTU
One leg		6 FTU
One foot		2 FTU

Figure 17.1 Approximate number of fingertip units (FTUs) required to treat various anatomical sites once. Long CC, Finlay AY. The finger-tip unit—a new practical measure. *Clin Exp Dermatol* 1991; **16**:444–7.

- Contact allergy.
- Disguise or worsening of infections.

Systemic or generalised side-effects are rare but can happen, especially if using very potent or potent topical corticosteroids over large areas of inflamed skin (delicate skin) for a prolonged time. These include:

- Rebound phenomenon: worsening on withdrawal of treatment.
- Tachyphylaxis: topical corticosteroids lose their efficacy despite frequent use.
- Glaucoma.
- Cushing's syndrome.
- Growth retardation in children.

Specific points to note are as follows:

- Be careful about similar-sounding names for topical drugs and read the labels and prescriptions carefully: clobetasone (Eumovate®) is *moderate potency*, while clobetasol (Dermovate®) is *very potent*.
- Prescribing ointments instead of creams helps minimise risk of contact allergic dermatitis due to additives in creams (of course, patient preference counts!).
- Document a start date and an end date for topical corticosteroids (dependent on frequency and potency used).
- Avoid superpotent topical corticosteroids in psoriasis: there is a risk of causing the rebound phenomenon and destabilising the psoriasis, which may lead to a dermatological emergency.

Corticosteroid-sparing agents: calcineurin inhibitors

Topical corticosteroids are very effective for inflammatory dermatoses, in particular atopic eczema, but their continuous use in the long term for disease control can be detrimental. Corticosteroid-sparing agents (calcineurin inhibitors), namely pimecrolimus and tacrolimus, are good alternatives. They allow breaks from the continuous use of topical corticosteroids. Acting as immunomodulators, they have the added benefit of not being associated with tachyphylaxis, rebound effects or irreversible local side-effects, which are seen with topical corticosteroids.

The UK National Institute for Health and Care Excellence (NICE) has recommended the use of calcineurin inhibitors as a second-line treatment for moderate-to-severe atopic eczema, including in children aged two years and above. Topical tacrolimus (0.03% and 0.1%) ointment and pimecrolimus 1% cream are particularly good to treat atopic facial eczema, seborrhoeic dermatitis and sebopsoriasis. Unlike topical corticosteroids, calcineurin inhibitors do not cause atrophy and so are suitable for use on sensitive sites such as periocular and perioral areas, the neck and flexures. Other clinical indications include genital lichen sclerosus, vitiligo, discoid lupus and oral lichen planus. Twice-a-day treatment is well tolerated if patients are warned about the initial burning sensation after application, which usually wears off over a few days.

Topical antibiotics, antivirals and antifungals

Topical antibiotics are used to treat acute superficial bacterial skin infections. Before prescribing, consider the causative organism being targeted and the use of antiseptic shampoos, emollients and soap substitutes to reduce bacterial colonisation. For localised impetigo, both mupirocin and fusidic acid creams are at least as effective as oral antibiotics. Topical antibiotics are also indicated following skin surgery, for infected eczema sometimes in combination with topical corticosteroids (Table 17.5), and in acne and rosacea (see below). Repeated use of topical antibiotics can result in antimicrobial resistance.

Topical antivirals only have a role in treatment of mild ocular herpes or herpes labialis in individuals with a robust immune status. Always aim to start treatment as soon as clinically suspicious, ideally within five days of onset of symptoms. Oral or parenteral antivirals should be used for other viral clinical presentations (e.g. herpes zoster, genital herpes simplex).

Fungal infections, in particular tinea infections caused by dermatophytes, are common presentations in general practice and dermatology outpatients. These include tinea corporis ('ringworm' affecting trunk and limbs), tinea capitis (scalp), tinea cruris ('jock itch' affecting groin and genitalia), tinea unguium (fingernails or toenails), tinea manuum (hands) and tinea pedis (feet). Terbinafine and naftifine are effective for tinea cruris and tinea corporis. The azoles provide similar clinical and mycological cure rates. For fungal nail infections (onychomycosis), high-quality evidence supports the effectiveness of topical efinaconazole, while moderate-quality evidence supports ciclopirox 8% hydrolacquer and tavaborole. Topical 30% resin lacquer and topical 5% amorolfine lacquer provided similar efficacy for treating dermatophyte onychomycosis. However, oral terbinafine was significantly more effective in terms of mycological cure and clinical outcome than either topical therapy at the 10-month follow-up. Be aware of misdiagnosis with inappropriate treatment of nail changes due to psoriasis or trauma.

Consider the following:

- Inappropriate or incorrect use of antibiotics can lead to antimicrobial resistance.
- Aim to start antiviral therapy as soon as possible (within five days).
- Watch out for tinea masquerading as 'worsening eczema despite treatment with topical corticosteroids' (i.e. tinea incognito).

Acne and rosacea

Both acne and rosacea can have a significant impact on the quality of life of patients and are associated with high burden of disease. Acne is characterised by the presence of comedones, and can present with a combination of papules, pustules and sometimes nodules and cysts.

Table 17.5 Topical corticosteroid combinations

Corticosteroid combinations	Examples
With antiseptics	Betamethasone valerate with clioquinol cream and ointment (Betnovate C®)
	Fluocinolone acetonide with clioquinol cream and ointment (Synalar C®)
With antibiotics	Hydrocortisone with fusidic acid cream (Fucidin H®)
	Betamethasone valerate with neomycin cream and ointment (Betnovate N)
	Fluocinolone acetonide with neomycin cream and ointment (Synalar C)
With antifungals	Hydrocortisone with clotrimazole cream (Canesten HC®)
	Hydrocortisone with miconazole cream and ointment (Daktacort®)
	Betamethasone dipropionate with clotrimazole cream (Lotriderm®)
With antibacterials and antifungals	Hydrocortisone, chlorhexidine and nystatin cream and ointment (Nystaform HC®)
	Hydrocortisone, benzalkonium, nystatin, dimeticone cream (Timodine®)
	Clobetasone butyrate, oxytetracycline and nystatin cream (Trimovate®)
With calcipotriol	Betamethasone with calcipotriol ointment and gel (Dovobet®)
With salicylic acid	Betamethasone dipropionate and salicylic acid ointment and scalp application (Diprosalic®)
Mouth preparations (e.g. for aphthous ulcers)	Betamethasone soluble tablets
	Hydrocortisone 2.5 mg muco-adhesive buccal tablets or hydrocortisone oromucosal tablets

Start treatment early in inflammatory disease to prevent scarring. Mild-to-moderate acne can be treated with a range of topical non-antibiotic antimicrobials (azelaic acid, benzoyl peroxide), retinoids (especially for comedonal acne) and antibiotics (Table 17.6). Rosacea can be papulopustular, can have a red or telangiectatic component involving the centrofacial area, and may be complicated by rhinophyma (involving localised lymphoedema and hypertrophic sebaceous glands) or eye signs (ocular rosacea). Comedones are not seen in rosacea. Topical metronidazole, azelaic acid and ivermectin are effective treatments for rosacea. Topical ivermectin is acaricidal to the commensal demodex mites implicated in rosacea. Brimonidine gel and topical oxymetazoline work well for facial redness on a temporary basis (up to 12 hours) by acting as vasoconstrictors. For ocular rosacea, topical ciclosporin ophthalmic emulsion has demonstrated effectiveness and improved quality of life.

Photodamage

Photodamage is the skin damage that occurs on areas of frequent and chronic exposure to sunlight and can start to accumulate even before teenage years. Clinical manifestations include premature skin ageing or wrinkling, uneven and irregular pigmentation (e.g. lentigines) and freckles ('ephelides'). Photodamage may lead to precancerous lesions and skin cancers such as basal cell carcinomas, squamous cell carcinomas and malignant melanomas.

Prevention

Prevention is always better than cure! The best way to protect oneself and patients from sun damage and its consequences is to take measures early in life and proactively. Wearing long-sleeved clothing when outdoors, avoiding the sun between 11 am and 3 pm and wearing a broad-brimmed hat (instead of a cap) are all sensible approaches. (A cap does not protect the ears and the back of the neck, where skin cancers can lurk!) Remember, there is no such thing as a safe tan.

Sunscreens and sunblock

Sunscreens and sunblock have become popular and are widely used by the public. They have a role in the prevention of photo-immunosuppression with consequent development of precancerous lesions and skin cancers such as squamous cell carcinoma and melanomas. They also help delay signs of photoageing. Sunlight is partially blocked or reflected by some sunscreens, while others may chemically absorb specific wavelengths. With a hugely commercialised market, it can be confusing deciding which products to use.

Table 17.6 Selected topical formulary (up-to-date information can be found at www.bnf.org.uk)

Preparation types and comments	Examples
Barrier products	Petrolatum
	Drapolene® cream
	Metanium® ointment (for nappy rash)
	Zinc and castor oil ointment
Cleansing agents	Potassium permanganate (Permitabs®) one tablet in 4 litres of water (to soak affected parts)
	Chlorhexidine acetate 0.05%
	Chlorhexidine gluconate 4% (Hibiscrub® solution)
Antibacterials	Mupirocin (Bactroban® cream, ointment and nasal ointment)
	Fusidic acid (Fucidin® cream and ointment)
	Polymyxin and bacitracin (Polyfax® ointment)
	Chlorhexidine and neomycin (Naseptin® cream)
Antifungals	Amorolfine (Loceryl® nail lacquer)
	Clotrimazole (Canesten® cream)
	Miconazole (Daktarin® cream)
	Ketoconazole (Nizoral® cream)
	Terbinafine (Lamisil® cream)
	Tioconazole (Trosyl® cutaneous solution)
Antivirals	Aciclovir (5% cream) (may help in recurrent herpes simplex infections)
	Aciclovir eye ointment (alongside systemics for ophthalmic zoster)
Wart treatments	Salicylic acid: 26% Occlusal® solution, 50% Verrugon® ointment
	Salicylic acid and lactic acid: (Salactol® paint, Salatac®, Cuplex® gel) daily (for all sites)
	Glutaraldehyde (Glutarol® solution)
	Formaldehyde (Veracur® gel)
	Consider duct tape: it is easy to apply
	Aggressive cryotherapy
Scabies treatment	Permethrin (Lyclear® Dermal Cream)
	Malathion (Derbac-M® Liquid)
Pediculosis treatment	Permethrin (Lyclear Creme Rinse)
	Malathion (Derbac-M Liquid)
Other shampoos (leave on for five minutes before rinsing)	Selsun® (contains selenium sulfide, can treat pityriasis versicolor)
	Nizoral® (contains ketoconazole, can treat seborrhoeic dermatitis and pityriasis versicolor)
	Dermax® (contains benzalkonium chloride)

Table 17.6 (Continued)

Preparation types and comments	Examples
Antipruritics	Calamine lotion
	Crotamiton (Eurax®) cream
	Menthol 1% in aqueous cream
	Doxepin (Xepin® cream)
Antiperspirants	Aluminium chloride hexahydrate 20% (Driclor® solution)
	Glycopyrronium bromide 0.05% solution by iontophoresis for palms and soles
Keratolytics	Salicylic acid 2–4% in white soft paraffin or emulsifying ointment
	Lassar's paste
	Urea preparations
	Propylene glycol (20% in aqueous cream)
Depilatories	Eflornithine 11.5% (Vaniqa®) cream
Mouth preparations	
Topical analgesics	Benzydamine hydrochloride (Difflam® oral rinse)
	Chlorhexidine gluconate 1% (Corsodyl® mouthwash)
For fungal infections	Miconazole (Daktarin® oral gel)
	Nystatin (Nystan® oral suspension)
Topical immunomodulators	Pimecrolimus (Elidel® cream 1%)
	Tacrolimus (Protopic® ointment 0.03%, 0.1%)
Treatment of skin cancer and precancers	
5-Fluorouracil	Efudix® cream
	Actikerall® (fluorouracil 0.5%, salicylic acid 10%)
Imiquimod	Aldara® cream
Diclofenac	Solaraze® gel
Acne treatments	
With antibacterial	Benzoyl peroxide
	Benzoyl peroxide and potassium hydroxyquinoline (Quinoderm® products)
With antibiotics	Clindamycin (Dalacin-T® solution or roll-on)
	Benzoyl peroxide and clindamycin: 3%/1% or 5%/1% (Duac® once-daily gel)
	Erythromycin and zinc acetate (Zineryt®)
With azelaic acid and salicylic acid	Azelaic acid (Skinoren® cream, Finacea® gel)

(Continued)

Table 17.6 (Continued)

Preparation types and comments	Examples
With retinoids (contraindicated in pregnancy and lactation)	Adapalene gel (Differin® gel or cream)
	Adapalene and benzoyl peroxide (two strengths: 0.1%/2.5% and 0.3%/2.5%) (Epiduo® gel)
	Topical tretinoin
	Isotretinoin and erythromycin (Isotrexin® gel)
	Tretinoin (Retin-A products)
Other	Nicotinamide gel
Rosacea treatments	
Papulopustular rosacea	Ivermectin cream (1%)
	Metronidazole (Metrogel®, Rozex® cream)
	Azelaic acid (Finacea® gel)
Facial erythema in rosacea	Brimonidine tartrate (brimonidine gel, Mirvaso® gel)
	Intranasal oxymetazoline 0.05% solution
Ocular rosacea	Ciclosporin 0.05% ophthalmic emulsion

Weller RB *et al. Clinical Dermatology*, 5th edn. Chichester: Wiley, 2015.

It is important to emphasise that products should provide broad-spectrum protection, covering both ultraviolet A (UVA) (320–400 nm) and ultraviolet B (UVB) (290–320 nm) radiation. In the UK, the National Health Service (NHS) guidance when choosing a sunscreen is to look for a sun protection factor (SPF) of at least 30 to protect against UVB and at least four-star UVA protection. There are several products available on the market such as titanium dioxide (E45 Sun range) and combinations of cinnamate, oxybenzone and titanium dioxide (Sunsense Ultra®, RoC Soleil-Protect®, Uvistat range). Be aware of allergic contact dermatitis to sunscreen ingredients, which may need further investigation with patch or photopatch testing.

What is meant by SPF?

Sun protection factor or SPF is a measure of effectiveness of the sunscreen against UVB rather than UVA. It is calculated as the time taken to sunburn skin protected by sunscreen divided by the time taken to sunburn non-protected adjacent skin. SPF depends on the UV filter composition, its concentration and the vehicle (e.g. gel, cream, spray) used in the sunscreen. Helpful apps such as SunSmart educate and guide the public on measures to take for protection against sun damage.

Treatment

Photodamaged skin occurs due to a cumulative effect of sun exposure. This includes episodes of sunburn and tanning, which can lead to the development of precancerous and cancerous lesions. Topical therapies, including 5-fluorouracil (5-FU) and imiquimod, can be effective in treating precancerous and early cancerous lesions, and provide good cosmetic outcomes.

The chemotherapy agent 5-FU is used to treat actinic keratosis, Bowen's disease, porokeratosis and superficial basal cell carcinomas. 5-FU is an antimetabolite that blocks DNA replication and synthesis by inhibiting the action of thymidylate synthase. 5-FU is degraded by 80–90% in the body via an enzyme called dihydropyrimidine dehydrogenase (DPD), which is encoded by the *DPYD* gene. Genetic mutations in *DPYD* can lead to reduced or absent DPD activity. Even partial reduction of DPD activity can result in severe systemic side-effects, including severe neutropenia with the use of topical 5-FU. Despite discontinuation of treatment, patients may present with lethargy, painful mucositis and fever, and the effects can last for up to four weeks. In these rare cases, supportive treatment and haematology or oncology consultation are advisable.

Most patients respond well to topical 5-FU therapy and it is usually applied twice daily for three weeks, but you may have to titrate according to the patient's tolerance, condition and site of treatment. It is vital to explain to patients and warn them that the affected areas being treated will likely have a very brisk and florid inflammatory response, with redness, then vesiculation, erosion, ulceration, necrosis and finally epithelisation. Explain to patients that the skin can take over three weeks to heal after discontinuation of the treatment. For large areas, suggest application in sections or the patient may feel too sore to continue. Provide a patient information leaflet on 5-FU.

Topical imiquimod (5% Aldara®) is another treatment option for actinic keratosis and superficial basal cell carcinoma. It is also used for external genital warts. The dose and frequency vary according to the diagnosis and patient tolerance. The usual regimen to treat actinic keratosis is once daily for two weeks, then repeat treatment after a two-week treatment-free interval, and finally assess the response eight weeks after the second course. For superficial basal cell carcinoma, apply imiquimod five nights each week for 6 weeks and assess the response 12 weeks later. For extragenital and perianal warts apply three times a week until lesions resolve (up to 16 weeks). Local side-effects can include redness, crusting, oedema and exudate. Patients may also experience flu-like symptoms such as headache and fatigue. Other treatments for actinic keratosis include topical diclofenac (3%) gel (Solaraze®) applied twice daily for 60–90 days.

Psoriasis

Psoriasis is an immune-mediated chronic inflammatory skin disease that can often have systemic manifestations. Topical treatments need to be cosmetically acceptable for patients so they continue to comply and adhere to treatment regimens. For chronic thick plaque psoriasis, salicylic acid, coal tar preparations, calcipotriol or dithranol at different strengths (0.1–2%) are effective treatments (Table 17.7). Combinations with moderate

Table 17.7 Topical preparations for psoriasis

Psoriasis	
	Calcitriol (Silkis® ointment): low irritancy and can be used on face and flexures
	Calcipotriol–betamethasone (Dovobet®) ointment, gel or foam
	Dovonex® cream or ointment
	Tacalcitol (Curatoderm®)
	Diprosalic® ointment
	Salicylic acid ointment
With salicylic acid	Lassar's paste (with zinc oxide)
Dithranol	Micanol range 1%
Tar applications	Exorex® lotion, Psoriderm® cream
Calcineurin inhibitors	Topical tacrolimus or pimecrolimus (face, genitalia, intertriginous areas)
Scalp psoriasis	
Tar	Alphosyl 2 in 1® shampoo
	Polytar® liquid, shampoo
	Exorex® lotion
	T-Gel® shampoo
	Psoriderm® scalp lotion
Tar + salicylic acid combinations	Sebco® scalp ointment
	Cocois® ointment
	Capasal® shampoo
Corticosteroids	Betamethasone (Betnovate® 0.1% scalp application)
	Diprosalic scalp application with salicylic acid
	Dovobet gel (calcipotriol and betamethasone)
	Clobetasol propionate (Etrivex® shampoo)
Vitamin D analogues	Calcipotriol scalp solution
	Dovobet gel (calcipotriol and betamethasone)

and potent topical corticosteroids are tolerated better, with fewer adverse effects. Avoid long-term use of potent or superpotent corticosteroids in generalised body psoriasis, as stopping them can lead to a rebound phenomenon and an acute unstable psoriasis (e.g. acute pustular psoriasis), resulting in a dermatological emergency. Calcineurin inhibitors such as topical tacrolimus and pimecrolimus are good corticosteroid-sparing agents, particularly when treating facial psoriasis or sebopsoriasis, or in the case of genital or intertriginous skin involvement.

Calcipotriol is a vitamin D analogue used as first-line topical treatment for stable plaque psoriasis affecting up to 40% of body surface area (though for such extensive disease systemic therapy would normally be considered). It tends to irritate the skin, so alternative treatments are preferred for facial psoriasis. Hypercalcaemia due to the calcitriol content is rare if used within the maximum recommended doses of 100 g weekly of Dovonex® (equivalent of 5 mg calcipotriol) or 60 mL of scalp solution (equivalent of 3 mg calcipotriol). When using both body and scalp treatments together, the dose of calcipotriol should not exceed 5 mg weekly.

To use dithranol (Dithrocream®), start at the lowest strength to avoid irritation, apply to the psoriasis plaques only and use as short-contact therapy (e.g. 30–60 minutes once per day). Patients could start at a daily application of 10 minutes, then wash off and increase by 10 minutes every day if tolerated. Fair skin tends to be more sensitive than darker skin, so consider stopping treatment early if patients are unable to tolerate. Aim to build up to the optimum therapeutic effect over four weeks. Dithranol can stain the clothes and be irritating to the skin, so tolerance and adherence can be variable.

For nail psoriasis, the evidence for the use of topical treatments is inconclusive and of poor quality.

For scalp psoriasis, the plaques tend to go along the hairline, and the shedding of visible scales on dark clothing and bedclothes is particularly embarrassing and distressing for patients. For enhanced effectiveness and if the patient tolerates it, apply Cocois® or Sebco® ointment as an overnight application, cover the scalp with a shower cap and wash the hair the following morning. Warn the patients about the risk of stained bedclothes with overnight use. There is a helpful stepwise approach on how to treat scalp psoriasis from the British Association of Dermatologists (see Further reading).

What are 'Specials'?

NHS hospital and general practice pharmacies stock a limited range of products licensed for topical therapies. As dermatologists, we often rely on unlicensed topical treatments, which were historically formulated in local pharmacies, also known as 'Specials'. These products have been prepared and used on patients for many decades and the evidence data is largely empirical. They can include different strengths of topical corticosteroids in combination with other active constituents, such as dithranol, tar or salicylic acid, which are often prepared in different bases or concentrations. To allow for a reasonable standardisation of the hundreds of different mixtures that have been used, the British Association of Dermatologists (BAD) has published a booklet on 'Specials' (see Further reading). The booklet provides the indications and various treatment regimens. Do familiarise yourself with what is available and the costs versus benefits of the different products, particularly as they often have a short shelf life.

Conclusions

Topical therapies have the great advantage of reaching the skin directly as the target organ. Their usefulness as first-line treatment for most inflammatory skin disorders, as well as on photodamaged skin, should not be underestimated. It is vital to be familiar with the different preparations of topical treatments, and their indications and side-effects. This will allow you to prescribe and discuss management plans with patients with great confidence. If these are used appropriately, with care and reassurance, patients may be able to avoid or delay the need for systemic therapies and their increased risks and side-effects.

Pearls and pitfalls

- Some emollients can also be used as soap substitutes, but be aware that they can be very slippery in baths and showers.
- Warn patients about the risk of fire hazard with paraffin-based products. Dressings and clothing in contact or soaked with these products are easily ignited by a naked flame ('like a wick'). Patients should keep away from fire or flames and should not smoke when using these preparations.
- Once-a-day application of topical corticosteroid improves adherence compared to twice daily, and is usually enough to give benefit.
- Avoid giving more than 200 g of mildly potent, 50 g of moderately potent or 30 g of potent corticosteroid per week for more than four weeks in an adult patient.
- Inappropriate or incorrect use of antibiotics can lead to antimicrobial resistance.
- Do not miss tinea incognito masquerading as 'worsening eczema despite treatment with topical corticosteroids'.
- Use of topical corticosteroids will eventually worsen both acne and rosacea.
- Remember, there is no such thing as a safe tan, and watch out for allergic contact dermatitis caused by ingredients in sunscreen products.
- Efudix causes a marked inflammatory reaction: avoid or warn against use on the face before an important event such as a holiday or family event.
- Avoid superpotent topical corticosteroids in psoriasis: there is a risk of causing the rebound phenomenon and potentially leading to a dermatological emergency.

SCE Questions. See questions 24 and 25.

FURTHER READING AND KEY RESOURCES

Chi CC, Wang SH, Wojnarowska F *et al*. Safety of topical corticosteroids in pregnancy. *Cochrane Database Syst Rev* 2015; (10):CD007346. doi:10.1002/14651858.CD007346.pub3.

Foley K, Gupta AK, Versteeg S *et al*. Topical and device-based treatments for fungal infections of the toenails. *Cochrane Database Syst Rev* 2020; **1**(1):CD012093. doi:10.1002/14651858.CD012093.pub2.

Kirtschig G, Middleton P, Bennett C *et al*. Interventions for bullous pemphigoid. *Cochrane Database Syst Rev* 2010; (10):CD002292. doi:10.1002/14651858.CD002292.pub3.

Santer M, Ridd MJ, Francis NA *et al*. Emollient bath additives for the treatment of childhood eczema (BATHE): multicentre pragmatic parallel group randomised controlled trial of clinical and cost effectiveness. *BMJ* 2018; **361**:k1332.

Schmitt J, von Kobyletzki L, Svensson A, Apfelbacher C. Efficacy and tolerability of proactive treatment with topical corticosteroids and calcineurin inhibitors for atopic eczema: systematic review and meta-analysis of randomized controlled trials. *Br J Dermatol* 2011; **164**:415–28.

Zuuren EJ, Fedorowicz Z, Christensen R *et al*. Emollients and moisturisers for eczema. *Cochrane Database Syst Rev* 2017; **2**(2):CD012119. doi:10.1002/14651858.CD012119.pub2.

Textbook

Weller RB, Hunter HJA, Mann MW. *Clinical Dermatology*, 5th edn. Hoboken, NJ: Wiley-Blackwell, 2015.

Useful websites

British Association of Dermatologists. Patient information videos (including 'Treating scalp psoriasis' and 'How to use topical corticosteroids'). Available at: https://www.bad.org.uk/for-the-public/patient-information-videos.

British Association of Dermatologists. Specials. Available at: www.bad.org.uk/specials.

National Institute for Health and Care Excellence. Tacrolimus and pimecrolimus for atopic eczema. Available at: https://www.nice.org.uk/guidance/ta82/chapter/1-Guidance.

SunSmart. Available at: www.sunsmart.com.au.

Registered trademarks

Actikerall®, Curatoderm®, Solaraze®, Unguentum M®, Vaniqa®, Almirall, Uxbridge, UK

Aldara®, Meda Pharmaceuticals, Bishop's Stortford, UK

Alphosyl 2 in 1®, Lyclear®, Omega Pharma, London, UK

Aquadrate®, Hydromol®, Naseptin®, Occlusal®, Permitabs®, Quinoderm®, Timodine®, Alliance Pharmaceuticals, Chippenham, UK

Aveeno®, Aveeno, Skillman, NJ, USA

Bactroban®, Betnovate®, Corsodyl®, Dermovate®, Drapolene®, Driclor®, Eumovate®, Isotrexin®, Lamisil®, GlaxoSmithKline, Brentford, UK

Canesten HC®, Diprobase®, Bayer, Reading, UK

Capasal®, Dermax®, Dermol®, Dithrocream®, Doublebase®, Glutarol®, Psoriderm®, Salactol®, Salatac®, Dermal Laboratories, Hitchin, UK

Cetraben®, Genus Pharmaceuticals, Huddersfield, UK

Cocois®, RPH Pharmaceuticals, Jordbro, Sweden

Cuplex®, Crawford Pharmaceuticals, Old Stratford, UK

Daktacort®, Nizoral®, Janssen-Cilag, High Wycombe, UK

Daktarin®, McNeil Products, Maidenhead, UK

Dalacin-T®, Trosyl®, Pfizer, Sandwich, UK

Derbac-M®, GR Lane Health Products, Gloucester, UK

Differin®, Epiduo®, Etrivex®, Loceryl®, Metrogel®, Mirvaso®, Rozex®, Silkis®, Galderma, Watford, UK

Difflam®, Efudix®, Elidel®, Mylan, Hatfield, UK

Diprosalic®, Elocon®, Lotriderm®, Organon Pharma, London, UK

Dovobet®, Dovonex®, Finacea®, Fucidin H®, Locoid®, Protopic®, Skinoren®, Zineryt®, Leo Laboratories, Hurley, UK

Duac®, Stiefel, Brentford, UK

Emollin®, CD Medical, Bolton, UK

Epimax®, Aspire Pharma, Petersfield, UK

Eucerin®, Beiersdorf, Hamburg, Germany

Eurax®, Metanium®, Oilatum Plus®, Polytar®, Zeroderm®, Thornton & Ross, Huddersfield, UK

Exorex®, Teva, Harlow, UK

Hibiscrub®, Regent Medical, Manchester, UK

Mometasone®, Glenmark Pharmaceuticals, Watford, UK

Nystaform HC®, Veracur®, Typharm, Norwich, UK

Nystan®, Vygoris, London, UK

Polyfax®, PLIVA Pharma, Castleford, UK

RoC Soleil-Protect®, RoC Skincare, Bristol, UK

Sebco®, Derma, Newcastle upon Tyne, UK

Selsun®, Sanofi, Reading, UK

Sunsense Ultra®, Ego Pharmaceuticals, Knutsford, UK

Synalar®, Reig Jofre, Barcelona, Spain

T-Gel®, Neutrogena, Maidenhead, UK

Trimovate®, Ennogen Healthcare, Dartford, UK

Verrugon®, Optima Health and Nutrition, Swansea, UK

Xepin®, Cambridge Healthcare Supplies, Wymondham, UK

18

Systemic therapy

Sarah H. Wakelin and Mahbub M.U. Chowdhury

Introduction

The ability to safely and effectively prescribe systemic therapy is an essential skill for the trainee dermatologist to acquire. Keeping up to date with the expanding range of new drugs, especially biologics and small molecules, is a challenge. Another issue is lack of experience with drugs that are infrequently prescribed. This chapter provides a broad overview of systemic therapy of skin disease. For further advice, the reader should consult the *British National Formulary* (BNF)/*BNF for Children*, *Martindale: The Complete Drug Reference*, British Association of Dermatologists (BAD) guidelines, specialist textbooks, the manufacturer's summary of product characteristics and the Medicines and Healthcare products Regulatory Authority's (MHRA) e-medicines. The doctor–patient relationship forms the bedrock of good communication and the ability of the prescriber to tailor treatment to best suit the patient's needs.

General considerations

Consent

The recent General Medical Council (GMC) guidance on consent emphasises the importance of 'meaningful dialogue' between doctor and patient. This is applicable to all aspects of patient care, including prescribing. As well as choosing an appropriate drug, the prescriber needs to be able to explain to the patient (and/or their caregiver – which applies throughout

Dermatology Training: The Essentials. Edited by Mahbub M.U. Chowdhury, Tamara W. Griffiths and Andrew Y. Finlay.
© 2022 The British Association of Dermatologists. Published 2022 by John Wiley & Sons Ltd.
Companion website: www.wiley.com/go/chowdhury/dermatologytraining

this text) about common and rarer serious adverse effects and how the drug will be monitored. This helps patients share in the therapeutic choice and give informed consent to treatment. The BAD has several patient information leaflets on systemic drugs, which are updated regularly and are an invaluable resource for patients and prescribers. The information given to the patient should be documented in their medical records and they should receive clinic correspondence written in clear and simple terms.

In all but an emergency situation, and especially for drugs with potentially serious adverse effects, such as oral isotretinoin, the patient should have sufficient time to carefully review this information and the opportunity to raise concerns or questions. Hasty prescribing of potentially harmful systemic therapy may amount to a breach of the practitioner's duty of care, thereby putting them at risk of a clinical negligence claim in the event of harm to the patient. On the contrary, inaction or under-treatment is also suboptimal for patient care; it takes expertise and skill to navigate these boundaries and you will gain confidence as you progress through training and gain clinical experience.

Therapeutic options

The approach to prescribing should take into account several considerations: patient factors, prescriber factors, the dermatological condition to be treated, the proposed drug to be prescribed and external factors (Table 18.1). Treatment must be tailored to the patient's individual needs. The negative impact of severe or chronic skin disease on the patient's quality of life should not be underestimated and documentation relating to this is helpful to justify clinical decisions made (Chapter 8). An appropriate balance between potential benefit and risk should be sought. This clinical skill is honed with experience and in situations that are not straightforward. Hence, discussion with colleagues and reflective practice can be invaluable. Drugs new to the market are invariably expensive and prescribers may be restricted by prescribing policies, especially the National Institute for Health and Care Excellence (NICE) and BAD guidelines, as well as local formularies.

Avoiding error

Medication errors and unsafe medication practices are a leading cause of avoidable injury and harm in healthcare. The World Health Organization's (WHO) third global patient safety challenge, 'Medication Without Harm', launched in 2017, aimed to reduce severe avoidable medication-related harm by 50% over the following five years. This challenge is targeted at all involved, including the prescriber, pharmacist, patient, other healthcare professionals and those responsible for healthcare systems. Double-checking when prescribing or administering medicines is important to avoid medication errors.

Check that it is the:

- Right medicine.
- Right patient.
- Right dose.
- Right route.
- Right time.

Table 18.1 Examples of factors to consider when prescribing systemic therapy

Patient	
	Patient preferences
	Age, sex
	Social circumstances including employment
	Comorbidity and past medical history
	Medication history
Prescriber factors	
	Knowledge
	Experience
	Previous critical incidents
	Prescribing bias
Dermatological condition	
	Severity
	Treatment guidelines
	Expected response to proposed treatment
Proposed systemic therapy	
	Efficacy
	Route of administration
	Dose and formulation
	Pharmacogenetics
	Toxicity
	Cost
	Licence status
External factors	
	Clinical governance (e.g. National Institute for Health and Care Excellence, guidelines, protocols, licensing authorities)
	Financial

Standardised pro formas for initiating and continuing drug treatment and monitoring can be helpful in preventing errors and omissions. They provide accessible data for audit and evidence of good medical care, and facilitate nurse-led prescribing and monitoring.

Drug monitoring

Appropriate monitoring is a key aspect of safe prescribing when starting a drug and throughout its continuation. Shared-care arrangements between primary and intermediary or secondary care have several advantages, including ease of patient access and fewer hospital visits, but there needs to be a clear and written agreement on what tests need to be done and when, and who is responsible for acting on the results. It is important to pay attention to significant trends in blood parameters, even if these remain within the normal reference ranges, for example declining white blood cell count.

Licensed, unlicensed and 'off-label' prescribing

Prescription drugs that are authorised by the MHRA according to the terms described in the summary of product characteristics, known as the product 'label', are considered to be 'licensed' for that indication. If the drug is prescribed outside those terms, for example with a different indication, dose or age group, then the prescription is said to be 'off-label' or 'unlicensed' for that indication. UK doctors may also prescribe unauthorised ('unlicensed') products, if they are licensed elsewhere or have been manufactured in the UK by a licensed manufacturer as a 'special'. Unlicensed and 'off-label' prescribing is not uncommon in general dermatological practice, for example the use of double or triple recommended doses of antihistamines in urticaria, or prescribing methotrexate to manage chronic and extensive eczema. It is particularly relevant in the paediatric population, where licensed indications for various dermatological diseases are limited, and also for uncommon dermatoses where no licensed option exists.

Be aware when your prescribing is 'off-label' or unlicensed, as responsibility is increased given the manufacturer will have no liability in the event of an adverse effect. The patient should also be informed of 'off-label' use of medications, as this may cause initial alarm, particularly to worried parents in the paediatric population. However, if you are able to clearly and calmly justify your decision-making process, explaining for example that no licensed alternative exists and that it is within the boundaries of mainstream dermatological practice, then most patients will be reassured. This is necessary as part of the transparent and meaningful dialogue for shared decision making required between clinician and patient and should be documented in the medical record. Gaining confidence in understanding nuances in the risk–benefit ratio for safe and effective 'off-label' prescribing of systemic medications comes with time and clinical experience. If in doubt, seek senior advice.

Prescribing in special situations

Special considerations apply to children, older people and those with renal or hepatic impairment, and in pre-conception, pregnancy and lactation. Detailed advice in these situations can be found in the *BNF* and *BNF for Children*. Particular care needs to be taken when prescribing for frail, older people and those taking multiple medications.

Individual drugs

Regularly updated guidelines on the safe use of individual drugs are produced by societies such as the BAD, the Royal College of Physicians and the American Academy of Dermatology. Be aware that recommendations for doses and monitoring may vary between different authorities. This chapter provides a general overview of individual drugs, but for detailed prescribing information the reader should refer to specialised texts.

Antimalarials

The most commonly used antimalarial drug in dermatology is hydroxychloroquine (HCQ), which is used to treat all forms of lupus, including discoid lupus erythematosus. It is also licensed for use in photosensitivity disorders including porphyria cutanea tarda. Other dermatological uses include sarcoid and lichen planopilaris. Chloroquine is rarely used in dermatology because it has a higher risk of ocular toxicity than HCQ. Mepacrine (quinacrine) is unlicensed and prescribed infrequently. Antimalarials are disease-modifying drugs. They have been used for over a hundred years and remain a cost-effective and safe option for many patients. Their precise mechanism of action is not clearly understood, but they inhibit various immunological processes including low-affinity antigen presentation, cell activation and inflammatory mediator release without causing clinical immunosuppression.

Formulation, doses and duration

HCQ is available as 200-mg tablets and the usual daily dose is 200–400 mg, with a maximum of 6.5 mg/kg/day. Mepacrine is usually given at a dose of 50–100 mg/day. It causes yellow discoloration of the skin, which may be severe at higher doses.

All antimalarials have a slow onset of action and usually require 6–8 weeks before clinical benefit is evident. Many patients with cutaneous lupus erythematosus or photosensitivity disorders only require treatment during the sunnier spring and summer months and can take a drug holiday during the winter.

Monitoring and side-effects

The most common adverse reaction is gastrointestinal upset, which may limit tolerance. The side-effect of greatest concern with HCQ (and chloroquine) is retinopathy, which may be commoner than previously reported and is usually irreversible. This has led to new guidelines in 2020 from the Royal College of Ophthalmologists for ocular screening. The risk of retinopathy is increased in patients taking HCQ at a dose of more than 5 mg/kg/day and with prolonged treatment (> 5 years). It is also increased in renal impairment and women taking tamoxifen. Damage to the retinal pigment epithelium produces a characteristic 'bull's eye' maculopathy and central visual loss. Patients who are likely to need long-term treatment should have a baseline ophthalmology examination within 6–12 months of starting treatment, with specialist retinal photography and scans. Those who continue HCQ for more than five years should be monitored annually. The availability of this specialist eye screening is not uniform across the UK at present in spite of the recommendations.

Antimalarials may induce severe flares in patients with psoriasis and should therefore generally be avoided. They may also cause severe cutaneous adverse reactions, including toxic epidermal necrolysis and drug rash with eosinophilia and systemic symptoms (DRESS). There is a small but significant risk of bone marrow suppression with antimalarials, so routine bloods should be checked every three months.

Interactions

Potential drug interactions include an increased risk of ventricular arrhythmia when chloroquine or HCQ is given with amiodarone or moxifloxacin. Efficacy of anticonvulsant drugs may be reduced and ciclosporin levels can be increased.

Apremilast

Apremilast is a relatively new systemic treatment licensed for moderate-to-severe chronic plaque psoriasis, psoriatic arthritis and Behçet's disease in adults. It inhibits phosphodiesterase type 4 (PDE4) and has anti-inflammatory actions. Its main role in dermatology is as an alternative to standard systemic psoriasis therapies or where these cannot be used because of intolerance or contraindications. In practice, most patients who fulfil these criteria and have severe disease will progress to a biological therapy. However, apremilast is a useful alternative in those who prefer oral treatment without the need for routine blood monitoring. It can be used in combination with methotrexate and ultraviolet phototherapy, and safety is not affected by mild-to-moderate renal impairment and hepatic impairment.

Starting and continuing treatment

An initial dose of 10 mg daily is gradually increased over a week up to the recommended dose of 30 mg twice daily. Gastrointestinal side-effects are common, especially anorexia, nausea, vomiting and diarrhoea. These usually occur early in treatment and may be severe. Weight should be monitored in those with a low body mass index. Insomnia and psychiatric adverse effects with depression and suicidal ideation have been reported. Patients should be warned about this possibility and advised to stop treatment if affected by adverse mood change.

Interactions

Several drug interactions may occur, including reduced apremilast levels when taken with strong cytochrome P450 3A4 enzyme inducers such as rifampicin, phenytoin, carbamazepine and St John's wort. Apremilast is contraindicated in pregnancy as animal studies have shown toxicity.

Azathioprine

Azathioprine (AZA) is a synthetic purine analogue that was originally developed as an immunosuppressant. It is a pro-drug, and following absorption it is rapidly hydrolysed to 6-mercaptopurine. This then undergoes enzymatic metabolism to form active metabolites, thioguanine nucleotides (TGN) and inactive metabolites. The main deactivating pathways are regulated by the enzymes thiopurine methyltransferase (TPMT) and xanthine oxidase. Genetic polymorphisms and drug interactions can reduce the activity of these pathways, leading to accumulation of potentially toxic levels of TGN and then to myelotoxicity. TPMT activity should be measured before starting AZA to reduce the risk of this serious adverse effect, but it does not require continued monitoring as this will not change in an individual patient.

AZA is often prescribed with prednisolone, serving as a steroid-sparing drug. It is licensed as a treatment of pemphigus, systemic lupus erythematosus and dermatomyositis. It is also frequently used to treat bullous pemphigoid and chronic actinic dermatitis.

Starting and continuing treatment

AZA may be given as a single or divided oral dose. The starting dose is usually 0.5–1 mg/kg/day, which can be increased up to 3 mg/kg/day according to baseline TPMT levels and the full blood count (FBC). It is contraindicated in patients with low or absent levels of TPMT. The drug has a slow onset of action over about 6–12 weeks.

Monitoring and side-effects

The major toxicities of AZA are myelosuppression and hepatitis. FBC and liver function tests should be performed at baseline and weekly for the first four weeks of treatment. After this, the frequency of blood tests can be reduced to three monthly. Careful attention should be paid to any decline in the neutrophil count, as this may herald severe neutropenia. Patients often experience nausea at the start of treatment and this may be reduced by prescribing the AZA in a divided dose. Long-term treatment with AZA carries a high risk of causing non-melanoma skin cancer, as the drug brings about UV-induced DNA damage. There is also an increased risk of lymphoma. Measurement of the metabolites of AZA, 6-TGN, may be useful to assess adherence and guide dosage in patients who fail to respond.

Interactions

Allopurinol inhibits xanthine oxidase, leading to accumulation of 6-TGN and myelotoxicity. Other drugs that may cause bone marrow suppression should also be avoided, including trimethoprim and co-trimoxazole.

Ciclosporin

Ciclosporin is a calcineurin inhibitor and immunosuppressant that impairs T-lymphocyte activation by inhibiting production of interleukin (IL)-2. Originally developed to prevent transplant rejection, it has been licensed for decades as a treatment of severe psoriasis and for short-term treatment of severe atopic dermatitis. Its rapid onset of action is of benefit in treating erythrodermic and pustular psoriasis. It is also used to treat other inflammatory dermatoses, including pyoderma gangrenosum and vasculitis. The main adverse effects of concern are hypertension and nephrotoxicity.

Starting and continuing treatment

Ciclosporin is usually administered orally twice a day. Microemulsion formulations are generally used due to more reliable gastrointestinal absorption. The brand should be specified and not switched, to avoid variations in bioavailability.

The initial dose is usually 2.5–3.0 mg/kg/day, increased up to 5 mg/kg/day if necessary. The drug is best given in short intermittent courses of 3–6 months to avoid renal toxicity. In practice it is often used for longer periods, as patients are reluctant to stop an effective treatment.

Monitoring and side-effects

Baseline investigations include routine bloods, fasting lipids, and hepatitis and HIV serology. Regular monitoring of blood pressure and renal function (estimated glomerular filtration rate, eGFR) are required throughout treatment, with tests done every two weeks for the first two months. A rise in creatinine of 25% above baseline or a fall in eGFR of more than 25% necessitates dose reduction. Hypertension should be treated, preferably with a calcium channel blocker or angiotensin receptor blocker. Nifedipine should be avoided due to the risk of gum hyperplasia with ciclosporin.

Other adverse effects include nausea, paraesthesia, cramps and hypertrichosis. Long-term treatment is associated with an increased risk of non-melanoma skin cancer and there may also be a higher risk of lymphoma.

Interactions

A large number of interactions with ciclosporin are documented in the *BNF*. Notable ones include macrolide antibiotics, which increase the plasma concentration of ciclosporin; non-steroidal anti-inflammatory drugs (NSAIDs), which can increase nephrotoxicity; and rifampicin, which decreases the plasma concentration. Grapefruit juice increases ciclosporin levels and should therefore be avoided.

Colchicine

Colchicine is an ancient herbal remedy obtained from the autumn crocus. It is licensed as a treatment for gout and is occasionally used in dermatology for its anti-inflammatory actions. The main effect is on neutrophil chemotaxis and motility. Uses include neutrophilic dermatoses, immunobullous diseases, Behçet's disease and leucocytoclastic vasculitis. It has a narrow therapeutic index and is highly toxic in overdose. Elderly or frail patients may be more susceptible to toxicity, manifesting as gastrointestinal, renal, hepatic, cardiac and haematological complications.

Starting and continuing treatment

The usual starting dose for skin disease is 0.5 mg daily, increasing up to 1.5 mg in divided (500 μg) doses. The duration is dependent upon the clinical situation.

Monitoring and side-effects

Routine blood tests should be checked at baseline, with monthly FBC and liver and renal function tests every three months. Mild gastrointestinal upset is common. Bone marrow suppression, myopathy and neuropathy may occur.

Interactions

There are several potential interactions with drugs that affect the cytochrome P450 3A4 enzyme system. Macrolide antibiotics increase the risk of colchicine toxicity and colchicine increases the plasma concentration of ciclosporin. Statins and fibrates increase the risk of acute myopathy.

Cyclophosphamide

Cyclophosphamide is an alkylating agent that is mainly used in the treatment of haematological malignancies, connective tissue disease and systemic vasculitis. It is metabolised *in vivo* to active metabolites that produce an immunosuppressive, cytotoxic and bone marrow-suppressive action. Cyclophosphamide suppresses B cells more than T cells. It is rarely prescribed by dermatologists, but it can be used to treat severe recalcitrant immunobullous diseases, especially pemphigus, pyoderma gangrenosum and advanced mycosis fungoides. This drug has serious toxicities and requires careful prescription and monitoring.

Starting and continuing treatment

Cyclophosphamide can be given orally or intravenously. Low doses are used orally in dermatology, for example 50–200 mg/day. High-dose intravenous pulses are sometimes given in combination with dexamethasone. The drug dose should be adjusted if renal impairment or haematological toxicity, especially leucopoenia, occurs.

Monitoring and side-effects

Routine blood tests are checked at baseline, with a dose reduction if there is renal impairment and in patients aged over 60 years. Treatment should be stopped if the white blood cell count is lower than 4×10^9 cells per litre and only restarted when the blood count has recovered. Bladder toxicity with haemorrhagic cystitis is a serious adverse effect and a high fluid intake should be maintained throughout treatment. Prolonged treatment also increases the risk of bladder cancer.

Conception and pregnancy

Cyclophosphamide is a teratogen and should not be used in pregnancy. Prolonged therapy may also cause irreversible loss of fertility. Expert advice should be obtained for people of reproductive age to discuss sperm and oocyte banking.

Dapsone

Dapsone (4,4′-diaminodiphenylsulfone) is used globally in the treatment of leprosy. It is also licensed for the treatment of dermatitis herpetiformis and is widely used in dermatology to treat other immunobullous diseases and neutrophilic dermatoses. Its exact mechanism of action in these dermatoses is unclear, but it is thought to impair neutrophil function (chemotaxis and myeloperoxidase activity) and release of inflammatory mediators.

Starting and continuing treatment

For most dermatological conditions, the starting dose is 50 mg daily for the first week, increasing thereafter according to clinical response. The minimum effective dose is usually 1–2 mg/kg and doses should not exceed 300 mg/day. The response in dermatitis herpetiformis is characteristically very rapid, with relief of pruritus and improvement in lesions after a few days. Symptom control may be achieved with a low dose.

Monitoring and side-effects

Dapsone shortens erythrocyte survival due to oxidation of glutathione. This inevitably leads to haemolysis and a fall in haemoglobin concentration and is dose related. Patients with glucose-6-phosphate dehydrogenase (G6PD) deficiency are likely to experience severe haemolysis, so G6PD level should be checked before starting dapsone. Deficiency is most common in people of African, Asian, Middle Eastern and Mediterranean descent. Dapsone also causes methaemoglobinaemia, which may present with shortness of breath and blue lips. Patients with underlying cardiorespiratory disease may not tolerate a reduction in haemoglobin, experiencing angina or breathlessness. Other adverse effects include a hypersensitivity syndrome or DRESS (Chapter 16), neuropathy, rashes and depression. Agranulocytosis has been reported rarely and is usually gradual in onset, but may occur suddenly. Regular monitoring of routine blood tests is required at weekly intervals for the first month, then at longer intervals when the dose is stabilised.

In patients who are intolerant of dapsone, another sulfonamide, sulfapyridine, may be considered. This drug is currently unlicensed in the UK. The usual starting dose is 500 mg twice a day, increasing if needed to 4 g per day. Adverse effects include crystalluria and nephrolithiasis.

Dimethyl fumarate

Dimethyl fumarate (DMF) is a component of fumaric acid esters, which have been used in dermatology, especially in Germany, since the 1960s. It has recently been licensed in the UK as a treatment for moderate-to-severe plaque psoriasis in adults, following its approval as a treatment of relapsing forms of multiple sclerosis. Following oral intake, DMF is metabolised rapidly to its primary active metabolite, monomethyl fumarate, which has immune modulatory and antioxidative effects that are not fully understood. They include an overall shift from a proinflammatory Th1/Th17 response to an anti-inflammatory or regulatory Th2 response.

Starting and continuing treatment

DMF gastroresistant tablets are taken in an escalating regimen starting with 30 mg per day, increasing weekly up to a maximum of 240 mg three times per day if needed for disease control. The slow escalation is aimed at improving tolerability.

Monitoring and side-effects

Flushing and gastrointestinal upset with nausea, diarrhoea and abdominal pain are very common in the first months of treatment and may lead to treatment withdrawal. DMF often causes a fall in the white blood count, especially lymphopenia. The FBC should be checked at baseline and regularly during treatment. If the lymphocyte count falls below 0.07×10^9 cells per litre, treatment must be stopped and patients should be monitored until their lymphocyte count has returned to normal. There have been rare cases of serious opportunistic infection, in particular progressive multifocal leucoencephalopathy, in association with DMF-containing products, and persistent lymphopenia is a risk factor for this serious neurological disease. Renal function and urinalysis should also be checked at baseline and during treatment due to a risk of renal damage. DMF is contraindicated in pregnancy as animal studies have shown harm.

Glucocorticosteroids

The introduction of systemic glucocorticosteroid ('steroid') therapy was a major advance in dermatology in the 1950s and these drugs still have an indispensable role in the treatment of inflammatory dermatoses. The most frequently used systemic steroid is oral prednisolone: prednisolone is the active metabolite of prednisone, used widely in the USA. Other systemic steroids include hydrocortisone, methylprednisolone and dexamethasone. Glucocorticosteroids (GCS) act on intracellular glucocorticoid receptors to alter transcription of a range of genes, with multiple downstream effects that include anti-inflammatory, antiproliferative and immunosuppressive actions and vasoconstriction. Synthetic GCS have a glucocorticoid component and most, except dexamethasone, have additional mineralocorticoid activity (Table 18.2).

Starting and continuing treatment

Systemic GCS are usually given orally, but may be given parenterally (intravenously, intramuscularly) if necessary. Prednisolone has a plasma half-life of up to 4 hours, but is biologically active

Table 18.2 Comparative efficacy of glucocorticosteroids

	Equivalent anti-inflammatory dose
Prednisolone	5 mg
Hydrocortisone	20 mg
Methylprednisolone	4 mg
Dexamethasone	0.75 mg

up to 36 hours, so dosage is usually once a day. It should be taken first thing in the morning to minimise the suppressive effect on endogenous cortisol synthesis. The appropriate dose is determined by bodyweight and disease severity. A typical starting dose for skin disease is 0.5 mg/kg/day and it rarely exceeds 1 mg/kg/day. If treatment is needed for more than a week, the dose is usually tapered, rather than abruptly stopped, to reduce the risk of a flare. A key principle is to use the minimum dose that suppresses the disease and for the minimum period of time. Alternate-day dosing may reduce adrenal suppression (see later).

Methylprednisolone is given by intravenous infusion at a dose of 500 mg to 1 g daily for five days ('pulsed therapy') in an attempt to get a rapid onset of therapeutic effect in patients with severe or refractory disease. A depot intramuscular preparation of methylprednisolone may be useful when adherence to oral therapy is a problem, but the drawback of depot therapy is that the drug cannot be withdrawn if adverse effects occur.

Dexamethasone has insignificant mineralocorticoid activity. It can therefore be a useful option where high doses of prednisolone are required, but when fluid retention would be problematic.

Hydrocortisone, which is short acting (plasma half-life 1–2 hours, biological half-life up to 12 hours), is used intravenously for emergencies such as anaphylaxis and where there is short-term inability to take oral medication, for example perioperatively.

Complications of high-dose GCS include neuropsychiatric effects, hyperglycaemia, electrolyte shifts, hypertension, acute hepatotoxicity, thromboembolic disease and sudden cardiac death due to arrhythmias and myocardial infarction.

Monitoring and side-effects

GCS have a range of adverse effects (Figure 18.1). With long-term therapy, patients should be monitored for hyperglycaemia, hypertension and weight gain, with growth retardation also monitored in children. The risk of peptic ulceration and gastrointestinal bleeding with GCS is greatest when co-prescribed with NSAIDs, including aspirin. In these circumstances, prophylaxis with proton pump inhibitors such as omeprazole should be considered. Enteric coated formulations do not prevent adverse

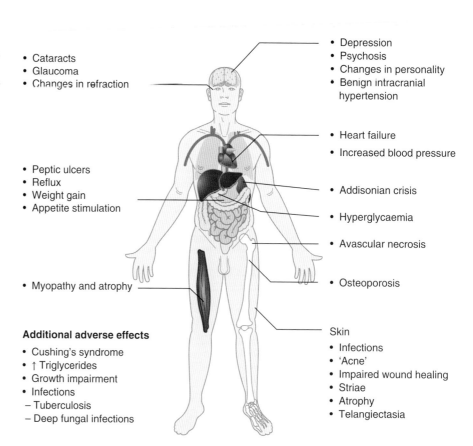

Figure 18.1 Corticosteroid side-effects extend to every body system. Chowdhury MMU *et al. Dermatology at a Glance*, 2nd edn. Chichester: Wiley, 2019.

- Cataracts
- Glaucoma
- Changes in refraction

- Peptic ulcers
- Reflux
- Weight gain
- Appetite stimulation

- Myopathy and atrophy

Additional adverse effects
- Cushing's syndrome
- ↑ Triglycerides
- Growth impairment
- Infections
  - Tuberculosis
  - Deep fungal infections

- Depression
- Psychosis
- Changes in personality
- Benign intracranial hypertension

- Heart failure
- Increased blood pressure

- Addisonian crisis

- Hyperglycaemia

- Avascular necrosis

- Osteoporosis

Skin
- Infections
- 'Acne'
- Impaired wound healing
- Striae
- Atrophy
- Telangiectasia

gastrointestinal effects as these are due to systemic rather than local actions of the drug.

GCS have an adverse effect on bones, causing bone loss and increased fracture risk rapidly after initiation therapy. The fracture risk increases with dose and duration of therapy and is seen for vertebral and non-vertebral fractures, including hip fractures. It is partially independent of bone mineral density. Algorithms for computing the 10-year probability of major osteoporotic fracture include the FRAX tool, which is recommended by NICE. These can then guide use of bone-protection therapy. In general, women age ≥ 70 years, or with a previous fragility fracture or taking large doses of glucocorticoids (≥ 7.5 mg prednisolone or equivalent per day), should be considered for bone-protective therapy with a bisphosphonate. Bone-protective therapy may also be appropriate in some premenopausal women and younger men, particularly in individuals with a previous history of fracture or receiving high doses of glucocorticoids. Lifestyle measures to improve bone health include increasing physical activity, stopping smoking, reducing alcohol intake to ≤ 2 units per day and ensuring adequate dietary calcium intake and vitamin D, with supplements if needed.

Systemic GCS therapy lasting more than three weeks may lead to suppression of the hypothalamic–pituitary–adrenal axis. Treatment should therefore be withdrawn gradually to allow recovery, particularly after reaching a daily dose of 7.5 mg prednisolone, which is similar to the normal physiological level of cortisol. Patients taking oral GCS for more than a month require higher doses during periods of acute illness to prevent an acute adrenal crisis.

Interactions

GCS antagonise the therapeutic effect of a number of drugs, including antihypertensives, hypoglycaemics and diuretics. They also increase the risk of peptic ulcer disease when given with NSAIDs. The anticoagulant efficacy of coumarin may be enhanced by high doses of corticosteroid, so closer monitoring is required. High doses of GCS reduce the immune response to vaccines, so live vaccines should be avoided.

Intravenous immunoglobulins

Intravenous immunoglobulin (IVIg) is a blood product obtained from the pooled human plasma of up to 10,000 donors. A complex manufacturing process is required to screen for infections and to optimise safety. High-dose IVIg has immunomodulatory actions that have led to its successful use in several dermatological diseases, in particular severe immunobullous disease, systemic vasculitis and connective tissue diseases, especially dermatomyositis. It is also a treatment of choice for Kawasaki disease. It is of particular value when high-dose immunosuppressant treatment would be contraindicated by sepsis or malignancy. It is an expensive treatment and a funding request usually needs to be granted for its use in dermatology.

Starting and continuing treatment

IVIg is usually given at monthly intervals at a dose of 2 g/kg bodyweight given over two to five consecutive days. Common side-effects include headache, fatigue and febrile infusion reactions. Serious adverse effects include thromboembolism, pulmonary oedema, aseptic meningitis and anaphylaxis. Patients with selective IgA deficiency should be given a special IgA-depleted preparation, because of the risk of severe allergic reactions or anaphylaxis.

Methotrexate

Methotrexate (MTX) is a derivative of folic acid and is classified as an antimetabolite cytotoxic agent with immunomodulatory but not immunosuppressive actions. Its efficacy at the low doses used in dermatology may be more related to anti-inflammatory actions on white blood cells. The only licensed indication in dermatology is severe psoriasis, but MTX is also widely used off-label as a treatment of severe atopic dermatitis, connective tissue diseases, immunobullous diseases and sarcoid. MTX is considered the 'gold standard' traditional systemic treatment for psoriasis and is widely prescribed by dermatologists; it is also licensed to treat psoriatic arthritis. Pustular and erythrodermic psoriasis usually respond within a few weeks, while a slower response is typical in chronic plaque psoriasis. The main adverse effects of concern are hepatotoxicity and bone marrow suppression.

Starting and continuing treatment

The 2016 BAD guidelines recommend a starting dose of 5–15 mg weekly in healthy adults, with lower doses in those with renal impairment as the drug is excreted renally. MTX is usually given orally, but subcutaneous formulations exist in a range of doses that patients can be taught to self-administer (with special precautions for safe disposal of the medication and injection device). The dose can be increased up to 25 mg per week in adults, and once disease control or clearance is achieved the lowest maintenance dose should be used. Efficacy should be reviewed after 3–4 months and a switch from oral to subcutaneous treatment considered if the response is inadequate.

Monitoring and side-effects

A comprehensive screen of baseline tests should be carried out before starting MTX, such as FBC, liver and renal function tests, hepatitis and HIV serology. Varicella zoster virus immune status should be checked with measurement of antibodies if the patient does not give a clear history of chickenpox. Serial measurement of serum procollagen 3 peptide (P3P) levels should also be undertaken three monthly throughout treatment to monitor for drug-induced liver fibrosis. P3P levels are elevated in children due to growth and are increased in inflammatory arthritis and after fracture. Routine monitoring with serial liver biopsies is no longer recommended and has been surpassed by safer non-invasive methods of assessing liver fibrosis, including Fibroscan®. Liver enzymes are not a reliable indicator of MTX hepatotoxicity, which can progress silently with normal routine blood results, so special tests are essential.

Nausea is a common adverse effect and may be improved by taking folic acid on non-MTX treatment days. This can also reduce the risk of bone marrow toxicity related to folate deficiency. Mucosal ulceration is a warning sign of MTX myelotoxicity and may be accompanied by cutaneous necrosis. Myelotoxicity may be either acute or chronic. MTX toxicity or overdose requires emergency treatment with folinic acid rescue. Weekly blood tests are needed at treatment initiation and dose escalation, but once stabilised these can be reduced to every 3–4 months. It is important that trends in values as well as absolute levels are monitored to detect the earliest signs of potential toxicity. Regular monitoring of renal function is essential with dose reduction if renal function is impaired. Pulmonary fibrosis is a rare complication in dermatology patients and baseline chest radiology is not routinely recommended in those without underlying lung disease.

Interactions

Aspirin, NSAIDs, ciclosporin and probenecid increase methotrexate levels by decreasing renal clearance. Sulfonamides, trimethoprim and phenytoin increase methotrexate's antifolate activity, with potential toxicity.

Conception and pregnancy

MTX is a teratogen, so women of childbearing age should use adequate contraception while taking it and for at least three months after ceasing. It is also excreted in breast milk, so should not be used when breastfeeding. MTX may impair spermatogenesis and men are advised to delay fathering children for at least three months after their last dose.

Special point

MTX is one of the commonest drugs associated with harm due to prescribing, dispensing and monitoring errors. In addition, patients may take the wrong dose if it is dispensed in different tablet sizes (10-mg and 2.5-mg tablets) and they can confuse MTX and folic acid tablets because of similarities in their appearance, with serious consequences.

Mycophenolate mofetil

Mycophenolate mofetil (MMF) is another immunosuppressant drug used in dermatology, following its successful use in transplant medicine. However, all dermatological use is off-label. MMF may be given as monotherapy or as a steroid-sparing drug and is mainly used to treat immunobullous diseases and connective tissue diseases. It has also been used to treat severe psoriasis and atopic dermatitis. MMF inhibits *de novo* purine synthesis, which impairs T-lymphocyte proliferation and B-lymphocyte antibody synthesis.

Starting and continuing treatment

The usual starting dose is 500 mg twice daily, increased after a month, if needed, in 500-mg increments. The usual maintenance dose is 1 g twice a day, with a maximum dose of 1.5 g twice a day.

Monitoring and side-effects

Myelosuppression is usually mild and dose related with anaemia and neutropenia. Regular monitoring of the FBC is required weekly for the first four weeks, then twice a month for two months and every month in the first year. The commonest adverse effects involve gastrointestinal upset, especially at higher doses. They include nausea, diarrhoea, abdominal pain and constipation, and rarely peptic ulceration, gastrointestinal bleeding and perforation. The risk of common and opportunistic infections is also increased, so influenza and pneumococcal vaccines should ideally be given at least two weeks before starting MMF.

Interactions

The absorption of MMF is reduced by concurrent treatment with antacids and cholestyramine. There is an increased risk of agranulocytosis when MMF is co-prescribed with clozapine.

Conception and pregnancy

MMF should be avoided in pregnancy as it is a teratogen. Women of childbearing age should use adequate contraception and a pregnancy test should be checked before starting treatment.

Retinoids

Four systemic retinoids are licensed for use in skin disease in the UK: acitretin, alitretinoin, isotretinoin and bexarotene. They are derivatives of vitamin A and exert their effects through binding to and activating the retinoic acid receptor (RAR) and retinoid X receptor (RXR). These modulate gene expression with effects on keratinocyte proliferation, differentiation and apoptosis. They also have anti-inflammatory effects and affect growth factor and oncogene expression.

All synthetic retinoids are highly teratogenic, so great care must be taken when they are prescribed for women of childbearing potential, who must be engaged in the pregnancy prevention programme (PPP) throughout treatment. They also frequently cause dyslipidaemia with raised triglycerides. Asymptomatic mild hepatitis with elevated transaminase enzymes occurs frequently, but severe hepatitis is rare. Retinoids cross the blood–brain barrier and all members of this group have the potential to cause neuropsychiatric effects. Mucocutaneous and musculoskeletal adverse effects are common, but vary in frequency between different retinoids. Routine monitoring of all retinoids includes checking liver function tests and fasting lipids at baseline and at intervals during treatment.

Synthetic retinoids are fat-soluble drugs, so they should be taken with a meal containing fat for maximum bioavailability. Some retinoids (alitretinoin, bexarotene) may also affect thyroid function.

Vitamin A supplements should be avoided with all synthetic retinoids due to a risk of toxicity, and tetracyclines are also contraindicated due to an increased risk of pseudotumor cerebri. This is a rare but serious complication of all retinoid treatment. Symptoms include severe headache, nausea and visual disturbance.

Acitretin

Acitretin is mainly used to treat moderate-to-severe psoriasis. It is also licensed to treat Darier's disease and is the most effective systemic therapy for severe congenital ichthyoses. It is generally less effective than MTX and ciclosporin in the treatment of chronic plaque psoriasis, but may be preferred when immunosuppressants are contraindicated. Unlike most systemic therapies, it works well in combination with psoralen UVA or UVB phototherapy. The main side-effects are dryness of the lips and other mucous membranes and hair thinning. It potentially has a long half-life, due to storage of metabolites in fatty tissue, so pregnancy should be avoided during treatment and for at least three years after discontinuing. This means that it is not usually a suitable treatment option for premenopausal women.

Starting and continuing treatment

The usual starting dose in psoriasis is 25–30 mg daily or 0.5 mg/kg/day. Lower doses are used in Darier's disease. Doses can be increased up to 1 mg/kg/day, but tolerability is often limited by mucocutaneous adverse effects.

Alitretinoin

Alitretinoin is licensed for the treatment of severe chronic hand eczema in adults that has failed to respond to potent topical steroids. In order to be eligible according to NICE criteria, patients should have a Dermatology Life Quality Index score of at least 15. Chronic hand eczema is often multifactorial and allergic contact dermatitis should be excluded by patch testing before starting alitretinoin. It is the only drug specifically licensed for severe chronic hand eczema and is an effective treatment, with almost half of all patients achieving clear or almost clear hands in a large randomised placebo-controlled trial. The commonest adverse effect is headache, which can be helped by taking the medication at night. It has a relatively short half-life and women of childbearing potential should follow a PPP as for oral isotretinoin (see later).

Starting and continuing

The usual starting dose is 30 mg once daily. If side-effects are not tolerated the dose can be reduced to 10 mg daily, and this lower dose is recommended for patients with diabetes,

hyperlipidaemia and risk factors for cardiovascular disease. A treatment course lasts for up to six months, when in the UK treatment funding is usually discontinued.

Prescribing and dispensing errors may occur, as acitretin and alitretinoin are 'sound-alike' drugs, so extra care should be taken to avoid confusing them.

Isotretinoin

Oral isotretinoin is widely prescribed by dermatologists to treat acne, which is one of the commonest skin diseases globally. For the last 40 years it has been by far the most effective treatment for acne. It is licensed as a treatment of severe or cystic acne where there is a risk of scarring and when there has been an inadequate response to standard topical agents and oral antibacterial therapy. It is also used when acne is associated with severe psychological upset. Isotretinoin is frequently prescribed to adolescent and young adult women at an age when they are most fertile, so great care needs to be taken to avoid pregnancy, as even small doses can lead to profound foetal harm (retinoid embryopathy). All women of childbearing potential should therefore be enrolled on a PPP. The MHRA has produced a thorough and systematic checklist for the PPP outlining the risks of harm to an unborn child, as well as the possibility of contraceptive failure. This is presented as a list of points that must be signed (as acknowledged and understood) by the patient and countersigned (as explained) by the prescriber before treatment is started. This includes the need to use effective contraception for a month before treatment, during treatment and a month after completion. Long-acting reversible contraceptives have the advantage of being highly reliable and lack the risk of user error associated with contraceptive pills and barrier methods.

Minor adverse effects such as dry lips are almost inevitable and a sign that the drug is working, as a reduction in sebum production is one of its mechanisms of action. Dry skin is common, especially on the dorsal hands and forearms, and underlying atopic eczema may worsen as a result. Other common adverse effects include epistaxis, dry eyes and myalgia, especially after strenuous exercise. Retinoid therapy has been associated with mood change and depression. Cases of suicide have been attributed to the use of oral retinoids, in particular isotretinoin. Although many patients report an improvement in mood and self-esteem as their skin clears, the possibility of a serious deterioration in mental health needs to be discussed and documented. The possibility has been raised of long-term sexual adverse effects in males, including erectile dysfunction and loss of libido, and although the true prevalence of this is unclear, patients should be informed of this before treatment.

Starting and continuing treatment

The usual starting dose is 0.5 mg/kg/day. Lower doses may be used in patients with severe acne to reduce the risk of a flare. Macrocomedones can be treated with light cautery before starting isotretinoin, as they will not otherwise respond. The dose should be gradually increased to 1 mg/kg/day if tolerated, aiming for a treatment duration of 16–24 weeks. Lower doses may increase tolerability but extend the risk period for teratogenicity in women. Prescriptions are only valid for seven days and should be limited to a month's duration in women, with evidence of a negative pregnancy test before repeat ongoing prescription. A final post-treatment pregnancy test should also be checked five weeks after completing treatment.

Bexarotene

Bexarotene is mostly used in specialist centres for the treatment of advanced cutaneous T-cell lymphoma or mycosis fungoides in adults.

Thalidomide

Thalidomide has a notorious history, as it caused severe congenital abnormalities with phocomelia when taken in early pregnancy as a sedative and antiemetic. Interest in this drug and its derivatives has rekindled in recent years following the finding that it has significant anti-inflammatory, immunomodulatory and anticancer effects. Its actions include inhibition of tumour necrosis factor alpha synthesis. It is licensed as a treatment for myeloma and all dermatology use is off-label. Thalidomide is used globally to treat erythema nodosum leprosum and has also been reported to help a range of inflammatory skin diseases, including cutaneous lupus erythematosus, pyoderma gangrenosum, sarcoid, Behçet's disease and severe aphthous stomatitis. All patients must participate in a stringent PPP, which includes use of condoms by men because the drug is secreted in semen.

Starting and continuing treatment

Prescribing may be difficult due to regulatory issues and may require submission of an electronic authorisation form. The usual dose of thalidomide is 50–100 mg taken at night because of its sedating effects. The dose can be slowly increased over several months and titrated down when disease is controlled. Due to the high risk of serious adverse effects, thalidomide should be given for the minimum possible duration.

Monitoring and side-effects

In addition to teratogenicity, other serious adverse effects include an increased risk of venous and arterial thromboembolism, bradycardia and heart block. Peripheral neuropathy may occur with long-term use, presenting typically as painful distal paraesthesia. This may be irreversible. Patients should be asked about neurological symptoms and undergo nerve conduction studies every six months.

Biologic therapies

Biologic therapies are licensed for the treatment of severe psoriasis, eczema, urticaria, hidradenitis suppurativa and metastatic melanoma. They also have benefit in other inflammatory skin diseases such as pyoderma gangrenosum (Tables 18.3 and 18.4). Some are now also licensed for use in children and adolescents.

Table 18.3 Biologic therapies: indications and uses

Severe psoriasis or psoriatic arthritis
Severe atopic dermatitis
Chronic idiopathic urticaria
B-cell skin lymphoma
Metastatic malignant melanoma
Pemphigus
Hidradenitis suppurativa
Pyoderma gangrenosum
Sarcoidosis
Behçet's disease
Dermatomyositis
Vasculitis, e.g. Wegener's granulomatosis

Adapted from Chowdhury MMU *et al. Dermatology at a Glance*, 2nd edn. Chichester: Wiley, 2019.

These immunologically active proteins have highly specific structures and functions. They are monoclonal antibodies, recombinant cytokines or receptor binding proteins that reduce the relevant molecule or inflammatory response, for example tumour necrosis factor or T-cell receptors.

Due to their targeted actions, biologics are usually more effective than conventional systemic therapy, with fewer side-effects. However, their considerable expense and prescribing restrictions in particular NICE guidelines mean that they are only accessible by patients with the most severe disease (e.g. psoriasis with Psoriasis Area and Severity Index > 10 and Dermatology Life Quality Index > 10) and where conventional treatment has failed or is contraindicated. The newest psoriasis biologics have high efficacy, with many patients achieving clear or almost clear skin in clinical trials, though real-world data suggests they may be less effective in practice.

Pre-treatment screening is essential (depends on the summary of product characteristics recommendations as below), including history of infections such as tuberculosis (chest X-ray, blood assay), hepatitis and HIV, and exclusion of systemic lupus (anti-nuclear antibodies, anti-dsDNA), demyelinating conditions and heart disease. The main side-effects are serious infections such as tuberculosis reactivation, injection-site reactions, anaphylaxis, potential cancers and demyelination and heart disease.

As this is a rapidly expanding and changing field with new biologic treatments and their biosimilars, it is essential to refer to updated guidelines. The BAD guidelines are regularly updated with evidence-based recommendations.

Janus kinase (JAK) inhibitors

Many of the cytokines that are implicated in the pathogenesis of atopic dermatitis signal directly through the JAK–STAT (signal transducer and activator of transcription) pathway: IL-4, IL-5,

IL-6, IL-12, IL-13 and IL-23. There are four members of the JAK family of enzymes: JAK1, JAK2, JAK3 and tyrosine kinase 2 (Tyk2). JAK inhibitors are small molecules so can be taken orally. They target the JAK family of enzymes, with variable selectivity. Oral JAK inhibitors include baricitinib (blocks JAK1/2), which is now licensed in the UK as an effective, safe option for moderate-to-severe atopic dermatitis. These drugs are well tolerated and are also licensed in some countries for use in psoriasis, alopecia areata, androgenetic alopecia and rheumatoid arthritis. Adverse effects include diarrhoea, headache, increased risk of infection, venous thromboembolism, transaminitis and lipid abnormalities.

Table 18.4 Biologic therapies: mechanisms of action and indications

Condition	Mechanisms of action
Moderate-to-severe psoriasis and psoriatic arthritis	
Adalimumab	Fully humanised anti-TNF monoclonal Ab
Infliximab	Chimeric (25% mouse) anti-TNF human–mouse monoclonal Ab
Etanercept	Fusion protein binds soluble and receptor-bound TNF
Secukinumab	Human IgG1 monoclonal Ab selectively binds to and neutralises IL-17A
Ustekinumab	Human monoclonal Ab binds to p40 protein subunit preventing IL-12/IL-23 binding to T-cell receptors
Ixekizumab	Human monoclonal Ab binds IL-17A and blocks pro-inflammatory cytokines and chemokines
Brodalumab	Human monoclonal IgG2 Ab binds human IL-17 receptor A
Guselkumab, tildrakizumab, risankizumab	Recombinant human (or humanised from mouse) monoclonal IgG1Ab binds to IL-23 p19 subunit and blocks pro-inflammatory cytokines
Moderate-to-severe eczema	
Dupilumab	Ab binds IL-4/IL-13 receptor alpha subunit; inhibits inflammatory response
Urticaria	
Omalizumab	Recombinant humanised monoclonal Ab selectively binds to IgE receptor and inhibits IgE binding to mast cell receptor; also used in asthma
B-cell skin lymphomas, pemphigus	
Rituximab	Potent B-cell-depleting chimeric IgG1 anti-CD20 Ab
Metastatic malignant melanoma	
Ipilimumab	Anti-CTLA-4 protein receptor human monoclonal Ab, blocks cytotoxic T cells, which are immune checkpoint inhibitors of T-cell activation
Nivolumab, pembrolizumab	Anti-PD1 receptor protein, down-regulates T cells and immune system, used if positive BRAF V600 mutation; used with ipilimumab if no BRAF mutation
Vemurafenib, dabrafenib, encorafenib	BRAF protein inhibitor, used if positive BRAF V600 mutation; used with MEK protein inhibitors
Trametinib, binimetinib, cobimetinib	MAPK kinase/MEK protein inhibitor, used if positive BRAF V600 mutation

Ab, antibody; CTLA, cytotoxic T-lymphocyte-associated protein; IL, interleukin; MAPK, mitogen-activated protein kinase; MEK, MAPK kinase; PD, programmed cell death protein; TNF, tumour necrosis factor. Adapted from Chowdhury MMU *et al. Dermatology at a Glance*, 2nd edn. Chichester: Wiley, 2019.

Conclusions

Prescribing and monitoring systemic drugs confidently and safely can only be learnt by clinical experience and, if needed, discussion with experienced practitioners who have prescribed these treatments previously.

There are some general principles that are useful to consider when prescribing systemic therapies. It is important to refer to the most up-to-date BAD or other national guidelines and to refer to the drug's summary of product characteristics to inform clinical decision making, and find clear guidance for pre-screening of drugs. Try to explain complex information clearly to patients, for example consider doing this in a specialised biologic clinic with allocated time. Using written patient information sheets and decision aids for risks, benefits, comparative data and evidence-based clinical experience is useful to save time and provide clear information.

Be honest when communicating with patients if prescribing a new or off-label drug and inform patients if you have not prescribed a drug previously. If needed, look up details and information prior to discussing again with patients. An open discussion is essential to alleviate any patient (or prescriber) anxieties and misunderstandings, and this will enable safe clinical practice with good shared decision making with patients.

Pearls and pitfalls

- Standardised pro formas for initiating and continuing drug treatment and monitoring can be helpful in preventing errors and omissions.
- Shared-care arrangements between primary and intermediary/secondary care can improve patient access to treatment and tests, but protocols should be agreed in advance to ensure patient safety.
- Extra care needs to be taken when prescribing systemic drugs for frail, older people, those with comorbidities and patients taking multiple medications.
- Thiopurine methyltransferase activity should be measured before starting azathioprine to reduce the risk of severe neutropenia.
- Check G6PD levels before starting dapsone, as deficiency can lead to severe haemolysis. This is most common in people of African, Asian, Middle Eastern and Mediterranean descent.
- Systemic glucocorticosteroid therapy lasting more than three weeks may lead to suppression of the hypothalamic–pituitary–adrenal axis.
- Care should be taken with prescribing of methotrexate, as the weekly regimen combined with daily folic acid, and differing tablet sizes and similar appearance, have been associated with serious error and harm. Patients should be carefully monitored for haematological and hepatic toxicity.

SCE Questions. See questions 21–23.

FURTHER READING AND KEY RESOURCES

Aronson JK, Ferner RE. Unlicensed and off-label uses of medicines: definitions and clarification of terminology. *Br J Clin Pharmacol* 2017; **83**:2615–25.

Fernandez JM, Fernandez AP, Lang DM. Biologic therapy in the treatment of chronic skin disorders. *Immunol Allergy Clin North Am* 2017; **37**:315–27.

Mahil SK, Ezejimofor MC, Exton LS et al. Comparing the efficacy and tolerability of biologic therapies in psoriasis: an updated network meta-analysis. *Br J Dermatol* 2020; **183**:638–49.

Smith CH, Yiu ZZN, Bale T et al. British Association of Dermatologists guidelines for biologic therapy for psoriasis 2020: a rapid update. *Br J Dermatol* 2020; **183**:628–37.

Tharp MD, Bernstein JA, Kavati A et al. Benefits and harms of omalizumab treatment in adolescent and adult patients with chronic idiopathic (spontaneous) urticaria: a meta-analysis of 'real-world' evidence. *JAMA Dermatol* 2019; **155**:29–38.

Wollenberg A, Barbarot S, Bieber T et al. Consensus-based European guidelines for treatment of atopic eczema (atopic dermatitis) in adults and children: part II. *J Eur Acad Dermatol Venereol* 2018; **32**:850–78.

Textbooks

Brayfield A, ed. *Martindale: The Complete Drug Reference*, 39th edn. London: Pharmaceutical Press, 2017.

Lebwohl MG, Heymann WR, Coulson I, Murrell D, eds. *Treatment of Skin Disease: Comprehensive Therapeutic Strategies*, 6th edn. Amsterdam: Elsevier, 2021.

Wakelin SH, Maibach HI, Archer CB. *Handbook of Systemic Drug Treatment in Dermatology*, 3rd edn. Boca Raton, FL: CRC Press, 2021.

Useful websites

American Academy of Dermatology. Clinical guidelines. Available at: https://www.aad.org/member/clinical-quality/guidelines.

BAD. Patient information leaflets. Available at: https://www.bad.org.uk/for-the-public/patient-information-leaflets.

British National Formulary and *British National Formulary for Children*. Available at: www.bnf.org.

Electronic Medicines Compendium. Available at: https://www.medicines.org.uk/emc.

FRAX®. Fracture Risk Assessment Tool. Available at: https://www.sheffield.ac.uk/FRAX.

General Medical Council. Decision making and consent. Available at: https://www.gmc-uk.org/ethical-guidance/ethical-guidance-for-doctors/decision-making-and-consent.

Royal College of Ophthalmologists. Hydroxychloroquine and chloroquine retinopathy: recommendations on monitoring.

Available at: www.rcophth.ac.uk/wp-content/uploads/2020/12/Hydroxychloroquine-and-Chloroquine-Retinopathy-Monitoring-Guideline.pdf.

Royal College of Physicians. Osteoporosis: assessing the risk of fragility fracture – NICE guideline. Available at: https://www.rcplondon.ac.uk/guidelines-policy/osteoporosis-assessing-risk-fragility-fracture-nice-guideline.

WHO. Medication Without Harm. Available at: https://www.who.int/patientsafety/medication-safety/en.

19

Skin surgery

S. Walayat Hussain

Introduction

Dermatology is not a purely 'medical' specialty. It is unique among physicianly specialties as it not only encompasses a major medical component, but it also includes both paediatrics and a significant surgical element. The majority of any department's workload now relates to the diagnosis and management of suspected skin cancer. Competence in dermatological surgery is therefore an integral facet of dermatology training. Starting out in skin surgery can be very daunting, as this may be your first real experience of hands-on operating. It is essential there is adequate support and supervision available during the sessions you are allocated, particularly in the first few weeks of your dermatology surgery training.

Consider reading the 'Principles of skin surgery' chapter in *Rook's Textbook of Dermatology* (see Further reading), as this provides a more detailed account of what a dermatologist should know about skin surgery. The British Society for Dermatological Surgery (BSDS) website is also a very useful resource and there are some helpful introductory dermatology surgery textbooks to be read early in training.

Dermatology Training: The Essentials. Edited by Mahbub M.U. Chowdhury, Tamara W. Griffiths and Andrew Y. Finlay.
© 2022 The British Association of Dermatologists. Published 2022 by John Wiley & Sons Ltd.
Companion website: www.wiley.com/go/chowdhury/dermatologytraining

Preparation for skin surgery

Dermatological surgical procedures fall into four categories:

- Diagnostic (e.g. punch biopsy of a rash).
- Therapeutic (e.g. excision of a skin cancer).
- Cosmetic (e.g. blepharoplasty).
- Corrective (e.g. revision of a scar if it causes functional compromise).

It is crucial that both the patient and the operator have a clear understanding of which category of skin surgery is being undertaken at any given time. It is also essential that you always work within the level of your training and competence. It is far better to leave a wound open (and seek senior help) than to try to start a procedure or reconstruction you are not comfortable with and cannot complete with expected good outcomes for you and the patient.

Discussion of the surgical procedure with the patient (Table 19.1)

It is absolutely crucial to take time to explain the planned procedure to your patient, why it is needed and what it entails. The majority of all dermatological surgery complaints arise from miscommunication. The patient may not have received enough information to fully understand the likely outcome of any surgical intervention, resulting in dissatisfaction due to having a 'different expectation' of the outcome of their procedure.

Too often the term 'minor surgery' is used when referring to dermatological surgery. There is no such thing as 'minor' surgery or 'minor' operations! Avoid using the term altogether and refer only to skin surgery or dermatological surgery.

Obtaining adequate consent is fundamentally important. Following the Montgomery ruling, it is expected that you do the following:

- Explain the procedure, provide written information and ask the patient to read it.
- Discuss the risks of the intervention. Common and rare risks should be discussed; also ensure you discuss site-specific risks such as ectropion and eye swelling, which are associated with any periocular procedure.

Table 19.1 Patient preparation

Explain:

What you are going to do
Why you are going to do it
What the **risks** are
What **alternatives** are available
What the likely expected **outcomes** are

- Discuss what alternative options are available (if any).
- Document that you have given the patient the opportunity to ask questions.

Updated General Medical Council (GMC) guidance on decision making and consent was published in 2020. Ensure you have read and understood this, as ultimately this is the standard against which you will be judged should a complaint arise (Table 19.2).

Pre-operative medical history

Most departments will use a pro forma in clinic and the following key points should be addressed:

- Any previous surgery: assess the risk of scar hypertrophy or keloid formation, especially in a keloid-prone site such as the upper back, chest or upper arms – the 'cape' distribution.
- Smoking history: smoking reduces skin blood flow. The risk of graft and flap failure is much higher in people who smoke than in those who do not. Ask the patient to stop smoking and refer to a smoking cessation clinic if needed.
- Anticoagulant and antiplatelet medication (including non-prescribed 'herbal' treatments): each department will have its own guidance in place pertaining to 'blood-thinning' medication and surgery. Ensure you are familiar with your local guidance. The BSDS has published excellent comprehensive guidance on this topic. As a general rule, the risk of post-operative bleeding associated with a dermatological surgical procedure is less than any potential adverse consequence of stopping such medication (such as a myocardial infarction or stroke).
- Do not forget about haematological dyscrasias, which may result in low and dysfunctional platelet counts.
- Implantable devices: these will influence your choice of method to establish haemostasis (e.g. bipolar should be used in a patient with a pacemaker). Comprehensive up-to-date guidance on this may be accessed on the BSDS website.

Table 19.2 General Medical Council guidance on consent: the key principles

Support patient decision making
Listen to your patient and those close to them
Share information that is relevant to your patient
Understand the different roles you and your patients play in decision making
Respect your patients' decisions
Recognise the importance of the decision-making process
Presume, assess, maximise and review capacity
Involve your patient as much as possible in discussions and decisions about their care, even when they cannot make a decision
Involve others when making decisions where patients are unable to do so

Table 19.3 Surgical checklist

Pre-op

- Introduce the team
- Positively identify the patient (i.e. ask them to tell you their name, date of birth and address) – ensure labels match all details of the patient
- Confirm with the patient the type of procedure they understand they are having and check this with the booking form and medical records
- Positively identify the site of the lesion(s) to be treated with the patient and other team members using a mirror, medical images and hospital records – if there is any doubt, do not proceed
- Note any allergies, implantable devices and blood-thinning medication

Post-op

- All sharps accounted for and disposed of safely (operator's prime responsibility)
- Ensure histology sample and labels match patient details and procedure performed
- Record procedure accurately in medical records as soon as practically possible
- Provide verbal and written aftercare instructions to patient (or carer), including who to contact with any post-operative concerns
- Clear work area of all records and specimen samples before calling for next patient (to avoid mix-ups)

Other important factors that should be considered relate to the post-operative period. For example, operating on the dominant hand of an individual will impact on their activities of daily living and their job; any post-operative dressing near the eye will preclude the individual driving. For an elderly patient, always consider if they will need someone to look after them after the planned procedure. A surgical checklist should always be used before starting any skin surgery procedure (Table 19.3).

The skin biopsy

This is the commonest skin surgery procedure performed (Figure 19.1) and ultimately your choice of biopsy method will be determined by what you want to know (Tables 19.4–19.6). The more tissue your dermatopathologist receives, the better the diagnostic yield, but clearly this needs to be balanced with the morbidity (scarring and functional impairment) caused by the procedure itself.

Have a clear idea in your mind what you are trying to achieve with the biopsy. For example, if when querying a panniculitis you fail to include deep fat in your biopsy, then this is subjecting the patient to a valueless procedure and is a waste of your time; performing a superficial shave biopsy will not enable a dermatopathologist to confidently distinguish between a squamous cell carcinoma (SCC) and a keratoacanthoma. As a general rule, pigmented lesions should not be biopsied but excised whenever

Figure 19.1 Types of skin biopsy. Finlay AY, Chowdhury MMU. *Specialist Training in Dermatology.* © 2007 Mosby Elsevier.

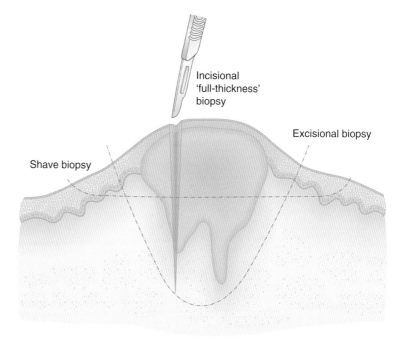

possible. Exceptions would be for suspected lentigo maligna or other clinical scenarios where excision may confer significant morbidity in large ill-defined lesions. In these situations the clinically most suspicious area should be sampled.

Table 19.4 Punch biopsy

Advantages
- Quick
- Easy to process in the pathology lab
- Suitable for biopsies of rashes and tumours
- Defects easy to suture

Limitations
- Depth – may be unsuitable in panniculitis, morphoea and some cases of vasculitis
- Difficulty in assessing depth of tumour invasion
- May in theory lead to embedding of tumour fragments deeper in the skin
- Sampling error

Table 19.5 Shave biopsy

Advantages
- Quick
- Heals secondarily with no suture requirements

Limitations
- Depth
- Unsuitable for rashes, vasculitis, panniculitis or assessment of tumour invasion, e.g. Bowen's disease versus squamous cell carcinoma

---

Table 19.6 Incisional biopsy

Advantages
- Provides the dermatopathologist with the best biopsy sample, e.g. useful to examine the edge of an ulcer or a rash to compare with 'normal' adjacent skin
- The full thickness allows examination of the fat and deep blood vessels, which is useful in suspected infiltrative diseases and granulomatous disorders and diseases of connective tissue and fat

Limitations
- Will often leave a significant scar, which may be difficult to suture (especially for an ulcerated lesion)
- More time-consuming than a rapid punch biopsy

Local anaesthetics

Lidocaine is the most widely used drug for local anaesthesia of the skin. Concentrations of 1% and 2% are available with adrenaline (1:80,000 and 1:200,000) or without adrenaline (i.e. plain lidocaine).

The maximum safe dose of subcutaneous lidocaine is 3 mg/kg without adrenaline and 7 mg/kg with adrenaline. Lidocaine 1% contains 10 mg of lidocaine per mL. Remember that for the most commonly used local anaesthetic preparation (1% xylocaine or lidocaine with 1:200,000 adrenaline) the safe maximum amount is 0.7 mg/kg of the patient's bodyweight. A 70-kg person should therefore have no more than 49 mL of 1% lidocaine with 1:200,000 adrenaline.

Adrenaline prolongs the duration of anaesthesia and causes vasoconstriction, two very useful properties. A 1:1000 solution of adrenaline contains 1 mg/mL; 1:100,000 contains 1 mg adrenaline per 100 mL. It is seldom necessary for a general dermatologist to infiltrate more than 50 mL of 1% lidocaine with 1:200,000 adrenaline (250 μg), so the safety margin for adrenaline is high.

Large volumes of anaesthetic used in tumescent anaesthesia require a greater dilution of lidocaine and adrenaline. Adrenaline has alpha-1 (vasoconstriction), beta-1 (inotropic, chronotropic) and beta-2 (vasodilatation) properties. Its use in patients taking non-cardioselective beta blockers may give rise to unopposed alpha-1 vasoconstriction, leading to hypertension and reflex bradycardia.

Nerve blocks used commonly in dermatology are supraorbital and supratrochlear nerve blocks and infraorbital and mental nerve blocks. Familiarise yourself with the anatomy of these nerves. When performing a nerve block, all that is needed is to bathe the region of the nerve with anaesthetic; it does not need pinpoint precision. It is less painful for the patient if you use plain local anaesthetic (without adrenaline) when performing such blocks. Using a longer-acting agent such a bupivacaine for nerve blocks may be preferable, because it provides the patient with prolonged anaesthesia for larger procedures. Bupivacaine is an anaesthetic with slower onset (about 5–10 minutes) and long duration (5–8 hours). It can therefore provide post-operative pain relief as well and is available as 0.25% and 0.5% concentrations. The maximum safe dosage for bupivacaine is 2 mg/kg. It is not a problem to use adrenaline-containing local anaesthetic when performing a digital ring block; there is enough supportive data to prove that it is safe. The dermatological 'myth' that suggests it is unsafe should be forgotten. A total volume of 4 mL of anaesthetic on either side of the digit should not be exceeded to avoid ischaemia from direct compression. It is entirely safe and appropriate to use lidocaine with adrenaline for subcutaneous infiltration on the nose, ear and penis.

Injecting local anaesthetic

It is good practice to aspirate and check that there is no intravascular injection when administering local anaesthetic. When accidental intravascular injection occurs, there is sudden blanching in the distribution of the vascular network around the injection site, and you should therefore stop injecting immediately. The signs of minor toxicity of lidocaine include circumoral paraesthesia, tinnitus and dizziness, and sometimes a metallic taste. The injection of local anaesthetic can be uncomfortable and the application of topical local anaesthetic creams, such as EMLA, in children and needle-phobic patients can be helpful.

When injecting, a fine-gauged needle such as 27G or preferably 30G should be used. The skin to be injected should be pinched to decrease pain perception and the patient warned about the injection beforehand. Try to introduce the needle down a follicle (e.g. on the nose), with the bevel of the needle pointed downwards, and inject subcutaneously and not intradermally. The injection should be slow and the syringe aspirated frequently to check for intravascular injection. Distraction techniques such as tapping on the patient's forehead or simply talking to the patient can help lessen the discomfort of anaesthetic infiltration.

Multidose vials of local anaesthetic are widely used. They contain lidocaine, adrenaline, sodium metabisulfite (antioxidant) and also parabens (preservative). Lidocaine 2% is considered more painful than 0.5% preservative-free plain lidocaine. Adrenaline and sodium metabisulfite both significantly increase the discomfort associated with the injection. Warming the anaesthetic to 37 °C may cause less discomfort than using anaesthetic at 20 °C. Local anaesthetic remaining in a multidose vial must not be used to treat another patient because of the risk of cross-infection.

Type C pain fibres are anaesthetised more quickly than the larger pressure and proprioceptive fibres. Warn patients beforehand that they will feel pressure and joint movement and that this does not indicate failure of the local anaesthetic. Motor fibres are affected later on after the injection. It is important to warn patients who have had infiltrative anaesthesia on the face that they may not be able to raise the eyebrows or tightly close the eyes after injections in the temple region or that they may have drooping of the mouth for some hours after an injection in the cheek.

Anatomy

It is essential to have a sound knowledge of anatomy when performing dermatological surgery (Figure 19.2). On the face, the skin with the underlying fat lies on the superficial fascia, which is known as the superficial musculoaponeurotic system (SMAS). Above the zygoma this layer is known as the superficial temporal fascia, splitting to ensheath the frontalis, procerus, occipitalis and auricular muscles, and then extending up on the scalp as the fibrous galea. Below this fascia is the deep temporalis fascia covering the temporalis muscle. Below the zygoma, the SMAS is made up of parotid fascia, which is a fibrotic degeneration of the platysma muscle. The parotid fascia is in continuity with the platysma, risorius and depressor anguli oris muscles. The central facial and nasal muscles are devoid of a distinct aponeurotic

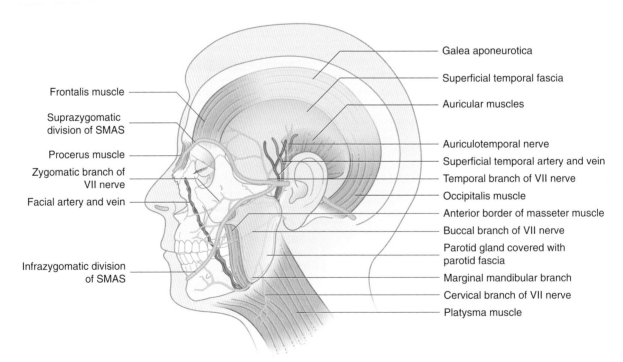

Figure 19.2 Diagram of the face to show the location of the branches of the facial nerve in relation to the fascia and the parotid gland, and the overlying facial and superficial temporal arteries. Finlay AY, Chowdhury MMU. *Specialist Training in Dermatology.* © 2007 Mosby Elsevier.

component. Knowledge of the SMAS helps predict the location and depth of important blood vessels and nerves. Axial blood vessels and sensory nerves to the upper face arise deeply and ascend to lie in the SMAS–fat interface. The superficial temporal artery is frequently seen on the temple and forehead. It lies on the superficial temporal fascia and is above the plane of the temporal branch of the facial nerve, which runs beneath this fascia upon the deep temporalis fascia. On the forehead, branches of the supratrochlear and supraorbital nerves run on the fascia above the frontalis muscle, along with branches of the supraorbital and supratrochlear arteries.

The facial nerve exits the skull through the stylomastoid foramen and enters the parotid gland at the midpoint of a line connecting the superior border of the tragus of the ear to the angle of the jaw. The temporal branch of the facial nerve exits the parotid gland, and rami are distributed over the middle third of the zygomatic arch. The medial part of the zygomatic arch is a safe area, as the nerve has now entered the orbicularis muscle. It is most vulnerable over a 25-mm section over the midpart of the zygomatic arch. Here the nerve is covered only by fascia, fat and skin. This area can be mapped out by (i) a line drawn from the tragus to the upper forehead crease and (ii) a second line drawn from the earlobe to the eyebrow (Figure 19.3a). The path of the ramus to the frontalis muscle is along a line drawn 0.5 cm below the tragus to 1.5 cm above the lateral eyebrow (Figure 19.3b). This ramus lies between the SMAS (superficial temporal fascia) and the deep temporalis fascia before it enters the frontalis muscle at its lateral border.

The superficial temporal artery and vein along with the auriculotemporal nerve emerge from the parotid gland and lie on the superficial temporal fascia. If working within no more than 1 cm anterior to a vertical line drawn from the scalp to the insertion of the anterior helix of the ear, the posterior ramus of the temporal branch is safe. The zygomatic and buccal branches of the facial nerve pass medially from the parotid gland on the masseteric fascia. The SMAS is very poorly developed here, and the nerves are covered by skin and fat, which however is quite deep at this site. The branches of the zygomatic and buccal nerves anastomose (i) just anterior to the masseter and (ii) at the point under the modiolus (the dimple). These two points correspond to the posterior and anterior borders of the buccal fat pad, respectively, which is seen when removing deeply invasive tumours over the mid cheek area. Rich anastomoses between these two branches account for frequent recovery if some of the branches are damaged.

Another important structure below the fat in this area is the parotid (Stenson's) duct. This leaves the parotid gland and continues anteriorly, before winding round the anterior border of the masseter muscle and piercing the buccinator muscle to enter the oral cavity by the second upper molar tooth. The parotid duct can be felt under your finger when you clench your teeth and palpate the anterior border of the masseter muscle. The duct can be mapped to a point where a line from the tragus to the upper lip crosses the anterior border of the masseter – the tragolabial line. At the point where the anterior border of the masseter muscle attaches to the mandible, the facial artery can

(a)

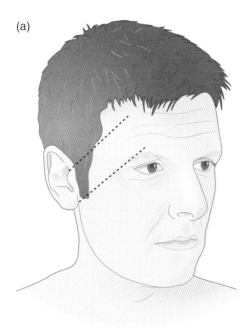

(b)

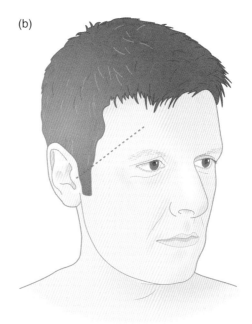

Figure 19.3 (a) The surface markings demonstrating the region within which the temporal branch of the facial nerve is at risk during surgery. (b) A line drawn from the tragus, across the temple, to the forehead indicates the path of the nerve as it supplies the frontalis muscle. Finlay AY, Chowdhury MMU. *Specialist Training in Dermatology.* © 2007 Mosby Elsevier.

be felt. Behind the artery lies the facial vein and in front of the artery lies the marginal mandibular nerve. The nerve at this point is vulnerable to injury. It is covered solely by a variable amount of platysma muscle, fat and skin. There is an anastomosis with the buccal nerve in only 10% of people. Injury to this nerve is very serious, as it innervates the lower-lip muscles, which are essential to achieve oral continence.

In the neck the posterior triangle is bounded by the clavicle inferiorly, the posterior border of the sternomastoid anteriorly and the anterior border of the trapezius posteriorly. The floor of the triangle consists of the splenius capitis muscle superiorly, and the levator scapulae and the posterior and middle scalene muscles inferiorly, which are covered by the pre-vertebral layer of the deep cervical fascia, which is itself covered by the superficial layer of the deep cervical fascia. Between these layers of fascia many important structures are located on the floor of this triangle: the lesser occipital nerve, great auricular nerve, transverse cervical nerve and spinal accessory nerve, which is the motor nerve to the trapezius and sternomastoid muscles.

Erb's point is located where a line perpendicular from the midpoint of a line drawn from the angle of the jaw to the mastoid crosses the posterior border of the sternomastoid muscle (Figure 19.4). The lesser occipital, great auricular, transverse cervical and spinal accessory nerves lie within an area 1 cm above and below this point. The spinal accessory nerve runs on the floor of the posterior triangle from approximately the junction

Figure 19.4 Diagram showing Erb's point and the danger zone for nerve damage.

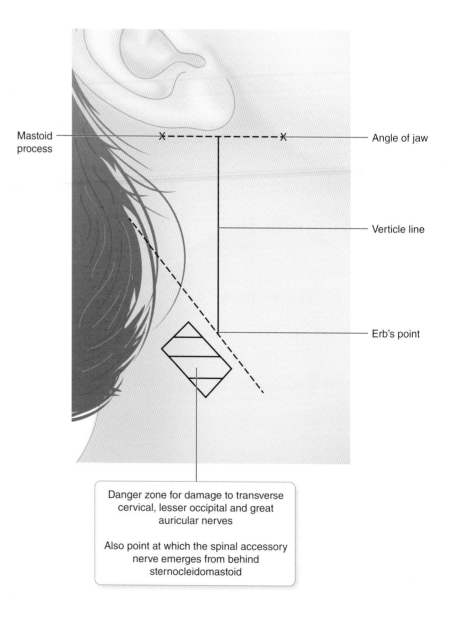

Mastoid process

Angle of jaw

Verticle line

Erb's point

Danger zone for damage to transverse cervical, lesser occipital and great auricular nerves

Also point at which the spinal accessory nerve emerges from behind sternocleidomastoid

of the upper one-third/lower two-thirds of the sternomastoid muscle, descending approximately obliquely to leave the triangle at the junction of the middle/lower third of the trapezius muscle.

The structures in the posterior triangle are covered by skin, fat and the superficial layer of the deep cervical fascia, which ensheaths the trapezius muscle posteriorly and the sternomastoid muscle anteriorly. These structures are safe providing the fascia is not breached. This can be breached when attempting to remove an epidermoid cyst in the posterior triangle or excising a deeply invasive malignant tumour. Damage to the spinal accessory nerve will result in shoulder drop due to paralysis of the trapezius muscle.

Other motor nerves you should be familiar with are the ulnar nerve at the elbow, where it runs 1 cm below and lateral to the medial epicondyle of the humerus, and the common peroneal nerve (lateral popliteal nerve) as it winds around the head of the fibula. The nerves at these points are very superficial and patients should be consented for potential damage to such structures.

Haemostasis

Superficial wounds

For haemostasis of superficial wounds, such as following shave excision or curettage, a styptic such as 20% aluminium chloride in 70% isopropyl alcohol can be used. This acts as a protein-precipitating agent. Driclor® is an alternative. Silver nitrate and Monsel's solution (ferric subsulfate) are seldom used now because of the small risk of tattooing of the skin.

Electrocautery

This is an effective haemostat. A current passing through a high-resistance metal such as platinum produces heat and the cautery tip is like a soldering iron. Electrocautery is now seldom used in clinical practice.

Diathermy

This is another technique for haemostasis. Surgical diathermy generates heat by:

- Resistance to current that passes through the tissues.
- Duration of application of the current (proportional to the square of the current).
- Current density, which is inversely proportional to the surface area of the electrosurgery tip.
- Heat from sparking. The temperature of an electric spark can be as high as 1000 °C. Sparking is achieved by activating the diathermy tip without making contact with the skin surface. This is known as electrofulguration (Latin *fulgur*, 'lightning'). This technique may result in slight surface damage and may cause scarring if superficial dermal damage occurs. The deeper tissues are not damaged, because charring acts as an insulating barrier.

Direct contact with the skin and the diathermy tip results in electrodesiccation. The heat generated from the current and the current density produces further heating (and therefore injury) at a deeper level than is achieved with fulguration.

With instruments such as the hyfrecator, fulguration or desiccation is achieved without attachment of another ('dispersive') electrode to the patient to disperse the current; that is, to 'ground' the patient. The patient therefore acts as a capacitor, storing electrical charge and shedding free electrons from the skin surface to the air, the couch, the operator and the assistant before going to ground. It is sometimes possible for the operator or assistant to discern a light shock or tingle if the patient is touched lightly. This is more likely at higher power settings or if the hand is ungloved or the tip of the finger is in contact with the patient, as a small surface area such as a fingertip allows discharge at a point like a lightning conductor.

Deeper wounds

Bleeding from the depth of a wound following excision is best dealt with immediately by placing firm pressure on the wound and slowly retracting the gauze to reveal the bleeding vessel. This can then be sealed with diathermy, and if this is not successful the vessel can be tied with an absorbable suture using a figure-of-eight knot.

Instruments now used widely for electrocoagulation in skin surgery do not have a dispersive electrode and are the 'bipolar' type. The tips of the coagulation forceps are insulated and AC current flows between the tips of the forceps that are grasping the tissue. The current density is high and the distance between the tip is small, so the tissue resistance is lowered. Tissue damage is much more localised.

Complications of electrosurgery instruments

During electrosurgery, complications such as burns or pacemaker interference can occur.

Burns

Burns occur due to:

- Poor surface contact with the dispersive electrode.
- Inadvertent contact with the earth or ground through metal on the operating table.
- Fire risk from alcohol-based antiseptics.

Pacemaker interference

The sensing function of a demand pacemaker may pick up stray electromagnetic radiation (EMR) from electrosurgical apparatus and interpret this as cardiac muscle myopotential, which could, in turn, inhibit generator function. In practice very few problems are encountered because modern pacemakers are insulated with titanium, which filters and screens stray EMR from machines such as microwaves and shavers. However, check and adhere to your department's policy pertaining to surgery in patients with cardiac devices.

Practical tips if a person has a pacemaker

- Contact your local cardiac department prior to the procedure and seek advice.
- Use short bursts of activity (less than 5 seconds).
- Avoid using the active electrode over the precordium in a patient with a pacemaker or on the skin over the pacemaker power source.

Needles and sutures

There are a great many needles and sutures to choose from and you are advised to read one of the standard texts or the BSDS annual surgery workshop manual for further information. The shape of the needles is commonly 3/8 of a circle. Compound curve (J-shape) needles are particularly useful in placing subcuticular buried stitches in confined areas. Small needles are 12 mm in length and are often attached to fine sutures used on the face; 19-mm needles are used for the trunk and limbs. Some sutures are attached to large 25-mm or 29-mm needles and are useful if large bites of skin are needed.

Modern needles are usually manufactured with either the inner or the outer surface of the curve honed to a sharp edge. These are known as cutting (inner surface) or reverse cutting (outer surface) needles. Reverse cutting needles are best for skin surgery, as this shape prevents the needle track from cutting in towards the wound edge during the passage of the needle. 'P' needles and 'Prime' needles have excellent points and are best used for skin surgery. Always hold the needle in the needle holder two-thirds from the tip. Do not grasp the needle near the swage where the suture is attached (a swaged needle is a prepacked eyeless needle attached to suture thread). This part of the needle is very weak and frequently detaches if handled with force.

Suture materials

There are two broad categories of suture: absorbable and non-absorbable.

Common absorbable sutures are either braided such as Vicryl®, or monofilament such as Monocryl™ and PDS™ (all from Ethicon, Somerville, NJ, USA). Vicryl retains 50% of its strength at 2–3 weeks, Monocryl retains 50% strength at 10 days and PDS retains 50% strength at 6 weeks.

Of the many non-absorbable sutures, the most commonly used are Ethilon™ (polyamide) or Prolene™ (polypropylene; both from Ethicon). Sutures are made in various thicknesses; the higher the number, the finer the thread. Many texts dictate which sutures should be used on which part of the body.

Table 19.7 Suture removal

All wound tension should be taken by your buried stitches. Leaving surface stitches in for > 7 days almost always results in unacceptable track marks on the skin. A guide for suture removal is as follows:

- Face: 4–7 days
- Trunk and limbs: 7 days (the only exception is for below-knee surgery, where track marks do not seem to form even if stitches are left in for 10 days)

In reality there is no absolute rule, as the extent and type of the repair will determine which type of suture is required. However, one of the commonest mistakes pertains to the length of time during which surface skin sutures are left *in situ*. The longer they are left in, the greater the risk of unacceptable 'track marks' on the skin (Table 19.7).

Surgical procedures

Punch biopsy (Figure 19.5)

Mark the skin to show the preferred axis of the scar. Stretch the skin at right angles to this. Rotate the punch while advancing down to its hilt. The plug will usually spring up attached to the fatty base. Support and lift the skin gently with a hook or forceps; do not crush the biopsy with the forceps. Cut the biopsy from its fatty base with scissors. The elliptical (fusiform) defect is then easily sutured. Fine 6/0 sutures on the face or 4/0 sutures on the limbs usually allow faster healing and a neater scar than leaving the wound to heal by second intention.

Shave biopsy/excision (Figure 19.6)

Gently scoring the margins of the lesion after local anaesthetic injection enables this procedure to be performed with excellent reproducible results. Stretching the skin with the non-dominant hand facilitates the use of the blade in creating a clean and even superficial shave on the skin. The procedure may be performed either by holding the scalpel parallel to the skin surface, or via the use of a Wilkinson blade (as shown). Haemostasis is often not required, but a topical styptic will cause less tissue damage in aesthetically sensitive areas, although light diathermy or cautery may be used.

Curettage (Figure 19.7)

Disposable ring curettes either 4 mm or 7 mm in size are universally available. One side of the circular blade is sharp and the other is relatively blunt. The sharp side is indicated by a mark on the handle. As the process of curettage is a superficial destructive process, it is advisable to adopt a 'backhand' technique with the curette 'away' from yourself, rather than towards you, as this

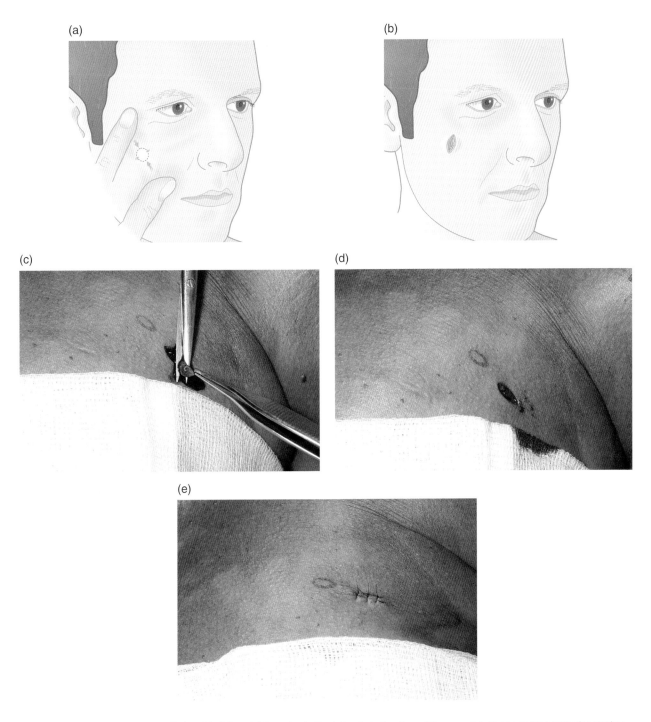

Figure 19.5 Punch biopsy – stretch the skin (a) at right angles to the intended direction of the scar (b). Remove the biopsy by cutting (c). Do not crush the specimen. The defect (d) is then sutured (e). (a, b) Finlay AY, Chowdhury MMU. *Specialist Training in Dermatology.* © 2007 Mosby Elsevier. (c, d, e) © Medical Illustration Cardiff and Vale UHB.

maintains a superficial plane. Hold the curette sharp side down, as you would a pencil between the middle finger, forefinger and thumb, stretching the skin between the hands. Pull the curette gently but firmly at an angle of about 45 degrees across the tumour from one margin to the next, separating it from the underlying skin. The action should be gentle, seeking out the plane of least resistance. A double cycle of curettage and cautery may be considered a therapeutic procedure for low-risk lesions such as small, well-defined nodular basal cell carcinomas (BCCs), well-differentiated SCCs or Bowen's disease.

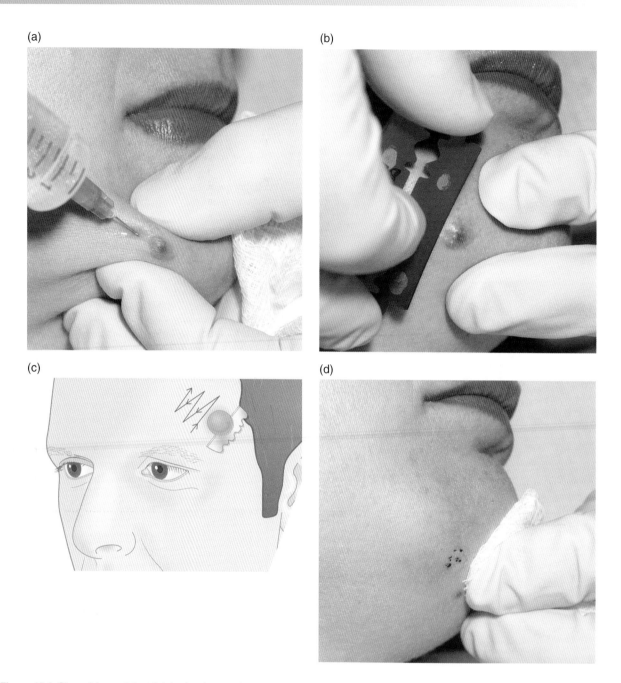

Figure 19.6 Shave biopsy. Inject (a) the local anaesthetic deeply so as not to elevate the lesion. This minimises the risk of producing a depression on the surface. Hold the blade firmly (b) and cut continuously (c) to produce a flat defect (d). (a, b, d) © Medical Illustration Cardiff and Vale UHB. (c) Finlay AY, Chowdhury MMU. *Specialist Training in Dermatology*. © 2007 Mosby Elsevier.

Incisional biopsy (Figure 19.8)

This is similar in principle to taking a slice out of a cake and is a useful technique when histological examination of the entire dermis and dermis–fat interface is needed, for example in dermal infiltrative disorders such as lymphomas, morphoea, vasculitis, panniculitis or infiltrating carcinoma. Deep narrow wedges of the skin can be closed easily without tension. For tumours, it is better to use a large 25-mm 3/8 curve needle, which enters and exits wide and passes deep to the tumour. If possible, avoid passing the needle point deliberately through the body of the tumour. These sutures often pull through; that is, 'cheese wiring'.

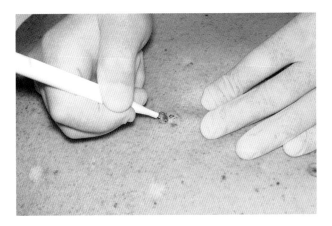

Figure 19.7 Ensuring the skin is stretched firmly facilitates a superficial cleavage plane during curettage. Note how the 'backhand' technique (away from the operator) allows a shallow wound to be created. © Medical Illustration Cardiff and Vale UHB.

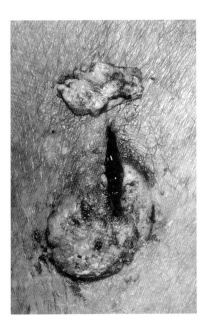

Figure 19.8 Full-thickness biopsy through the edge of the tumour. This allows assessment of invasion of the tumour as far down as the fascia. © Medical Illustration Cardiff and Vale UHB.

Excision (Figure 19.9)

The elliptical (fusiform) excision is the workhorse procedure for all dermatologists when dealing with skin lesions. It is imperative that the procedure is well planned. Remember: measure and plan twice, cut once! Degrease the skin with an alcohol wipe and clearly delineate the margins of what you are removing using magnification and good lighting. Think about what ideal orientation you want for the scar. Generally, it is best not to follow the principle of 'cutting something out' and 'seeing which way it

can be closed', as this will lead to suboptimal results. As the surgeon, it is best for you to try to orientate the scar where you know it will lead to a superior outcome. This also becomes an important aspect relating to patient consent, as if you do not know what the scar will look like (e.g. length, orientation), how can you adequately consent your patient?

To plan an excision, start by drawing the relaxed skin tension lines in the area you are working. On the face, ask the patient to wrinkle their nose or close their eyes or raise their eyebrows or purse their lips to define these areas more clearly. This gives the necessary information as to where you should intend to place the scar. Anaesthetising the skin will cause soft tissue distortion. This is why it is essential to have drawn the skin markings beforehand. The length-to-breadth ratio of a typical excision is usually 3:1. Patients are frequently surprised by the 'length' of a scar, and unless they are counselled appropriately pre-operatively, they may complain about the 'extent' of the surgery. Explaining why a scar is elongated should be part of your consent discussion and ideally occur in clinic, well before the patient attends for surgery. Aesthetically, a shorter scar does not necessarily predict a better cosmetic outcome. A longer scar that creates a better contour and avoids depressions and protrusions on the skin is superior to a shorter, bulky scar that is raised at the apices due to the standing cutaneous deformities (dog-ears).

Cut the skin with the cutting edge (i.e. the curvature/belly of the blade) perpendicular to the surface, using your non-dominant hand to stretch and support the skin. Trainees will often equate this to holding the blade-holder at 90 degrees, but this then does not optimise the blade's contact with the skin. Once you have incised to the depth of the desired tissue plane, remove the specimen with curved tissue dissection scissors. Use the scissors to perform blunt dissection, which will create less bleeding. The ellipse may then be lifted from the skin using a skin hook or fine Adson Micro Toothed forceps. To optimise wound closure and eversion, undermining should be performed. Blunt dissection with curved Metzenbaum tissue scissors should be used to undermine the wound edges; the plane of dissection will vary according to what you have excised and where on the body you are operating. Ensure meticulous haemostasis and use skin hooks to elevate the wound edges to ensure haemostasis also under the edges.

In order to maximise wound eversion and produce superior aesthetic outcomes, the first stitch should be a buried vertical mattress suture. This type of stitch is the single most important stitch to master, as it takes all the tension off the wound and is an everting stitch (Figure 19.9). If done correctly, this stitch should create a kidney-bean shape, rather than an oval shape, under the skin surface. Skin stitches should not be used to close any wound space; this is the function of the buried sutures (Figure 19.9c). Skin stitches are used to perfect wound edge alignment and should not be tied under any tension at all (Figure 19.9d). Interrupted skin stitches are less strangulating to the wound edges than a continuous running stitch, but occasionally the latter may be preferable if there is an increased risk of bleeding, for example in a patient on warfarin.

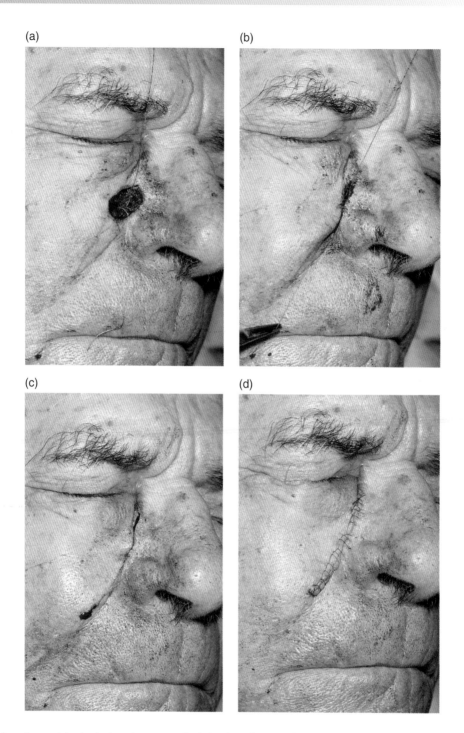

Figure 19.9 Note how the excision is designed pre-operatively to place the scar along the nose–cheek junction, enabling the patient to be fully informed pre-operatively about the site, length and orientation of the scar. (a, b) Meticulous placement of a buried vertical mattress suture takes all the tension off the wound, reduces the dead space and everts the wound edges. (c) Correctly placed buried sutures should enable complete wound approximation. (d) Surface stitches placed under no tension will allow optimal aesthetic outcomes (a–d) © Medical Illustration Cardiff and Vale UHB. (e) The correct sequence to position a buried vertical mattress suture. Adapted from the diagram by Riley Grosso, MD., Closing the Gap: Deep Sutures, Emergency Medicine Tamed, Taming The Sru.

(e)

How to insert a buried vertical mattress suture

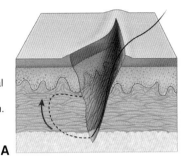

To start, the needle is inserted at the level of the deep fat or superficial fascia and exits at the dermoepidermal junction.

A

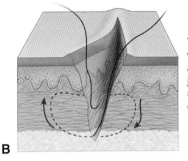

The needle is then rearmed with the driver and inserted at the dermoepidermal junction on the contralateral side and exited at the level of the superficial fascia.

B

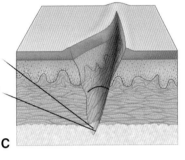

Crucial to this process is that the leading and trailing segments of the suture remain on the same side of the loop.

C

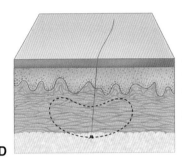

Using 3 or 4 throws, the knot is tied and buried at the level of the superficial fascia. The knot is cut leaving only 2-mm 'trails'.

D

Figure 19.9 (Continued)

Dissolvable sutures such as Vicryl Rapide™ (Ethicon) are commonly used, as their use avoids the patient having to return for suture removal, particularly important for example during the COVID-19 pandemic. However, it should be noted that such stitches will not dissolve in the expected time of 7–10 days unless they are kept moist, for example with petroleum jelly. Furthermore, Vicryl Rapide surface stitches can result in significant skin redness and inflammation, especially in younger patients.

Neither oral nor topical antibiotics should be routinely prescribed, except in cases where an ulcerated tumour has been excised. These tumours are frequently infected with coagulase-positive *Staphylococcus aureus* and carry a risk of post-operative wound infection. There is no significant risk of bacteraemia during skin surgery, and antibiotic prophylaxis for endocarditis is not required for routine dermatological procedures, even in a patient with a pre-existing heart lesion.

Wound care

The dressing is a matter of personal choice and every practitioner will have their own preference. There is no data to suggest that topical antibiotics are superior to normal petroleum jelly in reducing the incidence of skin surgery complications such as infection. It is common practice to apply petroleum jelly to the sutured wound (or chloramphenicol eye ointment if operating in the periocular region) in conjunction with a paraffin-impregnated mesh dressing such as Jelonet® or Bactigras® (both Smith and Nephew, London, UK), followed by an alginate dressing such as Kaltostat® (ConvaTec, Runcorn, UK) or Melgisorb® (Mölnlycke, Berchem, Belgium), covered with a non-adhesive dressing and secured with an adhesive tape. This can then be removed after 24–48 hours by the patient and petroleum jelly applied to the suture line 3–4 times daily until sutures are removed or they fully dissolve.

Safety and governance in skin surgery

All departments should have protocols and policies in place to ensure patient safety is maximised during skin surgery; make sure you are familiar with all of these. In most departments, a bespoke adaptation of the World Health Organization (WHO) safer surgery checklist will be used. Ensure at all times that you are treating the correct patient and providing the correct treatment at the correct site. Wrong-site surgery is a 'never event' that must be reported as a serious clinical incident when it occurs. The same investigation and root-cause analysis are mandatory whether the wrong limb has been removed or the wrong skin lesion has been biopsied. Numerous methods can help eliminate the risk of wrong-site skin surgery (Table 19.8).

Table 19.8 Avoiding wrong-site surgery

- Accurately mark and document the site of the lesion: use distance of lesion from two fixed anatomical landmarks
- Use accurate anatomical language in documenting lesion site. For example, anterior crus of right ear, rather than just stating right ear; soft triangle of left alar rim, rather than just stating left tip of nose
- Perform same-day surgery whenever possible
- Use photography to identify lesion
- Get patient to positively identify lesion to be treated, with a mirror if feasible
- Ensure all team members agree that the lesion that is marked is the correct lesion to be treated

You should not forget about your own safety and that of your staff when operating. You should ensure you have the appropriate level of personal protective equipment available for the procedure you are performing – this should include gloves, masks, eye protection and surgical gowns. When performing any plume-generating procedure (most commonly hyfrecation) you should ensure your operating facility has appropriate plume extraction devices available. It is also imperative that you are familiar with your department's protocols and guidelines pertaining to a needlestick injury and the spillage of any hazardous substance.

Surgical treatment of melanoma

The treatment of primary cutaneous malignant melanoma is wide excision. Any tumour suspected as being a melanoma should be excised with a small margin of normal skin to allow histological staging first. Punch biopsy, shave biopsy or curettage is not appropriate in cases of suspected melanoma. Re-excision of the scar is performed later – the margin depending on the Breslow thickness, as recommended by the BAD or national guidelines.

If you are excising a pigmented lesion, always orientate the scar in a manner that will enable a wider local excision should the histology confirm a melanoma. On the limbs, always excise lesions vertically towards the draining lymph node basin and not horizontally (i.e. excise up and down and not across the limb).

Surgical treatment of non-melanoma skin cancer

The standard treatment is excision. Other surgical and non-surgical treatments may also be used for treatment of skin cancer and are described in the appropriate BAD guidelines and Chapter 13.

For well-defined BCCs up to 2 cm diameter, a 4-mm margin will excise the tumour completely in 98% of cases. SCCs

deemed high risk either by virtue of their histological features or due to their size may require wider margins of excision. BCCs occurring on the ala nasi, alar base, pre- and post-auricular area and periocular area may extend more widely and deeply than is clinically suspected. Furthermore, non-melanoma skin cancers in these areas are considered at higher risk of incomplete excision, as smaller margins may be taken by the surgeon to enable closure of the subsequent surgical defect. Clearly this is not good practice and will lead to higher rates of incomplete excisions. Nodular BCCs greater than 2 cm in diameter and sclerosing (morphoeic, infiltrative) BCCs may also require wider margins. Remember that tumour growth is *not* symmetrical around the clinical margin: larger BCCs, those in high-risk facial locations and those that are ill defined, infiltrative or morphoeic are most appropriately treated with Mohs micrographic surgery.

It is best practice for all excised lesions to be examined histologically. The limitations of traditional histological tissue preparation for assessing adequacy of tumour excision are often not appreciated. Bread-loaf cross-sectioning (bread-loafing) permits very limited examination of the deep and lateral surgical margins.

Complete examination of the entire surgical margin of a 1-cm specimen using 5-μm sections would require 2500 'slices' to be examined. Typically three or four sections are therefore prepared for the pathologist, who will then examine 0.1% of the surgical margin. This explains why pathologists often report 'tumour appears completely excised', or 'appears completely excised in the planes of the sections examined', or 'tumour does not extend to the margins of the sections examined' (Figure 19.10).

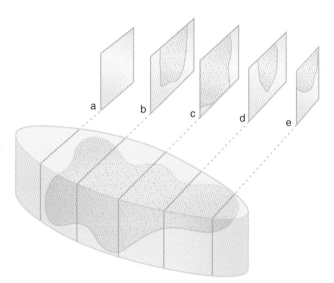

Figure 19.10 Ellipse of skin containing a tumour examined using 'bread-loaf' cross-sections. Examination at points c and e would have demonstrated tumour invasion of the surgical margin. If sections from points a, b and d had been examined, the pathologist's report would have concluded that the tumour appears to be completely excised. Finlay AY, Chowdhury MMU. *Specialist Training in Dermatology.* © 2007 Mosby Elsevier.

The incompletely excised tumour

All incompletely excised malignant tumours should be discussed in your local skin cancer multidisciplinary team (MDT) meeting.

If a tumour is incompletely excised, an MDT approach, even for a non-malignant lesion, will allow options to be discussed with a patient. It is not always appropriate to perform further treatment on a low-risk tumour, at a low-risk site, even if excised with an incomplete peripheral margin. Such lesions may never cause any issues in the future. With an ageing population, we need to ensure we are not just treating 'lesions' for the sake of it – that is why an MDT approach is always useful.

Your management approach should be informed by local guidelines and is likely to follow National Institute for Health and Care Excellence (NICE) Improving Outcomes Guidance pertaining to skin cancers.

Mohs micrographic surgery

Frederic Mohs, a surgeon from Madison, Wisconsin, USA, devised a margin-controlled method to ensure complete removal of skin cancers. The fleshy bulk of the tumour may first be removed by curettage to create a saucer-shaped defect. A further margin of skin encompassing the side and base of the wound is removed intact and the surgical margin is then prepared for horizontal sectioning (Figure 19.11). The section may be cut into either halves or quadrants (Figure 19.11) to permit easy tissue handling and mapping on a diagram of the anatomical site. These segments are then stained at their margins with different-coloured inks.

This technique enables the entire surgical margin to be examined. If tumour is seen in these horizontal sections, it *must* therefore have breached the surgical margin at that point. It is therefore possible to identify the area in the wound bed corresponding to this point in the histological section. Further skin is then removed from this area in the wound and sectioned horizontally again to check complete excision. This process is repeated until there is confirmation of no tumour remaining.

The technique ensures that all the tumour has been excised completely, yet minimises the amount of skin removed and is therefore tissue sparing.

Mohs surgery is unique in terms of a surgical procedure, as the surgeon acts as both the pathologist and reconstructive surgeon. There are therefore national and international standards of training and accreditation to ensure the competency of those practising the technique. In the UK, where competency is achieved via fellowship programmes, there are agreed national standards pertaining to training and provision of Mohs surgery, in addition to an external quality assurance programme for all Mohs centres in the UK.

Indications for micrographic surgery

It is usually performed for BCCs and some SCCs, mainly on the face. It is seldom needed on the limbs and trunk, where a

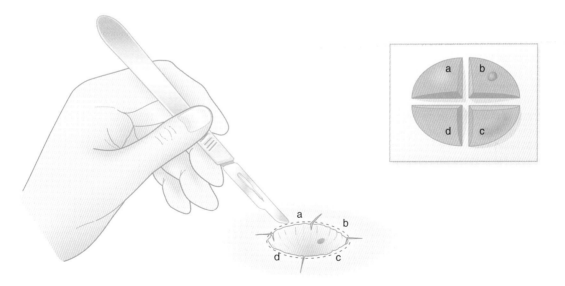

Figure 19.11 The tumour is debulked by curettage. A thin plate encompassing the entire margin and wound bed is excised. In this example there is residual tumour at the base of the wound. The tissue is divided into quadrants (inset) and the cut edges marked with dye. The surgical margin of the tissue is sectioned horizontally to include the epidermis and deep margins in the same plane and examined under the microscope. Any tumour seen must have breached the surgical margin at the point that can be accurately located in the wound. Further specimens are removed until the surgical margins are clear of tumour. Finlay AY, Chowdhury MMU. *Specialist Training in Dermatology.* © 2007 Mosby Elsevier.

generous margin of skin does not compromise repair, but the nail apparatus and genitalia may benefit from the tissue-sparing benefit of Mohs surgery (Table 19.9).

Table 19.9 Indications for Mohs micrographic surgery

- Tumours > 2 cm in diameter
- Tumours arising in periorbital, perinasal, perioral and periauricular regions
- Ill-defined lesions
- Recurrent tumours
- Morphoeic or infiltrative histology or with perineural spread

Surgical reconstruction

Following the surgical excision of any skin lesion, the resulting defect must be repaired, with several options available (Table 19.10). Many of these are specialised surgical techniques requiring extra training. However, all dermatologists require an awareness of the basic principles of complex reconstruction.

It is important that skin closure does not result in tension and distortion at free margins such as the lower eyelid or the vermilion border of the lip. In such situations skin grafts or random-pattern flaps may be used. A flap is a unit of skin bearing its own blood supply (the pedicle), which is moved from one location to another by advancement, rotation or transposition. Random-pattern flaps are useful because they provide skin of good colour, texture and contour, in contrast to skin grafts. Well-chosen flap repairs give excellent cosmetic results and facilitate repairs not possible with other closure techniques (Figures 19.12–15).

Full-thickness skin grafts (FTSGs) are frequently used to repair defects. The donor site should be chosen that best fits the colour and texture of the recipient site. Pre- and post-auricular skin is a common donor site. For larger skin defects, skin may be taken from the supraclavicular or clavicular area. Split-thickness skin grafts may provide coverage for larger defects. Although their metabolic requirements are less than those of FTSGs, the aesthetic outcome is generally less satisfactory than with FTSGs (Figures 19.16 and 19.17).

Wounds healing by second intention can produce excellent results, particularly on the temple and post-auricular areas and if close to the inner canthus (Figure 19.18). Second intention healing should not be used near free margins, for example the

Table 19.10 Options for wound repair

- Primary repair
- Local skin flap
- Distant (pedicled) skin flap
- Skin graft (full thickness or split thickness)
- Granulation (second intention)

vermilion border, alar rim or lower eyelid margin, because contraction of the wound will result in distortion.

Nail surgery

Biopsy of the nail apparatus is an essential technique in dermatological surgery. If a subungual lesion is suspected, an X-ray of the distal phalanx will be helpful to exclude bone involvement and to determine subungual bony exostosis.

To perform nail surgery, you may need additional instruments, including nail splitters (anvil scissors) and a nail elevator (a Freer septum elevator is an excellent alternative).

The digit should be anaesthetised using a ring block technique. Haemostasis is important. For the finger, it is useful to apply a surgical glove to the patient's hand. The fingertip of the glove should then be snipped off and the glove rolled back to the metacarpal phalangeal joint. Alternatively, a broad strip can be cut from the cuff of a surgical glove and wound round the proximal digit tightly, before securing the tourniquet with artery forceps. Both these techniques are effective, and commercial tourniquet rings such as the T-RING® (Precision Medical Devices, Thousand Oaks, CA, USA) can also be used, as they are less strangulating on the digit and therefore less liable to induce neuropraxia (transient trauma-induced peripheral nerve injury akin to 'nerve concussion'), which may in rare cases last for several months after the event.

Avulsion of the nail

First, separate the cuticle from the nail plate. Insert the elevator under the nail, pushing up against the nail plate, and advance up to the lunula, which represents the distal part of the matrix. Nail adhesion to the nail bed is much less at this point. Free the entire nail, including the lateral horns under the proximal nail fold. Grasp the nail with nail-pulling forceps, a needle holder or artery forceps, and twist the nail to roll it free from its attachment under the nail fold. The nail can then be easily fully detached. The nail bed can now be examined. Any tumour arising in the nail bed can be biopsied. A 4-mm punch biopsy from the nail bed and a 3-mm punch biopsy from the matrix are usually considered as having low risk of causing scarring-related nail dystrophy. However, the patient needs to be informed of this risk, including pterygium formation, and consented accordingly. The risk of pterygium is reduced and healing enhanced if the nail plate is replaced and used as a biological dressing after biopsy.

Biopsy of the nail matrix and nail bed

Pigmented streaks arise usually from a melanocytic lesion in the matrix. To expose the matrix, the proximal nail fold will need to be reflected back by making incisions for approximately 5 mm from the lateral nail fold bilaterally. The matrix should be biopsied at the origin of the pigmented streak. For biopsies not exceeding 3-mm width, a punch biopsy will be sufficient. If larger biopsies are needed, a horizontal (transverse) fusiform biopsy should be taken that follows the curve of the lunula, and the

(a)

(b)

(c)

(d)

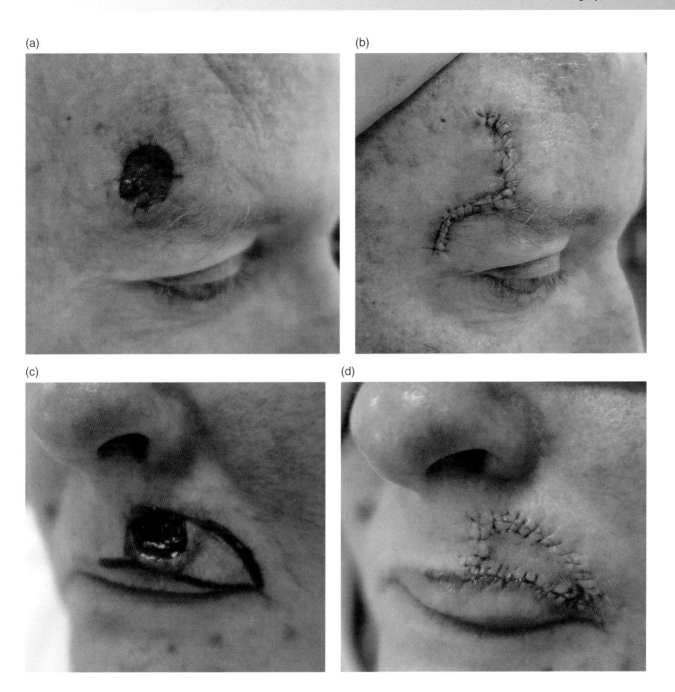

Figure 19.12 Advancement flap examples (Burow's and island pedicle flap). (a) Defect on the supra-eyebrow region of the right side of the forehead. (b) Burow's advancement flap avoids the eyebrow. (c) Upper cutaneous lip defect. (d) Island pedicle flap repair (also referred to as a V to Y closure).

defect repaired with absorbable sutures. This should avoid a permanent nail defect post-operatively.

In severe nail dystrophy, the defect may arise in the bed or in the matrix. A longitudinal nail biopsy is the best investigation, without prior nail avulsion. It is helpful to administer the ring block first and then, to reduce the risk of infection and to soften the nail,

soak it for about 20 minutes in antiseptic solution before applying the tourniquet; remember to minimise the amount of time the tourniquet is applied. Using a size 15 blade, the nail plate and nail bed should be cut down to the periosteum from the free margin of the nail to a point approximately 5 mm proximal to the proximal nail fold. If possible, biopsy the lateral nail plate.

(a)

(b)

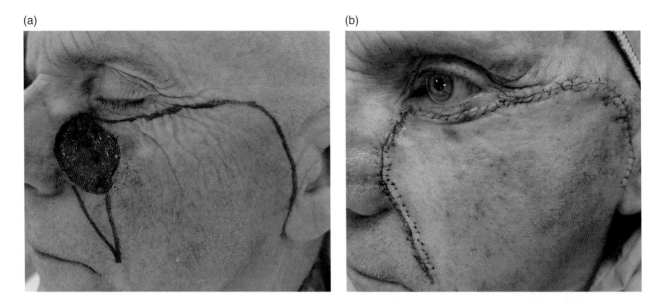

Figure 19.13 Rotation flap example. (a) Large medial cheek defect. (b) Cheek rotation flap enabling tension-free closure.

(a)

(b)

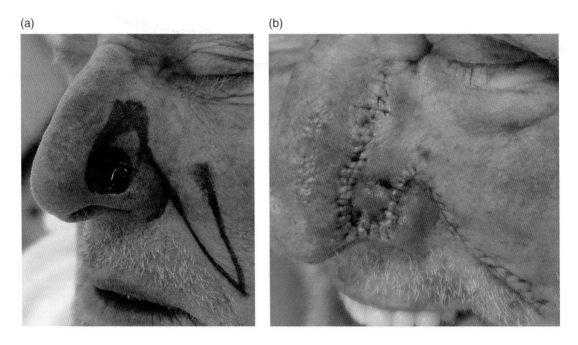

Figure 19.14 Transposition flap example. (a) Deep medium-sized nasal defect. (b) Nasolabial (cheek to nose) transposition flap.

The width of the biopsy should not exceed 3 mm. Remove the entire nail, nail bed and matrix with the overlying nail fold as a single unit, carefully supporting the biopsy with forceps while dissecting the tissue off the periosteum with sharp scissors. It can be helpful to orientate the specimen on a card prior to placing it into a biopsy cassette and then to put in the formalin fixative. The resulting defect should be repaired with vertical mattress sutures to ensure good approximation of the skin to the lateral nail plate.

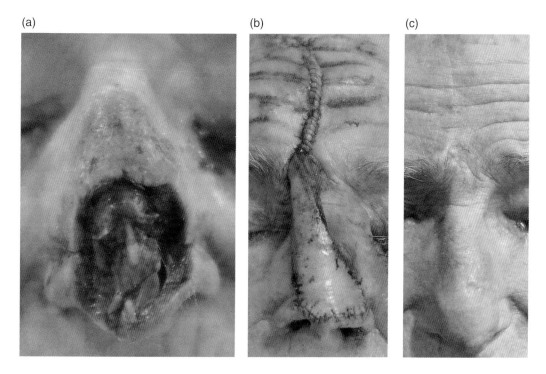

Figure 19.15 Interpolated flap. (a) Significant loss of distal nose after Mohs tumour extirpation. (b) Interpolated right-sided paramedian forehead flap used to resurface the defect. (c) Following flap division and inset, satisfactory restoration of volume and contour function.

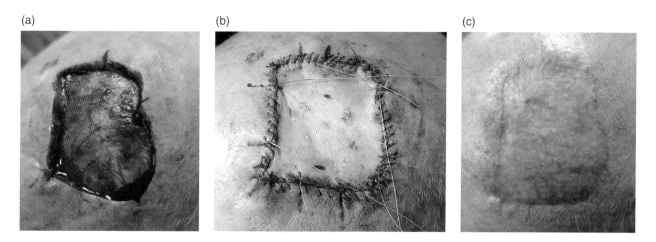

Figure 19.16 Full-thickness skin graft. (a) Large defect of the left frontal scalp. (b) Full-thickness skin graft harvested from the right clavicular region. (c) Outcome at 8 weeks.

Post-operative care

The digit will be painful for several days, so your patient should be advised to start regular analgesia immediately, as reflex sympathetic dystrophy has been described after nail surgery, the risk of which is increased with high levels of post-procedure pain. Apply a non-adherent dressing over paraffin-impregnated gauze. A high arm sling post-procedure reduces bleeding, swelling and pain and should therefore be encouraged. There is no routine requirement to prescribe antibiotics unless the lesion is clearly eroded.

(a)

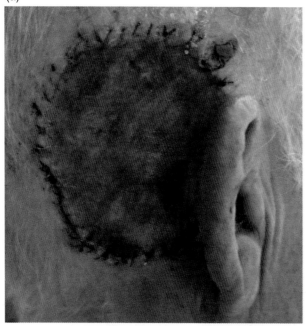

(b)

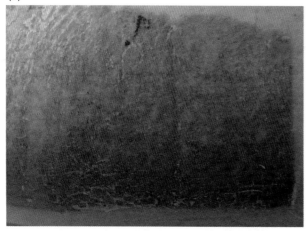

Figure 19.17 Split-thickness skin graft. (a) Large occipitoparietal split-thickness skin graft seen immediately after dressing removal at day 7. The graft has established a blood supply as indicated by its pink colour. (b) The donor site (lateral thigh) heals secondarily (shown two weeks post-procedure).

Cryosurgery (cryotherapy)

Cryosurgery is the deliberate destruction of tissue by cold in a controlled manner. Various refrigerants have been used over the years: surface temperature reductions obtainable with carbon dioxide (CO_2) are −79 °C, nitrous oxide −75 °C and liquid nitrogen spray −196 °C. Most cells are killed at temperatures of −25 to −30 °C, a temperature that can be readily achieved using liquid nitrogen spray cryosurgery.

Technique

The spray technique is most commonly used. The area to be treated can be marked with a skin marker to include a margin appropriate for the lesion that is being treated; that is, the lateral freeze line. The spray tip is held 5–10 mm from the surface and liquid nitrogen is directed at the centre of the field (Figure 19.19a). A visible ice field forms quickly and spreads laterally to the predetermined margin (Figure 19.19b). The freeze time *begins* as soon as the ice ball fills the designated area. By slight adjustment of the flow rate and distance to skin, the ice field will be prevented from extending beyond the boundaries. The spray tip should be moved continuously over the ice field in a zigzag or whorl pattern. It is essential to establish the ice ball as quickly as possible. This ensures that the −25 °C isotherm is at a deep level. Slow freezing produces very shallow injury. For example, using a cotton bud method of delivering liquid nitrogen, it is not possible to freeze colder than −18 °C beyond a depth of 2 mm. Use of a 'C' nozzle spray quickly freezes fields of 10–15 mm in size; 'B' nozzle spray is better used for larger areas up to 20 mm in diameter. Repeat-freezing produces greater tissue destruction than a single freeze. Before a second freeze is given, the treated area must thaw slowly back to body temperature. Significant cellular injury is caused by thawing. It is imperative to record accurately the freeze time used in the medical record, as cryosurgery is one of the commonest reasons for medicolegal complaints in dermatology.

Cryosurgery is painful. Most adults and children over 10 years of age may tolerate a single freeze up to 10 seconds. Consider using local anaesthetic (without adrenaline) if treating larger areas or using topical local anaesthetic cream, which may obviate the need for injection of local anaesthetic.

Liquid nitrogen spray cryosurgery can be a very effective treatment for carefully selected non-melanoma skin cancers, but, due to prolonged healing times and an inability to histologically confirm tumour clearance, it is being used far less commonly in clinical practice.

Pitfalls of cryosurgery (Table 19.11)

As noted, cryosurgery is one of the commonest causes of medicolegal complaints in dermatology. It is therefore essential that prior to administering the treatment, patients are adequately counselled about the treatment and the expected outcomes.

Patients should be forewarned about pain, swelling, blistering, hypo- or hyperpigmentation, delayed healing, incomplete treatment (requiring repeat treatment) and more rarely scarring and delayed healing (especially on the lower legs). Depending on what part of the body is being treated, the functional impact the treatment and subsequent recovery will have on activities, such as work and exercise, needs careful consideration prior to treatment.

Temporary unwanted effects are common, for example scar hypertrophy and milia. These settle without treatment. Impaired

(a)

(b)

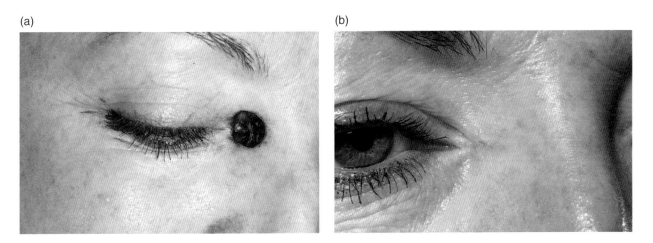

Figure 19.18 Wounds in concave areas may heal very well via granulation. This defect (a) arising in the medial canthus has produced a perfectly acceptable outcome (b) following second intention healing. © Medical Illustration Cardiff and Vale UHB.

(a)

(b)

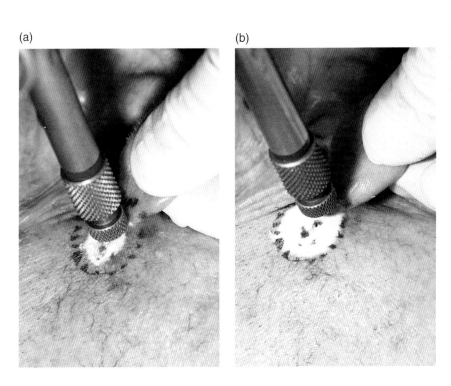

Figure 19.19 Cryotherapy. Hold the spray tip (a) 5–10 mm from the skin surface. The freeze time begins when the ice ball has filled the predetermined area (b). © Medical Illustration Cardiff and Vale UHB.

sensation may be noticed in the finger following digital cryosurgery and this may last for 12–18 months. Damage to hair follicles is frequently seen with longer freeze times, resulting in permanent alopecia and giving a poor cosmetic result. Melanocytes are very sensitive to cold injury; this will result in hypopigmentation and is usually permanent. It is more likely to develop after longer freeze times, but slight pigment loss may be seen following short freeze cycles. Cryosurgery should be performed with great caution in skin of colour, especially in type V and type VI skin.

Avoid collateral damage from splatter from the spray by using gauze or a non-adherent dressing, cut to shape if required.

Post-treatment care following cryosurgery

The patient may take aspirin, non-steroidal anti-inflammatory drugs or paracetamol. A light non-adherent dressing gives some comfort for the first 24 hours or so. Washing the cryosurgery wound

Table 19.11 Potential side-effects and pitfalls of cryotherapy

- Pain
- Blistering
- Hypo- or hyperpigmentation
- Scarring
- Prolonged healing
- Inadequate information to the patient before the procedure (leading to complaints)

does not hinder healing. If a blister forms and is under tension, it is best to burst this with a sterile needle. A thin film of an occlusive ointment such as yellow soft paraffin should then be regularly applied, with or without a non-adherent dressing (depending on the body site treated), until the area has healed.

How to stay out of trouble (Table 19.12)

Unfortunately, it is part and parcel of clinical practice that sometimes things go wrong, patients are unhappy and complaints arise. Patients get cross if they develop discomfort or restriction of activity post-operatively that they were not warned about beforehand. Communication is key! Spend time explaining the expected side-effects of all the planned treatment. Make sure the patient understands *why* they are having the test or treatment. Tell the patient what would happen if no investigation or treatment was carried out. This often convinces them about the need for treatment. Be certain of your diagnosis. It is very difficult to defend against any legal action or complaint when something has gone wrong if it was not at all necessary to do the test or treatment in the first place.

Do not work under pressure or in a hurry. Accidents occur more commonly when working too fast. Do not delegate treatment to inexperienced staff, who may feel reluctant to take on the job.

Table 19.12 Staying out of trouble

- Know your anatomy and danger zones
- Always work within your level of training
- If in doubt, do not proceed with a procedure, and seek senior help
- Ensure you are up to date with the latest GMC guidance on obtaining informed consent
- Do not rush, take your time and focus solely on the patient in front of you
- If you have made a mistake or misjudged a situation, you must be honest with your patient and explain what has happened (duty of candour)
- Ensure your records are accurate and legible and provide a clear outline of what you did and how you did it

Remember: if you are perceived as failing to exercise the skill you have or claim to have, you are in breach of duty of care and may be found to be negligent. Always work within the limits of your training, ability and experience. Never feel pressurised either by your peers or by the patient to perform a treatment you do not feel comfortable with.

The majority of claims arising from skin surgery do *not* result from incomplete excision of a lesion, excessive scarring, severing a nerve or vessel, post-operative infection, failure to obtain a histological diagnosis or failure to arrange the necessary follow-up. The majority of complaints are in fact due to 'miscommunication' and a perceived failure to convey the risks associated with a treatment. This essentially is failure to obtain informed consent. Extra time taken with your patient during the initial consultation will save you a lot of time in the long run.

Conclusions

Skin surgery can be extremely rewarding once the required basic skills have been mastered. Always treat every case with diligence and full concentration, making sure the proper environment and preparation are in place. Getting distracted can lead to avoidable mishaps, for example forgetting to dispose of used sharps leading to needlestick injuries. If faced with a surgical case beyond your current competencies, always ask for help. The only way to ensure progression is with adequate supervision to gain confidence in new procedures. This best and safe practice applies throughout all of our dermatology careers, no matter how experienced we are.

Pearls and pitfalls

- Avoid using the term 'minor surgery' when discussing any skin surgery procedure – just use the term 'skin surgery' or 'dermatological surgery'.
- Always work within the level of your competency and training, and remember that your first priority is to ensure you 'do no harm' to your patient.
- Adrenaline-containing local anaesthetics may be used when performing a digital ring block.
- The maximum volume (in mL) of 1% xylocaine with adrenaline 1:200,000 that may be administered to a patient equates to 0.7 mg/kg of their bodyweight (in kg). A 70-kg patient may therefore receive up to 49 mL of local anaesthetic if needed.
- Orientate the excision of any pigmented lesion on the limb vertically, towards the draining lymph node basin, to facilitate the subsequent wider excision in cases of confirmed melanoma.
- Remember that alcohol-containing antiseptics may pose a potential fire hazard if the vapour has not fully evaporated before hyfrecation is performed.

SCE Questions. See questions 31 and 32.

FURTHER READING AND KEY RESOURCES

Brown SM, Oliphant T, Langtry J. Motor nerves of the head and neck that are susceptible to damage during dermatological surgery. *Clin Exp Dermatol* 2014; **39**:677–82.

Hussain SW, Motley RJ, Wang TS. Principles of skin surgery. In: *Rook's Textbook of Dermatology* (Griffiths C, Barker J, Bleiker TO, Chalmers R, Creamer D, eds), 9th edn. Chichester: Wiley-Blackwell, 2016; Chapter 20.

Miller CJ, Antunes MB, Sobanko JF. Surgical technique for optimal outcomes: part I. Cutting tissue: incising, excising and undermining. *J Am Acad Dermatol* 2015; **72**:377–87.

Miller CJ, Antunes MB, Sobanko JF. Surgical technique for optimal outcomes: part II. Repairing tissue: suturing. *J Am Acad Dermatol* 2015; **72**:389–402.

Textbooks

Lawrence CM. *An Introduction to Dermatological Surgery*, 2nd edn. London: Churchill Livingstone, 2002.

Useful websites

British Society for Dermatological Surgery. Available at: www.bsds.org.uk. Note: Annual Surgery Workshop and Manual (updated yearly).

General Medical Council. Available at: www.gmc-uk.org.

National Institute for Health and Care Excellence. Improving outcomes for people with skin tumours including melanoma. Cancer service guideline CSG8. Available at: https://www.nice.org.uk/guidance/csg8.

20

Wound care and dressings

Mark Collier and Tamara W. Griffiths

Introduction

Wounds can be acute or chronic, and although there is no true definition, it is widely accepted that acute wounds progress through the normal stages of healing within four weeks, while chronic wounds take much longer and persist. Dermatologists create intentional wounds on our patients as a prerequisite of skin surgery, but this chapter will focus on the assessment and management of chronic wounds.

Stages of normal wound healing

In order for the clinician to understand chronic wounds, a basic understanding of the normal stages of wound healing is required.

Wounds should progress through four stages of healing in a timely and orderly fashion. Much of the research in chronic wound healing is currently focused on factors influencing progression through these stages. This research may help to understand some chronic wounds, which appear to get 'stuck' in a certain stage.

1. **Haemostasis**: tissue injury provokes immediate activation of the coagulation pathways, resulting in fibrin formation. This acts as a temporary plug to close the wound.
2. **Inflammation**: neutrophils initially clear the wound of debris, which may impair wound healing. Macrophages release cytokines, which provide the correct environment for promotion of new tissue formation. Additionally, they produce extracellular molecules that combine with others to produce a provisional matrix, which serves as a scaffold for dermal regeneration and epidermal migration and proliferation.
3. **Proliferation**: angiogenesis provides capillary loops within the provisional matrix, which give the wound its red granular appearance, hence the term 'granulation' tissue. Fibroblasts proliferate and migrate into the provisional matrix and synthesise collagen. Epithelial cell proliferation and migration then occur.
4. **Remodelling**: this transitory phase from granulation tissue to scar involves reorganisation and maturation of collagen fibres. During this phase, the wound is converted from approximately 20% normal, unwounded tensile strength to

Dermatology Training: The Essentials. Edited by Mahbub M.U. Chowdhury, Tamara W. Griffiths and Andrew Y. Finlay.
© 2022 The British Association of Dermatologists. Published 2022 by John Wiley & Sons Ltd.
Companion website: www.wiley.com/go/chowdhury/dermatologytraining

approximately 70–80% of the strength of normal skin. This process can last for up to 1–2 years after the wound has appeared to heal externally.

Leg ulceration

Chronic leg ulceration is a common problem and is likely to become more prevalent with our ageing population. The healthcare burden of leg ulcers is enormous in terms of both morbidity and finance. This cost can be partly addressed by expeditious treatment of leg ulcers by experienced clinicians in a multidisciplinary setting.

Until recently, many doctors perceived leg ulceration as a chronic, incurable problem, and the management of patients with leg ulcers has been largely neglected in both undergraduate and postgraduate medical teaching. As leg ulcers do not automatically fall under one specialist category, it has been left to clinicians in varying fields such as dermatology, diabetology and vascular and plastic surgery to develop subspecialist interests in the management of these patients.

Traditionally, nurses have shouldered the burden of work by becoming intrinsically involved with the patient management through regular contact with patients when applying wound dressings and bandaging. The specialist role of 'tissue viability nurse' has been developed to provide advice on the prevention and treatment of wounds of varying aetiologies throughout the hospital. It is optimal to work in a multidisciplinary team, particularly with complex or hard-to-heal wounds, and the focus must be on a holistic view of the patient and evidence-based, cost-effective management.

The cost of leg ulceration

An estimated 1.5% of the adult population have an ulcer, and about 80% of all leg ulcers are venous. Most of these patients are over 65 years old and it is likely that as the population ages, the prevalence will increase. Leg ulceration has a profound adverse effect on quality of life. Pain, restriction in physical and social functioning, and perceived poorer general health have been demonstrated at all ages. The financial implications of leg ulcer management are sizeable, estimated to be around £2 billion per year in the UK. This cost reflects nursing time, dressing and bandage costs and medical care, as well as loss of patient earnings.

In order to reduce patient morbidity and healthcare costs, dermatologists must play a role in both the multidisciplinary management of patients with leg ulceration and teaching and promoting good practices of wound care to other healthcare professionals. This section provides a practical approach to the management of patients with leg ulceration.

Assessment of leg ulcers

Most of the causes of leg ulceration, together with cofactors that can impair healing, are listed in Table 20.1. As ulcers are more common in older people, it is common to have multi-aetiological

ulcers with numerous cofactors present. Although the vast majority of leg ulcers in the community are primarily venous in origin, the aetiology of those presenting to outpatient dermatology clinics also includes more complex vasculitic, rheumatoid and multi-aetiological ulcers, as well as pyoderma gangrenosum and dermatitis artefacta. The other conditions mentioned in Table 20.1 are rare and should be considered when an ulcer cannot be categorised into one or more of the commoner causes, when the ulcer fails to respond to treatment, or in case of additional clinical signs or laboratory abnormalities.

Before considering what dressings to use in the management of leg ulceration, the cause(s) and any important cofactors that are thought to be delaying healing must first be elicited and addressed. This requires a full assessment of the patient including history, examination and investigation as appropriate.

History and examination

As leg ulcers often have multiple causes, a full history (Table 20.2) and examination are essential. If pyoderma gangrenosum is suspected, care should be taken to elicit the exact

Table 20.1 Aetiological factors and cofactors in leg ulceration

Causes of leg ulceration	Cofactors in leg ulceration
Venous insufficiency and dependency (70%)	Anaemia
Arterial occlusion (10%)	Old age
Diabetic (10%)	Infection
Other (10%)	Malnutrition
Pressure (decubitus)	Immunosuppressants and chemotherapeutic agents
Pyoderma gangrenosum	Drugs, e.g. non-steroidal anti-inflammatory drugs
Vasculitic ulceration	Psychosocial stress
Malignancy	
Sickle cell disease	
Hydroxyurea induced	
Hypertensive ulcer	
Dermatitis artefacta	
Infection	
Microcirculatory disorders	
Neuropathic diseases	
Clotting disorders	
Metabolic diseases	

way in which the ulcer started, as a history of pathergy or pustule formation can be extremely helpful diagnostically. Associated conditions such as rheumatoid arthritis or inflammatory bowel disease may also provide useful clues.

Table 20.2 History taking in leg ulceration

General

Occupation, e.g. standing all day

Date when ulcer started

How ulcer started

History of previous leg ulcers

Ulcer pain

Type and severity of pain

Impact of leg ulcers on life

Indicators of venous disease

Varicose veins

Surgery for varicose veins

Deep venous thrombosis

Fracture in affected limb

Joint surgery

Major surgery

Number of pregnancies

Indicators of arterial disease

Hypertension

Cerebrovascular accident, transient ischaemic attack

Ischaemic heart disease, myocardial infarction

Intermittent claudication

Rest pain

Diabetes mellitus

Smoking history

Other

Rheumatoid arthritis

Obesity

Anaemia

Mobility, e.g. unrestricted, walks in garden, walks around house, immobile

Medication

History and examination must include vascular assessment, as arteriosclerosis is common in older people and may be a cofactor if not a direct aetiological factor. It is helpful to measure the length and width of ulcers to allow progress to be monitored objectively. This is done by measuring the longest ulcer length and the longest perpendicular width (Figure 20.1).

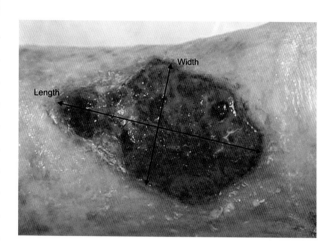

Figure 20.1 Ulcer healing can be monitored by measuring length and width as shown. © Betsi Cadwaladr University Health Board.

Handheld Doppler examination

In combination with a complete clinical assessment, Doppler ultrasound is used to confirm the presence or absence of arterial disease (Figure 20.2 and Table 20.3). A crystal in the Doppler probe transmits sound waves, which are reflected back by moving red blood cells. These are received by a second crystal and transmitted into audible sounds.

An ankle brachial pressure index (ABPI) of 0.9–1.0 is considered normal. In general, indices below 0.8 signify some arterial disease. More severe clinical symptoms such as rest pain are usually found with ABPI < 0.5, while readings between 0.5 and 0.8 may be associated with intermittent claudication. ABPI > 1.0 should be interpreted with caution as this may suggest calcification of vessels (see below). Further investigation may be required in these patients to assess the degree of arterial disease.

Pitfalls with handheld Doppler examination

There are certain clinical scenarios in which Doppler readings can be misleading, potentially resulting in inappropriate management with disastrous clinical outcomes (Table 20.4). Doppler results must therefore always be interpreted together with the clinical assessment and should be used to confirm clinical findings. A reading that is discordant with clinical findings should be considered aberrant until otherwise proven.

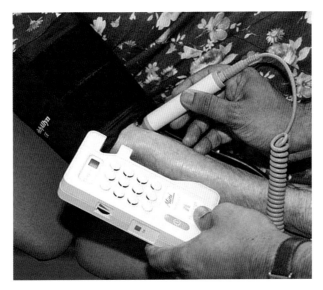

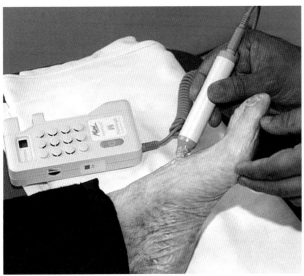
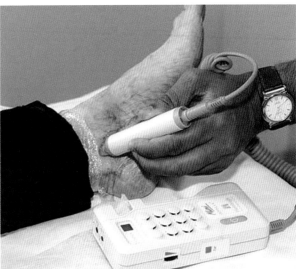

Figure 20.2 Handheld Doppler ultrasound examination. © Betsi Cadwaladr University Health Board.

Doppler waveforms

With more sophisticated machines, but using the same technique, a graphic waveform may also be produced that can be used as an adjunct to overall vascular assessment (Figure 20.3). This is particularly helpful for those patients in whom ABPI is artificially elevated due to the calcification of the vessels. A normal waveform is triphasic. If mild arterial disease exists proximal to the probe, waveforms become biphasic, with monophasic waveforms in the presence of more severe disease.

Pulse oximetry with blood pressure cuff

Pulse oximetry together with a blood pressure cuff can be used as an alternative to Doppler examination, and is a simple and easily maintained skill. Importantly, it is more reliable than Doppler in patients with significant oedema. The pulse oximetry sensor is applied to a digit and a blood pressure cuff is applied as for a normal Doppler. The cuff is inflated and deflated and the pressure at which the pulse oximetry signal is lost is recorded.

Table 20.3 Procedure for recording Doppler ankle brachial pressure index (ABPI)

1. Lie patient supine for 10–20 minutes (to negate effects of exercise on blood pressure) and explain procedure

2. Apply protection over any ulcers, e.g. with cling film

3. Apply correct size of cuff around upper arm

4. Locate brachial pulse and apply ultrasound gel

5. Angle the Doppler probe at 45–60 degrees and locate pulse

6. Inflate cuff until audible sound disappears

7. Release cuff slowly and record pressure at which signal reappears

8. Repeat the procedure on the other arm. Use the higher of the two brachial pressure measurements to calculate ABPI

9. Apply appropriate size of cuff to ankle immediately above the malleolus

10. Locate dorsalis pedis by palpation and apply ultrasound gel and probe as before

11. Inflate and deflate cuff as previously and record when signal reappears

12. Locate posterior tibial pulse and repeat procedure. Take the higher of the two readings to calculate ABPI

13. Perform the same procedure on the other leg

14. To calculate the ABPI, divide the highest ankle pressure (either the left or right ankle) by the highest brachial pressure obtained:

$$\frac{\text{Higher ankle pressure}}{\text{Higher brachial pressure}} = \text{ABPI}$$

The toe/finger oximetry index is similar to the Doppler ABPI, such that it is safe to apply high-compression therapy with a toe/finger index of > 0.8. If there is any doubt, compression bandaging can be applied and the signal checked with the leg horizontal and then elevated. Loss of signal or a significant drop in SpO_2 (oxyhaemoglobin saturation) indicates that further assessment is necessary before proceeding with compression.

Duplex ultrasonography

In some patients, further investigations may be helpful to understand the degree of arterial disease. Duplex ultrasonography can provide non-invasive, accurate information regarding the site and nature of vascular lesions. Its sensitivity is greatest above the knee, where it has comparable diagnostic capabilities to angiography in the assessment of arterial occlusive disease in patients with symptoms of peripheral vascular disease.

Table 20.4 Advantages and disadvantages of handheld Doppler

Advantages

Non-invasive

Easily performed

Outpatient procedure

Disadvantages

In approximately 10% of the older population and in patients with diabetes, calcification of the medial layer of the distal arteries occurs, rendering the arteries incompressible and so yielding a falsely elevated ankle brachial pressure index (ABPI)

Gross oedema can confound ABPI results

Inter-observer variability demonstrated in some studies

Lack of reproducibility demonstrated in some studies

Venous leg ulcers

Typically, patients with venous leg ulcers have a history of either deep venous thrombosis or varicose veins, or predisposing factors for these, such as multiple pregnancies, major abdominal operations or fractured limbs.

Venous leg ulceration can occur anywhere below the knee, although it is much more common over the malleolar area. Most venous leg ulcers occur over the medial malleolus, where there is a high proportion of perforator veins, which transmit the high pressure to the superficial venous system.

Clinical signs of venous hypertension seen below the knee (Figure 20.4) are:

- Peripheral oedema
- Varicose veins
- Venous flare
- Hyperpigmentation
- Atrophie blanche
- Leg ulceration
- Venous eczema
- Lipodermatosclerosis

Management involves demonstration of venous incompetence, either clinically or by investigations such as venous duplex scan. Once venous incompetence has been established, graduated compression of the affected leg is the treatment of choice, provided that clinical and Doppler examination has excluded significant arterial disease.

Compression therapy

Below-knee, graduated, high compression in the form of bandages or hosiery is the main treatment in the management of uncomplicated venous leg ulcers. Treatment reduces pain and

(a)

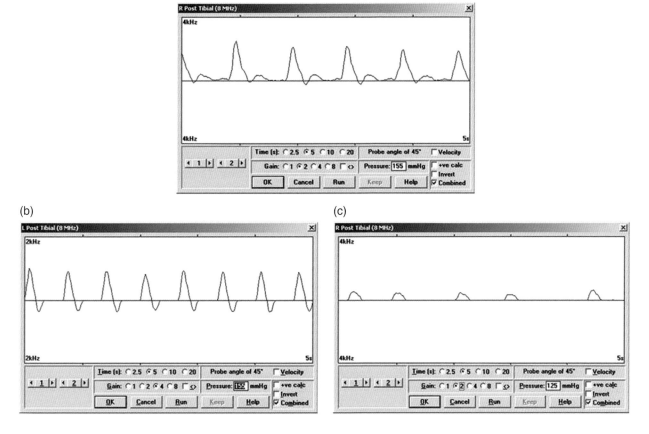

(b)　　　　　　　　　　　　　　　　　　　(c)

Figure 20.3 Doppler waveforms. (a) Triphasic waveforms. (b) Biphasic waveforms. (c) Monophasic waveforms. © Betsi Cadwaladr University Health Board.

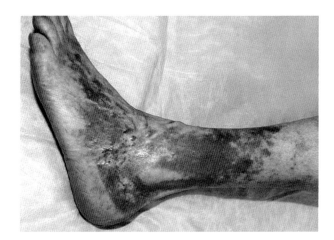

Figure 20.4 Varicosities and hyperpigmentation in a patient with venous hypertension. © Betsi Cadwaladr University Health Board.

oedema, and enhances quality of life through improved healing rates. High, multilayer compression has been shown to be more effective than low or single-layer compression. Inappropriate application of compression in the presence of arterial disease can result in reduction in blood flow, which can potentially lead to gangrene.

Prior to application of compression, a full vascular examination should be performed. This should include an arterial Doppler examination; however, this should not be taken in isolation. The Doppler result should be used to confirm the findings from your clinical examination.

When is it safe to apply compression?

There is currently no evidence to indicate at what level high compression may be safely applied to a limb; however, current opinion states that high compression should not be applied to a limb with an ABPI < 0.8. Modified or low compression, with close monitoring, may be used by experienced clinicians in patients with ABPI 0.6–0.8.

How can graduated compression be applied?

According to Laplace's law, the sub-bandage pressure applied is directly related to both tension in the bandage and limb circumference. Therefore, in a normal-shaped limb, a bandage applied with constant tension and overlap will achieve graduated compression with the greater compression being at the ankle. Recommended high compression is 40 mmHg at the ankle, reducing to 15–20 mmHg at the calf.

Laplace's law:

$$\text{Sub-bandage pressure} = \frac{\text{tension} \times \text{number of layers} \times \text{constant}}{\text{circumference of limb} \times \text{bandage width}}$$

Which bandage should I use?

There are many different bandage systems available, each with different properties (Figure 20.5). No studies have shown superiority of one specific bandage system over another. In general, high compression is better than low compression for the treatment of venous leg ulcers. Patient concerns such as bandage bulkiness, comfort and lifestyle should therefore be considered to aid concordance when applying compression bandaging.

Elastic bandages (e.g. Setopress®):

- Also known as long-stretch or highly extensible bandage.
- Produce sustained compression with high pressure at rest. When the calf muscles expand during walking, the bandage expands, producing slightly less but still high pressure.
- Able to accommodate changes in limb circumference when oedema reduced, i.e. bandages still effective when oedema has reduced.

Inelastic bandages (e.g. Comprilan®):

- Also known as short-stretch bandage.
- Provide a relatively rigid system that produces high compression during walking (when calf muscle contracts against the fixed bandage) but low resting pressures.
- Unable to conform to accommodate any reduction in oedema. This may result in bandages falling down if not changed frequently following initial application.

Multilayer bandaging (e.g. PROFORE™):

- Three or four layers, including padding and crêpe and a variety of inelastic or elastic and cohesive bandages.
- Can be bulky, leading to difficulty with footwear.
- Various bandaging combinations are available that have the advantages of both compression systems.

Arterial leg ulceration

Arterial ulceration usually presents as painful, punched-out ulcers on the dorsum of the foot, or as distal gangrene affecting the toes. However, a number of patients present with ulcers on the lower leg, often precipitated by trauma, which have a predominant arterial element. Again, these are usually painful and patients typically have a history of intermittent claudication with or without rest pain. Peripheral pulses are diminished or absent and the limb is often cold and dusky, with delayed capillary refill time. Exposed tendon may be visible in the base of the ulcer. These patients need a vascular surgical opinion to assess the extent of disease and operability. Dressings should aim to keep any exposed tendon moist to retain viability while not causing undue maceration. Excessive moisture within wounds that have

Figure 20.5 A selection of currently available compression bandages. © Betsi Cadwaladr University Health Board.

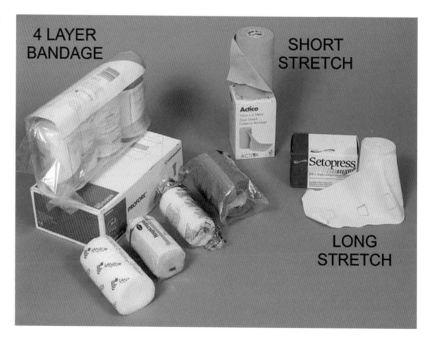

severely compromised arterial supply increases the risk of wet gangrene and ensuing amputation.

After correction of the underlying arterial problem, a full assessment is again required to assess suitability for compression if any venous incompetence is present (Table 20.5). Provided that adequate blood flow has been restored, graduated compression therapy can be used to expedite healing.

In those patients who are deemed unsuitable for surgical intervention or those in whom surgery has not been successful, management should be directed at pain relief, correction of other aetiological factors and cofactors, and prevention and prompt treatment of infection.

If the arterial insufficiency is such that healing is not expected, the aim of management should be to keep the wound dry and free of infection and thus avoid wet gangrene. Simple dressings such as Betadine® spray or iodine gauze are ideal for these wounds. Surgical debridement is contraindicated as this can lead to a larger area of ulceration that has no chance of healing.

Pressure ulcers

Pressure ulcers or bed sores are caused by sustained pressure that interrupts blood flow, resulting in local tissue necrosis. They usually occur over a bony prominence and can be exacerbated with concomitant shear forces. The incidence of pressure ulcers is recognised as a key indicator of the quality of patient care, and they remain a significant healthcare problem, with over 1300 new ulcers reported each month. Treatment of pressure ulcers costs the National Health Service more than £1.4 million every day.

As a result of these significant resource implications, a five-step approach to preventing and treating pressure ulcers has been developed as a reminder to all with responsibilities for caring for people at risk of pressure ulcer development (Table 20.6).

Diabetic foot ulceration

Although diabetic foot ulcers (DFUs; Figure 20.6) do not usually present to dermatologists, it is important to understand this condition so that problems can be prevented or treated at an early stage. DFUs are essentially pressure ulcers, which occur in patients who have lost protective sensation. They typically occur on either the plantar aspect of the foot or the dorsum of the toes and are usually caused by trauma or repeated friction. Because of their sensory neuropathy, the patient seldom notices this trauma and may not be aware of an ulcer developing until blood is seen on the carpet. Peripheral vascular disease can play an important role in causing DFUs, and patients presenting with ulcers at this site should be fully assessed from both the vascular and sensory points of view. Vibration is the first sense to be reduced in diabetic peripheral neuropathy.

Diabetic foot ulceration is often accompanied by infection. Early assessment by a healthcare professional with experience in management of DFUs is of paramount importance and prevention is key (Table 20.7). Basic management involves exclusion of foreign bodies and infection, including osteomyelitis, by clinical examination and X-ray. Pressure relief and treatment of any infection or vascular problems are essential.

Wound healing and management

At all times during the healing process, the patient should be involved in shared decision making to ensure maximum concordance and to enhance psychological wellbeing. Patient concerns such as pain and bulkiness of bandaging should be taken into consideration.

After identifying and addressing all aetiological issues and cofactors, the focus should be turned to wound bed preparation in order to facilitate wound healing. Wound bed preparation addresses the local factors thought to be most important in healing, namely debridement, bacterial balance and moisture control.

Debridement

When the term was first applied to surgery in the 1700s, debridement referred to the surgical removal of debris from open wounds. Since then, the meaning has been broadened to include other methods by which the wound is cleared of devitalised tissue that may harbour bacteria and impair wound healing (Figure 20.7). Debridement is an essential step in wound management. The selection of the most appropriate debridement technique for an individual wound varies during the lifetime of a wound and depends on the following (Table 20.8):

- Degree of necrosis.
- Patient preference.
- Size of wound and amount of exudate production.
- Aetiology of wound, e.g. avoid sharp debridement in pyoderma gangrenosum.
- Practitioner time constraints.
- Resources, e.g. availability of competent practitioners and equipment, access to theatre.
- Cost-effectiveness.
- Primary or secondary care setting.

Bacterial balance

Chronic infection delays wound healing and reduces tissue tensile strength. As there is no gold-standard test to identify wound infection, clinicians are dependent on their clinical skills taken together with information from wound swabs. Wound swab results only provide information about bacteria present on the wound surface. These bacteria are not necessarily responsible for delayed wound healing or infection.

Table 20.5 Assessment of leg ulceration

Type of leg ulcer	History	Examination	Investigation	Treatment
Venous	Varicose veins ± DVT. Pain and ankle swelling, worse at end of day, which is relieved with limb elevation	Ulcers typically below the knee. Peripheral oedema and signs of venous hypertension present	ABPI > 0.8	High-compression therapy. Consider venous surgery
Arterial	Ask about intermittent claudication, rest pain, smoking, diabetes, past history of CVA or IHD	Punched-out ulcers, typically on dorsum of foot, or distal gangrene. Peripheral pulses absent	ABPI < 0.5. Confirm presence of venous insufficiency	Vascular surgery assessment. Pain control
Mixed arteriovenous	Mixed symptoms as above	Ulcer may be circumferential	ABPI 0.5–0.8	Complete vascular assessment. Consider modified compression
Lymphoedematous	Legs chronically swollen. Usually bilateral	Non-pitting oedema with hyperkeratosis	ABPI > 0.8 (note: use wide cuff)	Foot hygiene to prevent cellulitis. High compression
Vasculitic	Painful, often rapidly enlarging ulceration. May be associated with rash or other vasculitis signs	Palpable purpuric lesions develop into necrotic purplish bullae that ulcerate. Look for rash elsewhere	Biopsy	Treat underlying cause
Pyoderma gangrenosum	Painful, rapidly expanding ulcer. May be at atypical site. May have underlying condition	Ragged undermined violaceous edge arising from pustule or nodule in some cases	Biopsy to exclude other causes such as infection. Investigate for underlying condition	High-dose steroids ± immunosuppressants often required
Infectious	History of trauma	Nodules or pustules may precede ulceration. Look for lymphadenopathy	Swab and/or tissue biopsy for culture	As indicated by investigation
Malignancy	Long-standing ulcer. Never decreasing in size	Can be unremarkable. May have rolled edges, e.g. basal cell carcinoma	Low threshold for biopsy from edge of ulcer, may require multiple biopsies	Surgical removal usually indicated

ABPI, ankle brachial pressure index; CVA, cerebrovascular accident; DVT, deep vein thrombosis; IHD, ischaemic heart disease.

Table 20.6 SSKIN is a five-step approach to preventing and treating pressure ulcers

Surface: make sure your patients have the right support

Skin inspection: early inspection means early detection

Keep your patients moving

Incontinence/moisture: your patients need to be clean and dry

Nutrition/hydration: help patients have the right diet and fluid intake

Table 20.7 Prevention of diabetic foot ulceration in patients with diabetes and loss of protective sensation

Advice	Reason
Attend for regular chiropody or podiatry	Toenails should be kept short to avoid trauma to surrounding skin
	Callus should be pared
	Appropriate footwear can be issued
	Early ulceration can be detected
Wear appropriate shoes	Ill-fitting shoes will cause pressure, callus and ulceration. The diabetic foot changes shape due to diabetic motor neuropathy
Regularly apply emollient to feet	Autonomic neuropathy causes dryness of the soles of the feet. This can cause cracks, which act as portals for infection
Look at soles of feet daily	Due to loss of protective sensation, patients will not be able to feel foreign bodies, blisters or ulcers
Check shoes daily for foreign objects	Checking footwear regularly prevents stones etc. from rubbing and causing problems

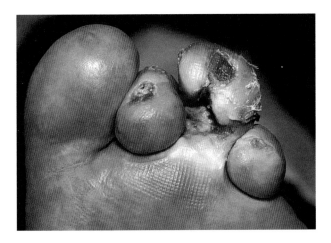

Figure 20.6 Diabetic foot ulceration. © Betsi Cadwaladr University Health Board.

Microbiologists advocate that the most accurate way to assess wound bacterial burden is to perform a quantitative biopsy. This involves removing a quantity of tissue, usually with a punch biopsy, and measuring the quantity of bacteria found per gram of tissue. However, this procedure is time consuming and invasive. In contrast, wound swabs are quick and easy to perform and can provide useful information in some cases. Note that this information should be used to support the clinical impression and not vice versa.

Although all chronic wounds have bacteria present within them, these bacteria are not always harmful. The state of these bacteria and their influence on the host are the most important considerations:

- **Contamination** refers to bacterial flora that has relocated to the wound from either the host or environment and that is not replicating. All wounds are contaminated.
- **Colonisation** occurs when these bacteria are replicating but causing no host injury. It has been suggested that a certain amount of bacteria in the wound may be beneficial to healing.

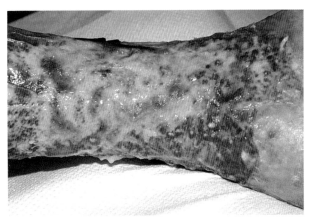

Figure 20.7 Debridement is an essential step in wound management. © Betsi Cadwaladr University Health Board.

- **Critical colonisation** is a term used to describe the pivotal stage that occurs when bacterial load results in arrest of healing without overt infection. Clinically there is delayed wound healing, with only very subtle clinical symptoms and signs. Signs of critical colonisation include increasing odour, pain and exudate, beefy red and friable granulation tissue and delayed healing.

Table 20.8 Methods of debridement

	Method	Advantages	Disadvantages
Sharp surgical debridement	Dead and devitalised tissue cut away by competent practitioner	Most effective method	Requires skilled competent practitioner and availability
			Analgesia often required
			Contraindicated in pyoderma gangrenosum
Autolytic debridement	This method uses the body's own enzymes to break down necrotic tissue. Devitalised tissue is softened and liquefied through the use of hydrating occlusive or semi-occlusive wound dressings, e.g. hydrogels, hydrocolloids, hydrofibre	Relatively inexpensive	Slow acting
		Easy to apply	Requires regular nursing input
		Painless	Requires frequent monitoring for bacterial infection
		Selective for necrotic tissue only	
		Available in primary and secondary care	
Larval therapy	Using potent proteolytic enzymes, the larvae liquefy and digest necrotic slough and bacteria	Fast acting	Unappealing to some patients
		Cost-effective	Training required in application
		Available in primary and secondary care	Contraindicated if wound is communicating with internal organs
Enzymatic debridement	Combination of proteolytic enzymes that break down fibrin and fibrinogen	Fast acting	Limited preparations available
		Selective for necrotic tissue only	Expensive
		Best used on large wounds	Preparation requires reconstitution
			Contraindicated in wounds with exposed structures
Mechanical debridement	Dead and devitalised tissue is removed by mechanical means such as high-pressure jets	Rarely used in chronic leg ulcer management	Can be non-selective, i.e. can remove viable tissue as well as necrotic tissue
			Requires equipment and trained practitioners

- **Wound infection** is defined as the presence of multiplying bacteria within a wound, which cause host injury. In most cases, this host injury is seen as an inflammatory soft tissue response with or without systemic inflammatory symptoms and signs.
- **Biofilms** are multicellular, dynamic communities of microorganisms held together by self-produced extracellular matrix. They exist as mixed strains of bacteria, fungi, yeasts, algae or other cellular debris, which adhere to the wound surface and inhibit fibroblast development, inflammatory response and the efficacy of antimicrobial therapy.

The use of antibiotics in patients who have contaminated or colonised wounds is not beneficial in promoting wound healing. Additionally, inappropriate antibiotic use contributes to antibiotic resistance. Biofilms are notoriously resistant to antibiotics due to the physiological attributes of their structure, including slower growth rate of organisms and reduced metabolic activity of cells.

When should I take a swab from a leg ulcer?

- When a wound appears infected, with surrounding tenderness, warmth, redness or pus. In this case, antibiotics can be started empirically and altered if necessary when the wound swab results are available.
- When critical colonisation of the wound is suspected clinically.
- When a wound is failing to heal despite correction of all other factors.

Should I use topical antibacterial agents or systemic antibiotics?

Systemic antibiotics are indicated for wound infection. The choice of antibiotic should be informed by the site, chronicity and nature of the wound, as well as by previous and current wound swab results. If current wound swab results are not available at the time of prescribing, antibiotics can be prescribed empirically based on the clinical nature of the wound and previous culture results. When culture results are available, the antibiotics can be changed if there is inadequate response to those already prescribed. In general, systemic antibiotic penetrance into wounds is not optimal. Courses of 10–14 days are usually required for wound infection.

Numerous topical antibacterial agents are now available in a plethora of wound dressings (Figure 20.8). These should be considered for use in wounds where critical colonisation is suspected or in chronic wounds that are failing to heal despite correction of all causes and cofactors. Antibacterial agents should be used for a maximum of 2–4 weeks. Preparations with neomycin and other potential sensitisers should be avoided if possible, particularly in venous leg ulceration.

Iodine is widely available as an antibacterial agent. The term 'iodine' is used generically, but there are two distinct preparations: povidone and cadexomer iodine. They are both composed of elemental iodine, but in cadexomer iodine, the iodine is released only on exposure to wound exudate and there is better evidence to support its clinical use as an antiseptic agent. Although iodine has been shown to be cytotoxic *in vitro*, numerous *in vivo* studies have shown acceleration of wound healing with its use.

Silver compounds have been used as bactericidal agents for over a century and act by interfering with bacterial electron transport. Sulfadiazine is silver with sulfonamide in an oil-and-water cream with slow release of the silver ions. 'Medical-grade' honey, which is filtered, gamma irradiated and produced under controlled hygiene standards, is also a broad-spectrum antibacterial agent. Bacterial resistance is much less likely to develop with iodine, silver or honey, compared to topical antibiotics.

Prontosan® is a wound cleansing solution that is purified water combined with the antimicrobial agent polyhexamethylene biguanide and the surfactant betaine. It is effective in cleansing and decontaminating wounds at risk of infection, by reducing bacterial burden and disrupting biofilms.

Moisture control

Why does the wound have to be moist?

The theory supporting moist wound healing is based on work in the 1960s by George Winter, a zoologist, who demonstrated faster wound healing in moist wounds compared to those left exposed to the air. But excess moisture around the wound can cause maceration, irritant dermatitis and skin necrosis, all of which delay wound healing.

How do I control wound exudate?

Refractory lower-limb oedema and critically colonised or infected wounds are the main reasons for excessive wound exudate. Addressing these factors will help to control the exudate. The use of more absorbent dressings and/or increased frequency of dressing changes can also be helpful.

Dressings

Wound dressings must be used in conjunction with treatment of the underlying ulcer cause. Failure to do this will almost inevitably result in failure to heal. Unfortunately, there is no 'one fits all' wound dressing, and many different dressings are available with the aim of providing optimum wound bed preparation. The challenge is to select the most appropriate of these treatments for a particular setting. Such treatment is highly patient dependent,

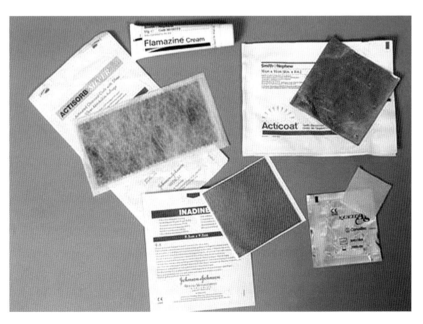

Figure 20.8 A selection of currently available topical antibacterial agents. © Betsi Cadwaladr University Health Board.

with decisions often being influenced not only by local wound factors, but also by systemic host factors.

Knowledge of the action and properties of different classes of modern wound products is paramount. Wound healing is a dynamic process and the selection process must take into account the stage of wound healing. Dressings should ideally be both clinically effective and cost-effective, and factors such as frequency of dressing changes, nursing time, patient comfort and patient concordance need to be considered at the same time as the ability of the dressing to maintain an optimum wound healing environment.

Classification of dressings

Most commonly used dressings are based on five main dressing classes (films, hydrogels, hydrocolloids, alginates and foams) (Figure 20.9). In a bid to create the optimum dressing, manufacturers create mixtures of these dressing types. Knowledge of the basic classification provides a foundation on which to build your understanding.

Films, e.g. Tegaderm™ (least absorbent):

- Rarely used in leg ulcer management.
- Provide an occlusive dressing with no absorptive capacity.
- Useful for superficial skin tears.

Hydrogels, e.g. Intrasite Gel®:

- Amorphous gel that donates fluid to wound. It hydrates slough, allowing easier removal.
- Used with dry necrotic or sloughy wounds.
- Available in gel or sheet form. Sheet form useful for soothing the symptoms of superficial blistering disease.
- Requires secondary dressing.

Hydrocolloids, e.g. DuoDERM®:

- Semipermeable film coated with sodium carboxymethylcellulose and outer plastic film impervious to liquids and bacteria.
- Interacts with wound fluid to form a gel that hydrates the wound.
- Used with superficial leg ulcers, pressure ulcers and dry necrotic areas.
- Easy to apply and no secondary dressing required.
- Useful as an occlusive dressing when dermatitis artefacta is suspected.

Alginates, e.g. Sorbsan®:

- Manufactured from a variety of alginate-rich seaweeds.
- Highly absorbent dressing. Some alginates have haemostatic properties.
- Hydrophilic gel is formed when alginate contacts wound exudate.
- Used in highly exudating wounds and ulcers.
- Wounds should be cleaned with normal saline to remove all traces of dressing fibres.
- Some require secondary dressing.

Foams, e.g. ALLEVYN® (most absorbent):

- Polyurethane foam covered by semipermeable film.
- Highly absorbent.
- Used in moderately or highly exudating wounds and cavities.
- May be adhesive or non-adhesive.
- Require no secondary dressings.

Charcoal dressings, e.g. CliniSorb®:

- Charcoal fibres manufactured to become microporous cloth sheets.
- Used to control odour in malodorous wounds.

Figure 20.9 A selection of currently available dressings. © Betsi Cadwaladr University Health Board.

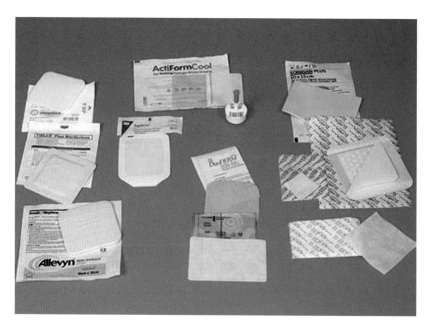

- Odour levels are reduced by activated charcoal and, in some cases, charcoal absorbs bacteria and wound toxins.
- Some dressings require primary dressing.

Non-adherent dressings for fragile skin, e.g. Mepitel®:

- Soft silicone dressing with skin-friendly adhesive.
- Available as a wound contact layer or with polyurethane foam backing.
- Used for non-exudating to moderately exudating wounds.
- Has the ability to conform to awkward areas.
- Useful for fragile areas of skin in blistering disorders such as pemphigus, pemphigoid and epidermolysis bullosa.

Negative-pressure wound therapy

Negative-pressure wound therapy (NPWT) is a method of suctioning fluid and debris from a wound to facilitate healing. A vacuum pump is connected via tubing to a closed seal dressing applied to the wound. Devices can be either fixed or portable. Initially used only in the acute setting, they are now more commonly utilised in primary care, though specialised nursing training is required for dressing changes. Some devices direct irrigation fluids or prescribed fluids, such as antimicrobial compounds, straight onto the wound bed. NPWT promotes increased microvascularity in the wound bed to stimulate granulation tissue and reduces exudate and bacterial load, as well as reducing dead space or fistulas within the wound.

The benefits of NPWT are that it can:

- Increase microvascularity of the wound bed with stimulation of granulation tissue.
- Increase wound-healing cytokines and chemokines as a result of improved vascularity.
- Reduce 'dead' spaces and fistulas within the wound.
- Reduce exudate and bacterial load within the wound.

Why is the wound failing to heal?

When wounds fail to heal, the clinician must question whether the diagnosis and treatment are correct. Skin cancer developing in the edge of a wound does not always have characteristic signs. A high index of suspicion and a low threshold for biopsying wounds should be adopted if wounds fail to heal in the expected timeframe. Wounds should be measured at each review to monitor progress. Correct management should address the underlying cause of the ulcer as well as cofactors that may hinder healing. If the wound fails to heal despite correct diagnosis and treatment, poor patient concordance must be considered.

Blistering diseases

Management of superficial ulceration secondary to blistering diseases follows the standard principles of wound healing management. Where possible, the underlying aetiology should be identified and addressed. To facilitate healing, blistered areas should be kept clean and pain relief should be addressed.

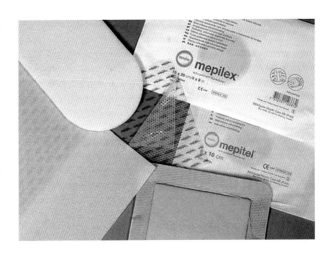

Figure 20.10 Wound dressings used for fragile skin. © Betsi Cadwaladr University Health Board.

Slitting of blisters and allowing release of fluid can help relieve discomfort and will also allow identification of new blistered areas to monitor ongoing disease activity. Where possible, blisters should not be deroofed, as the necrotic skin overlying the denuded area acts as a protective layer that impedes bacterial invasion. Low-adherent silicone dressings, such as Mepitel® and Mepilex®, are recommended for painful, raw areas (Figure 20.10). For pain relief on larger sensitive areas, hydrogel sheets can be useful. Blisters on the legs of elderly patients may heal more quickly if pedal oedema is reduced. In more severe cases, the use of pressure-relieving mattresses will help to reduce friction and shear.

Conclusions and the future

With the ageing population and likely increase in chronic wounds, particularly leg ulcers, it is important that all dermatologists are skilled in their assessment and management. Fundamental to this is an understanding of the basic principles and stages of normal wound healing, and treatments that will facilitate or promote this. It is particularly important to make evidence-based clinical decisions on the use of antibiotics to prevent unnecessary treatment and the risk for increasing drug resistance and allergy. Furthermore, be mindful of possible contact allergy in patients who use numerous products over long periods. It is likely your expertise within the multidisciplinary team will be required for hard-to-heal or recalcitrant wounds, to exclude skin cancer or other underlying diagnosis, such as pyoderma gangrenosum, vasculitis or dermatitis artefacta.

Underlying pathophysiological processes in abnormal wound healing are still largely unknown. Wound healing is a complex, orchestrated system dependent on a number of cell types and mediators, and a sophisticated temporal sequence. It is clear that macrophage activity is a key player in the transition from inflammation to proliferation, and blood-clot-derived cytokines and growth factors are crucial for neovascularisation. Further understanding will promote new treatment options, for example autologous platelet-rich plasma. Another topic of interest is tissue engineering in skin wound repair, which seeks to recreate an environment that promotes cell survival and proliferation, and differentiation of clinically viable tissue, including matrix scaffolding to promote cell adhesion and migration. Study of the pathophysiology of exaggerated wound healing such as keloid formation, where transforming growth factors are implicated, is critical in the identification of novel therapeutic options for treatment of this common fibroproliferative disorder.

Nurses, general practitioners, physicians and surgeons alike must all have skills in wound management; a multidisciplinary team approach is optimal. As dermatologists we have much to offer and must play our role in both patient care and academic progress within the field.

Pearls and pitfalls

- Normal wound healing is a complex process dependent on interplay between a multitude of cell types and mediators.
- Leg ulcers, particularly venous, and pressure ulcers contribute to a major healthcare burden requiring a multidisciplinary team approach.
- Compression bandages in arterial disease can lead to vascular occlusion and gangrene, therefore full assessment prior to treatment is required.
- Avoid prolonged use of topical antibiotic or antiseptic treatments to prevent contact allergy.
- Maintain a high index of suspicion for cutaneous malignancy in slow-to-heal wounds; other differential diagnoses include pyoderma gangrenosum and dermatitis artefacta.

SCE Questions. See question 45.

FURTHER READING AND KEY RESOURCES

Atkin L, Bućko Z, Conde Montero E *et al*. Implementing TIMERS: the race against hard-to-heal wounds. *J Wound Care* 2019; **28** (3 Suppl. 3):S1–S49.

Franks P, Barker J, Collier M *et al*. Management of patients with venous leg ulcers: challenges and current best practice. *J Wound Care* 2016; **25** (Suppl. 6):S1–67.

Guest JF, Ayoub N, McIlwraith T *et al*. Health economic burden that different wound types impose on the UK's National Health Service. *Int Wound J* 2017; **14**:322–30.

Luker K, Cullum N, Duff L. The development of a national guideline on the management of leg ulcers. *J Clin Nurs* 2000; **9**:208–17.

Malone M, Bjarnsholt T, McBain AJ *et al*. The prevalence of biofilms in chronic wounds: a systematic review and meta-analysis of published data. *J Wound Care* 2017; **26**:20–5.

Mekkes JR, Loots MAM, van der Wal AC *et al*. Causes, investigation and treatment of leg ulceration. *Br J Dermatol* 2003; **148**:388–401.

Nelson EA, Adderley U. Venous leg ulcers. *BMJ Clin Evid* 2016; **2016**:1902.

Singer AJ, Tassiopouls A, Kirsner RS. Evaluation and management of lower-extremity ulcers. *N Engl J Med* 2017; **377**:1559–67.

Smith JJ, Guest MG, Greenhalgh RM, Davies AH. Measuring the quality of life in patients with venous ulcers. *J Vasc Surg* 2000; **31**:642–9.

Sorg H, Tilkorn DJ, Hager S *et al*. Skin wound healing: an update on the current knowledge and concepts. *Eur Surg Res* 2017; **58**:81–94.

Textbooks

Cowan T, ed. *Wound Care Handbook 2020–2021*. Salisbury: Mark Allen Group, 2020.

Flanagan M, ed. *Wound Healing and Skin Integrity: Principles and Practice*. Chichester: Wiley-Blackwell, 2013.

Useful websites

Diabetes UK. Diabetes complications: foot ulcers. Available at: http://www.diabetes.co.uk/diabetes-complications/diabetic-foot-ulcers.html.

Guidelines. Pressure ulcers: prevention and management. Available at: https://www.guidelines.co.uk/NICE/Pressure-ulcers.

National Institute for Health and Care Excellence. Leg ulcer infection: antimicrobial prescribing (NICE guideline NG152). Available at: https://www.nice.org.uk/guidance/ng152.

National Institute for Health and Care Excellence. NICE guidance (UK guidelines on relevant evidence-based and cost-effective practice). Available at: https://www.nice.org.uk/guidance.

National Institute for Health and Care Excellence. Wound management products and elasticated garments. Available at: https://bnf.nice.org.uk/wound-management.

Tissue Viability Society. Available at: www.tvs.org.uk.

World Union of Wound Healing Societies. Available at: https://wuwhs2022.org

Wounds International. Available at: www.woundsinternational.com.

Wounds UK. Available at: www.wounds-uk.com.

Registered trademarks

ALLEVYN®, Smith and Nephew, Hamburg, Germany
Betadine®, Mundipharma, Cambridge, UK
CliniSorb®, CliniMed, High Wycombe, UK
Comprilan®, BSN Medical, Hull, UK
DuoDERM®, ConvaTec, Runcorn, UK
Intrasite Gel®, PROFORE™, Smith & Nephew, Watford, UK
Mepilex®, Mepitel®, Setopress®, Mölnlycke, Milton Keynes, UK
Prontosan®, B. Braun Medical, Sheffield, UK
Sorbsan®, Aspen Medical Europe Ltd, Ashby-de-la-Zouch, UK
Tegaderm™, 3M, Bracknell, UK

21

Cosmetic dermatology

Tamara W. Griffiths

Introduction

Cosmetic dermatology can be a polarising subject, but it is important for all dermatologists to have a basic understanding of some key concepts. Skills and proficiency can be developed further if desired, but the young dermatologist ought to bear in mind this should be 'in addition to' and not 'at the expense of' other aspects of mainstream medical, surgical and paediatric dermatology.

The absence of clear regulation of this diverse and complex sector can lead to poor decision making not only in patients, but also in practitioners. A heightened awareness of ethical standards, core principles and your own personal and professional boundaries is imperative. Engagement in private cosmetic practice during training is strongly discouraged, with medical indemnity being particularly relevant. If you are involved, this must be thoroughly discussed and explored with your educational supervisor, and noted at your annual review.

Listen to your gut instinct as you would with any other area of clinical practice; if something seems wrong or you are unsure, take time out to reflect and discuss with colleagues. Be aware of subconscious bias or conflicted interests, particularly when financial gain is involved. Transparency must continue at appraisals beyond training.

Common dermatological conditions

The General Medical Council (GMC) definition of a cosmetic intervention is any procedure or treatment carried out with the primary objective of changing an aspect of a patient's physical appearance. This in itself creates ambiguity when applied to dermatology. There are several dermatological conditions that may be variants of physiological normal or mild manifestations of skin disease that can fall under the 'cosmetic' label. These include (but are not limited to) vitiligo, melasma, post-inflammatory hyperpigmentation, solar lentigines, seborrheic keratoses, rosacea, acne vulgaris and scarring, milia, benign facial naevi, epidermoid cysts, cherry angiomata, hirsutism and androgenic alopecia.

Although the emotional response by the medical profession to the concept of 'cosmetic' ranges from trivialisation to vilification, a more rational approach may be to view it as a continuum that can be fluid depending on a number of variables such as the site, severity, psychological impact and available resources. In the public sector, dermatologists must follow national guidance on procedures of limited clinical value, but more flexibility exists

Dermatology Training: The Essentials. Edited by Mahbub M.U. Chowdhury, Tamara W. Griffiths and Andrew Y. Finlay.
© 2022 The British Association of Dermatologists. Published 2022 by John Wiley & Sons Ltd.
Companion website: www.wiley.com/go/chowdhury/dermatologytraining

in the private setting tailored to the individual needs of the patient. When executed well, cosmetic procedures can add a challenging, creative and rewarding dimension to dermatological practice.

Furthermore, dermatologists are well placed to lead in the cosmetic arena due to our depth and breadth of knowledge, procedural proficiency and academic approach. In fact, most non-surgical cosmetic procedures commonly used today, such as chemical peels, botulinum toxin injections, autologous fat transplantation, dermal filler injections and many laser- and light-based therapies, were pioneered by dermatologists for the treatment of skin disease. It must be emphasised that the change in indication from disease to 'cosmetic' does not reduce the inherent risk of the procedure itself.

Skin ageing and rejuvenation

In the early 1990s, investigation into skin wrinkles and how to get rid of them was elevated to a scientifically rigorous evidence-based approach, following the serendipitous observation that topical retinoic acid (tretinoin) used to treat acne in adult women also smoothed wrinkles at the corners of their eyes (the 'crow's foot' area). The seminal research output from John Voorhees' department at the University of Michigan resulted in the recognition of retinol as a household name.

The pathophysiology of accelerated skin ageing due to cumulative sun exposure, called photoageing or photodamage (Figure 21.1), is now well understood. Histological changes associated with degradation of dermal collagen and elastin correlate to clinical signs of solar elastosis, coarse wrinkling and skin laxity. Ultraviolet radiation-induced free radical production contributes to cellular damage associated with skin ageing.

Routine full-skin examination of patients can highlight changes to the novice dermatologist. One can typically note smooth, minimally wrinkled skin on sun-protected sites such as the abdomen and buttocks, even in patients who demonstrate dramatic signs of photoageing, such as Bateman's purpura (Figure 21.2) on the forearms, and cutis rhomboidalis nuchae and poikiloderma of Civatte (Figure 21.3). There is evidence that other environmental factors such as smoking and pollution can further accelerate photodamage.

Irregularities in pigmentation are also associated with skin ageing and an undesirable appearance. Brown macules and patches due to melasma, solar lentigines and flat seborrhoeic keratoses can all play a role, and may take precedence over wrinkles, particularly in patients with skin of colour (Figure 21.4). Increased vascularity from spider naevi, telangiectasia and erythematotelangiectatic rosacea are also relevant in some patients.

Cosmeceuticals

The range of topical cosmeceutical products available to address skin ageing can be overwhelming, particularly as claims used in advertising may not correlate to the methodical

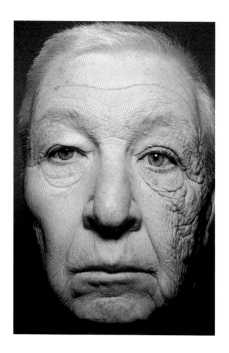

Figure 21.1 A 69-year-old US truck driver with extensive asymmetrical wrinkling and solar elastosis on the left side of his face due to ultraviolet A penetration through window glass while driving. Gordon JRS, Brieva JC. Unilateral dermatoheliosis. *N Engl J Med* 2012; **366**:e25.

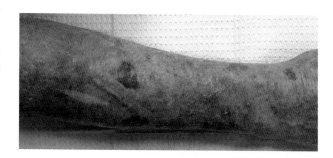

Figure 21.2 Bateman's purpura on the forearm. Chronic sun damage results in dermal atrophy and skin fragility, with easy rupture of superficial blood vessels and tearing. Dyer JM, Miller RA. Chronic skin fragility of aging: current concepts in the pathogenesis, recognition, and management of dermatoporosis. *J Clin Aesthet Dermatol* 2018; **11**:13–18.

evidence-based approach we use in other areas of our dermatological practice. Think critically about the level of evidence used for a particular active ingredient and its cutaneous target or mechanism of action, whether penetration has been demonstrated, and whether *in vivo* human studies have been performed. Understand that products appeal to consumers at both an emotional and a rational level and, when giving advice, try to be factual rather than judgemental.

5-Fluorouracil and photodynamic therapy, used to treat actinic keratoses and Bowen's disease, have been shown to repair

(a)

(b)

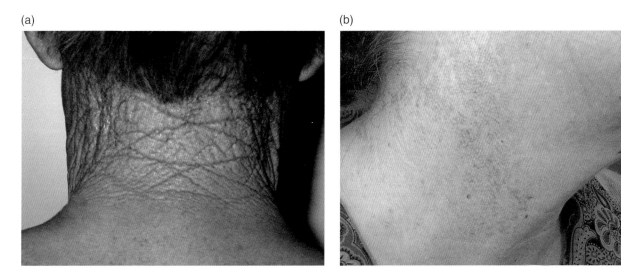

Figure 21.3 Photodamage on the neck. (a) Cutis rhomboidalis nuchae: note yellowish solar elastosis and rhomboid-shaped wrinkles on the sun-exposed site in contrast to the relatively smooth skin on the sun-protected upper back. *Source*: DermNet New Zealand Trust. (b) Poikiloderma of Civatte: note pigmentation changes in sun-exposed sites, but sparing the chronically sun-protected skin under the chin. *Source*: DermNet New Zealand Trust.

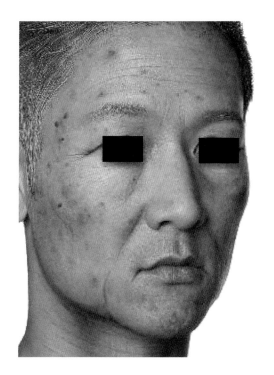

Figure 21.4 Solar lentigines in a Chinese man: pigmentation is more prominent as a sign of photodamage compared to wrinkling. Flament F *et al*. Distinct habits of sun exposures lead to different impacts on some facial signs of Chinese men of different ages. *Clin Cosmet Investig Dermatol* 2019; **12**:833–41.

dermal matrix with subsequent cosmetic rejuvenation. Likewise, systemic medications used as adjunctive therapy in the medical patient with widespread and difficult-to-manage actinic damage (e.g. nicotinamide, low-dose isotretinoin and acitretin) have also been used for cosmetic repair of photoageing.

Skin rejuvenation

There are a number of interventional procedures that can help repair dermal changes associated with photodamage, including light- and laser-based therapies, chemical peels, and physical modalities such as microneedling. The premise supporting these therapies is that damage to dermal collagen by whatever means results in a wound-healing response and subsequent extracellular matrix repair. Therefore, as a rule of thumb, increased damage and post-procedural recovery time are directly correlated to potential improvement, but they also increase the risk of scarring or infection.

A myriad of laser treatments exists to address signs of photoageing, including pigmentation and rhytides, depending on the target chromophore (Chapter 22). Devices can be classified as ablative and non-ablative laser, and also include other light sources such as light-emitting diodes and intense pulsed light. The gold standard for laser rejuvenation remains ablative CO_2 and Er:YAG lasers, though non-ablative lasers have some dermal impact without disruption of the epidermis, therefore reducing the scarring risk and healing time. Fractionated lasers deliver energy in localised vertical columns, creating microscopic treatment zones that alternate with areas of epidermal sparing.

Microneedling uses physical disruption rather than light energy to create wounding, and can be used as a roller device, stamp device or automated pen. It is sometimes used in conjunction with pre-application of platelet-rich plasma derived from the patient's own serum. Evidence for significant impact is lacking for photoageing, though some data support the use of platelet-rich plasma and microneedling in the treatment of androgenic alopecia.

Chemical peeling, also called chemo-resurfacing, is an ancient technique involving the application of chemical agents that are caustic to skin cells, resulting in damage and regeneration. The chemical agents can be classified depending on penetration depth as superficial (reaching epidermis to papillary dermis), medium (affecting papillary to upper reticular dermis) and deep (targeting mid reticular dermis) (Figure 21.5).

Common peeling agents include alpha-hydroxy acid, salicylic acid, trichloroacetic acid, Jessner's solution (resorcinol, lactic acid and salicylic acid) and tretinoin. Deep phenol peels have now largely been replaced by the use of laser and light therapies, as well as other devices such as radiofrequency and ultrasound therapies. The choice of peeling agent(s), duration of application, number of treatments and interval between these can be tailored to the patient and relevant problem, which includes photodamage, epidermal lesions, rhytides, scars and dyschromias. As with other skin rejuvenation modalities, the greater the potential repair, the greater the risks such as scarring, infection and dyschromias.

Facial aesthetics and non-surgical interventions

Facial ageing is a complex process where overall appearance is impacted by interactions at multiple anatomical levels. As dermatologists we focus on the skin, but understanding age-related changes at the level of the subcutaneous fat, muscle and bone is paramount for effective rejuvenation.

Additional considerations include heterogeneity in patient populations. Patients with skin of colour are sometimes perceived mistakenly as a uniform population, a concept that is becoming

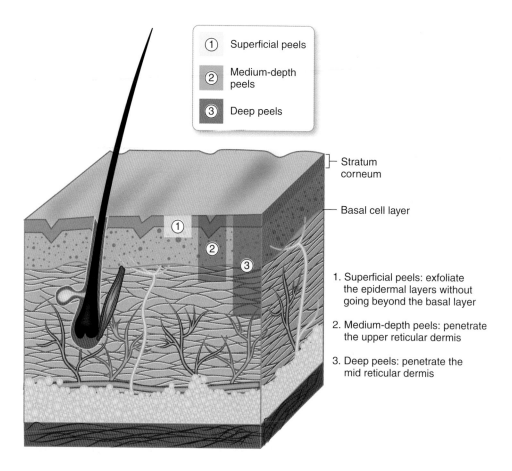

1. Superficial peels
2. Medium-depth peels
3. Deep peels

Stratum corneum

Basal cell layer

1. Superficial peels: exfoliate the epidermal layers without going beyond the basal layer

2. Medium-depth peels: penetrate the upper reticular dermis

3. Deep peels: penetrate the mid reticular dermis

Figure 21.5 Chemical peel depths. Adapted from Dr Raul Cetto, Medium Depth Peels, 19 Mar 2018. Aesthetics Media Ltd.

even more irrelevant due to increasing interracial diversity. Significant facial morphological variation exists between different ethnicities, as do cultural influences on what is considered to be desirable or beautiful. You must be cognisant in cosmetic practice, as in mainstream dermatological practice, of these underlying and contextual issues, and tailor management to the individual with shared decision making and fully informed consent.

Dermal fillers

The hallmark of facial ageing is loss of volume. Subcutaneous fat pads, which are partitioned into discrete compartments, atrophy with time and become malpositioned, which results in flattening of the midface. The facial fullness of youth deflates, with formation of hollowness, shadows and contour irregularities (Figure 21.6).

The most popular treatments used to address these changes are 'dermal' fillers, although they are in fact predominantly placed deep in the skin or even supraperiostally to re-volumise the deflated face (Figure 21.7). A number of products are now commercially available, but UK medical insurers usually only cover the handful of products approved by the US Food and Drug Administration (FDA). In comparison, there are hundreds of products available in the UK and Europe classified not as pharmaceutical agents, but as medical devices or even cosmetic injectables. This results in a much lower threshold for subsequent entry of new products onto the market.

Temporary fillers consisting of hyaluronic acid (HA) are favoured in facial aesthetics, due to the potential for reversal using hyaluronidase should an adverse event occur. The duration of action of most HA dermal fillers is typically six months, though there is evidence that perceived benefit may last longer, perhaps due to fibroblast stretching and stimulation of intrinsic collagen production.

HA is a natural component of the skin, and injectable fillers consist of long chains of HA. The cross-linking of these varies among products, as do the particle size and concentration. They are marketed as a pre-filled syringe containing a clear, colourless gel of varying viscosity, with or without lidocaine. HA products are commonly injected in the face, such as in the cheeks, lips, marionette lines (vertical sulci that develop from the corner of the mouth to the chin) and nasolabial folds. A good understanding of facial anatomy and safe technique is required to mitigate the risk of product embolisation and vascular occlusion. Other sites include the infraorbital tear trough region and hands, and HA can also be used to treat depressed acne scars.

Medical indications include lipodystrophy, atrophy from anti-HIV therapy, lupus profundus and linear morphoea. Cosmetic injection of filler implants to the breasts and buttocks is not approved by regulatory bodies, nor are they licensed for these sites; deaths have occurred due to the quantity of product used and subsequent large vessel embolism.

Other types of dermal fillers include calcium hydroxyapatite and poly-L-lactic acid (PLLA), which have longer duration than HA fillers but are less widely used. Permanent fillers such as polymethyl methacrylate (PMMA) have fallen out of favour due to long-term complications such as chronic foreign-body reactions.

Botulinum toxin

The combination of increased skin laxity and subcutaneous volume loss results in a disproportionate impact from underlying muscular activity. Dynamic lines form with facial expression, in a perpendicular direction to the vector of the muscle movement. With repeated contraction and relaxation, a permanent crease develops in the skin, which can persist even at rest.

Botulinum toxin, a neuromodulator that acts by blocking acetylcholine release at the neuromuscular junction, inhibits muscular activity, hence softening lines associated with facial expression. It is produced by the bacterium *Clostridium botulinum*, and two strains, A and B, are used medically. The onset of action is after 2–7 days and the blockade is permanent, but new nerve endings sprout after several months, allowing for resumed muscular activity. There are a number of commercial botulinum toxin products available, each product with its own storage, dilution and unit conversion profile (Table 21.1).

Table 21.1 Four types of botulinum toxins available in the UK, with unit conversion ratio of one Botox® unit compared to other products

Generic name	Trade name	Unit conversion
Ona-botulinum toxin A	Botox® or Vistabel®	1 unit
Abo-botulinum toxin A	Dysport® or Azzalure®	3 units
Inco-botulinum toxin A	Xeomin® or Bocouture®	1 unit
Rima-botulinum toxin B	Myobloc® or Neurobloc®	100 units

Bocouture®, Merz Pharma, South Elstree, UK; Botox®, Vistabel®, Xeomin®, Allergan, Irvine, CA, USA; Dysport®, Azzalure®, Galderma, Watford, UK; Myobloc®, Solstice Neurosciences, Malvern, PA, USA; Neurobloc®, Sloan Pharma, Bertrange, Luxembourg.

Common sites of treatment include the glabella (procerus muscle, corrugator muscle) (Figure 21.8), forehead (frontalis muscle) and periorbital crow's foot lines (orbicularis oculi muscle). More sophisticated techniques to address eyebrow shape, lower-face contouring (masseter muscle, depressor anguli oris muscle, mentalis muscle) and neck areas (platysma muscle) are used by experienced practitioners. Patient assessment is critical, making note of baseline asymmetry and ptosis, and includes examination of the patient both at rest and with facial animation. A thorough working knowledge of facial muscular anatomy and the relationships between muscle groups is fundamental for effective treatment.

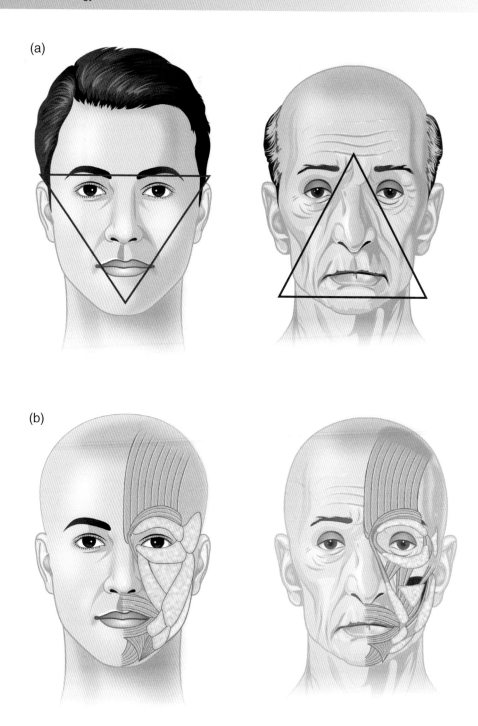

Figure 21.6 (a) Clinical appearance of volume deflation with age, and change of overall facial shape from an inverted to an upright triangle. (b) This effect is caused by changes in facial fat pads, which atrophy and become malpositioned with time.

Botulinum toxin use in non-facial sites to modify larger muscle groups such as the shoulders, arms and calves has been described, and is particularly popular in Asia and the Far East, but the risk of functional impairment must be noted. Furthermore, botulinum toxin injections to address dermatological conditions such as seborrhoeic dermatitis, rosacea and psoriasis have also been reported, although they are not part of standard practice.

(a)

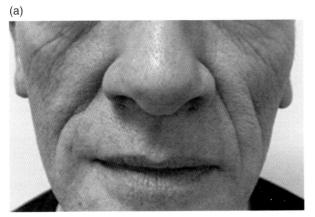

(b)

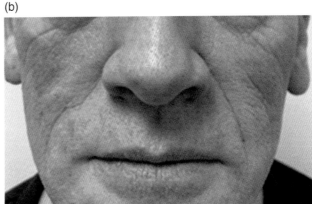

Figure 21.7 (a) Before and (b) after hyaluronic dermal filler injections to a patient with significant volume loss to the midface. © Tamara W. Griffiths.

Lifestyle and mental health

Facial bones, like long bones, atrophy with age. The negative space of the orbits expands, the maxilla flattens and the mandible shrinks. The net effect is reduction of bony scaffolding to support soft tissues, which contributes to facial sagging and drooping. Lifestyle and other factors that may help include cessation of smoking, vitamin D and calcium supplementation if required, and appropriate dental care.

It is important to be aware of the patient's psychological and mental health. Body dysmorphia is not uncommon, and it should be addressed sensitively as in general dermatological practice (Chapter 15). Even in the absence of body dysmorphia, patients who seek cosmetic interventions may be emotionally vulnerable. They may be blinkered about a desired outcome and therefore have unrealistic expectations or be unable to fully process the potential for a poor outcome. Astute clinical skills and experience, as well as constant vigilance, are required to detect and manage such situations. The potential for benefit may be less and the risk for dissatisfaction may be greater in the cosmetic patient.

Conversely, boosting the patient's satisfaction with their physical appearance can enhance confidence and improve mood. These are linked to healthier lifestyle choices such as exercise and healthy eating, as well as reduction in social isolation. As with any intervention, the risk–benefit ratio must be evaluated for each patient individually.

Other non-surgical treatments

Body sculpting treatments and lipolysis are increasing in popularity, but are less mainstream compared to facial botulinum toxin and dermal filler procedures. Deoxycholic acid injections are FDA approved for use in submental fat. The mechanism of action of these 'fat-busting jabs' is a detergent-like effect that disrupts cell membranes resulting in adipocytolysis, and is accompanied by a temporary phagocytic inflammatory response including oedema and tenderness. Unregulated use in larger areas, such as the abdomen, lacks safety and efficacy data.

Cryolipolysis devices are used for non-invasive body contouring, and exploit the premise that adipocytes are more susceptible to freezing than other skin cells. Fat cell death is again associated with an inflammatory phagocytic response. Radiofrequency and ultrasound technologies are used for skin tightening on non-facial sites. Successful application of any machine-based treatment requires practitioner expertise and careful patient selection.

Complications and contraindications

Although 'cosmetic' procedures are performed in the private sector, complications and adverse events often fall at the door of the National Health Service (NHS). Dermatology and plastic surgery, along with allied surgical specialties such as ear–nose–throat, ophthalmology and maxillofacial surgery, encompass the key clinicians responsible for diagnosing and managing patients who fall into this niche area of complication management.

A further layer of complexity exists as the patient may have received unsatisfactory care from the original practitioner (clinician or non-clinician), who at best may have been unable to effectively diagnose and treat the adverse event, but at worst may have absolved themselves of any obligation to a 'client' with complications. The patient may have a level of anger, guilt, remorse or shame about the course of events. For optimal care and in order to develop a level of trust, you must acknowledge and then diffuse these emotions in a professional and empathetic manner, reassuring the patient that you remain non-judgemental and are there to help.

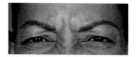

Pre-treatment

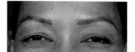

Week 4

Figure 21.8 Before and after botulinum toxin injections to the glabellar region (procerus muscle and corrugator muscle). Carruthers JD *et al*. DaxibotulinumtoxinA for injection for the treatment of glabellar lines: results from each of two multicenter, randomized, double-blind, placebo-controlled, phase 3 studies (SAKURA 1 and SAKURA 2). *Plast Reconstr Surg* 2020; **145**:45–58.

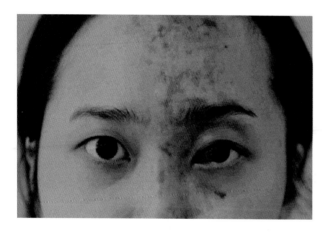

Figure 21.9 Complication of dermal filler injection for augmentation rhinoplasty causing occlusion in the distribution of the superior trochlear and angular arteries. Lee JI *et al*. Skin necrosis with oculomotor nerve palsy due to a hyaluronic acid filler injection. *Arch Plast Surg* 2017; **44**:340–43.

Networking with clinical meetings and multispecialty multidisciplinary teams is useful to discuss complex cases. A national database of adverse events would help identify worrying trends. Medicines and Healthcare products Regulatory Agency (MHRA) yellow card reporting can also facilitate this; however, treatments may not involve prescription medications, they may be device related, or the patient may not be aware of the specific product used, and so this safety net is not as effective as for other areas of medicine.

Complications associated with skin rejuvenation depend on the modality of treatment used. Particular care must be taken in patients with skin of colour due to the risk of pigmentary disruption. The range of complications associated with chemical peels,

and laser, light or other types of devices include infection, herpes simplex virus reactivation, burns, scarring, post-inflammatory hypo- or hyperpigmentation, and eye damage to both patient and practitioner.

Common side-effects of dermal fillers include pain, bruising, redness, swelling and itching. Infection (including low-grade biofilm or atypical mycobacterium), foreign-body granuloma, product migration and vessel embolisation with subsequent necrosis and scarring are uncommon (Figure 21.9). Thankfully, permanent blindness due to retinal artery occlusion (from retrograde flow in anastomosing vessels) and anaphylaxis are very rare, but must be discussed during the consent process. They are considered medical emergencies requiring immediate and urgent action.

Avoid dermal filler injection in patients with active autoimmune disease, due to increased risk of inflammatory nodule or granuloma formation. If nodule formation does occur, consider biopsy and culture for atypical mycobacterium. Antibiotics that also have anti-inflammatory properties may be indicated, such as doxycycline. Oral prednisolone or even surgical extrusion of the product may be necessary. Hyaluronidase can be used to dissolve unwanted HA product, but in itself can cause problems such as an allergic reaction, or overcorrection with consequent damage to normal tissue.

The duration of action of botulinum toxin is usually limited to approximately 3–4 months, therefore any untoward events such as unsatisfactory cosmetic outcome, asymmetry, and ptosis of the brow (from over-injection of the frontalis muscle) or eyelid (due to diffusion into the levator palpebrae superioris muscle) will spontaneously improve. Alpha-adrenergic eyedrops, such as apraclonidine, can aid the recovery of the eyelid ptosis by stimulating Muller's muscle to raise the upper eyelid. Muscle weakness in the lower face can be more problematic, with speech difficulties and other functional problems, for example drinking from a straw or whistling. Again, due to the temporary duration of treatment action, these will also resolve, although they may be highly distressing to the patient in the meantime.

Other potential adverse events associated with botulinum toxin are injection related, such as pain, headache, bruising and infection. Contraindications include history of neurological disease such as myasthenia gravis, Lambert–Eaton syndrome or motor neurone disease. Incidents of respiratory depression and death have occurred with the use of 'black market Botox' due to the greatly increased strength of the illegal product.

There are a range of adipocytolytic treatments used. Some have a thorough safety and efficacy record established for reduction of submental fat, but off-label use and the use of other unlicensed products on large areas of the body can result in severe inflammation, infection, necrosis, scarring and surface irregularities. Device-based cryolipolysis can result in unintended cold-injury necrosis.

A risk common to all cosmetic interventions is patient dissatisfaction, therefore establishment of a good doctor–patient relationship with realistic patient expectations is critical. Be aware you may need to impose a cooling-off period for the over-eager patient, and do not get drawn into performing a procedure if it makes you feel uncomfortable. General contraindications to all cosmetic interventions include body dysmorphia, pregnancy and breastfeeding, skin infection, keloidal scarring and allergy to products. Bleeding disorders are a relative contraindication, as are blood thinners and calcium channel blockers, due to increased risk of bruising.

Regulation

Regulation is an important consideration in this area of clinical practice. In 2008, the UK's Department of Health and Social Care (DHSC) proposed deregulation of non-surgical treatments, including class 4 lasers and intense pulsed light therapy, provided the indication was solely cosmetic. As a result, those engaging in this type of practice and the premises where they worked fell under minimal and *ad hoc* scrutiny. Those with no healthcare background or training at all were permitted to perform procedures on any clients, in any setting, giving rise to peripatetic practitioners and the infamous 'Botox parties'.

The situation was complicated by blurred boundaries between 'cosmetic' and 'medical', with particular concern about missed pathology and inappropriate management of disease or adverse events. There were a number of UK and European attempts to improve standards and regulation, but it was the Poly Implant Prostheses (PIP) silicone breast implant scandal affecting over 47,000 women in the UK and approximately 300,000 worldwide that catalysed further action.

In 2013, the DHSC commissioned the Review of the Regulation of Cosmetic Interventions led by Sir Bruce Keogh, Medical Director of the NHS, to investigate issues in the cosmetic surgery sector, focusing on invasive procedures such as breast augmentation. However, it shone a brighter spotlight on the dysfunctional non-surgical cosmetic sector, which was responsible for over 75% of the UK cosmetic intervention market share.

The subsequent course of events led to some improvement, with standardisation and quality assurance, primarily involving educational frameworks for all groups of learners, including non-clinicians. Furthermore, specific professional clinical standards were agreed, developed by the UK Cosmetic Practice Standards Authority (CPSA) with multistakeholder input. Mandatory regulation remains unsupported by the DHSC and indirect 'light touch' regulation has ensued, acting as a lever to promote good practice and to provide some transparency and clarity for the general public. The Joint Council of Cosmetic Practitioners (JCCP) voluntary register enforces compliance with CPSA standards, though other registers exist.

Unfortunately, with voluntary registration, concern exists for the emergence of a two-tier system: those who join a register demonstrating they comply with agreed standards, and those who continue to practise 'under the radar'. Therefore, if you wish to develop a cosmetic practice, membership on a voluntary register is important not only to declare that your practice is aligned with recognised standards, but also as an act of solidarity to support good practice across the sector for improved transparency and patient care. Furthermore, in 2016 the GMC published general guidance for all doctors engaging in cosmetic practice, and you should familiarise yourself with these recommendations. You must declare any cosmetic practice with medical indemnifiers, as well as detailing it within your scope of practice during Annual Review of Competency Progression (ARCP) or annual appraisal.

Conclusions

Gaining competence in non-surgical cosmetic procedures is less well supported in many countries compared to other areas of dermatological practice, largely due to the lack of learning opportunities. However, our specialist skill set provides a more than adequate foundation on which to develop these competencies, and the importance of doing so is underscored by the expansion of training requirements. Dermatologists are the key clinicians responsible for diagnosing and managing complications even at the hands of others, so a working knowledge of popular cosmetic treatments and associated adverse events is essential.

Our specialty provides a unique perspective, combining the clinical expertise and academic rigour required not only to provide the highest standard of practice, but also to lead in the pursuit of new knowledge and research. After all, today's mainstream 'cosmetic' treatments were pioneered by dermatologists for treatment of disease, and management of even the most mainstream cutaneous pathology will usually have a cosmetic component to it.

Finally, dermatologists must play a role in monitoring standards of practice and horizon scanning for future problems in the sector, to safeguard patients and the public. Improved data collection on adverse events and harm to patients will strengthen the argument for tighter regulation in what currently remains a disjointed and confused sector. However, when executed well, cosmetic dermatology can provide a stimulating, creative and highly rewarding addition to mainstream dermatological practice.

Pearls and pitfalls

- When recommending a topical cosmeceutical agent, understand the active ingredients and their target: stratum corneum and epidermal maturation, dermal repair, pigmentation (melanin or haemoglobin) or prevention (sunscreen, antioxidants).
- Facial ageing involves changes that occur in the skin, the subcutaneous fat, and muscle and bone. An integrated approach to rejuvenation will give the most natural results, and holistic facial assessment is critical.
- Maintain an evidence-based approach to cosmetic practice, but be aware that the level of evidence available is often much lower than with medical treatments.
- Be vigilant for body dysmorphic disorder or other underlying psychological issues in cosmetic patients.
- A good doctor–patient relationship based on trust and respect is key to a successful cosmetic practice. Reflect on your own practice and remain aware of unconscious bias or conflict of interest.

SCE Questions. See questions 36 and 37.

FURTHER READING AND KEY RESOURCES

Bangash HK, Eisen DB, Armstrong AW *et al*. Who are the pioneers? A critical analysis of innovation and expertise in cutaneous noninvasive and minimally invasive cosmetic and surgical procedures. *Dermatol Surg* 2016; **42**:335–51.

Sundaram H, Liew S, Signorini M. Global aesthetics consensus: hyaluronic acid fillers and botulinum toxin type A – recommendations for combined treatment and optimising outcomes in diverse patient populations. *Plast Reconstr Surg* 2016; **137**:1410–23.

Vanaman M, Guillen Fabi S, Carruthers J. Complications in the cosmetic dermatology patient: a review and our experience (part 1). *Dermatol Surg* 2016; **42**:1–11.

Vanaman M, Guillen Fabi S, Carruthers J. Complications in the cosmetic dermatology patient: a review and our experience (part 2). *Dermatol Surg* 2016; **42**:12–20.

Textbook

Draelos Z. *Cosmetic Dermatology*, 2nd edn. Oxford: Wiley Blackwell, 2016.

Useful websites

Cosmetic Practice Standards Authority. Available at: www.cosmeticstandards.org.uk.

Department of Health and Social Care. Review of the Regulation of Cosmetic Interventions. Available at: https://www.gov.uk/government/publications/review-of-the-regulation-of-cosmetic-interventions.

General Medical Council. Guidance for doctors who offer cosmetic interventions. Available at: https://www.gmc-uk.org/ethical-guidance/ethical-guidance-for-doctors/cosmetic-interventions.

Health Education England. Non-surgical cosmetic procedures. Availableat:https://www.hee.nhs.uk/our-work/non-surgical-cosmetic-procedures.

22

Laser therapy

Raman Bhutani and Manjunatha Kalavala

Introduction

The term 'laser' is an acronym for light amplification by the stimulated emission of radiation. Lasers have been used in dermatology since the 1960s to treat a wide variety of conditions, including vascular and pigmented lesions, tattoos and scars. They have also been used to resurface and correct age-related skin changes and to remove unwanted hair. Cutaneous laser surgery was revolutionised by the concept of 'selective photothermolysis', introduced by Anderson and Parrish in the 1980s. The demand for laser surgery has increased substantially because of the relative ease with which many lesions can be treated, combined with a low incidence of adverse post-operative sequelae. Although not every dermatologist needs to be proficient in the use of lasers, it is important for all to be able to guide and advise their patients regarding appropriate laser therapies.

Fundamentals of laser therapy

The basic components of a laser system are the laser medium, optical cavity and pumping system (Figure 22.1). Lasers are usually named after the constituents of the laser medium. This may be a gas (e.g. argon or CO_2), a liquid (e.g. rhodamine, used in pulsed-dye laser, PDL), a solid (e.g. alexandrite, Er:YAG, Nd:YAG and ruby lasers) or solid state (diode laser) (Table 22.1). The atoms in the laser medium are 'pumped' to an excited state by an external source of energy. This means the electrons surrounding the nucleus move from their resting orbit to an orbit of higher energy further from the nucleus. This excited state is unstable and electrons spontaneously return to their resting state and emit the absorbed energy as they do so. The energy released by this process, termed 'spontaneous emission', is discharged as light, which travels in bundles of energy known as photons. When a majority of atoms in the medium exist in an excited state, this is termed a 'population inversion'. At this point

Dermatology Training: The Essentials. Edited by Mahbub M.U. Chowdhury, Tamara W. Griffiths and Andrew Y. Finlay.
© 2022 The British Association of Dermatologists. Published 2022 by John Wiley & Sons Ltd.
Companion website: www.wiley.com/go/chowdhury/dermatologytraining

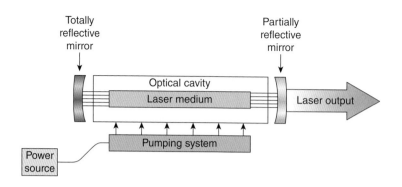

Figure 22.1 The components of a laser system. Adapted from Finlay AY, Chowdhury MMU. *Specialist Training in Dermatology.* © 2007 Mosby Elsevier.

Table 22.1 Abbreviations used concerning lasers

CO_2	Carbon dioxide
CW	Continuous wave
Er:YAG	Erbium-doped yttrium aluminium garnet
IPL	Intense pulsed light
KTP	Potassium titanyl phosphate
LP	Long pulsed
Nd:YAG	Neodymium-doped yttrium aluminium garnet
PDL	Pulsed-dye laser
QS	Quality-switched

the photons will travel along the long axis of the optical cavity and are increasingly likely to collide with atoms that are in an excited state. Stimulated emission occurs when an electron in an already excited state absorbs a photon of light and emits *two* photons of light while returning to the resting state orbit. Stimulated photons have identical wavelength and frequency. Reflecting mirrors are placed at either end of the cavity so that light travels back and forth within the cavity, promoting further amplification. One of the mirrors is only partially reflective, allowing a small portion of the light to travel out of the cavity as laser light, through a delivery system for transmission to the operator hand piece. Delivery systems may take the form of fibre-optic cable or articulated arms.

Properties of laser light

Laser light can be defined by three properties:

- **Monochromaticity**: laser light is of a single discrete wavelength determined by the laser medium. Cutaneous lesions contain targets or chromophores such as water, melanin, haemoglobin or tattoo ink. Chromophores can be specifically targeted by laser light of certain wavelengths (Figure 22.2).
- **Coherence**: the waves are in phase in time and space.

- **Collimation**: laser light is a narrow, intense beam of light capable of propagation across long distances without divergence. This 'collimated' light can be focused into small spot sizes, allowing for precise tissue destruction.

Selective photothermolysis

Laser light may be absorbed, reflected, transmitted or scattered by the skin (Figure 22.3). For there to be any clinical effect, light must be absorbed by components of the skin. Once this happens, three basic effects can occur: photothermal, photomechanical or photochemical. The most common reactions in laser therapy are photothermal and photomechanical. Photothermal effects happen when a chromophore absorbs light energy at its optimal wavelength; the absorbed energy is converted to heat, destroying the target. If the heat causes very rapid localised tissue expansion, this can induce acoustic waves and photomechanical destruction. In contrast, photodynamic therapy depends on photochemical effects that result from interactions between light and applied photosensitisers or between light and the normal chemical constituents of skin.

The theory of selective photothermolysis describes how controlled destruction of a targeted lesion is possible, while still protecting nearby normal tissue from thermal damage. The theory's key concept is that the laser pulse duration should be equal to or shorter than the thermal relaxation time of the intended target (definitions of key terms are given in Table 22.2). To achieve selective photothermolysis, a suitable wavelength that is preferentially absorbed by the target tissue or chromophore is selected. Fluence must be sufficient to achieve destruction of the target within the allotted time. Therefore laser parameters (spot size, wavelength, pulse duration and fluence) can be tailored for specific cutaneous applications to effect maximal target destruction with minimal collateral thermal damage. Consideration must also be given to the depth of the target structure. In general, the depth of penetration of laser energy increases with increasing wavelength.

Lasers are also classified according to the pulse characteristics of the beam (Table 22.3). Pulsed and quasi-continuous wave systems are better adapted for cutaneous laser surgery because, on

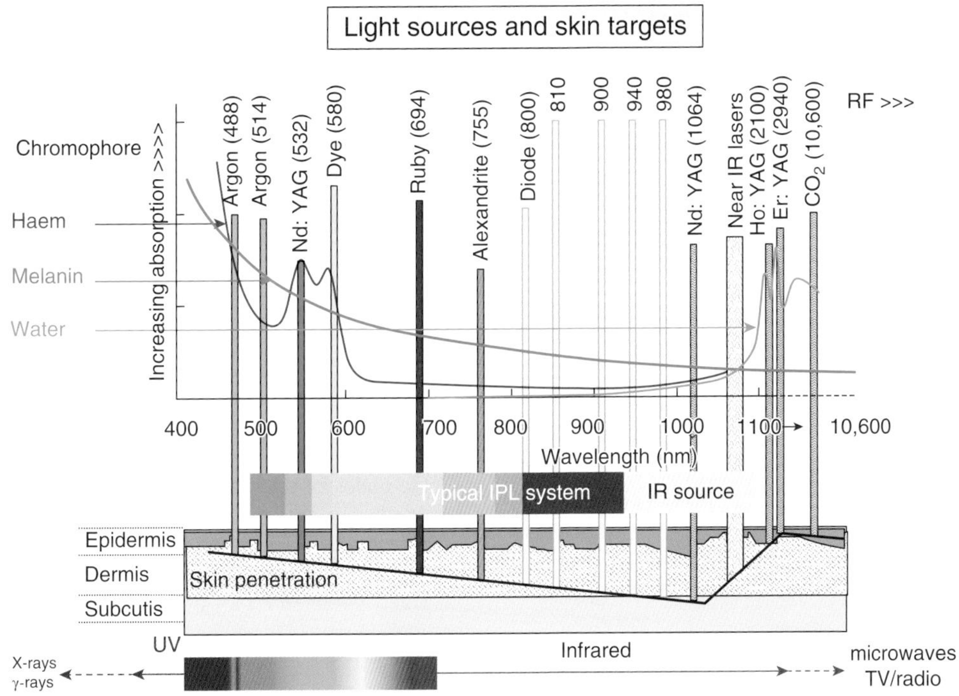

Light sources and skin targets

Chromophore >>>>

Haem

Melanin

Water

Increasing absorption >>>>

Argon (488)
Argon (514)
Nd: YAG (532)
Dye (580)
Ruby (694)
Alexandrite (755)
Diode (800)
810
900
940
980
Nd: YAG (1064)
Near IR lasers
Ho: YAG (2100)
Er: YAG (2940)
CO_2 (10,600)
RF >>>

400   500   600   700   800   900   1000   1100→   10,600

Wavelength (nm)

Typical IPL system   IR source

Epidermis
Dermis   Skin penetration
Subcutis
UV

X-rays
γ-rays

Infrared   microwaves
TV/radio

Figure 22.2 Diagrammatic representation of the absorption spectra of principal cutaneous chromophores. IPL, intense pulsed light; IR, infrared; RF, radiofrequency; UV, ultraviolet; YAG, yttrium aluminium garnet.

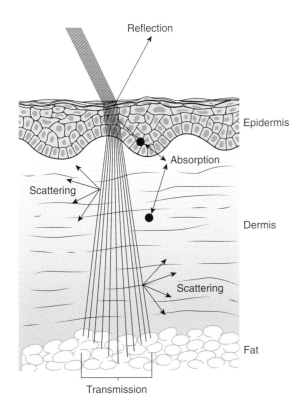

Reflection

Epidermis

Absorption

Scattering

Dermis

Scattering

Fat

Transmission

Figure 22.3 Laser–tissue interactions. Adapted from Finlay AY, Chowdhury MMU. *Specialist Training in Dermatology*. © 2007 Mosby Elsevier.

Table 22.2 Definition of key terms

Pulse duration: exposure duration of the target tissue to laser light at a set energy density (fluence); measured in milliseconds

Thermal relaxation time (TRT): time required for the targeted site to cool to one half of its peak temperature immediately between the pulses of laser radiation

Fluence: energy absorbed by target tissue in J/cm^2

the basis of the principles of selective photothermolysis, the thermal relaxation time of most cutaneous chromophores is very short. The pulse width is adjusted so that it approximates to the thermal relaxation time of the target chromophore. Spot size can be altered, taking into account the size of the target area being treated. A bigger spot size results in greater depth of penetration, greater clinical reaction and less scattering of the laser beam. If transferring from large to small spot size, higher fluence is required to achieve the same clinical effect (and vice versa).

Cooling

By cooling the epidermis, higher fluences and therefore higher temperature elevations are possible in the targeted structures in the dermis, while preserving the epidermis. This is particularly important in skin of colour to reduce the likelihood of dyspigmentation. Almost all cooling strategies will provide some pain relief. Cooling can be before the laser pulse (pre), during the pulse (parallel) or after the pulse (post). Cooling methods include:

- Contact pre-cooling with an aluminium roller, ice or gold gels, chilled sapphire window cooled to 4°C, or copper plate.
- Cold air.
- Cryogen spray cooling.

Table 22.3 Laser classification

Continuous wave lasers: emit a constant beam of light, e.g. CO_2 laser

Quasi-continuous wave lasers: interrupted emission of continuous waves, e.g. potassium titanyl phosphate, copper vapour, copper bromide, krypton and APTD (argon-pumped tunable dye) lasers

Pulsed laser systems: emit high-energy laser light in ultra-short pulse durations with relatively long intervening interval

1. Long pulsed: pulse durations of 450 microseconds to 40 milliseconds,e.g. pulsed-dye laser

2. Very short pulsed: pulse durations of 5–100 nanoseconds, e.g. Q-switched ruby, alexandrite, Nd:YAG

3. Super-pulsed: produce very short pulses in a repetitive pattern, e.g. modified CO_2 lasers

4. Pico-laser: pulse duration of less than 1 nanosecond

Anaesthesia

Most laser procedures are associated with some discomfort. The sensations described range from mild warmth to the 'the snap of a rubber band' or 'frying pan splatter', to 'severe burning pain'. In many cases, topical anaesthetic preparations such as a eutectic mixture of local anaesthetics (EMLA) or Ametop® (tetracaine;Alliance Pharmaceuticals, Chippenham, UK) alleviate most of the discomfort. For more invasive and extensive treatments, the pain can be quite intense, requiring the use of local or general anaesthesia, analgesics and/or anxiolytics.

Laser safety

Laser light can cause permanent retinal damage and vision loss. Therefore, eye protection in the form of optically coated glasses or specific goggles for the particular laser being used is required for all persons present in the room during laser treatment. If the patient's goggles obstruct the treatment area in the periorbital area, use of an anodised external metal eye cup can

be used to protect the patient's eyes. If the eyelids are to be treated, an eye shield should be placed on the eye, using topical anaesthesia, to protect the globe. The door to the treatment room must be kept closed and locked with an external warning sign during laser firing to protect innocent intruders or passers-by from possible injury.

Accidental fires can occur in the presence of circulating oxygen, leading to ignition of surgical tubing, sponges, clothes or drapes. To minimise these risks, oxygen sources, if present, should be turned down or off; saline-soaked drapes or clothes should be used intraoperatively; exposed hair-bearing areas should be kept moist; and alcohol-based skin preparations should be strictly avoided. In addition, lasers should be kept in the standby mode when not in use to avoid inadvertent firing.

Electrical hazards can be reduced by dedicating a specific electric outlet for each laser and by avoiding the use of extension cords.

There is a risk of infection during laser treatment. Smoke and aerosolised fragments have been reported to contain human papilloma virus, HIV p24 antigen, other viruses and cellular materials. A smoke evacuator, with clean filters and tubing, minimises infection risk.

Patient selection and counselling

The patient should be informed about all aspects of the procedure as well as its risks and benefits, and written consent should be obtained before the procedure. In general, side-effects and complications include blistering, crusting, pigmentation abnormalities (hyperpigmentation and hypopigmentation) and scarring. Treatment of vascular lesions may result in a variable degree of short-term purpura, especially with PDL.

Pre-operative laser evaluation should include a basic medical history, incorporating documentation of medications and allergies. The history taking should include questioning about abnormal scarring, excessive sun exposure, allergic or inflammatory conditions, herpes simplex virus (HSV) outbreaks, immune disorders, or cosmetic procedures within the involved area.

- If the patient has Fitzpatrick skin type I–III, ensure that the patient has not tanned recently. Sunscreen (with a minimum sun protection factor of 50) should be used for at least six weeks prior to and the whole duration of the treatment. This is important, because epidermal melanin may interfere with laser treatment and increase the risks of scarring and hypo- or hyperpigmentation.
- Patients who have been on oral retinoids within the previous six months may have increased risk of scar formation and poor healing.
- Photosensitivity reactions normally only occur following exposure to ultraviolet (UV) radiation. It is exceptionally rare for

photosensitising medication to cause a reaction to light above 500 nm, and most laser or light sources used have higher wavelengths than this. If the patient is taking a known photosensitising medication, the advice is to treat a test patch before proceeding to full treatment.

- Oral antiviral prophylaxis should always be considered for patients with a history of HSV infections undergoing ablative laser treatment. The patient can be placed on appropriate preoperative prophylactic antiviral therapy before initiation of therapy. If active HSV infection is present on the day booked for laser treatment, the treatment should be postponed until the area has healed completely.
- Obtain photographs at baseline and at regular intervals to monitor progress.
- It is important for patients to understand the importance of good wound care after a laser procedure. Written post-operative instructions should be provided.

Practical points to consider when using lasers

- Perform laser test spots on all patients prior to treating an entire lesion to determine the treatment parameters.
- To establish initial parameters, read the user manual and consult experienced laser surgeons who have been working with the particular laser being used.
- Begin with the lowest energy fluence. At subsequent treatments fluence can be increased by small increments of 0.5–1.0 J as necessary. Remember, using too high an energy fluence can result in thermal injury and scarring.
- Position the laser hand piece at a 90-degree angle, perpendicular to the skin surface.
- Ensure that the hand piece is held at the appropriate distance from the patient (each laser will have a specific spacer device).
- Try to deliver the pulses close to one another without significant overlap. While a small amount of overlap (10%) will generally not have an adverse effect, repeatedly delivering multiple pulses to the same area can result in unwanted thermal injury and scarring.
- In patients with skin of colour, lasers having longer wavelengths are generally safer, as they spare injury to the epidermis to a greater degree than shorter-wavelength lasers and hence reduce the risk of post-inflammatory dyschromia.

Therapeutic applications of laser therapy

Laser systems currently available and their cutaneous applications are listed in Table 22.4. In a single centre, it is unlikely that all lasers will be available and it is important to know the strengths and limitations of the available laser systems. Treatment of some common skin conditions is discussed briefly here.

Treatment of vascular lesions

Cutaneous vascular lesions are one of the most common indications for laser treatment in dermatology. The target chromophore is oxyhaemoglobin, which has absorption peaks in the range of yellow-green light at 418 nm, 542 nm and 577 nm. Laser light with 'shorter' wavelengths, such as PDL (585 nm), is well absorbed by oxyhaemoglobin. Such lasers are therefore often favoured in order to target the superficial blood vessels of vascular lesions. The longer the wavelength of laser light, the less is absorbed by epidermal melanin, another chromophore. Therefore, the longer the wavelength, the higher the proportion of laser light that penetrates into the dermis. As a consequence, lasers with longer wavelengths, such as Nd:YAG (1064 nm), are used for the coagulation of large, deep dermal vessels and have a lower risk of post-inflammatory dyschromia in patients with skin of colour. As vascular lesions often contain blood vessels at various depths, using lasers of different wavelengths during a course of several treatments can be helpful in achieving the desired clinical effect.

PDLs are the laser of choice for most congenital and acquired vascular lesions because of their superior clinical efficacy and low risk profile. PDL treatments are performed with fluences ranging from 3 to 10 J/cm^2 and a spot size of 2–10 mm with no more than 10% overlap. Shorter pulse durations are often used to minimise collateral damage in the skin, but they can lead to rapid heating of vessels and vessel rupture, contributing to post-treatment temporary purpura. Other laser and light systems that are currently used to treat vascular lesions include intense pulsed light, frequency-doubled Nd:YAG (KTP), diode and alexandrite lasers.

Common indications for vascular lasers include both congenital and acquired conditions:

- Congenital: port-wine stain and haemangiomas.
- Acquired: facial telangiectasia, rosacea, leg veins, hereditary haemorrhagic telangiectasia, spider angioma, venous lakes, pyogenic granuloma, cherry angioma, poikiloderma of Civatte, angiofibroma, blue rubber bleb naevus syndrome, keratosis pilaris rubra, resistant periungual warts, angiokeratoma and red hypertrophic scars.

Treatment of pigmented lesions and tattoos

Most benign epidermal and dermal pigmented lesions respond to high-energy Q-switched (QS) red and infrared lasers. The chromophore is melanin. Superficially located pigment is best treated with shorter-wavelength lasers (e.g. 532-nm QS Nd:YAG). For removal of deeper pigment, longer-wavelength lasers are needed (e.g. 755-nm alexandrite, 1064-nm QS Nd:YAG). Traditional ablative lasers (10 600-nm CO$_2$, 2940-nm Er:YAG) utilise water as the chromophore to eliminate skin pigmentation by non-selective vaporisation of the epidermis and superficial dermis.

The management of melanocytic naevi is controversial. Laser treatment should only be undertaken if there is no doubt about the nature of the lesion. The main concern in treating melanocytic naevi with lasers is the possibility that this may increase

Table 22.4 Therapeutic applications of lasers

Laser type	Wavelength (nm)	Indications for treatment
Potassium titanyl phosphate	532	Pigmented lesions, vascular lesions
Nd:YAG, frequency-doubled	532	Pigmented lesions; red, orange and yellow tattoos
Pulsed-dye laser	510	Pigmented lesions
	585/595	Vascular lesions, hypertrophic and keloid scars, striae, verrucae, non-ablative dermal remodelling
Ruby	694	Green, black and blue tattoos
Alexandrite	755	
Q-switched		Pigmented lesions, blue and black tattoos
Normal mode		Hair removal, leg veins
Diode	800–810	Hair removal, leg veins
Nd:YAG	1064	
Q-switched		Pigmented lesions; blue, black and green tattoos
Normal mode		Hair removal, leg veins, non-ablative dermal remodelling
Nd:YAG, long pulsed	1320	Hair removal, non-ablative dermal remodelling
Diode, long pulsed	1450	Non-ablative dermal remodelling, acne
Er:glass	1540	Non-ablative dermal remodelling
Er:YAG (pulsed)	2490	Ablative skin resurfacing, epidermal lesions
CO_2 (continuous wave)	10 600	Actinic cheilitis, verrucae, rhinophyma
CO_2 (pulsed)	10 600	Ablative skin resurfacing, epidermal and dermal lesions
Intense pulsed light source	515–1200	Superficial pigmented lesions, vascular lesions, hair removal, non-ablative dermal remodelling

the risk of future malignant transformation, although there is no evidence to support this. Also, any future malignant change could be more difficult to detect clinically, leading to a diagnostic delay and the potential for criticism and/or litigation.

Appropriate indications for laser therapy include:

• Epidermal lesions: lentigines, freckles, café-au-lait macules, naevus spilus, pigmented seborrhoeic keratosis.
• Dermal lesions: naevus of Ota, naevus of Ito, blue naevus, drug-induced pigmentation, acquired dermal melanosis (e.g. lichen planus pigmentosus).
• Mixed epidermal and dermal pigmentation: melasma, post-inflammatory hyperpigmentation, Becker's naevus, junctional naevus.

In tattoo removal, the target chromophores are small particles of tattoo ink within macrophages or scattered extracellularly throughout the dermis. For optimal pigment removal, the choice of laser is based on the absorption spectra of the ink colours present within the tattoo. Black and blue pigments are best treated with QS Nd:YAG (1064 nm); alternatives could be QS alexandrite (755 nm) or QS ruby laser (694 nm). Green inks respond well to QS ruby laser (694 nm) as red light has high absorption by green chromophore. Red inks respond well to 532-nm QS Nd:YAG laser. Picosecond alexandrite and Nd:YAG lasers have been used for blue and black pigmentation as they are less painful and more effective at lower fluence than QS lasers. White, yellow and fluorescent tattoos are unlikely to respond to treatment and should be treated with caution.

In resistant cases, ablative lasers can be used to stimulate transepidermal elimination of pigment and physical removal of tattoo pigment. In general, professional tattoos are more difficult to treat than amateur tattoos, because more pigment is used with deeper placement in the skin. Ingredients found in professional tattoos that give them specific colours are carbon and iron oxide (black), cobaltic aluminate (blue), chromium oxide (green), mercury sulfide or cadmium selenide (red), cadmium sulfide or ochre (yellow) and titanium dioxide and zinc oxide (white). Complications of laser treatment of these tattoos include

Table 22.5 The Kirby–Desai scale to estimate the number of laser treatments needed for tattoo removal

Phototype	Location	Colour	Ink amount	Scarring	Layering
I: 1 point	Head and neck: 1 point	Black only: 1 point	Amateur: 1 point	No scar: 0 points	None: 0 points
II: 2 points	Upper trunk: 2 points	Mostly black with some red: 2 points	Minimal: 2 points	Minimal: 1 point	Layering: 2 points
III: 3 points	Lower trunk: 3 points	Mostly black and red with some other colour: 3 points	Moderate: 3 points	Moderate: 3 points	
IV: 4 points	Proximal extremity: 4 points	Multiple colours: 4 points	Significant: 5 points	Significant: 5 points	
V: 5 points	Distal extremity: 5 points				
VI: 6 points					

Points are assigned depending on six parameters: Fitzpatrick skin phototype, location of the skin, colour of ink, amount of ink used in the tattoo, scarring and tissue change, and presence or absence of tattoo layering. The physician should calculate the total number of points to estimate the number of treatment sessions needed for laser removal (plus or minus 2.5). Based on Kirby W *et al. J Clin Aesthet Dermatol* 2009; **2**:32–7.

dyspigmentation and local or systemic allergic reactions. 'Paradoxical darkening', where darkening occurs immediately after treatment, can occur with tattoos containing iron oxide or titanium dioxide, secondary to chemical reduction of ferric oxide or titanium dioxide. The Kirby–Desai scale estimates the number of treatment sessions needed, based on Fitzpatrick skin type, location, pigment colour, amount of ink used, scarring, and damage to the tissue and ink layer. This scale can be a useful aid during patient counselling (Table 22.5).

Treatment of hypertrophic scars, keloids and striae

When treating scars, PDL produces marked improvement in redness, pliability, inflammation and abnormal sensations (dysaesthesia) during early stages of scar formation, and generally targets hypervascularity of the scar. Fractional CO_2 laser can be used at a later stage of scar progression when improvements in stiffness, contour and pliability are desired.

Keloids and very thick or proliferative hypertrophic scars may require prior or simultaneous use of intralesional corticosteroid, or 5-fluorouracil injections to reduce the thickness, followed by vascular laser to improve residual redness. Significant clinical improvement of early striae can be achieved using low-fluence PDL irradiation. However, mature striae are less likely to respond.

Laser photo-epilation

Melanin content is much higher in melanin-bearing structures, such as the hair shaft and in matrix cells, than in the hair follicle. Melanin captures energy from the laser and distributes it to the surrounding follicular structures. This results in the destruction of the hair matrix and hair bulge stem cells. Lasers and intense pulsed light (IPL) sources with wavelengths in the red or near-infrared region (600–1200 nm) effectively target melanin within the hair shaft, hair follicle epithelium and heavily pigmented matrix. LP ruby (694 nm), LP alexandrite (755 nm), pulsed diode (800 nm), QS and LP Nd:YAG (1064 nm) and IPL (590–1200 nm) sources are currently used for laser photo-epilation. These lasers are all 'long pulsed' (LP) as opposed to QS, working via a photothermal response. The longer the wavelength, the smaller the absorption coefficient, meaning that less absorption occurs in the epidermal melanin, resulting in greater penetration. Longer-wavelength lasers provoke less of the thermal injury that can cause pigmentary change. They are therefore less likely to cause dyspigmentation in skin of colour. Hence, LP ruby (694 nm) and LP alexandrite (755 nm) are suitable for Fitzpatrick skin types I–IV and LP Nd:YAG (1064 nm) is suitable for skin types III–VI.

The most common medical indications for photo-epilation include hirsutism associated with polycystic ovarian syndrome, pilonidal sinus, hidradenitis suppurativa, pseudofolliculitis barbae, hairy intraoral flaps, transgender requirements and genital gender reaffirming surgery.

Skin reactions (e.g. pain, transient inflammation and perifollicular oedema) are common. Acneiform rash, persistent urticaria, long-term hyperhidrosis and paradoxical hypertrichosis are also reported side-effects.

Cutaneous resurfacing lasers

CO_2 and erbium:YAG lasers are the long-established lasers that ablate skin by heating up abundant water in the dermis and epidermis. These lasers are used as both conventional ablative and fractionated resurfacing devices. They are commonly used for cutaneous resurfacing, with the main indications for treatment being photodamaged facial skin, photoinduced facial rhytides (fine creases), dyschromia, vascular changes and skin laxity.

Fractionated lasers emit numerous narrow, evenly placed pixelated microscopic columns of laser light, creating an array of microscopic thermal zones of injury. The reservoir of undamaged skin adjacent to sites of such laser injury facilitates rapid re-epithelialisation by migration of viable cells into the wounded areas, resulting in prompt and predictable epidermal healing with collagen remodelling. The risk for complications is also lower than with traditional ablation, and so fractionated lasers are commonly used for facial rejuvenation and acne scars.

Eradication of benign, pre-malignant and malignant lesions can also be achieved with ablative laser systems. Benign conditions such as seborrhoeic keratoses, dermatosis papulosa nigra, verrucae vulgaris, xanthelasma, sebaceous gland hyperplasia, syringoma, neurofibroma, rhinophyma and trichoepithelioma can be successfully treated. Symptomatic control can be achieved of localised resistant areas of Darier's disease, Hailey–Hailey disease and hidradenitis suppurativa. Treatment of pre-malignant and malignant skin lesions may be considered, including actinic cheilitis, superficial basal cell carcinoma and Bowen's disease. Ablative laser resurfacing is associated with significant morbidity until complete re-epithelialisation occurs.

Complications of ablative laser therapy

- **Post-treatment redness**: this often lasts for up to 14 days after ablative laser treatment. Occasionally the redness may be prolonged, lasting 3–6 months for no obvious reason, but it may be associated with higher fluence, multiple passes during treatment or secondary infection. If there is evidence of secondary infection, a skin swab for culture and sensitivity should be taken and antibiotics started. If there is persisting redness, consider the use of vascular lasers.
- **Infection**: increasing pain, serous drainage, erosion or crusting suggests infection. Infected or 'impetiginised' wounds should be treated with appropriate oral and topical antibiotics, after taking a swab for culture and sensitivity. Prophylactic antivirals should be considered for patients who are prone to reactivation of HSV infection, especially before full-face ablative treatment. Candida infection, although rare, can present with prolonged redness and pruritus.
- **Dyspigmentation**: transient post-inflammatory pigmentary change is often seen, especially in skin of colour. It tends to resolve spontaneously, but may require application of hydroquinone, a skin-lightening agent, along with careful sun protection, including the use of broad-spectrum (ultraviolet A and B) sunscreen. Hypopigmentation or depigmentation can occur if there is thermal injury of melanocytes. This pigmentary change can be prolonged or occasionally permanent: it may not be evident until several months after treatment and more commonly occurs in darker skin types.
- **Acneiform eruptions** and milia can develop in the post-operative period.

- **Contact dermatitis** is uncommon, but if suspected requires withdrawal of any suspected medicament and appropriate investigation. The compromised skin barrier in the treated area adds to the risk of contact dermatitis.
- **Scarring** (both atrophic and hypertrophic) can occur after treatment, especially at the high-risk sites of the nasal ala and jawline. The likelihood of scarring can be reduced by ensuring appropriate laser settings and by careful perioperative screening, such as exclusion of procedures on keloid-prone skin and performing a laser test spot.

Conclusions

Lasers have revolutionised medical and cosmetic dermatology, providing safe and reliable means for treating a wide variety of cutaneous pathologies. Laser surgery is constantly evolving with technological innovations. It is essential to remain updated with this ever-changing and expanding specialty. As a beginner it can be daunting to learn how to operate a laser system, and working with an experienced laser operator is essential. You are encouraged to attend a laser safety course and always to read the user manual to familiarise yourself with a specific laser.

Pearls and pitfalls

- The initial consultation visit should include discussions about realistic patient expectations. Detail the potential adverse outcomes and the need for multiple laser treatments, explain variable response at certain anatomical locations, incomplete response and chances of recurrences.
- Failure to establish the correct diagnosis and suitability for laser treatment before starting treatment can result in an adverse outcome with medicolegal complications.
- A representative area for a laser patch test with selected laser parameters should always be treated to assess skin reaction, patient response and cosmetic outcome.
- Initial and periodic digital photographic documentation should be performed in order to guide and assess the treatment efficacy.
- Using longer wavelengths, longer pulse durations, low fluences and more efficient cooling systems minimises adverse outcomes in patients with skin of colour.
- Prophylactic antivirals should be considered for patients who are prone to reactivation of HSV infection, especially before full-face ablative treatment.
- Incomplete control of background inflammation prior to initiation of vascular or ablative laser treatment can risk rebound inflammation, scarring and pigment change.

SCE Questions. See questions 70–72.

FURTHER READING AND KEY RESOURCES

Alexiades-Armenakas MR, Dover JS, Arndt KA. The spectrum of laser skin resurfacing: nonablative, fractional, and ablative laser resurfacing. *J Am Acad Dermatol* 2008; **58**:719–37.

Alster TS, Khoury R. Treatment of laser complications. *Facial Plast Surg* 2009; **25**:316–23.

Anderson RR, Parrish JA. Selective photothermolysis: precise microsurgery by selective absorption of pulsed radiation. *Science* 1983; **220**:524–7.

Chan HH, Wong DS, Ho WS et al. The use of pulsed dye laser for the prevention and treatment of hypertrophic scars in Chinese persons. *Dermatol Surg* 2004; **30**:987–94.

Gold MH, Berman B, Clementoni MT et al. Updated international clinical recommendations on scar management: part 1 – evaluating the evidence. *Dermatol Surg* 2014; **40**:817–24.

Gold MH, McGuire M, Mustoe TA et al. Updated international clinical recommendations on scar management: part 2 – algorithms for scar prevention and treatment. *Dermatol Surg* 2014; **40**:825–31.

Graber EM, Tanzi EL, Alster TS. Side effects and complications of fractional laser photothermolysis: experience with 961 treatments. *Dermatol Surg* 2008; **34**:301–7.

Hultman CS, Edkins RE, Lee CN et al. Shine on: review of laser- and light-based therapies for the treatment of burn scars. *Dermatol Res Pract* 2012; **2012**:243651.

Hultman CS, Yoshida S. Laser therapy for hypertrophic scars and keloids. https://www.uptodate.com/contents/laser-therapy-for-hypertrophic-scars-and-keloids.

Kelly KM, Choi B, McFarlane S et al. Description and analysis of treatments for port-wine stain birthmarks. *Arch Facial Plast Surg* 2005; **7**:287–94.

Kirby W, Desai A, Desai T et al. The Kirby–Desai scale: a proposed scale to assess tattoo-removal treatments. *J Clin Aesthet Dermatol* 2009; **2**:32–7.

Reish RG, Eriksson E. Scars: a review of emerging and currently available therapies. *Plast Reconstr Surg* 2008; **122**:1068–78.

Seidi N, Jagdeo J. Tattoo removal. Available at: https://www.uptodate.com/contents/tattoo-removal.

Vrijman C, van Drooge AM, Limpens J et al. Laser and intense pulsed light therapy for the treatment of hypertrophic scars: a systematic review. *Br J Dermatol* 2011; **165**:934–42.

Useful website

Cosmetic Practice Standards Authority. Available at: www.cosmeticstandards.org.uk.

Section 5

Subspecialty dermatology

23

Cutaneous allergy

Deirdre A. Buckley and Mahbub M.U. Chowdhury

Introduction

The skin has evolved over millions of years to provide an almost perfect defence between the body and the outside environment. The latter had remained largely stable over an unimaginable period of time. However, since the Iron Age, the outside environment has changed dramatically and it now contains thousands of chemicals never encountered during our evolution. The immune mechanisms 'designed' primarily to defend against microbes and other hostile organisms have been confused into attacking a myriad of new chemicals, resulting in inflammation of the skin, in other words allergic contact dermatitis (ACD). As our ancient skin-defence mechanisms react against the twenty-first-century environment, it is our job to identify which chemicals and exposures are to blame and to help calm the 'friendly fire' of our confused defences.

In addition to true allergens, the majority of the vast number of substances that provoke irritant contact dermatitis (ICD) were almost completely absent for most of our biological history. For example, soap was invented 'only' 5000 years ago by the Babylonians, so until then we lived in a soap-free world.

The clinical challenges of managing people with cutaneous allergy combine detective work, a special knowledge of the environment, and an understanding of specialised investigation techniques and methods of protection. This unique combination of skills can lead to very satisfying and rewarding clinical outcomes for your patients in the patch test clinic.

Not all cutaneous reactions to exposure to external agents will conform to a classic irritant or allergic dermatitis pattern. Many morphologically different skin reactions can occur. These include acne, urticaria, lichenoid eruptions, hyper- or hypopigmentation and dermatitis (eczema). An example of irritant dermatitis would be exposure of the skin to acids or bases including soaps. The reaction is due to direct local damage to the skin rather than an allergy. In an allergic reaction the skin is sensitised to an agent, for example nickel, and subsequent exposure to this agent tends to cause ACD.

Dermatology Training: The Essentials. Edited by Mahbub M.U. Chowdhury, Tamara W. Griffiths and Andrew Y. Finlay.
© 2022 The British Association of Dermatologists. Published 2022 by John Wiley & Sons Ltd.
Companion website: www.wiley.com/go/chowdhury/dermatologytraining

The mechanism of the reaction differs between ACD and ICD. ACD is a type 4 or 'delayed hypersensitivity' reaction, while ICD is the result of localised toxic effects of an irritant on the skin. To complicate matters, in chronic forms both ICD and ACD can look quite similar clinically, are difficult to differentiate and often may coexist, for example in the case of hand dermatitis.

ICD accounts for approximately 80% of all contact dermatitis, while ACD accounts for the remaining 20%. This is often in contrast with what you or your patient may think, as patients frequently suspect an allergy.

Allergy tests include prick testing (for immediate-type allergy: type 1 or acute hypersensitivity reaction) and patch testing (for ACD: type 4 or delayed hypersensitivity reaction).

Occupational skin diseases

Occupational skin diseases account for 35% of all occupationally related diseases. The different manifestations of these skin diseases can have a significant impact on workers' quality of life, with physical, psychological and financial hardships.

ICD and ACD are the most common occupational skin diseases, with atopy as an important cofactor; over 2000 occupational allergens are known.

Occupational contact dermatitis

Occupational contact dermatitis can be caused by irritants (e.g. direct contact with caustic agents) or allergens (e.g. rubber glove allergy).

ICD can be divided into several types:

- **Acute ICD** results from a single contact with a strong chemical substance causing an acute strong reaction similar to a burn, for example a reaction to a caustic cleaning chemical.
- **Acute delayed ICD** is a delayed reaction, with the ICD developing 8–24 hours after the initial contact, for example alkaline cement 'burns'.
- **Cumulative ICD** is the most frequent type of ICD and results from repeated exposure to irritants such as soaps, shampoos, detergents and mild acids and alkalis. This can result in erythema, dryness and cracking, and irritant hand dermatitis. For example, in hairdressers and bar workers a frequent clinical picture is of dermatitis starting under the rings and in the finger web spaces, and usually spreading over the dorsa of the hands. During the COVID-19 pandemic, cumulative ICD was very frequent in healthcare workers (and the public), associated with frequent handwashing.
- **Pustular and acneiform ICD** can follow exposure to oils, greases and tars. Atopic patients and people who have previously had acne are most prone. It can also be seen following repeated occlusion from a helmet or mask, such as the mask-related acne that occurred in healthcare and other workers during the COVID-19 pandemic.

The diagnosis of ICD is usually made by the history (exposures, type of occupation), by typical clinical features (e.g. dryness, web space dermatitis, absence of vesicles) and by exclusion of ACD. The commonest manifestation of ICD is hand dermatitis, which is discussed later in this chapter.

Allergic contact dermatitis

ACD occurs much less frequently than ICD, but is of great importance. It can often force a worker to change jobs, as protective measures frequently fail. ACD must be differentiated from atopic dermatitis, psoriasis, pustular eruptions, herpes simplex and zoster infections, fungal infections and ICD. Patch testing must be thorough, as patients may not realise that they have had contact with potential allergens, and testing to the patient's own items is essential. Examples of allergens encountered in various occupations are shown in Table 23.1.

Occupational contact urticaria

Occupational contact urticaria accounts for 5–10% of occupational skin disease. It is important not to miss this clinically; it can be confirmed with appropriate investigations such as prick testing, specific IgE tests and repeat open application tests (ROATs).

Contact urticaria (CU) is a transient weal-and-flare reaction appearing after contact with certain specific chemicals (haptens) and proteins. These reactions develop within 10–60 minutes of the skin contact and resolve within 2–24 hours. CU can be missed if it worsens pre-existing dermatitis or urticaria, and has two main mechanisms: immunological (IgE mediated) and non-immunological. It is more frequent in those with atopy. Certain occupations and hobbies convey an extra risk of CU (Table 23.2).

CU caused by natural rubber latex has been well documented in association with glove use in healthcare workers and any other workers who wear latex gloves throughout the day (Table 23.3). The cutaneous reactions vary from mild erythema with itching at the site of contact to severe vesicular and delayed exacerbations of eczema. Anaphylactic reactions, occasionally leading to death, have been associated with prolonged mucosal contact with latex proteins, such as surgical gloves being used within the abdominal cavity. The most useful element of the history in establishing CU to latex is whether the individual can blow up a party balloon without symptoms. If they can do this, allergy to latex is much less likely. Since 1995 there has been a dramatic reduction in latex allergy, due to banning of powdered latex gloves in hospitals. There is now better awareness in workers, strict implementation of latex avoidance policies, and vigilant occupational health departments who refer early to dermatology cutaneous allergy experts for advice and investigation. Chlorhexidine is now a much more common cause of intraoperative anaphylaxis. Polyethylene glycols have been recently recognised as a source of CU, especially those of higher molecular weight.

In general, the most common type of CU is non-immunological, requiring no previous sensitisation. With sufficient provocation, nearly all exposed persons will develop a reaction. It is due

Table 23.1 Examples of allergens encountered in various occupations

Occupation	Allergens
Agriculture workers	Rubber, oats, barley, animal feed, veterinary medications, cement, plants, pesticides, wood preservatives
Bakers and confectioners	Flavours and spices, orange, lemon, essential oils, dyes, ammonium persulfate and benzoyl peroxide
Bartenders	Orange, lemon, lime, flavours, preservatives
Beauticians	Methacrylates, cyanoacrylates, fragrances, dyes
Butchers	Nickel, sawdust, animal proteins
Cleaners	Rubber gloves, preservatives, fragrances
Construction workers	Chromates, cobalt, rubber and leather gloves, resins, woods
Cooks and caterers	Foods, onions, garlic, spices, flavours, rubber gloves, sodium metabisulfite, lauryl and octyl gallate, formaldehyde, preservatives
Dentists and dental technicians	Local anaesthetics, mercury, methacrylates, eugenol, disinfectants, rubber
Electricians	Fluxes, resins, rubber
Electroplaters	Nickel, chromium, cobalt
Embalmers	Formaldehyde
Florists and gardeners	Plants, pesticides, rubber gloves
Foundry workers	Phenol- and urea-formaldehyde resins, colophonium
Hairdressers	Dyes, persulfates, nickel, perfumes, rubber gloves, formaldehyde, preservatives
Homemakers	Rubber gloves, foods, spices, flavours, nickel, chromates, polishes, preservatives
Jewellers	Epoxy resin, metals, soldering fluxes, cyanoacrylates
Massage therapists	Fragrances in essential oils, preservatives
Mechanics	Rubber gloves, chromates, epoxy resin, antifreeze, cyanoacrylates
Medical personnel	Rubber gloves, anaesthetics, antibiotics, antiseptics (e.g. chlorhexidine), phenothiazines, formaldehyde, glutaraldehyde, chloroxylenol, fragrances, cyanoacrylates, methacrylates
Metalworkers	Nickel, chromates, additives (e.g. fragrances and preservatives) in some cutting oils
Office workers	Rubber, nickel, glue
Painters	Turpentine, cobalt, chromates, polyester resins, formaldehyde, epoxy resin, adhesives, isothiazolinones
Plastics workers	Hardeners, phenolic resins, polyurethanes, acrylics, plasticisers, sodium metabisulfite
Printers	Methacrylates, nickel, chromates, cobalt, colophonium, formaldehyde, turpentine
Rubber workers	Rubber chemicals, dyes, colophonium
Shoemakers	Glues, leather, rubber, turpentine, octylisothiazolinone
Tannery workers	Chromates, formaldehyde, tanning agents, fungicides, dyes
Textile workers	Formaldehyde resins, dyes, chromates, nickel

Table 23.2 Causes of occupational contact urticaria

Antimicrobials: chlorhexidine, triclosan, sodium hypochlorite, chloroxylenol (Dettol) – healthcare workers, patients, cleaners

Ammonium persulfate – bakers, hairdressers

Natural rubber latex – healthcare workers, dentists, vets

Animal proteins: cow dander, semen, insects, bait maggots, cockroaches – farmers, fishers, animal keepers, veterinary workers

Acrylates/epoxy resins – electronics workers, dentists, beauticians

Foods: milk, fish (squid), chapatti flour, wheat and barley (beer), raw fruits and vegetables, garlic – chefs, bar workers, food industry workers

Enzymes: proteases, papain, alpha-amylase – pharmaceutical industry and manufacturing workers

Table 23.3 Latex allergy

Risk factors: occupation, multiple surgeries, mucosal exposure, hand eczema, atopy, latex-fruit syndrome, e.g. cross-reaction with avocado, banana, kiwi, chestnut and raw potato

Investigations: specific IgE for Hev b1, b3, b5, b6; prick test to latex solution and to a latex balloon; glove use test (if diagnosis is uncertain, previous reactions are mild and prick test is negative)

Table 23.4 Causes of non-immunological and immunological contact urticaria

Non-immunological contact urticaria (NICU)

Myroxolon pereirae (Balsam of Peru), benzoic acid, sodium benzoate

Cinnamic alcohol, cinnamal

Sorbic acid

Menthol

Foods: raw fish, meat, vegetables

Nettle (*Urtica dioica*)

Animals: caterpillars, moths, jellyfish, sea anemones

Immunological contact urticaria (ICU)

Natural rubber latex

Antibiotics: penicillins, cephalosporins, gentamicin

Foods: apple, potato, shellfish, squid, pork, beef, lamb

Animals: e.g. animal dander and saliva, cow placenta, cockroaches

Plants: e.g. grass pollen

Hair cosmetic products: ammonium persulfate, *para*-phenylenediamine (PPD), *para*-toluenediamine (PTD)

Sunscreen: benzophenone-3

Antimicrobials: chlorhexidine, benzoic acid, parabens

Metals: nickel, aluminium, platinum

Table 23.5 Contact urticaria syndrome

Stage 1: Localised urticaria

Stage 2: Generalised urticaria

Stage 3: Urticaria plus extracutaneous symptoms, e.g. conjunctivitis, rhinitis, gastrointestinal, angio-oedema

Stage 4: Systemic anaphylactic shock

Based on Süß H *et al. Contact Dermatitis* 2019; **81**:341–53.

to release of vasoactive substances (histamine, prostaglandin, leukotrienes, substance P) without the involvement of immunological processes. The reaction remains localised and does not cause systemic manifestations or generalised urticaria. The concentration, substance and skin site will determine the reaction strength. Substances known to trigger this type of CU include alcohols and *Myroxolon pereirae* (Balsam of Peru) in healthcare workers (this balsam's constituents are cinnamic acid, cinnamal and sodium benzoate); sorbic acid; fruits and vegetables in cooks; and nettles, caterpillar hair, moths and other insects in gardeners. Other more exotic exposures triggering non-immunological CU include corals, jellyfish and sea anemones. Some immediate cosmetic reactions, such as itching, papules and erythema, represent non-immunological CU to sorbic acid and sorbates, benzoic acid and benzoates, cinnamates, and/or menthol in cosmetics (Table 23.4).

Immunological (allergic) CU is caused by an antigen–antibody type 1 IgE-mediated hypersensitivity reaction and requires previous sensitisation. Raised serum-specific IgE antibody levels have been demonstrated in immunological CU. Causes of immunological CU include natural rubber latex; medications including antibiotics (e.g. penicillins, cephalosporins and gentamicin); foods (e.g. potato, apple, flour, fish and meat); animal and plant products (e.g. animal dander and saliva, cow placenta,

cockroaches and grass pollen); cosmetics (e.g. hair bleaching products and rarely *para*-phenylenediamine); sunscreens (e.g. benzophenone-3); antimicrobials and antiseptics (e.g. benzoic acid, parabens and chlorhexidine); metals (e.g. aluminium, nickel and platinum salts); and chemicals (e.g. isocyanates) (Table 23.4).

The stages of the CU syndrome were well described in 1975 by Maibach and Johnson (Table 23.5). The contact urticant (antigen) penetrates the epidermis and reacts with specific IgE antibodies on dermal mast cells with early-phase release of histamine, serotonin and mast cell proteases. This is followed by late-phase mediators such as the cytokines interleukin (IL)-4, IL-5, IL-13; chemokines; and newly synthesised mediators such as prostaglandin 2 (PGD2), platelet activating factor (PAF) and leukotrienes C and D. This sequence of mediator release will determine the degree of skin symptoms, including redness and oedema. Other symptoms may include conjunctivitis, rhinitis, asthma and angio-oedema. Anaphylactic shock is extremely rare, but can occur, for example with immediate immunological CU to hair dyes and perming agents.

Protein contact dermatitis may be a manifestation of immunological CU, presenting with chronic hand and fingertip eczema associated with urticarial and vesicular flares. Burning and stinging occur within a few minutes of handling the allergen, such as grains (barley, wheat), enzymes (proteases) and foods (garlic, raw potatoes and other fruits and vegetables, raw meat, raw fish and shellfish). The eczema then flares a few hours later and lasts for days. The mechanism is likely to be a combined immediate type 1 and delayed type 4 allergic reaction to proteins. Prick-to-prick tests with the specific raw food are positive, and patch tests with delayed readings are negative. Most patients with protein contact dermatitis can consume, without symptoms, the same food when cooked. Gloves should be worn when handling the raw food.

The identification of occupational skin disease such as contact allergy and CU needs a high level of clinical acumen and detailed occupational history taking, clinical examination and appropriate investigations such as patch testing. Testing for CU includes blood tests for specific IgE and/or prick tests. In addition, patch test chamber testing (open or closed; with or without prior scratching of the skin at the test site) on non-affected and affected skin can be done sequentially. Readings are carried out at 20 minutes, 1 hour and 48 hours. Testing of several controls is important with new allergens.

Identification and avoidance of the main causative allergens are essential, in addition to supportive measures such as non-sedating antihistamines, topical corticosteroids and calcineurin inhibitors. Rarely, in cases of anaphylaxis where the allergen cannot be avoided, an adrenaline pen for emergency use may be required.

Prick testing

This test is primarily used to detect allergens involved in the occurrence of type 1 or acute hypersensitivity reactions. The classic example of this is a contact urticarial reaction to an allergen such as a nut or latex. Prick testing to allergens such as house dust mites, moulds, pets and pollen is used in the investigation of asthma and hay fever. Prick testing to foods such as cows' milk protein, eggs, soya, wheat, fish, shellfish and nuts is used to investigate type 1 food allergy.

In the dermatology clinic, prick testing is used most commonly in the assessment of suspected latex allergy and to investigate protein contact dermatitis, where raw foods such as vegetables, fruit, meat and fish cause immediate itching and vesiculation of palms and fingers, and a delayed flare of pre-existing hand eczema. In type 1 hypersensitivity the antigen (allergen) binds to a specific IgE antibody on the surface of the dermal mast cells. This causes degranulation of the mast cells and release of histamine and other vasoactive substances, leading to dermal oedema (a 'weal'), surrounded by a reddish flare.

Technique

In prick testing, an individual sterile lancet for each allergen is used to gently prick the skin through a drop of solution containing the allergen. This allows a very small quantity of allergen into the dermis. The test is usually carried out on the forearm, although with young children the back may be more suitable so they cannot see what is happening. The test is not painful and results are available within 10–20 minutes. If testing with an allergen that is known to trigger anaphylaxis, ensure full resuscitation facilities are available.

Solutions containing antigens are available commercially for a number of allergens, including latex, house dust (and other) mites, animal fur, feathers, moulds, trees, grasses, weeds and numerous food products. In most cases, clinics have purified commercial liquid forms of the allergen, but sometimes, for example in the case of foods, the patient may be asked to bring in a fresh sample for more reliable results. Different foods (for example nuts, raw vegetables, fruits, meat and fish) can be brought into clinic in labelled small plastic containers with lids to prevent cross-contamination.

Interpretation of prick tests

A positive prick test occurs when the skin at the site of introduction of the allergen becomes pruritic and red with subsequent development of a weal (Figure 23.1). The weal reaches its maximum size in about 15–20 minutes and the reaction fades within a few hours. The larger the weal, the more likely that the patient is allergic to the allergen, but weal size does not predict the severity of the clinical reaction. Every patient should also be tested to a negative and a positive control. The negative control is a physiological saline solution, to which a response is not expected. However, if a patient reacts to the negative control, then this will indicate that the skin is, for whatever reason, extremely sensitive (for example has active urticaria or dermographism) and that the results need to be interpreted with the utmost care. The positive control solution is histamine, to which everyone is expected to react.

A negative response to a prick test solution usually indicates that the patient is not sensitive to that allergen. Negative reactions may, however, occur if the patient is taking antihistamines or other medications that block the effect of histamine. Patients should be asked to avoid taking any antihistamines a few days prior to the test to minimise false negatives. The skin in some elderly people may not be capable of reacting, and some unexplained negative reactions occur, despite a clear clinical history of immediate hypersensitivity on exposure.

(a)

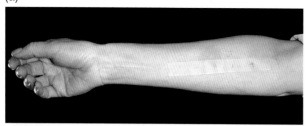

(b)

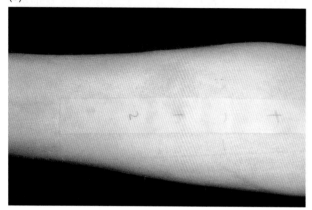

Figure 23.1 (a) Positive prick test to latex. (b) Close-up view of a positive reaction. © Medical Illustration Cardiff and Vale UHB.

For reasons not yet fully understood, prick testing with commercially available food allergens is less reliable than with some other commercial allergens such as house dust mite and pollens. False negative reactions can occur to the commercial liquid despite concomitant positive reactions to the fresh food. Testing with the actual food (e.g. fresh fruits, vegetables and nuts) is done as a prick-to-prick test, where the lancet is first pricked through the skin or outer surface of the fruit, vegetable or nut, and then into the patient's skin. This may be carried out instead of using a commercial solution, or in parallel with the testing solution.

A blood test to look for specific IgE (formerly known as a RAST test or radioallergosorbent test) can be used instead of a prick test in the following scenarios:

- The patient has a significant risk of a severe anaphylactic reaction, so prick testing would be considered unsuitable (for example, a history of severe latex allergy or an anaphylactic reaction to insect venom).
- Extensive eczema makes prick testing impractical.
- Antihistamine medication cannot be stopped because of the severity of the symptoms.
- Unusual and rare allergens are suspected.

A positive specific IgE test may help to confirm the allergy in the presence of a typical history. Unfortunately, the finding of raised specific IgE (often to multiple allergens) is common in many atopic patients with raised total IgE, without apparent clinical significance. Such results should be interpreted with extreme caution. Conversely, a negative specific IgE test cannot completely exclude an allergy in the presence of a suggestive clinical history, and a prick test may also become necessary. Occasionally both specific IgE and prick testing may be negative in a patient with a highly suggestive clinical history, in whom the allergy may be confirmed by double-blind placebo-controlled challenge to the specific allergen.

Patch testing

Jadassohn first described the technique of patch testing 100 years ago. Since then, the technique has been continually improved and further developed, with many more allergens identified and tested. Patch testing is the gold standard for diagnosing ACD and the concept remains the same today. Allergens are applied to the skin, in a controlled fashion, in order to reproduce any possible allergic contact reaction and thus diagnose ACD.

ACD can affect people of any age group, and the frequency of allergy to specific allergens can vary depending on previous or current exposure. Often multiple exposures are required to induce sensitisation, a process that can happen gradually over many years. Fragrance allergy becomes more frequent in people regardless of sex with increasing age, and hence the cumulative effect of repeated exposures. Nickel allergy is more common in women than in men because of their greater exposure to jewellery. Similarly, there is variability in different regions due to different habits and government legislation, for example allergy to preservatives in cosmetics. The work environment plays an important role, as workers can be exposed to different agents and can be sensitised. These occupational contact allergies can be quite specific and unique to these work groups (Table 23.1).

One series of allergens could not possibly cover all possible clinically relevant allergens. In addition, the relevant allergens vary according to country, occupation and hobbies, and also with the body site affected. Some indications for patch testing are listed in Table 23.6.

Table 23.6 Indications for patch testing

Atopic dermatitis refractory to standard treatment
Hand dermatitis
Other dermatoses, e.g. discoid, stasis, seborrhoeic (if refractory to treatment or unusual distribution)
Specific-site dermatitis, e.g. eyelids, foot, perineal, fingertip, lip, axillary
Occupational dermatitis
Clear history of reacting to a product

Table 23.7 Important history points in patch testing clinic

Site of onset of dermatitis
Duration and spread of dermatitis
Relieving or exacerbating factors, including holidays and work
Past history
Atopy, psoriasis, suspected nickel or perfume allergy
Presence of vesicles or blisters
Response to any treatments
Occupational details
Potential allergen or irritant exposures
Personal protection, e.g. gloves, overalls
Handwashing frequency
Barrier creams and soaps
Hobbies (adults and children)
Potential exposures, e.g. oils, glues, plants, gloves in sport

It is essential to take a good history, and the clinician should ask questions about exposures at work and home, including hobbies. A standardised questionnaire or pro forma may facilitate a thorough history that does not miss relevant exposures (Table 23.7). The aim is to reach a provisional diagnosis prior to patch testing. This should be a stimulating intellectual challenge for you as the clinician and is part of the 'magic' of patch testing. The potential reward for you and your patient is to formally identify the suspect substance through patch testing. This provides the patient with the prospect of complete cure, and you the clinician with the satisfaction of having helped your patient, while confirming your pre-patch test theory. If an unexpected and/or additional substance tests positive, the task of identifying potential sources of exposure and assessing clinical relevance provides a further challenge. Hence, the more one learns about patch testing and other allergens, the more rewarding and interesting it becomes. There is no substitute for time spent in clinic with an enthusiastic and experienced patch testing expert.

Technique

Patch testing aims to reproduce, in miniature, an eczematous eruption. The perfect patch test should give no false positives or false negatives and no adverse reactions or sensitisation to the allergens. The technique initially varied considerably in different centres. However, now the recommended series, methodology of testing and interpretation of positive tests are standardised, using guidelines from the British Society for Cutaneous Allergy (BSCA) and the European Society of Contact Dermatitis (ESCD). The BSCA and British Association of Dermatologists (BAD) jointly recommend minimum service standards for patch test units.

Individual allergens are bought commercially and are placed (by squeezing from a tube or dropping from a bottle) in 'chambers' (concave disks). Finn Chambers® (SmartPractice, Phoenix, AZ, USA; Figure 23.2), 8-mm aluminium disks that provide good occlusion because of their design, are commonly used. They are available in strips of 10 on an adhesive tape (Scanpor) backing. Other similar brands of chamber made from plastic with a square design are also available. A group of filled chamber strips containing a particular group ('series') of allergens constitutes a prepared patch test series. The relevant allergen series to be tested are selected according to the history, occupation and location of the problem, for example a hairdressing series in a hairdresser with hand dermatitis. Preparing patch test allergens is time-consuming and requires space and concentration, and is best carried out by a skilled and experienced nurse.

The ideal concentration of the allergen chosen should be below the irritant concentration but above the allergic concentration. As the irritant threshold can vary in different populations, the standardised strength used in the patch tests has been reached by trial and error over many years. Despite the best

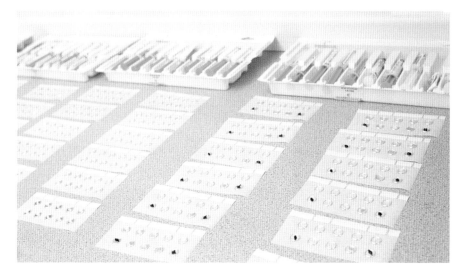

Figure 23.2 Finn Chamber allergens ready to be applied to the back.
© Medical Illustration Cardiff and Vale UHB.

efforts to quantify the 'right' concentration, false positives and false negatives may still occur. This is inevitable, as there is a range of thresholds within the normal population and this may also vary with skin colour. Skin of colour may be more prone to follicular and papular irritant and allergic reactions, with persistence of post-inflammatory hyperpigmentation and lichenification in some cases.

New or unknown allergens should ideally be tested in 10–20 control individuals. Reference textbooks may need to be consulted to determine the appropriate diluent and concentration for safe testing. Unidentified chemicals from the workplace should not be tested without seeking further information as to suitability for testing, such as from material safety data sheets. It should be documented in the case notes for each patient that they have been offered a patient information leaflet on patch testing, which they have read and understood, ideally the joint BSCA/BAD patient information leaflet. This will also inform the patient that their results may be recorded on an electronic patient record and that an anonymised database of results may be used for national audit to determine trends for allergen positivity, for example allowing uncommon allergens to be removed from test series.

After the appropriate patch test series have been adequately prepared, they should then be placed onto the skin, usually of the upper back (Figure 23.3). The patient should not (i) be pregnant or breastfeeding; (ii) have extensive eczema or sunburn on the test area; (iii) have had phototherapy within the last six weeks; or (iv) have applied topical corticosteroids to the patch test sites for 72 hours. Systemic corticosteroids (prednisolone 15 mg/day

or more) and other immunosuppressive agents should be avoided (if possible) during testing. Antihistamines should be continued, particularly in patients who are dermographic or have spontaneous urticaria, as the patient may otherwise become concerned about an adverse reaction to patch testing due to the formation of spontaneous weals. However, antihistamines should be avoided if testing for CU, or if prick testing.

Placement of the patch test series requires some training. As they need to remain on the back for two days, the patches are placed on the back with the adhesive tape to which the chambers are already stuck and then reinforced with more low-irritant adhesive tape such as Scanpor®. A diagram mapping where the patch tests are placed is recorded for future reference.

The patient is then asked to keep the back as dry as possible, avoiding excessive sweating and vigorous exercise, to ensure the patches remain secure until the second visit. It is a good tip to advise patients to wear dark clothing to avoid staining, with a shirt that buttons up the front, to avoid loosening of patches while dressing and undressing. When the patient returns two days (48 hours) later, the patches are inspected to check whether they have remained in place, and whether there was adequate contact between the chambers and the back.

As the patches are removed their position is re-marked in order to identify the location of particular allergens, using a skin marker pen. Any positive reactions are scored according to the international grading system (Table 23.8). The patient is then asked to keep their back dry until the final reading, which can be performed between three days and two weeks after initial application of the

(a)

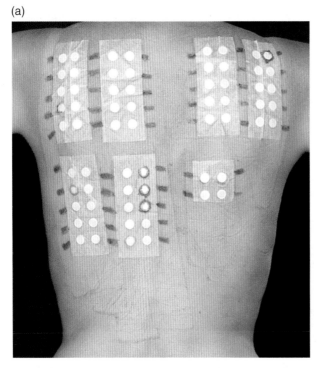

(b)

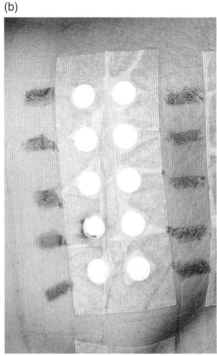

Figure 23.3 (a) Patches applied to the patient's back. (b) One set of 10 allergens applied to the back. © Medical Illustration Cardiff and Vale UHB.

Table 23.8 Scheme for interpretation of patch testing results

–	Negative reaction
?	Doubtful reaction
+	Weak reaction (palpable, non-vesicular)
++	Strong reaction (oedematous or vesicular)
+++	Extreme reaction (ulcerative or bullous)
IR	Irritant reaction
NT	Not tested

allergens, most commonly at day 4. At the second reading, the diagram map is used and any positive palpable reactions are read and graded. This grading is less straightforward in skin of colour, with difficulty detecting redness and more varied irritant reaction patterns, for example follicular or papular rather than a wrinkled rough glazed appearance.

If photopatch testing is being carried out, a photoallergen series is applied in duplicate to the patient's back, at the same time as the other series are being applied. When the patient returns two days later, the patches are removed and one set of photoallergens is irradiated with 5 J/cm² of ultraviolet A. Any differences between the two sets of photoallergens are noted on day 4. If an allergen shows an equally strongly positive reaction with or without irradiation, then the patient has contact allergy to that hapten. If the irradiated set shows a stronger reaction, the patient has contact and photocontact allergy to the hapten. If the reaction appears only on the irradiated side, the patient has photocontact allergy alone.

Positive reactions are caused by previous allergen exposure, which could have been at any time in the patient's life, and so may or may not be relevant to the current presenting problem. It is important to remember that a patient may have contact with these allergens at home, at work or in a recreational setting. Often the relevance is not clear at first and may require some detective work by the patient and clinician. Nevertheless, the names and information sheets of the positive allergens should be given to the patient. These information sheets are available online from the BSCA. The patient should try to avoid the positive allergens, although 100% avoidance may be impossible, for example for fragrances and preservatives.

In a perfect situation, only true positive and relevant reactions should occur and all allergens would be identified. However, practically, recording and interpreting the results may be difficult, as there may be false positive, doubtful positive or irritant reactions. Moreover, an important allergen may have been missed in the patch testing, if it was not identified from the initial clinical history.

In doubtful relevance, a repeat open application test is recommended. The test material, for example a leave-on cosmetic, can be applied by the patient to the skin of the antecubital fossa twice daily for two weeks, without any covering. In most cases of contact allergy, an itchy papular dermatitis will develop.

Occasionally, patients are unable to attend on one or both of their planned visits for readings. Patients should then be asked to arrange removal of the allergens carefully after 48 hours, and, if possible, to arrange clear overview photographs of their back and close-up photographs of each group of 10 allergens. These photographs may be used by the clinician for a 'virtual' reading. Although this is not as accurate as an actual reading (tests cannot be palpated, and repeat tests or more extensive test series cannot be added), it is a compromise solution in extenuating circumstances such as during the COVID-19 pandemic.

Patch test series and allergens

The International Contact Dermatitis Research Group (ICDRG) was founded in 1967 with the main aim of providing standardisation for routine patch testing. A standardised international patch test series was agreed in the 1960s, to test individual patients to the most common allergens encountered in the environment.

National groups have since been formed in many countries to develop local baseline or standard series relevant to the most frequent allergens encountered in that country. The North American Comprehensive Baseline series (80 allergens) and the European Comprehensive Baseline series (43 allergens) are the major standard series used around the world. The BSCA baseline series used in the UK (50 allergens) is shown, with brief details about the allergens, in Table 23.9. The BSCA facial (cosmetic) series (Table 23.10) and other series recommended by the BSCA, including fragrances, medicaments, steroids, hairdressing, methacrylates, shoe, rubber and photopatch, are available on the BSCA website.

Using a standard series has several advantages. Often, the patient omits an important part of the history, which they can later recall after the allergen is identified. Furthermore, if a patient is seen in another clinic, the attending doctor will know what allergens were tested and this therefore avoids miscommunication. Using a standard series allows comparative studies between different centres and potentially between different countries. The disadvantages include a possible downgrading of the importance of good history taking and potentially inducing sensitisation (low risk) to some of the additional allergens tested.

Extra series are frequently tested in addition to the baseline (standard) series, as deemed necessary by the investigator. Choosing these supplementary series depends on the patient's occupation, hobbies, habits and other exposures, and is facilitated by a very thorough history. There are many patch test series available commercially (Table 23.11). Allergens are available from several commercial companies, including Chemotechnique (Vellinge, Sweden) and allergEAZE (Bio-Diagnostics, Upton-upon-Severn, UK).

Recording and interpreting patch test results

This is usually the difficult part of the consultation and requires considerable skill and experience. Normally four days after the patch test series are put on the skin, the final results are read.

Table 23.9 2020 British Society for Cutaneous Allergy Baseline (Standard) Series (all diluted in petrolatum unless otherwise stated; aq. is aqueous, diluted in water)

	Reagent name	Concentration	Main uses
1	Potassium dichromate	0.5%	Tanning leather, cement
2	Neomycin sulfate	20.0%	Antibiotic in creams and drops
3	Thiuram mix	1.0%	Rubber accelerator, fungicides
4	*para*-Phenylenediamine	1.0%	Azo dye intermediate, hair dye
5	Cobalt chloride	1.0%	Metal
6	Caine mix III	10.0%	Local anaesthetic in creams, gel
7	Formaldehyde	2.0% aq.	Disinfectant, preservative
8	Colophonium	20.0%	Pine resin, adhesives, polishes
9	Quinoline mix	6.0%	Antimicrobial in creams, drops
10	*Myroxylon pereirae* (Balsam of Peru)	25.0%	Fragrance and flavouring agent
11	*N*-Isopropyl-*N*-phenyl-4-phenylenediamine	0.1%	Black rubber chemical
12	Lanolin alcohol	30.0%	Ointment base in creams
13	Mercapto mix	2.0%	Rubber additives
14	Epoxy resin, bisphenol A	1.0%	Resin in adhesives, paint
15	Parabens mix	16.0%	Preservatives in creams
16	4-*tert*-Butylphenol formaldehyde resin	1.0%	Resin in adhesives
17	Fragrance mix I	8.0%	Fragrances
18	Quaternium 15 (Dowicil 200)	1.0%	Formaldehyde releaser
19	Nickel sulfate	5.0%	Metal
20	Methylisothiazolinone/methylchloroisothiazolinone	0.02% aq.	Preservative in oils, cosmetics
21	Mercaptobenzothiazole	2.0%	Rubber chemical
22	Amerchol L101	50.0%	Lanolin product, emulsifier
23	Sesquiterpene lactone mix	0.1%	Plants
24	*p*-Chloro-*m*-cresol	1.0%	Fungicide in creams
25	2-Bromo-2-nitropropane-1,3-diol (Bronopol)	0.5%	Formaldehyde releaser
26	Cetearyl alcohol	20.0%	Emulsifier in creams
27	Sodium fusidate	2.0%	Antibiotic in creams, drops
28	Tixocortol-21-pivalate	1.0%	Hydrocortisone
29	Budesonide	0.1%	Non-halogenated topical steroids
30	Imidazolidinyl urea (Germal 115)	2.0%	Formaldehyde releaser
31	Diazolidinyl urea (Germal II)	2.0%	Formaldehyde releaser
32	Methyldibromoglutaronitrile (MDBGN)	0.3%	Preservative in coolants
33	Tree moss absolute	1.0%	Fragrance and lichen

Table 23.9 (Continued)

	Reagent name	Concentration	Main uses
34	4-Chloro-3,5-xylenol (PCMX)	0.5%	Preservative in coolants, creams
35	Carba mix	3.0%	Rubber chemical
36	Disperse blue mix 106/124	1.0%	Textile dye
37	Fragrance mix II	14.0%	Fragrances
38	Lyral	5.0%	Fragrance
39	Compositae mix II	2.5%	Plants
40	Methylisothiazolinone	0.2% aq.	Preservative in cosmetics, paints
41	Sodium metabisulfite	1.0%	Preservative in foods, creams
42	Linalool hydroperoxides	1.0%	Fragrance
43	Linalool hydroperoxides	0.5%	Fragrance
44	Limonene hydroperoxides	0.3%	Fragrance
45	Limonene hydroperoxides	0.2%	Fragrance
46	2-Hydroxyethyl methacrylate (HEMA)	2.0%	Acrylic and gel nails
47	Benzisothiazolinone	0.1%	Preservative in paint, detergents
48	Octylisothiazolinone	0.1%	Preservative in paints, leather
49	Decyl glucoside	5.0%	Surfactant
50	Lauryl glucoside	3.0%	Surfactant

The responses are seen and graded as positive (Figure 23.4), negative or irritant (Table 23.8). Interpret patch tests in skin of colour with care, as redness may not be obvious; careful palpation of the potential reaction sites is needed, as papules, swelling and warmth can be other classic signs of inflammation. Doubtful or uncertain reactions may need to be repeated to check reproducibility, including serial dilution testing. Testing of control patients may be necessary, and also repeat open application tests can be useful, as described earlier.

True positive reactions are likely to exhibit a crescendo effect, where the reaction appears or becomes more marked between the first and second readings. Irritant reactions in white skin tend to be well demarcated, red and flat, and show a diminishing effect between the first and second readings. Pustular reactions also usually indicate irritation and are common with metal allergens such as nickel and cobalt, occurring mainly in atopic patients. Some allergens are much more prone than others to cause irritant reactions, especially in atopic patients (Table 23.12).

To diagnose ACD, two significant steps should occur:

- Identify a positive reaction to the patch test.
- Demonstrate the clinical relevance.

Relevance can be determined through the process of reviewing exposures and products. Allergens may have past or current relevance. For example, a positive colophony (colophonium) patch test may have past relevance if the patient previously had a reaction to the adhesive of sticky plaster, but not current relevance if the present problem is unrelated. On the other hand, a positive colophonium patch test may be of current relevance in a patient with a generalised eczematous eruption who had cut a pine hedge the weekend before this developed.

It is worth keeping in mind that some allergens such as gold, neomycin and topical steroids may be late reactants (Table 23.13) and may become positive after more than four days, so in some cases it might be worth arranging for a further reading the following week. Where another visit is not possible, it is very useful to advise patients to take a photograph of their patch test sites if they develop a late reaction, both from a distance to locate the site that has become positive and in close-up, to show in detail the morphology of the reaction such as vesicles. Such photographs may be emailed to the clinician for interpretation.

Relevance may be inapparent if the patient has a reaction but no identifiable exposure to the allergen. There are a few particular allergens for which relevance can be hard to determine,

Table 23.10 2019 British Society for Cutaneous Allergy Facial (Cosmetic) Series (all diluted in petrolatum unless otherwise stated; aq. is aqueous, diluted in water)

Reagent name	Concentration
Panthenol	5.0%
Decyl glucoside	5.0%
Tosylamide/formaldehyde resin	10.0%
Octyl gallate	0.25%
Cocamidopropyl betaine	1.0% aq.
Propylene glycol	5.0%
tert-Butylhydroquinone (TBHQ)	1.0%
Dodecyl gallate	0.25%
Propyl gallate	1.0%
Hydroabietyl alcohol (Abitol)	10.0%
Benzyl alcohol	10.0%
3-(Dimethylamino)-1-propylamine	1.0% aq.
Triethanolamine (trolamine)	2.0%
Benzophenone-4	2.0%
Ethylenediaminetetraacetic acid (EDTA) disodium salt dihydrate	1.0%
Melaleuca alternifolia (tea tree, oxidised)	5.0%
Octocrylene	10.0%
Iodopropynyl butyl carbamate	0.2%
Oleamidopropyl dimethylamine	0.1% aq.
Sorbitan sesquioleate (Arlacel® 83)	20.0%
Coconut diethanolamide (Cocamide DEA)	0.5%
Propolis	10.0%
Lauryl glucoside	3.0%
Tocopherol acetate	10%

Table 23.11 Allergen series available

European Standard, BSCA Baseline (Standard) and International Standard Series
Bakery series
Corticosteroid series
Cosmetic (facial) series
Cutaneous adverse drug reaction series
Dental screening: also Dental materials for patients or staff
Epoxy series
European photopatch baseline and extended series
Fragrance series
Hairdressing series
Isocyanate series
Leg ulcer series
Medicament series
Metal series
Methacrylate series (adhesives, dental)
Methacrylate series (artificial nails)
Methacrylate series (printing)
Oil and cooling fluid series
Plant series
Plastics and glues series
Rubber additives series
Shoe series
Sunscreen series
Textile colours and finish series

Investigators should also be aware of possible adverse effects from patch testing (Table 23.15).

Patient education

Once relevant allergens are identified, the patient should be given written information on all of these chemicals. Complicating the information is the fact that many chemicals have numerous synonyms and can cross-react with other chemicals. The information sheets are available from books or commercially. Some departments have specific locally written ones that they use. The BSCA has produced comprehensive up-to-date patient information leaflets for its baseline, facial and medicament series allergens, which are available online from the BSCA website.

particularly if they are the only positive reaction (Table 23.14). Unexplained positive reactions also include some borderline irritant or doubtful reactions, and some reactions to mixes used to test a large number of allergens at the same time. For example, fragrance mix consists of eight allergens, but testing the individual eight allergens separately may not always give a positive reaction in those with a positive reaction to the mix. Although this may reflect a combined irritant effect of the allergens in the mix, studies suggest that testing the individual eight allergens at a higher strength (e.g. 2% in petrolatum) would improve the detection of true allergy to a fragrance constituent.

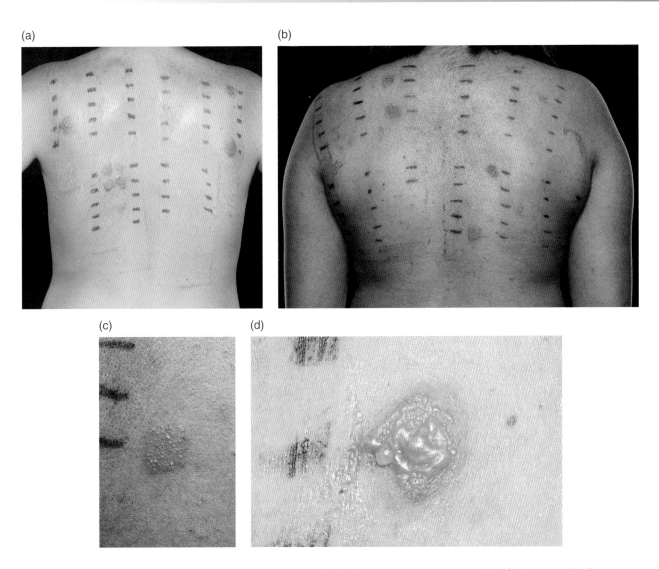

Figure 23.4 (a) Positive patch test reactions shown on the back. (b) Positive patch test reactions in skin of colour; note that less redness is seen. (c) Palpable and pustular positive reaction in skin of colour. (d) +++ (bullous) reaction to *para*-phenylenediamine base (PPD). © Medical Illustration Cardiff and Vale UHB.

Hand dermatitis

Hand dermatitis is most frequently a manifestation of ICD in a patient with an atopic tendency, but ACD can be superimposed on irritant and/or atopic hand dermatitis. A suggested management plan is shown in Figure 23.5.

Hand protection with gloves

Protective gloves are one of the key elements in the management of ICD and/or ACD and should be worn in the home and the workplace. The materials used for the manufacture of protective gloves are natural rubber, synthetic rubber (e.g. nitrile,

neoprene), textile fibres, leather and several polymeric materials, such as polyvinyl chloride (PVC). The actual protection afforded by gloves depends on the material used, its manufacturing quality, glove thickness, concentration of contactant, the duration of contact and environmental temperature and humidity. For example, (meth)acrylates used in nail bars penetrate vinyl gloves and hair perming agents penetrate nitrile gloves. ACD to rubber gloves is usually due to 'accelerator' chemicals such as thiurams and carbamates, added to natural rubber latex to speed up its processing into rubber items. Gloves are the commonest cause of rubber dermatitis and synthetic rubber gloves such as nitrile can also contain accelerators.

Gloves for industrial use are subject to tests to assess penetration, and gloves for medical use are tested for leakage through seams, pinholes and other imperfections. However, when users

Table 23.12 Allergens that commonly cause irritant patch test reactions

Metals

Nickel, cobalt, chromate

Preservatives

Parabens mix

Formaldehyde

Methylisothiazolinone

Methylchloroisothiazolinone/methylisothiazolinone mix

Benzisothiazolinone, octylisothiazolinone

Sodium metabisulfite

Thiomersal

Fragrances

Fragrance mix I

Myroxylon pereirae (Balsam of Peru)

Limonene hydroperoxides, linalool hydroperoxides

Surfactants

Decyl glucoside, lauryl glucoside

Rubber accelerators

Carba mix

Table 23.13 Late-reacting allergens (a delayed reading may be useful, e.g. day 7–10)

Neomycin

Gold

Tixocortol

Budesonide

2-Hydroxyethyl methacrylate

Table 23.14 Unexplained positive patch tests

Sodium metabisulfite

Cobalt (isolated reaction, when nickel and chromate are negative)

Thiomersal

Benzisothiazolinone

Table 23.15 Adverse effects of patch testing

Multiple severe reactions: 'angry back'

Flare of existing dermatitis: always warn patients

Pigment change (especially in skin of colour)

Blistering, necrosis, scarring

Active sensitisation (rare)

take the gloves on and off during the course of a working day, for example for changes in tasks or mealtimes, the chemicals covering the outside commonly contaminate the glove inner surface. This hastens the development of ICD or ACD caused by the occlusive effect of the glove. Patients need to be instructed how to remove gloves without contaminating themselves and reminded that if the gloves develop a hole or tear they should be discarded immediately.

Plastic or PVC gloves are useful for domestic tasks such as washing dishes and clothes.

Gloves should not be worn for more than 15–20 minutes at a time, if possible, and if water enters a glove it should be taken off immediately. Minimisation of the effects of contaminants may be achieved by turning the gloves inside out and rinsing them several times a week in hot running water before allowing them to dry completely.

Cotton gloves can be used under plastic gloves to soak up sweat, which may increase the occlusive effect (and possibly irritant potential) of gloves. Cotton liners should only be worn a few times before they are washed. Cotton gloves worn under rubber gloves in an attempt to protect the skin from an allergen such as a thiuram chemical are completely ineffective, and will themselves become contaminated with the allergen, which cannot be washed out. Cotton gloves can be very useful for 'dry' household chores. The patient should be told to purchase several pairs of plastic and cotton gloves at a time for use in the kitchen and bathroom and at work. Heavy-duty fabric gloves should be used when doing any gardening, 'do-it-yourself' and outdoor work, and gloves should be worn outdoors in cold weather to prevent the hands drying, cracking and chapping. It should also be remembered that the talcum powder (talc) or cornflour used in many gloves is also a skin irritant. If latex gloves are 'powdered', the powder absorbs latex, enhancing the overall latex exposure, increasing the risk of allergy development and acting as a vector for airborne exposure by inhalation.

Avoidance of irritants

Frequent wetting or washing of the hands at work or at home risks causing hand dermatitis, which is common in homemakers and carers. Other occupational groups particularly at risk are nurses, surgeons, dentists, caterers, cleaners, bartenders, hairdressers,

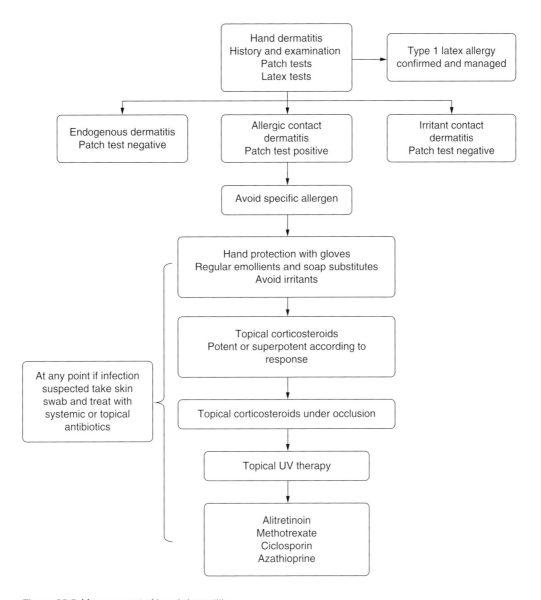

Figure 23.5 Management of hand dermatitis.

florists, mechanics and metalworkers. Eliminating the cause (or more often causes) of ICD is not easy.

All patients should be given a hand care information sheet with key points (e.g. the BAD patient information leaflet on 'How to Care for Your Hands') and asked to follow these guidelines fastidiously. Direct contact with detergents and other cleansing agents must be avoided, as these are strong irritants (Table 23.16). Skin cleansers used at work are also harsh on the hands and direct contact with them is best avoided altogether. The more explanation on irritant avoidance and emollient treatment the clinician gives the patient, the better the likely outcome, due to improved adherence.

The patient should be provided with a list of irritants that need to be avoided in the domestic situation (Table 23.16). This is important not only for those who perform traditional household tasks, but also for those doing more heavy-duty domestic chores such as car washing, painting and decorating.

Use of soap substitutes and moisturisers

Soap (solid or liquid) and water can be very irritating to the hands of a patient with dermatitis. Wearing of rings should be avoided if handwashing with soap. Soap and detergents remove lipids and amino acids from the skin and can cause alkali-induced damage

Table 23.16 Common skin irritants

Soaps and detergents
Shampoos and conditioners
Hair products such as hair lotions and hair dyes
Polishes including metal, wax, shoe, floor, car, furniture and window polishes
Solvents and stain removers such as white spirit, petrol, trichloroethylene and turpentine
Foods such as oranges, lemons, grapefruit, potatoes or tomatoes
Hand scrubs and 'wire wool'
Fibreglass

of the stratum corneum. Fatty acids in soaps may be directly irritant. Increased permeability of the horny layer and reduced water-holding capacity damage skin integrity. Hence, patients should be instructed always to use a soap substitute, such as a moisturiser. In addition, they should use lukewarm (preferably running) water when washing hands and dry the skin carefully with a clean towel, paying particular attention to the interdigital spaces where irritants can accumulate.

A moisturiser used as a soap substitute can either be a water-based paraffin-containing cream, a light gel-based moisturiser or a paraffin-based ointment. The choice of which to use depends on the patient's occupation and preference, as despite their efficacy ointment-based preparations may be impractical for some patients. If a patient chooses their own preferred emollient, this leads to increased patient adherence and hence greatly helps efficacy. The same emollient, or another of the patient's choice, should be used as a leave-on moisturiser each time the hands have been dried, applied directly to the skin to form a protective layer. Many patients benefit from having a gel-based moisturiser to use very frequently by day and an ointment-based one to use in the evenings, when not at work.

Moisturisers are widely available over the counter, which widens patient choice, and some moisturisers can be prescribed. The patient should be informed that some over-the-counter emollient products may contain many different allergens, including those described as 'natural' or 'plant based'. Fragrance-free moisturisers are preferable to reduce the risk of inducing fragrance allergy. The clinician should have available some emollient samples for the patient to try in clinic or at home. This allows patients to make an informed choice before purchasing or being prescribed an emollient.

Moisturisers are not only important in the treatment of established soap- or detergent-induced ICD, but also have a preventative role in the development of irritant dermatitis, both in experimental domestic situations and in real-life work contexts. Ideally, the patient should have available several large containers of moisturiser or soap substitute, which can then be placed next

to every sink both at home and at work. Smaller tubes to carry around in a bag or in the car are useful, and the patient can decant a suitable amount into a small liquid container, for use for instance during airline travel. The patient can be instructed to use the emollient preparation as a general moisturiser if required, and be reminded that these products are safe to apply to all areas of the skin, even in children. The patient should be instructed to apply emollient several times a day or whenever the skin feels dry or itchy, and on the hands after every handwash.

'Barrier creams' are a controversial area. They are intended to prevent or reduce the penetration and absorption of various hazardous materials into the skin, and to replace protective clothing in situations where personal protective equipment such as gloves, sleeves or faceguards cannot be safely or conveniently used. Some workplace 'barrier creams' contain potential sensitisers. Evidence for the efficacy of barrier creams is limited, and avoidance of irritants plus frequent use of emollients is preferable.

Prognosis and ongoing management

It is good practice to give the patient realistic advice about the prognosis of their hand dermatitis and the importance of continuing the suggested measures lifelong, especially in those with an atopic background. Caring for infants or elderly relatives, or an increase in housework, maintenance or gardening, is a common precipitating factor.

The patient should be told that it will take some months for their skin to return to below the irritant threshold and for clinical dermatitis to disappear. The skin will remain vulnerable for at least six months after the dermatitis appears to be completely healed, so they have to continue to follow the instructions given. For those with underlying atopy, especially in high-risk occupations such as nursing, the measures should be followed closely and indefinitely. A minority of patients may continue to develop problems despite following this advice and will require additional therapy.

Note that all patients with hand eczema must continue to use emollients frequently plus a soap substitute indefinitely.

Treatment of hand dermatitis (Chapters 17 and 18)

Topical corticosteroids

Topical corticosteroids are a key additional element in treating many patients with hand dermatitis. Issues to consider when assessing the patient include whether to treat with cream or ointment and what strength of topical steroid to use. Most corticosteroid creams are insufficiently lubricating, but corticosteroid ointments, the clinicians' preferred option, may be unacceptably greasy to some patients, and again a balance must be struck to increase adherence.

Different hand sites respond differently to the same strength of topical steroid. The choice of topical corticosteroid therapy depends on the location and severity of the dermatitis. Dermatitis of the back of the hands responds more readily than palmar dermatitis, due to the differences in stratum corneum thickness. Frequent use of a potent topical steroid may cause cutaneous atrophy on the dorsa of the hands or flexor aspects of the wrists, but on the palms this is extremely unlikely. Once-daily application of a topical steroid is sufficient, but, in some acute cases, twice-daily application may be useful for the first few days. Most clinicians would advise gradual reduction in frequency of application down to the minimum frequency necessary once the symptoms are controlled, for example once- or twice-weekly maintenance.

In patients unresponsive to standard regimes, corticosteroid penetration and hence efficacy can be increased approximately 10-fold by plastic occlusion. In hand dermatitis, occlusion can lead to rapid healing of fissures, and it dramatically improves psoriasiform and atopic hand dermatitis. However, if used continuously in the long term it can increase the risk of unwanted side-effects such as cutaneous atrophy on thinner skin sites, especially if combined with superpotent topical steroids. Occlusion of the hands is best accomplished by wearing thin plastic or cotton (not rubber) gloves overnight. This technique may be initially uncomfortable to the patient, but it is very beneficial after a few days. In patients with low-grade but very dry hand dermatitis, emollients alone can be used under occlusion to improve their efficacy. In acute vesicular hand dermatitis, a useful trick is to apply a superpotent topical steroid with an emollient on top and occlude with dampened cotton gloves for 30 minutes twice daily for a couple of days, before reverting to standard topical steroid and emollient regimens.

Topical and systemic antibiotics and antimicrobial agents

Hand dermatitis can become secondarily infected. Swabs from skin and nasal passages should be taken for culture and sensitivity, to determine appropriate antibiotic therapy. Some clinicians prefer to treat with a systemic antibiotic and a topical corticosteroid, although others favour topical antibiotic and corticosteroid combination treatment, in all but the most severely affected cases. Topical antiseptic soaks such as potassium permanganate pose no risk of antibiotic resistance. They are useful in acutely inflamed or infected hand dermatitis, where they combat infection, and in acute blistering hand dermatitis to help dry up any weeping or discharge.

Topical calcineurin inhibitors

Tacrolimus 0.1% ointment may be useful in patients with chronic and persistent dermatitis of the dorsa of the hands and the flexor aspect of the wrists. It avoids the need for continuous use of potent or superpotent topical steroids, and their associated risk of cutaneous atrophy. In contrast, on the palm, the efficacy of tacrolimus ointment is limited due to the thickness of the stratum corneum, and cutaneous atrophy at this site is highly unlikely.

Photochemotherapy (Chapter 25)

Psoralen ultraviolet A (PUVA) treatment is a useful option for unresponsive hand dermatitis. Either the psoralen is taken orally, or the hands are soaked in psoralen solution prior to the

UVA treatment. Twice-weekly hospital visits over several weeks are needed. If this is impractical in a rural or remote community, or for patients with heavy work commitments, then home UVA devices may provide a solution. PUVA of the hands has few side-effects, but the patient must understand that it does not lead to permanent remission and topical treatment must be continued regardless.

Systemic corticosteroids

In acute, severe vesicular hand dermatitis, a brief course of systemic corticosteroids may have a dramatic beneficial effect. The aim is to improve the dermatitis sufficiently for topical treatment to be tolerated and effective. One possible regimen is to use a tapering course of prednisolone, starting at 40 mg and reducing by 5 mg each day. In addition, topical corticosteroids and emollients should be used. In the most severe and painful cases topical treatment can be started after 24–48 hours, or as soon as the blistering and oedema start to decrease.

Oral retinoids

Alitretinoin is the only licensed systemic treatment for severe chronic hand dermatitis refractory to potent topical steroid treatment: a National Institute for Health and Care Excellence (NICE) requirement for use is a Dermatology Life Quality Index (DLQI) score ≥15. The recommended starting dose is 30 mg daily with food, which can be reduced to 10 mg daily if side-effects are troublesome. Treatment is for 12–24 weeks and courses can be repeated if relapse occurs. Patients with hyperkeratotic features are more likely to respond than those with pompholyx-type eczema. Strict contraceptive measures and enrolment on a pregnancy prevention programme are necessary for women of childbearing age.

Ciclosporin

Low-dose ciclosporin (up to 3 mg/kg/day) is a useful addition for the short-term treatment of severe chronic hand dermatitis in patients unresponsive to conventional therapy. However, it is contraindicated in patients with malignancy, hypertension or renal disease and requires regular, careful monitoring of full blood count, liver and renal function and blood pressure. The therapeutic effect is rapid and improvement may be seen within days.

Methotrexate

As well as its indication for psoriasis, methotrexate may also be used to treat severe atopic dermatitis, including hand dermatitis. Its safety profile is better than that of azathioprine, as it is not carcinogenic. Its use may be limited by gastrointestinal side-effects such as nausea, potential hepatotoxicity (especially in the obese or those with a high alcohol intake), potential bone marrow suppression and teratogenicity. It is contraindicated in women wishing to conceive; men wishing to father children also require a washout period of six months following its discontinuation.

Regular monitoring of full blood count and liver and renal function is required. It can take up to 12 weeks to be effective.

Azathioprine

Azathioprine can provide effective therapy of severe atopic dermatitis, although no controlled studies have been performed in hand dermatitis. Its therapeutic effects must be balanced against the drug's hepatotoxicity, potential for bone marrow suppression and gastrointestinal side-effects. Regular monitoring of full blood count and renal and liver function is required. Azathioprine increases the risk of skin cancer and hence it is important to advise patients to avoid sun exposure. It can take up to 12 weeks to be effective.

Dupilumab

Dupilumab is an injected 'biologic' treatment initiated only in hospital dermatology departments. It is recommended as an option for treating moderate-to-severe atopic dermatitis in adults (and children), if the disease has not responded to at least one other systemic therapy, such as ciclosporin, methotrexate, azathioprine or mycophenolate mofetil, or when these are contraindicated or not tolerated. It can cause persistent conjunctivitis in about 20% of patients. The onset of effect may be slow, but further improvement can take place over several months. Adequate improvement is defined as ≥50% reduction in the Eczema Area and Severity Index, and ≥4-point reduction in the DLQI from when treatment started. The NICE recommendation is that dupilumab should be stopped at 16 weeks if the atopic dermatitis has not responded adequately. It could potentially be used in patients with severe atopic hand dermatitis unresponsive to other systemic treatments.

Conclusions

Cutaneous allergy is an exciting field that requires great clinical acumen and a constant enquiring mind as a 'detective' to determine which allergens to test and their relevance for individual patients. New allergens are always emerging that may be the next cause of a cutaneous allergy epidemic, for example preservatives, cosmetic ingredients including fragrances, or (meth) acrylates. Databases and analysis of allergen trends in populations can allow us to influence industries to remove allergens, for example methylisothiazolinone removal from leave-on products. If needed, this may have to be enforced via legislation (e.g. the Nickel Directive to reduce nickel content in metal objects).

The concept of allergy can cause much confusion among clinical practitioners and patients in differentiating immediate, delayed, food, environmental and chemical contact allergies. Hence a clear understanding of mechanisms of action, likely clinical presentations and appropriate investigations will enhance your clinical practice as a dermatologist of the future.

Pearls and pitfalls

- Resuscitation facilities for prick testing must be available due to the risk of anaphylaxis, even though it is extremely unlikely.
- Prick tests are of no use in the investigation of chronic spontaneous urticaria.
- Beware over-interpreting irritant reactions as true positive patch tests, e.g. to formaldehyde.
- A detailed occupational history is essential, including details of any hobbies.
- Testing to patients' own items such as cosmetics is key.
- Interpret patch tests with care in skin of colour as redness may not be obvious; careful palpation of the potential reactions is needed.
- Patients should be encouraged to photograph and report any late reactions.
- For chronic hand eczema, explain simple management tips clearly with written information, e.g. frequent and long-term use of emollients and soap substitutes. This can continue long after the dermatitis appears to have healed.

SCE Questions. See questions 26–30.

FURTHER READING AND KEY RESOURCES

Adisesh A, Robinson E, Nicholson PJ et al. UK standards of care for occupational contact dermatitis and occupational contact urticaria. Br J Dermatol 2013; **168**:1167–75.

Amaro C, Goossens A. Immunological occupational contact urticaria and contact dermatitis from proteins: a review. Contact Dermatitis 2008; **58**:67–75.

Chowdhury MMU. Occupational contact urticaria. Br J Dermatol 2015; **173**:1364–5.

Johnston GA, Exton LS, Mohd Mustapa MF et al. British Association of Dermatologists' guidelines for the management of contact dermatitis. Br J Dermatol 2017; **176**:317–29.

Maibach HI, Johnson HL. Contact urticaria syndrome. Contact urticaria to diethyltoluamide (immediate-type hypersensitivity). Arch Dermatol 1975; **111**:726–30.

Solman L, Lloyd-Lavery A, Grindlay DJC et al. What's new in atopic eczema? An analysis of systematic reviews published in 2016. Part 1: treatment and prevention. Clin Exp Dermatol 2019; **44**:363–9.

Süß H, Dölle-Bierke S, Geier J et al. Contact urticaria: Frequency, elicitors and cofactors in three cohorts (Information Network of Departments of Dermatology; Network of Anaphylaxis; and Department of Dermatology, University Hospital Erlangen, Germany). Contact Dermatitis 2019; **81**:341–53.

Textbooks

De Groot AC, Weyland JW, Nater JP. *Unwanted Effects of Cosmetics and Drugs Used in Dermatology*, 3rd edn. Amsterdam: Elsevier, 1994.

Johansen JD, Mahler V, Lepoittevin J-P, Frosch PJ, eds. *Contact Dermatitis*, 6th edn. Berlin: Springer, 2021.

Lachapelle J-M, Maibach HI, eds. *Patch Testing and Prick Testing: A Practical Guide*, 4th edn. Berlin: Springer, 2019.

Wahlberg JE, Elsner P, Kanerva L, Maibach HI, eds. *Management of Positive Patch Test Reactions*. Berlin: Springer, 2003.

Useful websites

Bio-Diagnostics. AllergEAZE. Available at: http://www.biodiagnostics.co.uk/divisions/dermatology/allergeaze.

British Association of Dermatologists. Clinical guidelines (contact dermatitis and occupational contact dermatitis). Available at: https://www.bad.org.uk/healthcare-professionals/clinical-standards/clinical-guidelines#collapse270.

British Association of Dermatologists. Cutaneous allergy (patch testing). Available at: https://www.bad.org.uk/healthcare-professionals/clinical-services/service-guidance/cutaneous-allergy-patch-testing.

British Association of Dermatologists. Patient information leaflets (including 'Patch testing' and 'How to care for your hands'). Available at: https://www.bad.org.uk/for-the-public/patient-information-leaflets.

British Society for Cutaneous Allergy. Available at: http://cutaneousallergy.org.

Chemotechnique Diagnostics. Patch testing allergens. Available at: www.chemotechnique.se.

European Society for Contact Dermatitis. Available at: www.escd.org.

24

Photosensitivity

Tsui Chin Ling and Jean Ayer

Introduction

There exists an enigma surrounding photosensitivity disorders that causes some dermatologists to abandon the first principles of clinical medicine and prematurely refer patients on for a specialist opinion. This is explained, in part, by the lack of facilities for light testing in most units, even in teaching hospitals. At the other end of the spectrum is the uninformed and inexperienced clinician who is prepared to have a go at managing even the most complex and difficult photosensitivity syndromes without seeking specialist input. The ideal is found somewhere between these two scenarios. Clinicians who refer on without attempting to understand patients with photosensitivity should not forget that in most cases of photosensitivity, the diagnosis is made from a careful history, examination and a small number of simple (and widely available) investigations. Those clinicians who seldom or never refer on to specialist centres for investigation and monochromator light testing should be aware that in some cases, effective management of photosensitivity can only be achieved by understanding the diagnosis and the action spectrum of the disorder. Clinicians should also bear in mind that some patients who meticulously photoprotect may not have the classical signs and symptoms of photosensitivity, and certain disorders may not always present in a typical photodistribution.

There are several centres in the UK and Ireland with specialised facilities and expertise in light testing. Most centres accept tertiary referrals only, though some accept direct general practitioner referrals. This places the expertise for investigation of patients with photosensitivity within reach of most UK dermatology centres. It also provides easy access for training opportunities for junior dermatologists. Postgraduate photodermatology training courses for dermatologists and phototherapy courses aimed at healthcare professionals are also available.

Basic principles of photobiology

Photodermatology is the study of the effects of ultraviolet radiation (UVR) and visible radiation (light) on the skin. UVR and light comprise a tiny part of the electromagnetic spectrum, and consist of energy released during the transition of an electron from a higher to a lower energy orbit. The ultraviolet spectrum is subdivided, by convention, into UVC (100–280 nm), UVB (280–320 nm) and UVA (320–400 nm) (Figure 24.1). UVA is subdivided into UVAII (320–340 nm) and UVAI (340–400 nm), in order to reflect the fact that shorter-wavelength UVA behaves in a biologically similar manner to UVB. Visible light ranges from 400 nm (violet) to 700 nm (red). The primary source of UVR and light is, of course, sunlight. Artificial sources of UVR and light include low-pressure gas discharge lamps, medium-pressure mercury lamps, and high-pressure xenon arc lamps.

Dermatology Training: The Essentials. Edited by Mahbub M.U. Chowdhury, Tamara W. Griffiths and Andrew Y. Finlay.
© 2022 The British Association of Dermatologists. Published 2022 by John Wiley & Sons Ltd.
Companion website: www.wiley.com/go/chowdhury/dermatologytraining

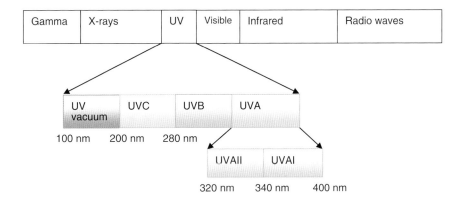

Figure 24.1 The electromagnetic spectrum, highlighting ultraviolet (UV) radiation. © Salford Royal NHS Foundation Trust.

At sea level, solar radiation consists of 95–98% UVA and 2–5% UVB, all the UVC having been absorbed by the ozone layer in the stratosphere. The depth of penetration into skin is determined by the wavelength of UVR. Most UVB is absorbed in the epidermis, while approximately 10–15% reaches the upper dermis, and the longer wavelengths of UVA penetrate deeper into the dermis. UVB provokes an inflammatory response and is responsible for 'sunburn'. UVA provokes much less inflammation than UVB and requires interaction with photosensitising agents in the skin in order to produce many of its biological effects.

Biological responses can only occur after UV and visible radiation are absorbed by molecules in the skin. These light-absorbing molecules, termed chromophores, may be DNA, urocanic acid and other intrinsic molecules, or exogenous agents such as an ingested photosensitising drug (e.g. tetracycline or psoralen). Whereas UVB can affect molecules directly, both UVB and UVA can also affect molecules indirectly through generation of free radicals and reactive oxygen species.

The action spectrum of a chromophore consists of those wavelengths of radiation most effective in generating a specific chemical or biological response. It is important, for example, to establish the action spectrum in solar urticaria, as this determination of the wavelengths causing the condition for an individual patient can guide the use of phototherapy.

The ultimate clinical effects of UVR and visible radiation may be acute, and include sunburn and various photosensitivity disorders, or chronic effects including photoageing and photocarcinogenesis.

Normal cutaneous responses to ultraviolet radiation

An understanding of normal skin responses to UVR and visible radiation is needed if abnormal responses are to be recognised. Central to this understanding is an appreciation of the range of these 'normal' responses as determined by racial variation in pigmentation of the skin and susceptibility to UV-induced inflammation.

Fitzpatrick skin phototype classification

The concept of sun-reactive 'skin phototyping' was created by Fitzpatrick in 1975 for a specific need: to be able to classify persons *with white skin* in order to select the correct initial doses of UVA for the treatment of psoriasis with psoralen–UVA. The classification depends on a patient reporting the degree to which they develop redness and tan in response to sunlight; the classification was later 'updated' to include other ethnic skin types. The Fitzpatrick categorisation continues to have some use when restricted to its original purpose, and to easily identify those people with white skin who are at high risk of skin cancer. However, the expanded Fitzpatrick phototyping now divides a range of skin tones into one of six phototypes, from skin type I to type VI (Table 24.1).

The Fitzpatrick classification was never intended to reflect the range of skin types or responses to UVR across the whole human race. An entirely different range of descriptors is needed

Table 24.1 Fitzpatrick skin phototype

Skin type	Typical features	Burning and tanning
I	Pale white skin, blue/green eyes, blond/red hair	Always burns, does not tan
II	Fair skin, blue eyes	Burns easily, tans poorly
III	Darker white skin	Tans after initial burn
IV	Light brown skin	Burns minimally, tans easily
V	Brown skin	Rarely burns, tans darkly easily
VI	Dark brown or black skin	Never burns, always tans darkly

Hon A/Prof Amanda Oakley, Fitzpatrick skin phototype, Dermatologist, Hamilton, New Zealand, 2012.

for that. Unfortunately, the Fitzpatrick classification has frequently been used inappropriately, as a descriptor of ethnic skin type (unrelated to phototype).

In practice, the skin phototype should be an *overall assessment* by the clinician taking into account the patient's burning and tanning ability, as well as patient characteristics of hair and eye colour and freckling. One method of assessing skin phototype adopted in Manchester is shown in Table 24.2.

Another widespread problem is that thinking among dermatologists has often focused on the sign 'erythema' (redness), instead of the underlying process of inflammation. The word 'erythema' (a clinical sign meaning 'red') has often been confused with 'inflammation' (a process). However, inflammation may or may not include the sign of redness, and redness may or may not be a sign of inflammation. The British Association of Dermatologists has produced guidance on describing skin conditions across a broad spectrum of skin tones to aid with this challenge.

In view of the poor reproducibility of skin phototype assessment, an objective method for summarising and grading different people's response to UVR was needed. The minimal erythema dose (MED) is the most widely used objective test to determine the acute (redness) response to UVB exposure.

There is an issue with the descriptor 'MED', as the objective of the test is really to determine the minimal detectable inflammation. Redness (erythema) is used as the key sign in this test, but there are other signs of inflammation such as other pigmentary changes or swelling, and in some darker skin types these may be more important. However, the MED is currently defined as the lowest dose of UVB to produce a just perceptible redness at 24 hours after testing with a graded series of UVB doses. The

MED is a measure of individual sensitivity to UVR, and differs from one individual to another. The 'standard erythema dose' (SED) is a standardised measure of redness caused by UV radiation currently being implemented in some tertiary centres. It is independent of skin type, and a particular exposure dose in SED may cause redness in fair skin, but none in darker skin. One SED is equivalent to an erythemal effective radiant exposure of 100 J/m^2.

When comparing MED assessment with skin phototyping, the two methods attempt to measure different aspects of the skin's response to UVB. The MED is a single snapshot of the redness response to a graded series of doses of UVB, while the skin phototype attempts to summarise a dynamic response and involves pigmentation as well as redness.

The time course of ultraviolet-induced inflammation

The acute skin response to UVB exposure is termed the sunburn reaction, and represents an acute inflammatory response. Sunburn is characterised by painful skin inflammation, with redness in some skin types, limited to sites of skin exposed to excess UVB. The onset of sunburn is typically delayed for 4–6 hours after sun exposure and peaks at 16–24 hours. Sunburn typically fades over 2–3 days, and in severe cases may then be followed by profuse exfoliation. The latent period between sun over-exposure and onset of signs of inflammation is thought to be explained by the time taken for damaged epidermal cells to mediate an acute inflammatory response in the dermis via cytokines and upregulation of expression of proinflammatory adhesion molecules.

History and examination of the photosensitive patient

Before proceeding to phototesting, the dermatologist should take a detailed history of the photosensitivity (Table 24.3). Understanding if and how the time of the year impacts the eruption is very relevant. A strong temporal association to sunlight significantly increases the probability of a photosensitive disorder, whereas the lack of seasonal variation reduces it. However, seasonality does not apply to short-lived photosensitivities, for example those that are drug induced. Furthermore, patients with very severe photosensitivity may be symptomatic all year round (though worse in sunnier months), and there are some photosensitivity conditions such as actinic prurigo that do not demonstrate marked seasonality.

The frequency of the eruption in relation to sun exposure is also important to understand. If an eruption occurs after *every* episode of photoexposure, a photosensitivity disorder is more likely. However, accurate history taking will require far more than simply putting this question to the patient, and it is important the dermatologist understands the concept of a provocation threshold. For example, some patients may have a high threshold and

Table 24.2 Suggested skin assessment questionnaire (Manchester). This is more descriptive about burning and tanning ability and less reliant on traditional phototypes of skin and eye colour

Please describe what happens to your skin if you go into the sun at 12 noon in June for 40 minutes without any sunscreen on exposed skin

Burn	Tan
Virtually always	Never/rarely
Usually	Light tan
Sometimes	Mid tan
Rarely	Heavy tan
Rarely and only after excessive exposure (naturally brown skin)	Skin darkens easily
Rarely/hardly ever (naturally dark brown/black skin)	Skin darkens very easily

Table 24.3 History taking: photosensitivity
Timing of eruption in relation to seasons
Frequency of eruption in relation to sun exposure
Latent period between sun exposure and onset of eruption
Duration of eruption
Appearance and distribution of eruption (review patient photographs)
Relieving factors
Exacerbating factors
Do sunscreens help or exacerbate photosensitivity?
Change in sensitivity with repeated sun exposure ('hardening response')
Drug history (prescribed and unprescribed)
Ingestion of exogenous psoralens

only intense photoexposure will provoke the condition. In photoaggravated eczema a longer duration of photoexposure (several hours to days) is required for provocation, and brief exposure may not trigger the rash. Some patients may report that sunlight in the UK provokes the eruption, whereas others may report it is only sun exposure when abroad. This may be due to the differences in the proportion of UVA (which is the most common wavelength associated with photosensitivity) and UVA exposure in different geographical regions.

The latent period after sun exposure may also provide clues to diagnosis. For example, a rash that occurs only a few minutes after exposure is more suggestive of solar urticaria or a drug-induced photosensitivity, whereas a period of a few days is more typical of photoaggravated eczema. Change in sensitivity with repeated sun exposure is also important. If the eruption occurs only at the start of summer with the first few sun exposures but then appears to improve, this may be due to photohardening and is quite common in polymorphic light eruption. Duration of the eruption is also a key question: does the eruption last for a few minutes, a couple of hours or a few days?

Ascertain whether there are exacerbating or relieving factors; the impact of sunscreen is a key question. If the eruption can be prevented or lessened by use of a sunscreen, it raises suspicion of a photosensitive condition. However, if an eruption only occurs following use of sunscreens, this may suggest photocontact dermatitis. If antihistamines help to prevent an eruption, this suggests solar urticaria. Always ask if sunlight transmitted through glass provokes the eruption, as this indicates that the action spectrum includes UVA and/or visible light.

If a drug-induced photosensitivity is suspected, confirm that the initial onset of the eruption began only after commencement of a new drug. Always ask whether the patient is taking any herbal, complementary or over-the-counter remedies; St John's wort is a common culprit. Increase your suspicion of a drug-induced photosensitivity if there is a quick onset of symptoms after UV exposure. The list of drugs that can cause photosensitivity is long and includes representation from a diverse range of pharmacological agents. The most common culprits include the tetracyclines, loop diuretics, antihypertensives and antipsychotics. The temporal relationship between the onset of photosensitivity and initiation of the drug should be carefully explored, and further information gathered from the referring clinician or general practitioner. The local hospital pharmacy and drug-information service can assist with cases where doubt persists.

Furthermore, certain foods contain exogenous psoralens and are known sensitisers if ingested in high amounts. These include limes, celery, carrots and figs. It is also worth noting that tonic water has photosensitising properties due to quinine content; patients are unlikely to be forthcoming with how much they may be consuming with their gin unless asked directly.

There is no substitute for seeing the eruption at its peak. However, the patient may attend the clinic some time after the eruption has resolved and it is important to try to ascertain the appearance and distribution of the rash. An open appointment to re-attend when the rash is present may be needed or, alternatively, good-quality digital photographs. Clear demarcation lines between exposed and covered skin may suggest photosensitivity, although an important differential would be airborne dermatitis. Certain conditions can be readily identified with photography, such as the weal-and-flare response typically seen in solar urticaria.

Once a careful history and clinical examination have been completed, it should be clear whether a photosensitivity disorder is a possible or even likely diagnosis. The possibility of a photoaggravated disorder, rather than a primary photosensitivity condition, should also be considered. Some photoaggravated conditions that can be confused with photosensitivity disorders are:

- Rosacea
- Seborrhoeic dermatitis
- Herpes labialis
- Lupus erythematosus
- Dermatomyositis

Where patients present with an eczematous eruption at exposed sites, the differential diagnosis to consider in the context of photocontact allergy includes other photosensitivity disorders and other eczematous disorders. In the history, it is important to establish what topical products the patient has used and whether there is a temporal relationship between their usage and the occurrence of the eruption. Photocontact allergy is unlikely in this context if the patient has not used a sunscreen. However, the ubiquitous inclusion of sunscreens in cosmetic products means that the patient may be unaware that they are applying such products. Contact dermatitis to airborne allergens may also cause confusion. Careful examination of the skin in airborne contact allergy will usually reveal involvement of the skin of the eyelids, under the chin and behind the ears. These are the sites typically spared by sun-mediated photosensitivity such as chronic actinic dermatitis or photocontact allergic dermatitis. However, these subtle signs are not always present, and trainees should be alert to other diagnoses in such patients. Finally, both atopic eczema involving exposed sites and seborrhoeic eczema should also be considered in the differential diagnosis of exposed-site dermatitis.

Phototesting

Phototesting is usually carried out to assist with establishing a diagnosis, and in some instances may help with the management of the disorder. Initial investigations generally available to most UK dermatologists include:

- Porphyrin screen (blood, urine, stool).
- Antinuclear antibodies, anti-SSA (anti-Ro), anti-SSB (anti-La) and/or antibodies to double-stranded DNA.
- Patch testing, which is important for chronic actinic dermatitis and in cases of airborne contact dermatitis that also affects exposed sites.

Other blood investigations typically undertaken in a photobiology unit include:

- Serum IgE (elevated in photoaggravated eczema and chronic actinic dermatitis).
- Human leucocyte antigen (HLA) typing: (HLA-DRB1*04:07 is present in 60% of cases of actinic prurigo).
- Vitamin D status (often low in photoprotected patients).

Full phototesting consists of:

- Monochromator testing.
- Photoprovocation testing.
- Photopatch testing.

Note that topical corticosteroids can suppress UV-induced inflammatory reactions. Prednisolone, even at an oral dose of only 10 mg daily, may suppress the abnormal photosensitivity of chronic actinic dermatitis. The effects of other immunosuppressants on phototesting have not been investigated; however, if a patient needs to be on immunosuppressive therapy, it is important to consider the possible impact of this on the results of phototests.

Indications for phototesting

The indications for referral for phototesting are as follows:

- To confirm the diagnosis in suspected congenital or acquired photosensitivity.
- To define the action spectrum of the photosensitive eruption in order to assist in its management.
- To reassess the severity of photosensitivity and range of provoking wavelengths in severe cases where this information would help with management.
- To help diagnose sunscreen allergies and identify a suitable sunscreen for use.
- To exclude photosensitivity, if necessary.

In practice, the following are the main conditions seen in photodermatology units (in approximate descending order of frequency):

- Polymorphic light eruption (PLE) (phototesting indicated for atypical presentation; not usually required for classical PLE).
- Chronic actinic dermatitis.
- Photoaggravated eczema and atopic eczema.
- Solar urticaria.
- Drug-induced photosensitivity.
- Photocontact allergy, usually to sunscreens.
- Actinic prurigo.
- Hydroa vacciniforme.
- Other photoaggravated dermatoses.
- Porphyrias.
- Genophotodermatoses.

Basic skills in interpretation of photoinvestigation procedures

Trainees should be able to describe the following phototest procedures, as well as read, record and interpret responses:

- Monochromator light testing.
- Photoprovocation testing.
- Photopatch testing.

As with patch testing, interpretation of results of phototests requires experience and may not always be straightforward. Of paramount importance is the interpretation of responses in the context of the detailed history and investigations that have already been obtained. For example, with solar urticaria the history is usually clear and the diagnosis can be made with confidence before the phototests. Immediate weal-and-flare responses to the photoprovocation confirm the diagnosis, usually fading in a few hours. The monochromator testing defines the action spectrum. Some patients with solar urticaria are sensitive to visible light as well as UV, and it is important to know they will not be adequately protected with conventional sunscreens (which provide little protection within the visible part of the spectrum). In contrast, a minority of patients with solar urticaria fail to urticate with monochromator light testing, despite a clear history and clinical features that are consistent with this diagnosis. This may be due to coexisting augmentary and inhibitory wavebands in the action spectrum of solar urticaria; however, the diagnosis may be made by exposure to natural UVR.

Monochromator testing

Monochromator light testing is an essential aspect of phototesting. The light source used is usually a 2500-watt xenon arc lamp (Figure 24.2). These lamps have an output that mimics sunlight. Skin exposure can be through a variety of UV filters in order to test at the desired waveband. Alternatively, the output of the lamp can be directed through a series of mirrors and water-cooled lenses into a monochromator and then directed onto the skin (usually the back) via a liquid light guide. The monochromator is a precision optical device designed to fractionate the light to allow exposure to

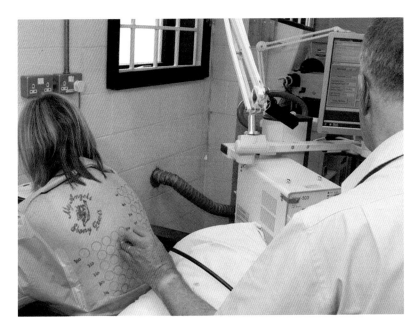

Figure 24.2 Monochromator light testing system. © Salford Royal NHS Foundation Trust.

a clearly defined waveband. The xenon arc lamp can also be used without filters as a solar simulator, where light exposure includes UVB, UVA, visible light and infrared. The wavelengths tested, and dose ranges used, vary between different photodermatology units. The dose ranges used may include UVB, UVA and visible wavebands, for example 300 nm, 320 nm, 330nm, 350 nm, 370 nm, 400 nm, 500 nm and 600 nm. The latter two visible-light wavebands are particularly relevant in patients suspected of sensitivity within the visible spectrum, for example in chronic actinic dermati-

tis, solar urticaria or the cutaneous porphyrias. It is abnormal for a positive response to occur in the visible range and abnormal to have urticarial responses in any range.

Photoprovocation testing

This is usually performed by exposure to broadband UVA only (Figure 24.3) or by broadband UVA plus visible optical radiation sources ('solar simulator') on a 5 × 5-cm square on the forearm of

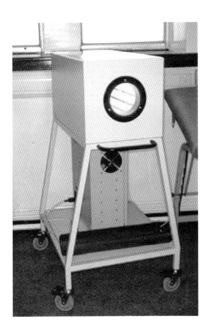

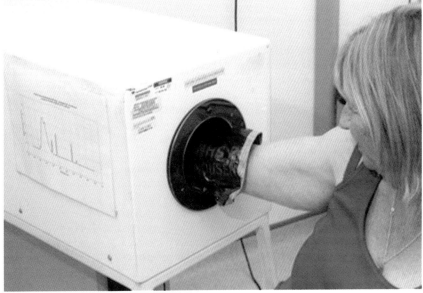

Figure 24.3 Ultraviolet A provocation. © Salford Royal NHS Foundation Trust.

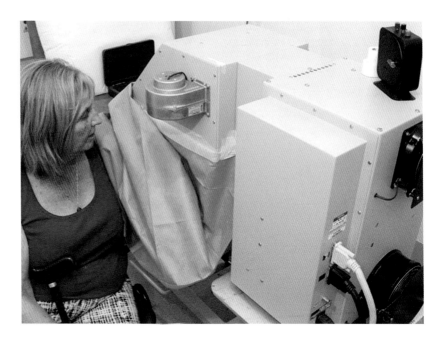

Figure 24.4 Solar simulator. © Salford Royal NHS Foundation Trust.

the patient (Figure 24.4). Repeated photoprovocation increases the yield for a positive provocation response, and the standard testing protocol should aim for three consecutive challenges. The tested area can also be extended to include the whole forearm if the first challenge was negative. The morphology of the artificially provoked rash helps with the diagnosis; a skin biopsy (with immunofluorescence studies where indicated) of the rash can further help confirm the diagnosis.

Photopatch testing

Where possible, photopatch testing should be offered as part of routine photoinvestigation. In addition to helping diagnose suspected contact and/or photocontact sunscreen allergy, it is also helpful to reveal any undiagnosed sunscreen allergies that may be contributing to the photosensitivity. Photopatch testing also helps to guide sunscreen choice for the patient.

As most of the relevant contact allergens are activated by UVA rather than UVB, the irradiation used in photopatch testing is to UVA (Figure 24.5). Typically, patients have two identical sets of the photocontact allergens applied in parallel to the left and right sides of the back. After two days these are removed. One side of the back is then covered with a suitable UV-opaque sheet, while the other side (including the site of application of the photopatch tests) is exposed to 5 J/cm^2 of UVA. In patients with significant photosensitivity to UVA, such as is seen in some cases of chronic actinic dermatitis, the dose of UVA used is reduced, for example to 2.5 J/cm^2 or less. The patient is asked to re-attend on three consecutive days for reading of the photopatch tests.

A typical positive photoallergic response is characterised by a positive response on the irradiated series, with a negative response to the same allergen on the non-irradiated side. Equal positive reactions on both sides indicate contact allergy alone. If positive responses are seen on both sides of the back, but with a stronger response on the UV-irradiated side, this suggests both contact allergy and photocontact allergy.

The most common cause of positive reactions on photopatch testing is currently to sunscreen products; however, photoallergic reactions to the topical nonsteroidal anti-inflammatory drugs (NSAIDs) ketoprofen and etofenamate are also common and should be included as part of the baseline photopatch test series. Patients who have photosensitivity on days when they have not used a sunscreen are more likely to have a primary acquired photosensitivity disorder or photoaggravated skin complaint rather than a photoallergy to their sunscreen. Patients who have used cosmetics or toiletries that have originated from outside the UK or European Union may still be exposed to

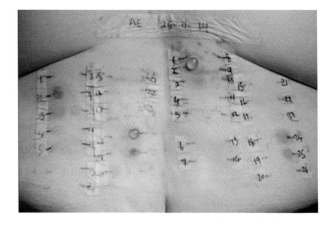

Figure 24.5 Photopatch test results with a range of responses. © Salford Royal NHS Foundation Trust.

potential photoallergens, such as musk ambrette, halogenated salicylanilide or 6-methylcoumarin (also found in fragrances, but now banned in Europe). As usage of these allergens varies from country to country, there is no single battery of allergens that is suitable for all photopatch testing. It is essential to test a patient's own products, especially if suspected to be causing a reaction. If multiple sunscreen allergies are demonstrated, it is advisable to refer patients on for full patch testing to investigate for coexisting contact allergies.

Patient counselling following phototesting

The diagnosis is often made after correlating symptoms with phototest findings. However, the diagnosis may not always be certain, due to poor patient history, lack of images or equivocal light test results. The phototests in isolation seldom provide the diagnosis, except where phototests demonstrate classical solar urticaria or chronic actinic dermatitis. Following detailed history and examination, the phototesting usually concludes the investigations and in most cases is followed by a working diagnosis and plan of management.

Patient counselling following phototesting includes:

- Verbal explanation about the diagnosis, supported with written information in the form of a patient information leaflet or website.
- Advice on physical photoprotective measures and correct application of sunscreens.
- Providing information about patient support groups.
- A management plan, including prescription of sunscreens. In photosensitivity disorders where the action spectrum is in visible-light wavelengths (e.g. some solar urticaria, erythropoietic protoporphyria), the Dundee sunscreen needs to be prescribed.
- A review appointment: this may be with the referring doctor or may require further photodermatology clinic review if diagnosis or management is not straightforward.

Standard photoprotective advice to patients should include behavioural adaptations, suitable clothing, hats or umbrella, sunscreen use, avoidance of midday sun and use of window UV film (a clear UVA-blocking film). It may take the patient several years before they fully adopt these measures. The range and diversity of the photodermatoses mean that 'counselling' requirements differ. For example, with PLE a simple explanation of the disorder and its management may suffice. For chronic actinic dermatitis a more detailed explanation is usually required, particularly in older people, who may have difficulty accepting the nature of the condition and the need for meticulous photoprotection. Similarly, in children with photodermatoses the 'counselling' is given to the parents, usually with the child in attendance. For severe congenital photosensitivity syndromes such as xeroderma pigmentosum or congenital erythropoietic porphyria, this is best managed by a multidisciplinary team. This ensures that sufficient expertise is present to provide the family with a clear understanding of the disorder and its implications, the management plan and the prognosis. Some patients may initially be in a state of denial, and

appropriate support and encouragement may be needed. In many patients whose photosensitivity is diagnosed and confirmed, it is usually an immense relief.

Photosensitivity disorders

'Photosensitivity' is an abnormal response to low doses of UVA and/or UVB and/or visible light. This is distinct from easy-burning individuals with Fitzpatrick skin type I, who are at one end of the normal spectrum of responses.

Classification of the photosensitivity disorders

Photosensitivity disorders can be classified broadly into idiopathic, genetic, biochemical, photosensitisation by exogenous drugs or chemicals, and photoaggravated dermatoses (Table 24.4). The clinical presentations vary widely due to the broad spectrum of pathology. They may occur as primary disorders or may be caused by an underlying systemic disorder. The severity of photosensitivity disorders may range from a transient acute eruption to a chronic disorder resulting in disfigurement.

The idiopathic photodermatoses

Polymorphic light eruption (PLE) is by far the most common of the idiopathic photodermatoses. It is defined as a recurrent pruritic skin eruption comprising papules and/or vesicles and/or plaques, which occurs on photoexposed sites following sun exposure and heals without scarring. PLE is the most common photosensitivity disorder in White populations; in Europe, the prevalence is estimated at 18%. The condition can occur in any age group including childhood, but typically the age of onset is in the second to third decades. More females are affected than males (ratio 3:1). A typical history is that of a recurrent skin eruption on photoexposed sites, occurring in early spring or summer, on sunny holidays, after recreational sunbed use or during winter sports.

UVA, which transmits easily through clear non-laminated glass, can trigger PLE during car journeys. In more severe cases, PLE can be provoked in bright winter sunshine. An exposure of 30 minutes to several hours of sunlight is needed to provoke the rash, which appears after a variable latent period, typically 3–24 hours but ranging from minutes to several days. Symptoms of pruritus, burning and tenderness are described; this settles after 3–10 days with no scarring. Some patients have symptoms of eye irritation or dry or burning lips, and it may also be associated with general malaise and systemic upset lasting a few hours to two days. As the summer progresses, symptoms may abate due to a 'hardening' phenomenon occurring in the skin phototypes with tanning ability.

There is a wide clinical spectrum of the morphology of PLE (Figure 24.6). In approximate order of decreasing frequency, these are papular, papulovesicular, vesiculobullous, plaque, erythema

Table 24.4 A classification of photosensitivity disorders

Idiopathic	Polymorphic light eruption
	Chronic actinic dermatitis
	Actinic prurigo
	Solar urticaria
	Hydroa vacciniforme
Genetic	Xeroderma pigmentosum
	Cockayne syndrome
	Trichothiodystrophy
	Rothmund–Thomson syndrome
	Bloom syndrome
	Smith–Lemli–Opitz syndrome
Biochemical	Porphyria cutanea tarda
	Erythropoietic protoporphyria
	Variegate porphyria
	Congenital erythropoietic porphyria
Photosensitisation by exogenous drugs and chemicals	Drug-induced photosensitivity
	Photoallergic contact dermatitis
	Phytophotodermatitis
Photoaggravated dermatoses	Photoaggravated atopic eczema
	Photoaggravated eczema
	Photoaggravated psoriasis
	Lupus erythematosus
	Jessner's lymphocytic infiltrate
	Dermatomyositis
	Erythema multiforme

multiforme-like, urticarial, purpura, pinpoint papular, haemorrhagic and 'PLE sine eruptione', where there is pruritus in photoexposed areas in the absence of a rash. The papular and papulovesicular forms are overwhelmingly the most common in the general population (up to 88% of cases). The pinpoint papular variant is most often reported in African American patients. Diffuse facial redness and swelling may sometimes occur with papular lesions elsewhere. PLE typically heals without scarring, although scarring may occur due to excoriation of lesions.

The typical sites of involvement are the photoexposed sites: V of chest, upper limbs, dorsum of hands and lower limbs. The face may be spared due to 'hardening' at this exposed skin site.

The sites particularly at risk appear to be those that are covered in winter and promptly exposed at the first sign of sunlight in spring or on a sunny holiday, for example the chest and arms. The typical histopathological change seen in PLE is a perivascular lymphocytic infiltrate, although this is not diagnostic as it is seen in other disorders. Management includes topical and oral corticosteroids, self-hardening techniques (by graduated exposure to natural sunlight in early spring), prophylactic phototherapy, and immunosuppression for individuals who are particularly severely affected.

Chronic actinic dermatitis (synonymous with actinic reticuloid, photosensitive eczema, photosensitivity dermatitis) is a severe form of chronic eczema of photoexposed sites. It is classically described in older White men, although it is now also recognised in younger, often female patients with darker skin types, particularly South Asians and people of Afro-Caribbean descent (Figure 24.7). In some instances it may develop into a pseudolymphomatous appearance (hence termed 'actinic reticuloid'). Phototesting in most cases demonstrates very low MED to UVB, UVA and sometimes visible light, and patch and photopatch testing may reveal sensitivity to multiple airborne allergens, for example Compositae plants, fragrances or colophony. Management is often challenging and may include use of immunosuppression as well as biologic therapy (e.g. dupilumab).

Solar urticaria is an uncommon form of urticaria. The action spectrum is mostly in the UVA and visible-light range, although UVB may also be implicated. In many patients, there may be a coexisting inhibitory UV spectrum that reduces or abolishes the urticarial response. Thus, in occasional patients in whom urticaria is readily provoked by daylight, no reaction can be induced using artificial light sources. Onset may occur at any age, with preponderance in the third decade. The female-to-male ratio is estimated to be 2:1. The clinical presentation is that of a burning sensation seconds to minutes after sun exposure, followed by signs of inflammation including redness and usually weals, and settling within two hours in most cases, or by 24 hours. Depending on the patient's action spectrum, indoor lighting and UVA sunbeds may also provoke solar urticaria. Photoprovocation testing often confirms the diagnosis (Figure 24.8), and establishing the action spectrum with monochromator testing can help with choice of sunscreens. In the absence of UVB photosensitivity, desensitisation phototherapy with narrowband UVB can be considered, but only after thorough phototesting. Omalizumab can be considered for solar urticaria that is unresponsive to antihistamines and desensitisation phototherapy.

Actinic prurigo is a photodermatosis affecting Native American and Canadian Inuit populations, and native populations from Mexico and Central and South America mixed with those of European descent. It occurs less commonly in those solely of European descent. In some populations it appears to be an autosomal dominant condition with incomplete penetrance. In the Chimila Indians in Colombia with actinic prurigo, it is associated with HLA-Cw4; in Mexicans, HLA-DRB1*04:07; and in Canadian Inuits, HLA-DRB1*14. In British White populations, HLA-DRB1*04:07 has been identified in 60% of patients. The exact action spectrum is unknown.

(a)

(b)

(c)

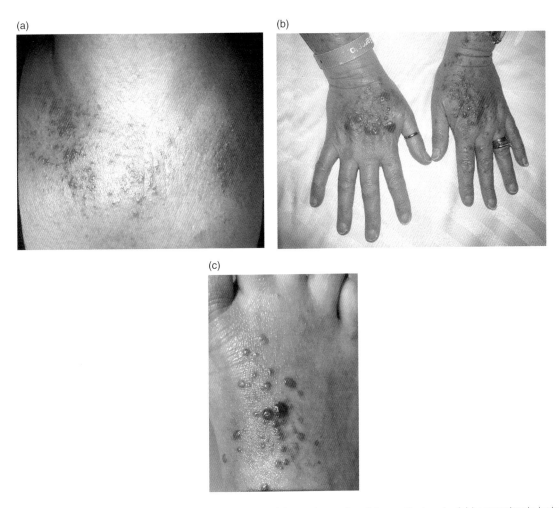

Figure 24.6 Polymorphic light eruption: (a) papules on the chest, (b) papules and vesicles on the hands, (c) haemorrhagic lesions on the foot. © Salford Royal NHS Foundation Trust.

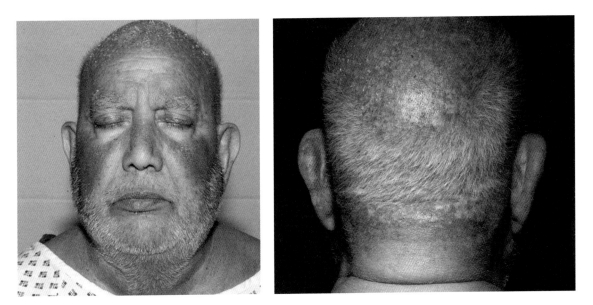

Figure 24.7 Chronic actinic dermatitis. © Salford Royal NHS Foundation Trust.

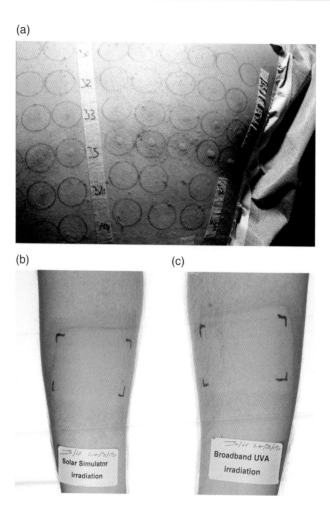

Figure 24.8 Solar urticaria photoprovocation: (a) with monochromator light testing, weal reactions occur within minutes and resolve within 1–2 hours; (b) to solar simulator; (c) to ultraviolet A. © Salford Royal NHS Foundation Trust.

The age of onset is usually around four or five years, with a female-to-male ratio of 2:1. Typically, the presentation is acute exudative facial eczema, prurigo-like lesions on the dorsal arms and hands, and excoriations, crusting, cheilitis and conjunctivitis (Figure 24.9). The presentation is less severe in the British population, with many patients presenting in adult life. The typical presentation is of chronic excoriated prurigo with eczematised nodules, lichenification and scarring, which may be pitted on the face. Covered sites are frequently affected and the relationship to UV exposure may not always be clear. Management may include prophylactic phototherapy, thalidomide and immunosuppressive therapy.

Hydroa vacciniforme is a very rare photosensitivity condition. It usually presents in childhood and remits by adolescence. There is no predilection for sex. It presents with papules and vesicles on the cheeks, nose and ears, and dorsa of hands. This is followed by haemorrhagic crusting, eventually healing with varioliform scarring (resembling variola or smallpox). Phototesting shows photosensitivity in the UVA spectrum, and the lesions can be provoked with UVA.

The genetic photodermatoses

The inherited photodermatoses are extremely rare. The underlying mechanism is a defect in DNA repair in all of these diseases, with the exception of Smith–Lemli–Opitz syndrome, where the defect is in cholesterol synthesis. In xeroderma pigmentosum (XP), Cockayne syndrome and trichothiodystrophy, the defect is in nucleotide excision repair, a part of the DNA repair pathway. In Rothmund–Thomson syndrome and Bloom syndrome, the defect is in the DNA helicases, which have a major role in DNA repair and recombination pathways. All patients with inherited photodermatoses have photosensitivity and require strict photoprotection.

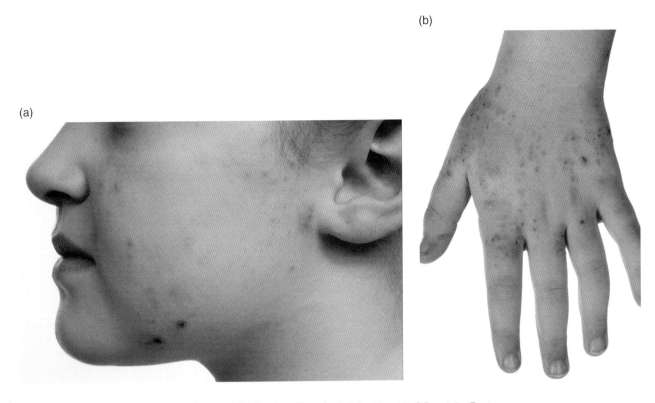

Figure 24.9 Actinic prurigo to (a) the face and (b) the dorsal hands. © Salford Royal NHS Foundation Trust.

The most common of these photodermatoses, XP, is an autosomal recessive disease that has no predilection for sex. Classical XP (Figure 24.10) occurs in 1 in one million of European and North American populations, and 1 in 100,000 people in Japan. The clinical manifestations consist of increased freckling, hyperpigmentation and severe sunburn response. There is a markedly increased incidence of skin tumours, especially of non-melanoma skin cancer, which are often evident before the age of five years. There are nine types of complementation groups, some of which are associated with ocular and neurological manifestations, and a reduced life span.

In XP variant, which constitutes about one-third of all cases of XP, the signs are less severe, skin tumours occur later, and neurological problems are not a feature. Phototesting in the classical type of XP shows pronounced sensitivity particularly to UVB, with a low MED and prolonged skin inflammation including redness, but phototesting in the variant type may be normal. The definitive test is a cell mutation study of cultures of the patient's fibroblasts, to assess the efficacy of DNA repair after UVR.

The cutaneous porphyrias

This category of photodermatosis is caused by an inherited or acquired enzyme defect in the metabolic pathway of haem,

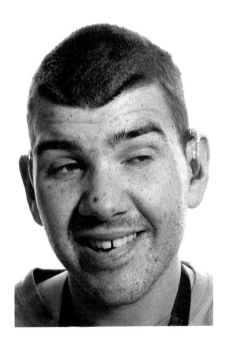

Figure 24.10 Xeroderma pigmentosum. © Salford Royal NHS Foundation Trust.

which results in accumulation of pathway intermediates causing skin photosensitivity and/or episodic neurovisceral attacks. Porphyria cutanea tarda (PCT), erythropoietic protoporphyria (EPP), variegate porphyria (VP) and congenital erythropoietic porphyria (CEP) all show varying degrees of photosensitivity. EPP typically presents in childhood, with crying within a few minutes of sun exposure. Further exposure will lead to skin inflammation including swelling or redness, and eventually scarring, which may be subtle clinically. PCT and VP present in adults with chronic features of photosensitivity, namely blisters and skin fragility, typically on the dorsa of both hands. Other associated signs are milia, hypertrichosis, pigmentation and sclerodermatous changes. Seasonal variation may not be present. VP has an additional complication with neurovisceral attacks. CEP (Günter's disease) is extremely rare. It presents in infancy with similar features to EPP, but much more severe symptoms and signs and with resultant severe scarring and mutilation.

Photosensitivity secondary to exogenous drugs and chemicals

Drugs can induce photosensitivity in several contexts: phototoxicity, pseudoporphyria, photoallergy, lupus erythematosus, lichenoid reactions and pellagra.

Phototoxic reactions may occur when certain photosensitising medications cause reactions on sun-exposed skin. A wide variety of drugs are reported to cause phototoxicity, including thiazides, loop diuretics, quinine, NSAIDs, antipsychotics, calcium channel antagonists, some antibiotics (e.g. the tetracyclines, fluoroquinolones and sulfonamides), antifungals, retinoids and psoralens. Phototoxic reactions have distinct patterns of presentation, which presumably reflect a wide range of photochemical events. These include an exaggerated sunburn, immediate inflammation, late-onset inflammation, increased skin fragility and blistering, and telangiectasia. Phototesting usually shows UVA sensitivity and sometimes also sensitivity to UVB or visible light.

Photoallergic contact dermatitis is a delayed-type hypersensitivity reaction, an immunologically mediated reaction. In contrast, phototoxicity is a non-immunological reaction that can occur in any individual exposed to a high enough dose of a phototoxic chemical and light of the appropriate wavelength. Phototoxic reactions typically occur within minutes of the first exposure, while a photoallergic reaction occurs only after subsequent exposure to the allergen and develops after 24–48 hours as an eczematous response. Most topical photoallergic reactions are due to sunscreens. The action spectra of both toxic and allergic photocontact dermatitis fall in the UVA range.

Phytophotodermatitis is caused by a psoralen-containing plant coming into contact with the skin, combined with UV exposure. It is a phototoxic reaction and not immune mediated. The presentation is often striking and related to the patient's outdoor activity and contact with plants. The signs of inflammation, including redness and blistering, which are usually bizarre, linear and/or angulated, may not appear for some days after the primary contact. It usually settles with post-inflammatory hyperpigmentation. The plants implicated include cow parsley, parsnip, celery, giant hogweed, lime and St John's wort (hypericin). The action spectrum is in the UVB/UVA region.

Photoaggravated dermatoses

This category includes a diverse range of dermatoses that can be induced or exacerbated by UV exposure, but may occur without it (Table 24.3). Management involves photoprotective measures and treatment of the underlying disease. The most commonly encountered photoaggravated dermatoses seen in photobiology clinics are photoaggravated eczema and lupus erythematosus (LE).

Photoaggravated atopic eczema occurs in about 10% of patients with atopic dermatitis and is increasingly recognised in patients of South Asian origin.

Both cutaneous and systemic LE are exacerbated by UVB and UVA. There are three main categories of presentation: cutaneous discoid LE, subacute LE and systemic LE. Cutaneous discoid LE can cause scarring, usually on the cheeks, and < 5% of cases will progress to systemic LE. Subacute cutaneous LE is associated with a pink-to-red, confluent polycyclic rash on the shoulders and is associated with positive anti-Ro antibodies in 60% of cases and anti-La in 80%. Systemic LE can present acutely with a 'butterfly rash' across the malar region or with a more diffuse sunburn-like reaction. The diagnosis of LE is supported by skin biopsy, immunofluorescence findings and serology.

Conclusions

Photosensitivity is often underdiagnosed due to lack of awareness among family physicians. It is distinct from burning in lighter skin types. Often patients adapt by drastic lifestyle measures to avoid sun exposure, and it is not unusual for patients to suffer silently for decades before being referred for further investigations. Improving disease recognition and clinical experience and expanding phototesting facilities are key to developing understanding in this area, as well as optimising quality of life in such patients.

Pearls and pitfalls

- Have a high index of suspicion for photosensitivity, as patients do not always offer a clear history of photosensitivity.
- In recalcitrant atopic eczema, consider a photoaggravated component to the disease.
- In skin of colour, be vigilant for photoaggravated eczema or chronic actinic dermatitis.
- Actinic prurigo is often misdiagnosed as eczema or nodular prurigo; the classical distribution includes covered sites such as the buttocks, as well as photoexposed sites.

- Very severe photosensitivity tends to occur all year round rather than having a clear seasonal variation, for example chronic actinic dermatitis, actinic prurigo and solar urticaria.
- A quick onset of symptoms after UV exposure suggests drug-induced photosensitivity; always take an accurate drug history including ingestion of non-prescribed treatments and supplements.
- Photoprotective advice should be tailored to the lifestyle and degree of severity of the patient's photosensitivity.

SCE Questions. See questions 66 and 67.

FURTHER READING AND KEY RESOURCES

Blakely KM, Drucker AM, Rosen CF. Drug-induced photosensitivity – an update: culprit drugs, prevention and management. *Drug Saf* 2019; **42**:827–47.

Choi D, Kannan S, Lim HW. Evaluation of patients with photodermatoses. *Dermatol Clin* 2014; **32**:267–75.

Diffey BL. What is light? *Photodermatol Photoimmunol Photomed* 2002; **18**:68–74.

Guitierrez D, Gaulding JV, Motta Beltran AF, Lim HW. Photodermatoses in skin of colour. *J Eur Acad Dermatol Venereol* 2018; **32**:1879–86.

Ibbotson SH, Allan D, Dawe RS *et al*. Photodiagnostic Services in the UK and Republic of Ireland: a British Photodermatology Group Workshop Report. *J Eur Acad Dermatol Venereol* 2021; doi: 10.1111/jdv.17632.

Petersen B, Wulf HC. Application of sunscreen – theory and reality. *Photodermatol Photoimmunol Photomed* 2014; **30**:96–101.

Textbook

Ferguson J, Dover JS, eds. *Photodermatology*. London: Manson Publishing, 2006.

Useful website

British Association of Dermatologists. Improving descriptors in dermatology. Available at: https://www.bad.org.uk/healthcare-professionals/inclusivity-and-representation/descriptors-in-dermatology.

25

Phototherapy and photodynamic therapy

Sally H. Ibbotson and Robert Dawe

Introduction

The use of light exposure to treat skin diseases is not a new concept, as the beneficial effects of sunlight for skin conditions, such as psoriasis, were recorded in Ancient Egypt and India. Light therapies used for skin disease are based on ultraviolet (UV) light and include UVB (290–320 nm), UVA (320–400 nm) and visible light (photodynamic therapy). The development of biologic and other therapies for psoriasis and eczema should not undervalue UV-based light therapy as a useful treatment option for a wide range of skin conditions in selected patients. Furthermore, photodynamic therapy (PDT) is an established non-surgical option for management of specific types of skin cancer and pre-cancer.

Dermatologists must be familiar with the range of light-based therapies available, and their indications, risks and benefits. It is also important to know how these services are set up and delivered, with good understanding of expected outcomes and current guidelines. Further reading, practical exposure and critical appraisal are encouraged in order to achieve the necessary knowledge, skills and competencies.

Phototherapy and photochemotherapy

What are phototherapy and photochemotherapy?

Phototherapy is the use of a phototherapy source (generally UV) alone and relies on chemicals within the patient's own skin to absorb the radiation, leading to the desired therapeutic effect. The commonest form of phototherapy is narrowband (NB)-UVB, with wavelengths of 311–313 nm. It has largely replaced broadband UVB as it excludes wavelengths that are not therapeutically beneficial, resulting in fewer side-effects. Broadband UVA

Dermatology Training: The Essentials. Edited by Mahbub M.U. Chowdhury, Tamara W. Griffiths and Andrew Y. Finlay.
© 2022 The British Association of Dermatologists. Published 2022 by John Wiley & Sons Ltd.
Companion website: www.wiley.com/go/chowdhury/dermatologytraining

is generally not used alone for phototherapy, although some specialist departments offer UVA1 phototherapy, which is long-wavelength UVA (340–400 nm).

Photochemotherapy is the use of UV to 'activate' an exogenous chemical that absorbs the radiation, resulting in the desired effects. The primary form of photochemotherapy is psoralen plus UVA (PUVA). Psoralen can be taken orally with the choice of two systemic drugs: 5- or 8-methoxypsoralen (MOP). Bath PUVA can be administered for whole-body treatment, or can be limited to the hands and feet in palmoplantar disease.

When taken orally, psoralen is a systemic drug that activates only with UVA exposure. This confines the main effects to the skin rather than affecting the whole body. However, the eye is also susceptible, and therefore UVA-filtered glasses must be worn during daylight hours after taking oral psoralen, in order to reduce the potential risk for cataracts. This is extended to 24 hours in children and high-risk patients, including those with pre-existing cataracts or atopic eczema. Patients may find this requirement to be prohibitive. Retinoid PUVA (RePUVA) is a therapeutic approach used in psoriasis, consisting of oral administration of a retinoid such as acitretin, combined with systemic PUVA. It can be considered as a treatment option in those with recalcitrant disease or used as a PUVA-sparing option.

How do phototherapy and photochemotherapy work?

These treatments are broadly immunosuppressive and cytotoxic. In inflammatory conditions such as psoriasis and eczema, the treatments work mainly through immunosuppression. In cutaneous T-cell lymphoma, their mode of action is primarily due to skin-directed cytotoxic effects. UVA used to activate the psoralen penetrates deeper than UVB. UVA1, available in specialised centres, is particularly effective in conditions that involve the deep dermis because of its greater depth of penetration and lower risk of skin inflammation. Paradoxically, phototherapy and photochemotherapy treatments can be used prophylactically for some light-induced conditions by desensitisation or 'hardening' the skin's response to UV.

Indications and contraindications

For most skin conditions, NB-UVB is the first-line phototherapy, with PUVA used as second line if NB-UVB is inadequate. Patients often do not understand the difference between these treatments, so it is important to explain that PUVA may still be effective even if they have not responded to NB-UVB previously.

Therapies can result in long-term clinical remission rather than merely suppressing disease during treatment. However, if relapses are relatively frequent, ongoing maintenance therapy is not appropriate.

Phototherapy and PUVA can be indicated for conditions such as psoriasis, atopic eczema, chronic spontaneous urticaria, mycosis fungoides, vitiligo, pruritus and nodular prurigo.

Paradoxically, it can also be used prophylactically for severe polymorphic light eruption, solar urticaria, erythropoietic protoporphyria and solar urticaria.

If NB-UVB phototherapy is ineffective, PUVA may be a good second-line option. The advantages and disadvantages of UVB compared to PUVA are detailed in Table 25.1. Where available, UVA1 is the phototherapy of choice for conditions with mainly dermal pathology, such as morphoea, widespread granuloma annulare, sarcoidosis and mastocytosis.

There are a number of situations where phototherapy and PUVA are potentially risky or may even be harmful (Table 25.2). They are contraindicated in patients with DNA repair genodermatoses, such xeroderma pigmentosum or Gorlin's syndrome. Previous skin cancers and a strong family history are a relative contraindication to PUVA, as high cumulative doses of PUVA are associated with cutaneous malignancy. Caution must also be noted in patients who have a previous history of immunosuppressive treatments such as ciclosporin or azathioprine, and their concomitant use should be avoided. There is less concern with NB-UVB and immunosuppressants; it is sometimes combined with methotrexate or topical tacrolimus.

Reactions from photosensitising drugs usually occur through a phototoxic mechanism, most commonly within the UVA range. However, as a general rule they are not relevant with the use of PUVA, because the additional photosensitising impact is inconsequential compared to that of the oral psoralen. Commonly used drugs that can potentially cause photosensitivity issues with NB-UVB are quinine, calcium channel blockers, non-steroidal anti-inflammatory drugs, thiazides, prochlorperazine, chlorpromazine and doxycycline.

Table 25.1 Advantages and disadvantages of UVB therapy compared with PUVA

Advantages

No oral or topical photosensitising drug is needed
No eye protection is necessary *following* therapy
The incidence of side-effects is lower
It is safe to use during pregnancy
Irradiation times are often shorter
In children it is safer than PUVA

Disadvantages

Treatment is usually given three times per week rather than two times per week, or three times every two weeks with bath PUVA
For some patients, duration of disease remission is shorter with UVB than with PUVA
It is less effective than PUVA in clearing psoriasis

Table 25.2 Contraindications to UVB therapy and PUVA

Relative contraindications to UVB therapy

Children

The elderly

Patients with skin phototype I (always burn, never tan)

Patients taking a photosensitising drug

Epilepsy induced by flashing lights

Those with photoaggravated skin disorders

Some patients with acquired photosensitivity (although narrowband UVB is sometimes used for this indication, it is always necessary to proceed with care)

Patients with skin conditions known to respond poorly (or relapse early) to narrowband UVB

Patients with cutaneous signs of chronic photodamage

Absolute contraindications to UVB therapy

Patients with a past history of skin cancer

Patients with genetic skin cancer syndromes (xeroderma pigmentosum, Gorlin's syndrome)

Patients unwilling or unable to comply with safety procedures (those in poor mental health or with learning difficulties)

Relative contraindications to PUVA

Children

The elderly

Patients with skin phototype I (always burn, never tan)

Patients taking a photosensitising drug

Intolerance of systemic psoralens (in which case topical PUVA could be tried)

Epilepsy induced by flashing lights

Those with photoaggravated skin disorders

Some patients with acquired photosensitivity (although PUVA is sometimes used for this indication, it is always necessary to proceed with care)

Patients with skin conditions known to respond poorly (or relapse early) to PUVA

Methodology

Narrowband ultraviolet B

The starting dose should be based on minimal erythemal dose (MED) testing, with results read after 24 hours, although they can also be read on the same day with a small test dose on the forearm. MED testing is performed for safety reasons to prevent burning, but may also allow the phototherapist to start at a higher initial dose if the test MED is higher than anticipated.

NB-UVB is usually given either two or three times weekly. Three times weekly may be more effective for psoriasis. The response to treatment varies greatly between individuals. On average, a course for psoriasis is 20–25 treatments, for eczema 25–35 treatments and for chronic urticaria 35–50 treatments. These total treatment numbers can be useful when discussing the duration of the treatment course with patients. Those who respond will see an improvement starting between 15 and 20 treatments, and if there is no improvement by then it may be necessary to consider alternative therapy such as PUVA. The main adverse effects of NB-UVB are a sunburn-like reaction and the possible but unproven increased skin cancer risk.

Psoralen plus ultraviolet A

The starting dose should be based on the minimal phototoxic dose (MPD), an important bioassay used to ensure therapeutic psoralen levels in the skin. Oral psoralens may have poor bioavailability and the MPD indicates adequate levels in the skin to provide effective treatment. Topical PUVA has a high risk of severe blistering phototoxic reactions and performing the MPD safeguards against this.

Psoralen plus ultraviolet A with psoralens applied undiluted

PUVA in combination with undiluted psoralen is used to treat limited areas of skin disease, such as occur in some cases of vitiligo. Psoralen emulsion or paint can be used by neat application to the affected skin. When treating the feet, the presence of fissuring or erosions may necessitate use of diluted psoralens to minimise stinging. Psoralen gel (methoxsalen 0.005%) is also available for the treatment of small areas of skin. It has a thicker consistency than either paint or emulsion, and is easier to apply to the required areas without inadvertent spread to adjacent skin. It is also usually tolerated by patients with sore and fissured skin. UVA irradiation is usually from hand and foot UVA units.

Bath psoralen plus ultraviolet A

A standard treatment regimen used in PUVA units throughout the UK involves mixing 30 mL of 1.2% 8-MOP lotion in 140 L of water for a final concentration of 2.6 mg/L. The patient then bathes in this solution for 10 minutes, taking care to gently swish the solution around, ensuring that all parts of the body are evenly exposed to the solution. The patient then emerges from the bath, dries the skin with a towel, and immediately enters the PUVA cabinet for exposure to UVA. The initial dose of UVA (typically 0.2–0.5 J/cm^2) is determined by prior MPD testing, with increments of 20–40%, depending upon skin response to previous treatments. Bath PUVA is commonly given in a twice-weekly regimen or three times every two weeks. There is no need for patients to shower or wash the skin following irradiation, as cutaneous absorption and binding dynamics suggest that no free psoralen remains on the skin surface. PUVA-induced erythema with topical psoralens peaks at 3–5 days, which explains why some PUVA units have changed from a twice-weekly regimen to three times every two weeks. This avoids the chance of giving further PUVA before the erythemal response of the previous treatment has peaked.

Systemic psoralen plus ultraviolet A

Some light therapy units do not have bath facilities and cannot offer bath PUVA. Systemic PUVA avoids the need for bath facilities. There is a choice of two different systemic psoralens, 8-MOP and 5-MOP. 8-MOP is more photosensitising and therefore more effective, but has a higher incidence of side-effects than 5-MOP. The greater photosensitising effect of 8-MOP may be a problem in more fair-skinned individuals and in vitiligo due to an increased risk of burning. Systemic psoralens are taken orally with a light meal two hours before treatment. The dose is determined by body surface area, at 25 mg/m^2 for 8-MOP and 50 mg/m^2 for 5-MOP. Eye protection that blocks natural UVA is required ideally for 24 hours after ingestion of psoralen, but at least until sunset on the day of ingestion as a minimum. UVA-filtered eyewear can be clear and colourless, as there is no need to block visible light.

The main adverse effect associated with oral psoralen is nausea. Taking it with a small amount of food can be beneficial, but a large meal could reduce bioavailability. 5-MOP has fewer gastrointestinal side-effects than 8-MOP, although it has a weaker photosensitising effect and is more expensive.

There is a risk of squamous cell skin cancer, which increases proportionally with the number of PUVA treatments, especially if there are more than 200 in total. This risk needs to be discussed in the wider context of alternative treatment options available to the patient.

Ultraviolet A1

This is a specialised form of phototherapy not widely available in the UK. If it is available where you work, you are advised to seek local advice. Similarly, if it is not available in your centre and you wish to refer a patient, seek advice from where it could be offered, particularly for any of the conditions mentioned earlier.

Consent

Prior to referral for phototherapy or PUVA, a full discussion about the range of treatment options should be reviewed with the dermatologist. If there is agreement to opt for phototherapy or PUVA, it is important to explain the risks and benefits of therapy, in addition to practical aspects of the treatment. This should be carried out by an appropriately trained and experienced member of staff, usually a senior phototherapist. Trainees should sit in on some sessions of this type in order to understand what information is covered. The implications of treatment need to be explained in detail and patient concerns addressed.

Signing a consent form before the start of treatment is required, but it is not legally binding and at best serves as a helpful reminder of the need to have a full and detailed discussion, including potential adverse events. As the dermatologist is ultimately responsible for the patient, it is best they obtain consent rather than delegating to the phototherapist administering the treatment, although there is regional variation particularly with NB-UVB.

Clinical governance

To help ensure the efficacy and safety of phototherapy and PUVA, consider participation in a clinical governance scheme. They assist centres to align practice with agreed standards, which is particularly important due to the complexity of phototherapy and PUVA services.

These schemes include Photonet – the National Managed Clinical Network for Phototherapy in Scotland. Support can also be obtained from other appropriate networks such as the South East of England Phototherapy Network. Other schemes are important in supporting centres to meet national UK standards based largely on the Photonet standards, but appropriate in the different UK countries. The Service Guidance and Standards for Phototherapy are accredited by the National Institute for Health and Care Excellence.

Patients should be offered annual review if they have received many treatments, such as more than 200 whole-body PUVA treatments or more than 500 whole-body NB-UVB treatments. Other indications include increased skin cancer risk, such as a history of immunosuppressive therapy with ciclosporin or azathioprine. This emphasises the need for vigilance to both patients and their primary care physicians. Patient education on adequate sun protection and self-skin checks is important. Historically, there was the idea of 'ceiling' doses or numbers of treatments that should never be exceeded. It is now recognised that risks increase continually; there is not a threshold below which there is no risk and above which the risk is unacceptable. It is important to discuss this with patients, and the numerical values noted above can be used as prompts for discussion.

Medical physics input

It is essential to ensure appropriate dosimetry and safety for patients and staff. Medical physicists can be invaluable in calibration and maintenance of phototherapy equipment and support protocols relating to clinical governance. The amount of input from a physicist with an interest in non-ionising radiation varies among dermatology departments. It is advisable that trainees working in departments without medical physics input attend a recognised course and seek opportunities to spend some time in a unit with integral medical physics support.

Setting up a phototherapy unit

When setting up a new unit or making changes to an existing unit, support from established centres and local networks is essential. Important considerations include:

- How will a service be organised to provide for the catchment area population? For example, should there be one main hospital centre or scattered satellite centres? Would supervised home phototherapy, as part of a hospital-based service, or self-administered phototherapy be part of the service?
- What are the most important phototherapies needed to serve the catchment area? The minimum will normally be whole-body NB-UVB and localised hand and foot PUVA, but local issues such as distance to the nearest whole-body PUVA centre need to be considered.
- What regimens will be followed? How will starting doses be determined? Here reference to national and local standards should help.

New developments

The phototherapies have been led by the development of new technologies. Natural sunlight (heliotherapy) was replaced by carbon arc and other lamps, which were in turn replaced by fluorescent lamps used both in broadband UVB and for the broadband UVA used in PUVA. Broadband UVB fluorescent lamps have subsequently been superseded by NB-UVB fluorescent lamps. It is expected that the fluorescent lamps will eventually be surpassed by ultraviolet light-emitting diodes (LEDs). These new sources will be easier to adjust, with the possibility of readily choosing different wavelength outputs for different conditions. Also, as the technology becomes more efficient with devices that are compact and easier to transport, home phototherapy is likely to become more widely available.

Photodynamic therapy

What is photodynamic therapy?

PDT involves oxygen-dependent photochemical light activation of a photosensitiser (Figure 25.1) in target tissue. This reaction is used in dermatology as a lesion-targeted topical treatment.

The term 'photodynamic reaction' was coined following the observation by Oscar Raab of the cytotoxicity of protozoa in the presence of acridine orange and daylight. In 1903, von Tappeiner and Jesionek reported on the beneficial effects of topical eosin and light exposure for a range of skin conditions, including skin cancers and lupus vulgaris. This formed the basis of PDT. After pioneering self-experimentation by Meyer-Betz in 1912 and studies in the 1970s by Dougherty using systemic porphyrin photosensitisers, topical PDT using porphyrin precursors was introduced by Kennedy and colleagues in 1990, with licensed use since 2003. Topical PDT is now widely used in dermatology. Systemic PDT is under evaluation and in limited use in the management of other malignancies, such as of head and neck, lung and brain.

How does photodynamic therapy work?

Topical PDT involves application of a pro-drug to the skin lesion or site to be treated. This is taken up and converted to a photosensitiser in the target tissue, prior to photochemical activation by light of appropriate wavelengths, in the presence of oxygen. The pro-drugs used in dermatology are porphyrin precursors: 5-aminolaevulinic acid (ALA) and methyl aminolaevulinate (MAL). These small molecules are taken up into lesional cells and metabolised via the haem cycle to the potent photosensitiser, protoporphyrin IX (PpIX), which is produced in mitochondria and is present at low levels in mammalian nucleated cells. Due to exogenous overload of ALA or MAL and the rate-limiting ferrochelatase enzyme step, PpIX accumulates in the target tissue (Figure 25.2). PpIX fluoresces in an oxygen-independent

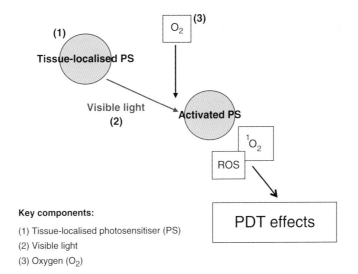

Key components:

(1) Tissue-localised photosensitiser (PS)
(2) Visible light
(3) Oxygen (O_2)

Figure 25.1 The essentials of photodynamic therapy. $^1O_2$, singlet oxygen; ROS, reactive oxygen species. © University of Dundee.

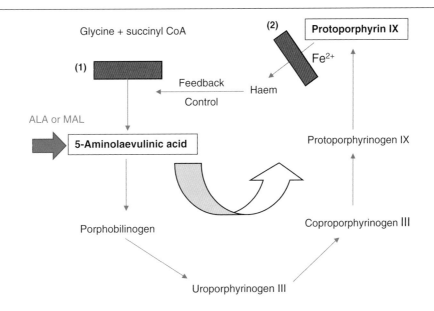

Haem cycle showing how overload of excess ALA or MAL leads to accumulation of protoporphyrin IX (PpIX) in the target tissue.

Rate-limiting steps (1) ALA synthase. (2) Ferrochelatase

Figure 25.2 'Porphyrin' photodynamic therapy – harnessing the haem cycle. ALA, 5-aminolaevulinic acid; MAL, methyl aminolaevulinate. © University of Dundee.

process, with crimson red fluorescence, which can be visualised using Wood's light showing lesion specificity (Figure 25.3).

After pro-drug application, preferential PpIX accumulation occurs in the diseased tissue (usually pre-malignant or malignant cells, although it also accumulates after pro-drug application to benign conditions such as psoriasis or viral warts). This mechanism of selectivity is not fully understood, but is likely multifactorial, including increased pro-drug uptake across abnormal lesional skin barrier, hyperproliferation, and possible relative iron deficiency and altered haem cycle enzymes in diseased tissue. This relative selectivity of PpIX accumulation is advantageous with respect to minimising damage to normal skin, which is also facilitated by targeted light delivery. PpIX absorbs light, particularly in the violet/blue part of the spectrum

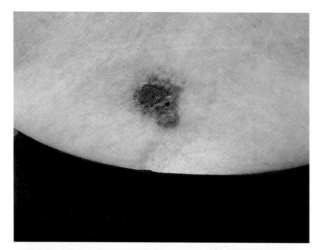

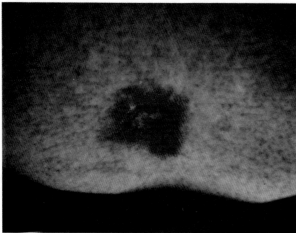

Figure 25.3 Wood's light examination showing lesion-specific crimson red fluorescence of protoporphyrin IX, three hours after pro-drug application to a superficial basal cell carcinoma. © NHS Tayside.

Table 25.3 Main indications for photodynamic therapy

Superficial, non-hyperkeratotic actinic keratoses on the face and scalp (includes field change carcinogenesis)
Bowen's disease
Superficial basal cell carcinoma
Thin nodular (1-2 mm) basal cell carcinoma if other treatments have failed or are not feasible

keratosis (AK), Bowen's disease (BD) and superficial basal cell carcinoma (BCC) are the main indications for PDT (Table 25.3).

In the UK, MAL (Metvix®, Galderma, Watford, UK; MAL 16% cream) and 5-ALA in nanocolloid emulsion (Ameluz®, Biofrontera Pharma, Leverkusen, Germany; ALA 8% gel) are licensed for use in topical PDT. MAL-PDT is approved for thin non-hyperkeratotic AK on the face and scalp, and BD and BCC (superficial and selected thin 1–2 mm nodular). Ameluz is also approved for similar AK and BCC indications. Metvix and Ameluz are also licensed for use in daylight PDT for mild-to-moderate AK on the face and scalp. There is a large evidence base for topical PDT, with many international multicentre randomised controlled studies comparing PDT with cryotherapy, 5-fluorouracil (5-FU), imiquimod and surgery. British Association of Dermatologists and other international guidelines and systematic reviews are available and should be read to understand the evidence base.

Topical PDT is at least as effective as, and in some studies superior to, standard comparators for AK, BD and superficial BCC. For AK, 5-FU has been shown to be the most effective first-choice therapy, and PDT is usually considered after failure to respond to or tolerate 5-FU. Efficacy rates of >75% are reported for AK treated with PDT, and similarly high efficacy rates can be achieved for BD and superficial BCC. Daylight PDT is of equivalent efficacy to conventional PDT for AK, but is much better tolerated. Longer-term recurrence after PDT may be up to 20–25%. This must be explained to patients, as it is higher than with surgical excision but comparable to other non-surgical treatments, and PDT is usually selected in settings where surgery would not be appropriate.

PDT is inferior to surgery for nodular BCC and is not advised unless surgery is not feasible. Furthermore, single-cycle PDT was shown to be inferior to imiquimod for both superficial and nodular BCC, but with fewer adverse effects. Imiquimod has not been compared to standard treatment with a double PDT cycle. Morphoeic BCC and invasive tumours, including melanoma and squamous cell carcinoma (SCC), should not be treated with PDT, as metastatic potential and high recurrence rates are concerns (Table 25.4).

Patient tolerance and satisfaction are high for PDT, with low incidence of significant adverse effects and excellent healing and cosmesis, likely consequent to treatment selectivity. The main adverse effect of PDT is pain or discomfort (Table 25.5), although this can be minimised by adjusting treatment regimens, as described later. Phototoxic inflammation after treatment is expected and is not usually limiting. Rarely, contact allergy to the pro-drug can occur; this can be confirmed on patch testing. PDT

(peak approximately 410 nm), although it also has absorption peaks in the red part of the spectrum (approximately 632–635 nm). Thus, light-induced photochemical activation of PpIX occurs during PDT, with type I and type II photo-oxidation reactions. The generation of reactive oxygen species, particularly singlet oxygen, initiates a cascade of events including activation of signalling pathways, pro-inflammatory changes, mitochondrial and membrane damage, and apoptosis and necrosis.

Dermatological indications

Topical PDT is suitable for treatment of superficial skin lesions, in particular dysplasia and non-melanoma skin cancers. As both photosensitiser accumulation and light delivery are limited to the epidermis and superficial dermis, thicker and deeper lesions should not generally be treated with PDT. In practice, actinic

Table 25.4 Relative contraindications to photodynamic therapy

Thick tumours, e.g. thick nodular basal cell carcinoma (histological thickness > 2 mm)
High-risk basal cell carcinoma, e.g. morphoeic or tumours at high-risk sites such as mid-face
Tumours with metastatic risk, e.g. squamous cell carcinoma and melanoma
Known allergy to pro-drug(s) or excipients
Patients with cutaneous porphyrias
Pregnancy

Table 25.5 Adverse effects of photodynamic therapy (PDT)

Pain/discomfort (common)
Erythema*
Oedema*
Urticaria*
Crusting or exudation*
Infection
Purpura/bruising
Contact allergy to pro-drug(s) or excipients
Scarring
Milia
Pigment loss or gain
Hair loss or gain
Photo-onycholysis
Erosive pustular dermatosis of scalp
Bullous pemphigoid

* Expected effects of a phototoxic insult.

Table 25.6 Advantages of photodynamic therapy

Highly effective for appropriate indications
Can be undertaken as an outpatient or at home
Lesion-specific treatment
Can be used for field carcinogenesis
Can be used in immunosuppressed patients
Well tolerated
Excellent cosmetic outcome
Low risk of scarring
High levels of patient satisfaction
Can be repeated if required
No evidence of cumulative toxicity

can be repeated as there is no evidence to suggest cumulative toxicity or carcinogenic risk. Indeed, there is some evidence that repeated PDT may have a prophylactic role in prevention of AK and SCC development, particularly in high-risk patients such as organ transplant recipients.

Specialist photodynamic therapy services

PDT services should be available to those involved in skin cancer management and accessible through affiliation with skin cancer multidisciplinary teams. Trainees should be aware of the indications and contraindications for PDT and of the need to account for individual patient and lesion factors when deciding on the most appropriate treatment option. Trainees should also be familiar with the advantages (Table 25.6) and disadvantages of PDT compared with other therapies for AK, BD and BCC, and also when PDT should not be used (Table 25.6). Trainees should familiarise themselves with the British Association of Dermatologists' service standards for PDT, as they are a useful guide for setting up and delivering a PDT service. They include standards for benchmarking, training, audit and governance processes. Other useful reading is the National Institute for Health and Care Excellence interventional procedures guidance for PDT.

Who should be referred for photodynamic therapy and clinical assessment?

Clinical assessment is essential, in order to ascertain the benefits, risks and appropriateness of PDT. Typically, there may be more than one treatment option, such as 5-FU, imiquimod or PDT. For example, a patient with AK with mild field change may initially use 5-FU, as evidence supports its superior efficacy as first treatment; PDT may be most appropriate for a patient with superficial BCC or BD who is unable to treat themselves at home; and a patient with superficial BCC who is able to self-treat may wish to use imiquimod.

Where feasible, confirmatory biopsy should be undertaken for BD and superficial BCC, but this may not be done, particularly if multiple lesions are present at sites of poor healing such as the lower leg. Of course, biopsy is essential if there is diagnostic doubt. PDT is particularly suitable for lower-leg BD, for multiple or large lesions of superficial BCC or BD, and for AK with non-hyperkeratotic field change on the face and scalp. It can also be used in patients who are immunosuppressed and may play an important role in this setting. Patients need to be counselled and made fully aware of the options. They must consent for treatment and for the time involved either in attending hospital or in self-treating with daylight PDT.

Method of administration

It is important to observe and supervise PDT treatments in a consultant-led clinic and to supplement knowledge acquired through independent study and ideally a photodermatology course. Assessment of PDT skills can be undertaken through direct observation of the procedure.

Conventional photodynamic therapy

A PDT cycle for AK usually involves a single treatment, whereas for BD and superficial BCC a PDT cycle involves two treatments at a one-week interval. Before application of the pro-drug (MAL or ALA), gentle surface preparation is undertaken using either a disposable ring curette or an abrasive pad to loosen and remove surface scale and crust. If lesions are hyperkeratotic, pre-treatment with salicylic acid may be required, although PDT is not licensed for hyperkeratotic AK. If nodular BCCs are treated with PDT, more thorough debulking may be required prior to PDT. A thin layer of MAL or ALA is then applied (about 1 mm thick) to the lesion or field, including the surrounding 5–10 mm of normal skin. The area is covered with an occlusive dressing for three hours, which is then removed and surplus cream or gel is wiped off. The lesional area is demarcated to include a 5-mm rim of clinically normal perilesional skin, and this may be guided by Wood's light examination of fluorescence to identify the irradiation field. Fluorescence will be photobleached by irradiation or dissipate within 24 hours due to the short half-life of PpIX.

While a range of light sources are available, red LEDs are generally used in conventional PDT (e.g. Aktilite®, Galderma; or RhodoLED®, Biofrontera Pharma), with a narrow spectrum of emission around 630–635 nm, to deliver a dose of 37 J/cm^2 (Figure 25.4). Alternative sources with a continuous spectrum in the range 570–670 nm may be used to deliver a dose of 75 J/cm^2. Irradiance must be kept below 150–200 mW/cm^2 to avoid thermal effects. The LEDs used in hospital PDT generally have irradiances of around 80–85 mW/cm^2. Battery-pack low-irradiance LEDs (approximately 7 mW/cm^2) for portable home use may also be effective, although they are not widely available in routine clinical care.

Only approved CE-marked lamps should be used, as they will have the necessary filters and mirrors to minimise heat, UV and blue light exposure. The manufacturer's user manual must be followed, maximum field size must not be exceeded, irradiance should be monitored and the correct light dose should be administered and measured, if a suitable detector is available. The light dose is determined by several factors, notably irradiance of the source, size of treatment field, distance between lamp and skin surface, and irradiation time. The patient and operator

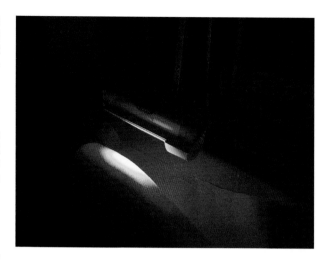

Figure 25.4 Conventional photodynamic therapy with red light-emitting diode irradiation. © NHS Tayside.

should wear protective goggles corresponding to the specific lamp spectrum during irradiation, as while red light exposure is not harmful, it can be uncomfortably bright. Healthy untreated perilesional skin does not need to be protected during illumination. Several lesions can be treated in the same session if they are within a single irradiation field.

Immediately after PDT, pain and phototoxicity can occur. Lesion response is assessed at three months, and lesions showing incomplete response may be re-treated using a further PDT cycle, with three-month follow-up after the last PDT cycle. Follow-up to at least one year after PDT for BD and BCC is desirable (Figure 25.5), and shorter-duration follow-up is usually needed for AK.

Daylight photodynamic therapy

Daylight PDT is increasingly used worldwide for patients with field carcinogenesis or superficial AK on the face and scalp, due to high levels of efficacy and tolerance. Daylight PDT can be used (in the UK) between April and October. It is essential to select patients who can comply with treatment and who have appropriate disease characteristics. A high sun protection factor (> 30) absorbent sunscreen should be applied to all exposed areas and allowed to dry, prior to surface preparation to remove surface scale, as described above. The pro-drug (MAL or ALA) is then thinly applied to the lesion(s) or field. Patients are advised to go outdoors into continuous daylight within 30 minutes of pro-drug application and expose the treatment areas to two hours of continuous unshaded light. After treatment the patient should go indoors, wipe off surplus cream or gel and stay indoors for the rest of the day, away from direct light. Mild discomfort during treatment may occur, and phototoxic inflammation is expected and may last a few days. Patients should be reviewed three months after daylight PDT and treatment can be repeated if there is a partial response.

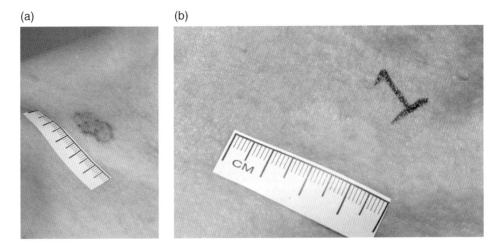

Figure 25.5 Conventional photodynamic therapy (PDT) for superficial basal cell carcinoma: (a) before PDT; (b) clear at one-year follow-up after PDT. © NHS Tayside.

Table 25.7 Factors influencing risk of photodynamic therapy-induced pain

Large treatment field
Severe field change with dysplasia
Specific body sites, e.g. face and scalp
Influence of disease unclear: actinic keratosis possibly more painful
Strong fluorescence

Table 25.8 Management of photodynamic therapy-induced pain

Methods that are practical and may be of benefit
Reassurance and distraction by the practitioner
Cooling water spray or fan
Pausing the treatment
Low-irradiance regimens, e.g. daylight or portable light-emitting diodes
Methods that are less practical or of limited benefit
Local anaesthesia, e.g. nerve blockade
Oral analgesia, e.g. paracetamol
Nitrous oxide (as used with oxygen during labour)
Transcutaneous electrical nerve stimulation (TENS)
Topical anaesthetics, capsaicin, morphine gel

Pain management during photodynamic therapy

Pain may be an issue during PDT and a mild degree of discomfort is to be expected. This used to be more problematic with higher-irradiance PDT regimens, but is now less of a problem and most patients tolerate PDT well. Awareness of factors that may influence risk of PDT-induced pain is important, as this may allow regimens to be adapted to minimise pain (Table 25.7). Low-irradiance PDT, such as daylight PDT, is extremely well tolerated without loss of efficacy. Other pain management measures may be of some limited benefit (Table 25.8).

Conclusions

Phototherapy and photochemotherapy (PUVA) are widely used in the treatment of primarily inflammatory skin disease, although indications expand well beyond this remit. Their success is reflected by the ever-expanding list of phototherapy units in the UK. Both forms of treatment can be dramatically effective and may transform a patient's life by managing or even clearing their skin disease. Acute and chronic adverse events can occur but should be uncommon. Expertise and clinical governance protocols are required for the safe and effective delivery of these treatments. The recognition of potentially serious adverse effects, in particular skin malignancy, has shifted the climate of opinion worldwide towards more controlled use of phototherapy and PUVA. PDT has emerged as a mainstream light-based therapy and is an established treatment for specific forms of non-melanoma skin cancer and dysplasia. Although dermatologists have personal opinions based on their education, training and experience, consensus has been reached through national guidelines and best-practice protocols. Dermatology trainees must be familiar with these and develop capabilities in the utilisation of phototherapy, PUVA and PDT in order to deliver the best care and offer a full range of treatment options to patients.

Pearls and pitfalls

- In order to prevent cataracts, patients who take oral psoralen must wear UVA-filtered eye protection from the time of psoralen ingestion. They must continue to wear it during daylight and indoor light exposure until sundown, or for up to 24 hours if they are at high risk.
- UVA penetrates more deeply into the skin than UVB, and therefore PUVA and UVA1 may be more effective in conditions with primarily dermal pathology.
- There is a higher correlation of skin malignancy with PUVA than with UVB.
- There is no cumulative toxicity with PDT and treatment can be repeated safely.
- Daylight PDT can be used in the UK from April to October and is an effective and convenient treatment in selected patients.
- Phototherapy, PUVA and PDT are complex services involving a variety of treatment indications, multidisciplinary healthcare providers and high specification equipment. Therefore it is important to adhere to protocols that comply with agreed standards.

SCE Questions. See questions 41 and 42.

FURTHER READING AND KEY RESOURCES

Bedair KF, Dawe RS. A retrospective review of factors associated with response to phototherapy and PUVA for atopic eczema. *Photodermatol Photoimmunol Photomed* 2021; **37**:153–6.

Boswell K, Cameron H, West J et al. Narrowband ultraviolet B treatment for psoriasis is highly economical and causes significant savings in cost for topical treatments. *Br J Dermatol* 2018; **179**:1148–56.

Collier NJ, Haylett AK, Wong TH et al. Conventional and combination topical photodynamic therapy for basal cell carcinoma: systematic review and meta-analysis. *Br J Dermatol* 2018; **179**:1277–96.

Dawe RS, Cameron HM, Yule S et al. A randomized comparison of methods of selecting narrowband UV-B starting dose to treat chronic psoriasis. *Arch Dermatol* 2011; **147**:168–74.

Hearn RM, Kerr AC, Rahim KF et al. Incidence of skin cancers in 3867 patients treated with narrow-band ultraviolet B phototherapy. *Br J Dermatol* 2008; **159**:931–5.

Ibbotson SH, Bilsland D, Cox NH et al. An update and guidance on narrowband ultraviolet B phototherapy: a British Photodermatology Group Workshop Report. *Br J Dermatol* 2004; **151**:283–97.

Ibbotson S, McKenna K. Principles of photodynamic therapy. In: *Rook's Textbook of Dermatology* (Griffiths C, Barker J, Bleiker T, Chalmers R, Creamer D, eds), 9th edn. Hoboken, NJ: Wiley, 2016; Chapter 22.

Ibbotson SH, Wong TH, Morton CA et al. Adverse effects of topical photodynamic therapy: a consensus review and approach to management. *Br J Dermatol* 2019; **180**:715–29.

Ling TC, Clayton TH, Crawley J et al. British Association of Dermatologists and British Photodermatology Group guidelines for the safe and effective use of psoralen-ultraviolet A therapy 2015. *Br J Dermatol* 2016; **174**:24–55.

Warburton KL, Ward A, Turner D, Goulden V. Home phototherapy: experience of setting up a new service in the UK's National Health Service. *Br J Dermatol* 2020; **182**:251–3.

Wiegell SH, Wulf HC, Szeimies RM et al. Daylight photodynamic therapy for actinic keratosis: an international consensus: International Society for Photodynamic Therapy in Dermatology. *J Eur Acad Dermatol Venereol* 2012; **26**:673–9.

Wong TH, Morton CA, Collier N et al. British Association of Dermatologists and British Photodermatology Group guidelines for topical photodynamic therapy (PDT) 2018. *Br J Dermatol* 2019; **180**:730–9.

Useful websites

British Association of Dermatologists. Photodynamic therapy (including the Photodynamic Therapy Service Guidance and Standards). Available at: https://www.bad.org.uk/healthcare-professionals/clinical-services/service-guidance/pdt.

National Institute for Health and Care Excellence. Photodynamic therapy for non-melanoma skin tumours (including premalignant and primary non-metastatic skin lesions). Available at: https://www.nice.org.uk/guidance/IPG155.

Photonet – the National Managed Clinical Network for Phototherapy in Scotland. Available at: www.photonet.scot.nhs.uk.

The South East of England Phototherapy Network. Available at: www.phototherapysupport.net.

26

Lymphoedema

Kristiana Gordon and Peter Mortimer

Introduction

Oedema, from the Greek word for swelling, represents increased extravascular tissue volume. Although the term has classical roots, the condition is highly relevant to modern dermatological practice, and it is crucial for trainees to understand the importance of these conditions, which not only create a significant burden to our healthcare system, but can also have potentially life-ruining consequences for patients. Fundamental to this is a review of the complex and often misunderstood lymphatic system.

The lymphatic system

The lymphatic system is an intricately linked and important part of the circulatory system. It consists of a large network of delicate, thin-walled vessels that drain into the lymphoid organs and tissues, carrying lymph fluid towards the heart. Unlike the cardiovascular system, it is not a closed system, and it provides an important accessory route to return interstitial fluid to the blood.

The system maintains the balance of body fluids via a network of capillaries and collecting lymphatic vessels, which drain and transport extravasated fluid, along with cellular debris and antigens, back to the circulatory system.

The lymph capillaries are blind-ended fingers, intermingling with tissues and at the arteriole–venule interface. Intraluminal valves ensure a unidirectional flow of lymph. It is important to note that most of the body's tissue fluids are drained by the lymph and not the venous system; the default position for all blood vessels is always filtration (Figure 26.1). This is due to the glycocalyx layer in the blood vessel wall, which maintains a relatively high osmotic pressure below the capillary endothelial layer so the osmotic gradient is less than needed for venous reabsorption.

Lymphoedema and chronic oedema

Lymphoedema is swelling due to a build-up of lymph fluid in the skin and subcutaneous tissues caused by inadequate lymph drainage, which plays a role in all forms of chronic oedema.

Dermatology Training: The Essentials. Edited by Mahbub M.U. Chowdhury, Tamara W. Griffiths and Andrew Y. Finlay.
© 2022 The British Association of Dermatologists. Published 2022 by John Wiley & Sons Ltd.
Companion website: www.wiley.com/go/chowdhury/dermatologytraining

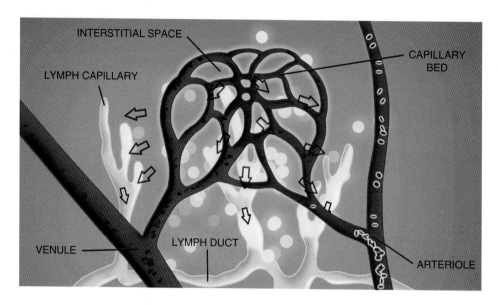

Figure 26.1 Blood vessels (red/blue) filter fluid from plasma into the tissue spaces (interstitium) from where it drains as lymph via the lymphatic vessels (yellow). Venous reabsorption occurs only transiently, and the default position is always filtration from blood vessels and fluid drainage via lymphatics. © Peter Mortimer.

Chronic oedema is an umbrella term, used for soft tissue swelling present for three months, and always indicates a problem with the lymphatic system. Either the lymph drainage is inadequate or lymph drainage is overwhelmed by too much fluid load, for example in venous oedema. Therefore, lymphoedema and chronic oedema are part of a continuum and chronic oedema should be managed in the same way as lymphoedema.

Lymphoedema presents most commonly as foot, ankle or leg swelling, but it can affect any peripheral tissue such as upper limb, torso, breast (e.g. following breast cancer treatment), genitalia (e.g. due to anogenital granulomatosis, a form of cutaneous Crohn's disease) and face (e.g. due to rosacea). This chapter focuses on chronic oedema and lymphoedema of lower limbs. You will often see swollen legs caused by chronic venous insufficiency or associated with inflammatory skin disease such as erythrodermic psoriasis or eczema.

Any chronic oedema can be of three types:

- **Low output failure**. This is where lymphatic flow is reduced due to failure of or damage to the lymphatic network, such as in cancer treatment-related lymphoedema and most types of primary lymphoedema. In this situation oedema develops because normal levels of capillary fluid filtration (lymph production) exceed the impaired lymphatic drainage.
- **High output failure**. When there is an increase in capillary filtration from whatever cause, lymphatic drainage increases until it reaches a transport capacity maximum. Capillary filtration then exceeds lymphatic drainage and oedema develops. This happens in venous oedema and also in heart failure and nephrotic syndrome.
- **Mixed**. Persistent high output failure can eventually lead to damage of the lymphatic system with reduction of lymphatic

transport capacity, creating a mixed picture and downward spiral. High capillary filtration continues but lymph drainage falls, for example in phlebolymphoedema.

Diagnosing lymphoedema

Lymphoedema following cancer treatment is relatively easy to diagnose because the cause is obvious: the removal of lymph glands. Lymphoedema generally starts as mild, reversible swelling, but at some point it becomes more permanent. A chronic build-up of lymph in the tissues eventually results in a more solid swollen texture. Characteristic thickened skin and induration of the subcutaneous tissues make pitting more difficult to elicit (but it is still present). The thickened skin makes it impossible to pinch and lift a fold of skin (Figure 26.2). This positive 'Stemmer sign' is pathognomonic of lymphoedema.

Elevation and diuretics can help to reduce lymph production (capillary filtration), but do not improve lymph drainage. Therefore, overnight elevation has little impact on lymphoedema (lymphatic failure), only reducing it by 10–15%, and diuretics are not effective. In contrast, a pure venous oedema (due to higher vascular fluid filtration) may reduce by up to 90% after a night in bed.

Types of lymphoedema

Primary lymphoedema occurs when there is an inborn weakness, usually genetically determined, in lymph drainage. Onset early in life or a family history suggests a primary lymphoedema. The discovery of causal genes has changed the way we approach diagnosis and management of primary lymphoedema.

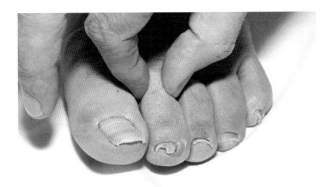

Figure 26.2 A positive Stemmer sign (otherwise known as Kaposi–Stemmer sign) is pathognomonic of lymphoedema. The thickened skin makes it difficult to pinch and lift up a fold of skin at the base of the second toe. © St George's Hospital.

Knowing the genetic cause enables better understanding of natural history, associated conditions, inheritance patterns and how these disorders develop.

Inherited lymphoedemas possess a germline mutation. Milroy disease, a specific congenital hereditary lymphoedema, is caused by mutations in the vascular endothelial growth factor receptor 3 gene (*VEGFR3*) (Figure 26.3). Testing for a mutation in *VEGFR3* in a blood or saliva sample can confirm the diagnosis. Some primary lymphoedemas develop from somatic mutations, which usually cause lymphatic malformations (e.g. lymphangioma). An extensive lymphatic malformation, with involvement of the main lymph draining pathways, can result in lymphoedema (Figure 26.4).

Secondary lymphoedema arises when damage occurs to lymph drainage routes such as from cancer treatment, infections such as filariasis, or accidental soft tissue trauma (e.g. road traffic accidents). Multiple factors can contribute to a secondary lymphoedema; for example, in breast-cancer-related lymphoedema, while the axillary intervention (surgery or radiotherapy) may be the main cause, obesity can be a contributing factor, as can chemotherapy, particularly with taxanes. The main causes of lymphoedema are presented in Table 26.1.

Chronic oedema: a multifactorial disease

The causes of chronic oedema may be multiple and complex, particularly in patients with several comorbidities. Age and obesity independently impair lymph drainage. A patient who is older, immobile and overweight and has some chronic right-sided heart failure will have multiple physiological factors contributing to swollen legs and the many skin problems that can result.

Rather than trying to pigeonhole one diagnosis, it makes more sense when confronted with swollen legs to consider factors influencing the physiology. What could be increasing fluid (lymph) production: high venous pressures (heart failure, venous disease), low plasma proteins (protein-losing states, liver disease) or inflammation (infection, inflammatory skin disease)?

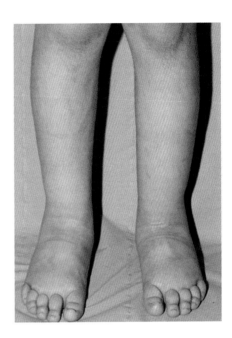

Figure 26.3 Milroy disease due to a mutation in the vascular endothelial growth factor receptor 3 gene (*VEGFR3*). © St George's Hospital.

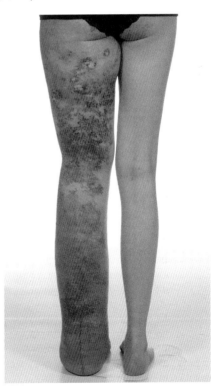

Figure 26.4 An extensive lymphatic malformation interrupting the main lymph drainage pathways within the limb, causing lymphoedema. The red 'birthmark' represents distended, malformed skin lymphatics containing blood. © St George's Hospital.

Table 26.1 Causes of lymphoedema and chronic oedema

Underlying cause	Examples
Primary lymphoedema, i.e. a genetically determined abnormality of the lymphatic system	Milroy disease
	Lymphoedema–distichiasis syndrome
	Klippel–Trenaunay syndrome
Malignancy and cancer treatment	Lymph node biopsy and clearance
	Radiotherapy
	Active or recurrent cancer
Infection	Filariasis
	Recurrent cellulitis
Inflammation	Acne, rosacea, eczema, psoriasis
	Cutaneous Crohn's disease
	Rheumatoid arthritis
	Pretibial myxoedema
Elevated venous pressures	Varicose veins, deep vein thrombosis
	Heart failure
	Obstructive sleep apnoea
Dependency	Immobility (e.g. after cerebrovascular accident or multiple sclerosis)
Medications	Calcium channel blockers
	Taxanes
	Corticosteroids
	Non-steroidal anti-inflammatory drugs
Damage to lymph pathways	Accidental trauma to the lymphatic system
	Surgical 'trauma'
Low protein states	Protein-losing enteropathy
	Liver disease
	Nephrotic syndrome
Obesity	

Could the chronic oedema be caused by impaired lymph drainage (damage to lymphatic system from surgery or infection, obesity, poor mobility or genetic predisposition)? Or could the oedema be caused by a combination of both high fluid filtration and declining lymph drainage?

Low plasma albumin can result from protein-losing states such as protein-losing enteropathy and nephrotic syndrome. Liver disease causes a failure of protein synthesis.

Renal failure generally does not cause oedema. Apart from nephrotic syndrome, kidney injury causes polyuria (salt and water loss), except in end-stage renal disease. Certain drugs can cause peripheral oedema, such as the calcium channel antagonist amlodipine, through a combination of impaired lymph drainage and higher orthostatic venous pressures. In sleep apnoea, high right-sided heart chamber pressures increase peripheral venous pressure, but also release hormones that provoke oedema through retaining salt and water.

Clinically you should consider systemic factors such as heart failure, medication and sleep apnoea. Check blood pro-brain natriuretic peptide, albumin and thyroid function. Consider the patient's lifestyle, such as poor mobility and sitting for long periods with the legs down, e.g. sleeping in a chair. Obesity is a major risk factor for lymphoedema and leaning forward in a chair results in the large abdominal girth pressing on the thighs and increasing intra-abdominal pressure, so obstructing both venous and lymph drainage. Getting the patient to try to move a little and more often (lymph drainage is totally dependent on movement and exercise), and also to recline to elevate the leg when resting in bed or a chair, can make a big difference.

Venous insufficiency

Venous disease causes oedema by producing too much fluid filtration into the legs, fluid that the lymphatic system does not have the capacity to drain. This is venous oedema. In chronic venous disease, whether from chronic venous (valvular) incompetence giving rise to varicose veins, post-thrombotic syndrome (post-deep vein thrombosis) or venous obstruction, venous pressures are raised and result in higher fluid (lymph) production. To avoid oedema, lymph drainage needs to compensate and drain this extra fluid. Oedema occurs frequently with chronic venous disease because lymph drainage fails.

Reasons for this lymph drainage failure include:

- Overload of lymph drainage capacity by excessive fluid pouring out of the venous system.
- A genetic weakness in lymphatic vessels (often associated with a genetic weakness in the veins because of the same embryological origin).
- Lymphatic vessel damage from thrombosis or infection.

Elevating the legs for a period of time drastically reduces venous pressures and should quickly ease the oedema. Treatment of the venous disease (e.g. endovenous ablation of varicose veins with laser or radiofrequency treatment) should reduce the fluid filtration by closing down the incompetent veins and so resolve the oedema. If this fails, the main reason for the oedema is likely to be poor lymph drainage. Phlebolymphoedema is a condition where lymphoedema has developed as a result of long-standing venous disease (Figure 26.5).

Asymmetrical chronic leg oedema

The combination of high lymph production and low lymph drainage can lead to very swollen legs. Asymmetrical swelling can occur due to worse lymph drainage or greater venous pressure on one side.

Swelling of just one leg means that the cause is likely to be confined to that lower limb or within the adjoining quadrant of the trunk, e.g. venous or lymphatic obstruction within the pelvis. Impaired lymph drainage or venous disease or both is likely to be the explanation. If acute there may be a deep vein thrombosis, in which case D-dimers should be checked, with or without an ultrasound examination. Obstructive pathology such as cancer in the abdomen or pelvis should be considered, so an ultrasound or CT scan may be indicated.

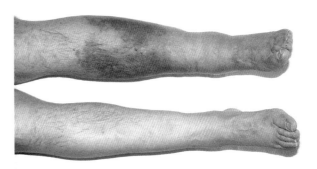

Figure 26.5 Phlebolymphoedema represents lymphoedema that has developed as a result of chronic venous hypertension. The high fluid filtration from the veins eventually exhausts lymph drainage. Signs of both chronic venous disease and lymphoedema coexist. © St George's Hospital.

Investigations

Most cases of lymphoedema are diagnosed on the history and clinical findings (Table 26.2). The use of imaging techniques is dependent on availability and expertise.

Lymphoscintigraphy is the clinical gold-standard test for the diagnosis of lymphoedema, but must be performed in a nuclear medicine department with a gamma camera. It involves injecting a radiolabelled protein or colloid, exclusively cleared by lymphatics, into the dermis or subcutis usually of the foot (for lower-limb examination). Measurement of uptake in regional lymph nodes and transit through the lymphatics permits both crude imaging of lymph drainage pathways and functional measurement of lymph flow. An abnormal scan has high specificity for lymphoedema (Figure 26.6).

Indocyanine green lymphography (ICGL) involves indocyanine green being injected intradermally into the web spaces between the toes. Using a near-infrared-sensitive camera, it enables in real time the visualisation of flow in the main lymphatic vessels within a limb. It can be undertaken in clinic and has become the investigation of choice before any lymphatic microsurgery.

Venous duplex Doppler ultrasound examination is the investigation of choice for suspected venous disease, but sustained venous hypertension simulating venous disease can be produced in patients who sit for long periods with legs dependent. Under these circumstances, signs of venous disease such as venous telangiectasia and reticular veins around the ankle, haemosiderin pigmentation, varicose eczema, lipodermatosclerosis, atrophie blanche, or even ulceration can be present, yet there may be no venous reflux on the Doppler ultrasound.

CT or **MRI** may prove useful in detecting the cause of any lymphatic obstruction, such as from a tumour.

Table 26.2 Lymphoedema consultation guide

Medical history: key facts

- Distribution and duration of the lymphoedema
- Exacerbating and relieving factors
- Is there a family history of lymphoedema (primary lymphoedema)?
- Activity status and reasons for any deterioration (e.g. recent cerebrovascular accident, severe arthritis)
- Do they go to bed at night (if not, they may have 'armchair legs')?
- Past medical history
  - Varicose veins and/or venous ulcers
  - Deep vein thrombosis
  - Recurrent cellulitis
  - Cancer, including treatments received (lymph node removal, radiotherapy, chemotherapy – particularly taxanes)
  - Cardiac failure
  - Hypertension requiring use of calcium channel blockers
  - Chronic inflammatory disease within region of swelling (e.g. rheumatoid arthritis, acne/rosacea, chronic eczema or psoriasis)

Physical examination: key findings

- Assess mobility status of the patient
- Obesity, especially of the abdomen, as it obstructs both lymph and venous drainage of the lower limbs by compression of the abdomen and groin/thigh region
- Distribution of lymphoedema, i.e. how many limbs affected, is there genital (patients are often embarrassed to mention genital swelling) or truncal involvement (sacral swelling can be a sign of heart failure or central lymphatic obstruction from malignancy)
- Pitting (if severe consider hypoalbuminaemia or heart failure)
- Cutaneous signs of venous hypertension (haemosiderin, venous flares, atrophie blanche, venous ulcers)
- Active cellulitis or its mimicker, lipodermatosclerosis (often bilateral)
- Tinea pedis (treat if present as it increases risk of developing cellulitis)
- Lymphadenopathy, especially within region of swollen limb(s)
- Could represent reactive lymphadenopathy from recurrent cellulitis; tropical infections such as filariasis (rarely seen in the UK); active or recurrent malignancy
- Presence of recurrent malignancy
- If heart failure is suspected from the history, then assess the jugular venous pressure, chest auscultation with or without brain natriuretic peptide level and echocardiogram
- Presence of chronic inflammatory disease (if history suggestive)

A **skin biopsy** can be consistent with, but not specific for, a diagnosis of lymphoedema. However, biopsy is the investigation of choice in lymphoedema caused by conditions such as Kaposi sarcoma or anogenital granulomatosis (cutaneous Crohn's disease).

Management

Patients with lymphoedema should be offered active treatment and not be expected to 'live with it'. Physical therapy can be very effective, although so far there is no drug therapy specific for lymphoedema and there is no surgical operation of proven benefit. Moderate-to-severe limb swelling should undergo a course of intensive treatment including manual lymphatic drainage,

multilayer lymphoedema bandaging and exercises, before transfer to long-term management with compression garments and exercises. Weight control is essential.

Unlike the blood circulation, which has the heart pumping it, lymph drainage requires muscle movement to stimulate lymph flow. Without movement lymph flow is slow. Compression from a bandage or stocking enhances the effect of movement on lymph flow. Massage can do the same.

Therapists trained in lymphoedema treatment techniques can provide intensive therapy using massage (manual lymph drainage) and multilayer compression bandaging. This bandaging involves toe bandaging as well as bandaging up to the thigh. This approach, combined with exercises, can have a dramatic effect within a few weeks on improving limb size and shape, as well as on the condition of the skin. Once swelling is improved

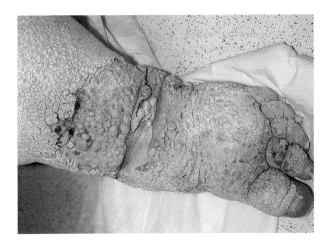

Figure 26.7 Papillomatosis and hyperkeratosis of a lymphoedematous lower limb. © St George's Hospital.

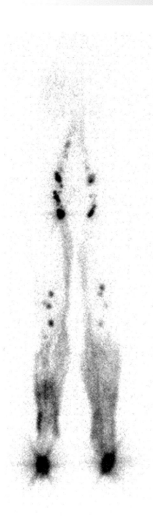

Figure 26.6 An abnormal lymphoscintigram characteristic of changes seen with a *FOXC2* mutation (lymphoedema–distichiasis syndrome). The images show reflux into the deep lymphatic system via the popliteal lymph nodes and into the skin. The legs appear in black profile because of lymphatic valve failure (similar to venous reflux in varicose veins). © St George's Hospital.

then control can be maintained through self-management techniques such as wearing compression garments and taking exercise. As obesity is a very significant risk factor for lymphoedema, weight control and general fitness are important.

Associated skin problems

Any chronic oedema, but particularly lymphoedema, can produce profound skin changes. Lymph accumulation in the skin produces marked epidermal and dermal hypertrophy. The skin thickening results in sclerotic, less pliable skin, which may demonstrate a positive Stemmer sign. Congested lymphatic vessels

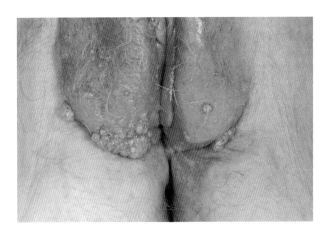

Figure 26.8 Lymphangiectasia of the labia on a background of genital lymphoedema as a result of cervical cancer treatment. © St George's Hospital.

within the dermis give rise to a cobblestone effect, which in time can form papillomatosis (Figure 26.7). Excess keratin production gives rise to hyperkeratosis.

In a more acute lymph congestion, dermal lymphatic vessels can bulge on the skin surface to resemble small blisters, or if grouped a 'frogspawn' appearance, so-called lymphangiectasia (not lymphangioma) (Figure 26.8). Appearances are identical to lymphangioma, where the 'lymph blisters' arise from deep dermal lymphatic obstruction from a lymphatic malformation (lymphangioma circumscriptum). If these lymphatic vessels break, copious lymph can weep onto the skin surface. This lymph leakage is called lymphorrhoea and is no different from tissue fluid discharge (as tissue fluid and lymph have the same composition). Fluid discharge from any wound can be considered the same as lymph. Use of emollients and compression form the basis of treatment for the hyperkeratosis and papillomatosis, as well as for lymphangiectasia and lymphorrhoea.

Skin infections are very common with lymphoedema because of the underlying local immunodeficiency caused by the impaired immune cell trafficking. Fungal and bacterial infections are common and can exacerbate the lymphoedema by compromising lymph drainage further, and thus lead to a vicious cycle of more infection and worse swelling.

Elephantiasis

Elephantiasis indicates lymphoedema with the characteristic skin changes and is the preferred term for diagnosis in tropical climates. Verrucous, cobblestone-like papules, nodules, or thickened plaques with non-pitting oedema are seen. Marked hyperkeratosis with both dermal and subcutaneous fibrosis can be seen on biopsy.

Filarial elephantiasis is caused by a mosquito bite introducing larvae that enter dermal lymphatics before developing into worms in the larger collecting lymphatic vessels close to the lymph nodes. This causes lymphatic obstruction. Non-filarial elephantiasis, otherwise known as podoconiosis, is caused by walking barefoot in soils containing silicates that penetrate the foot skin, leading to local dermal lymphatic damage and foot lymphoedema with profound skin changes (Figure 26.9).

In Western societies when severe skin changes of elephantiasis occur, caused usually by obesity and previous cellulitis, the term 'elephantiasis nostras verrucosa' is used, meaning warty lymphoedema due to Western society diseases.

Treatment of elephantiasis is the same as for lymphoedema, with improvement of lymph drainage through movement and compression essential.

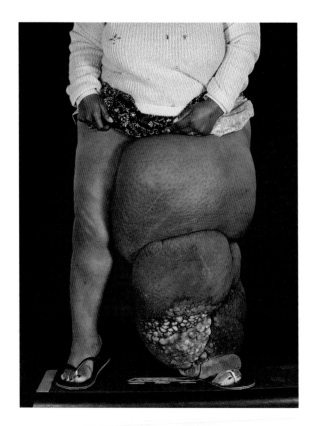

Figure 26.9 Elephantiasis skin changes in a patient with chronic lymphoedema of the left lower limb. © St George's Hospital.

Cellulitis

Compromised lymph drainage results in localised tissue immunodeficiency, as lymph drainage is important for appropriate immune cell trafficking. Disturbance to lymph drainage increases risk of infection, and subsequent eradication of infection can be difficult due to impaired local immunity.

Cellulitis is in the top 10 reasons for emergency admission to hospital and is often caused by underlying lymphoedema. Up to 50% of patients with lymphoedema experience one or more attacks of cellulitis. Acute cellulitis requires treatment with at least two weeks of antibiotics, or else recurrence develops due to inadequate treatment of the original infection. The treatment of choice is oral amoxicillin 500 mg 8-hourly, although most guidelines recommend flucloxacillin. If there is any evidence of *Staphylococcus aureus* infection, for example folliculitis, pus formation or crusted dermatitis, then flucloxacillin 500 mg 6-hourly should be prescribed in addition or as an alternative.

The risk of further bouts of cellulitis in lymphoedema is high. Patients who have had cellulitis are recommended to carry a two-week supply of antibiotics with them, particularly when away for any length of time. Amoxicillin 500 mg three times daily, erythromycin 500 mg four times daily or clarithromycin 500 mg twice daily are possible alternatives. Education on skin care is required to reduce portals of entry, especially via interdigital tinea pedis. Recurrent cellulitis may sometimes require lifelong prophylactic antibiotics and should be considered in patients with two or more attacks of cellulitis per year. Penicillin V 250 mg twice daily (500 mg twice daily if BMI $\geq$ 33 kg m^{-2}) should be the antibiotic of choice, with erythromycin 250 mg twice daily as an alternative.

Lipodermatosclerosis

People with swollen legs often appear to have bilateral cellulitis, but bilateral cellulitis is rarely due to infection and is more likely to be lipodermatosclerosis. This is a sclerosing panniculitis that can resemble erythema nodosum but is more diffuse, affecting the gaiter region of the lower leg, sometimes called the 'inverted champagne bottle' sign (Figure 26.10). Affected skin is red, indurated and tender with a woody feel. Over time the skin turns from red to pigmented brown.

Lipodermatosclerosis is frequently misattributed to venous disease, but it is often due to lymphoedema and is most commonly seen with a combination of venous hypertension and poor lymph drainage. To confuse matters further, infection such as cellulitis can complicate lipodermatosclerosis, and the only means of distinction may be systemic signs, such as fever or flu-like symptoms plus or minus raised inflammatory markers.

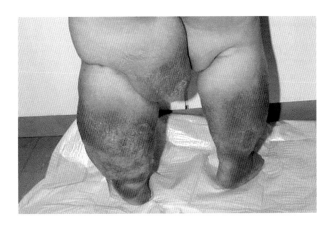

Figure 26.10 Lipodermatosclerosis represents an inflammatory change (without infection) of skin and subcutaneous tissues due to fluid congestion from lymphoedema, venous hypertension or both. © St George's Hospital.

accelerates wound regeneration, and stem cells appear important for this process. Analysis of lymphangiogenesis after full-thickness skin excision has revealed an essential role for vascular endothelial growth factor C. Lymphangiogenesis is required for local fluid homeostasis, granulation tissue formation, leucocyte trafficking and matrix remodelling. Poor lymph drainage results in oedema, fibrosis and lipid deposition, all of which could potentially impair wound healing. Defective healing of chronic wounds in diabetic patients can be attributed in part to a deficiency in lymphatic regenerative potential.

Stem cells promote lymphatic regeneration at the capillary level and functionally reconnect lymph nodes to the host lymphatic network. Stem cells significantly improve the wound healing process in the skin, and this is likely to be in part due to their stimulating effect on lymphatic vessel growth in wound granulation tissue.

Also, lymphatic dysfunction predisposes to infection through impaired immune cell trafficking and so may be a major contributor to infection rates in wounds, particularly leg, pressure and diabetic ulcers.

Stasis or varicose dermatitis, which is a venous pathology, can be distinguished on the basis of itch and scaling, but may coexist.

Treatment of lipodermatosclerosis involves reducing venous hypertension and improving lymph drainage through compression therapy and enhanced movement. The legs should be elevated when resting. Infection, i.e. conventional cellulitis, can complicate lipodermatosclerosis, so antibiotics may also be required.

Venous ulcers

Oedema is always seen in venous leg ulceration. It is called 'venous oedema', but do not underestimate the contribution of poor lymph drainage. In chronic leg ulceration both the dermal lymphatics in and around the wound and the main lymphatic channels within the leg become compromised, leading to higher rates of wound discharge, cellulitis and lymphoedema.

The treatment for venous ulcers is compression therapy, which improves lymph drainage as well as reducing ambulatory venous pressure and reducing the risk of cellulitis. The leg swelling and high wound discharge, manifestations of impaired lymphatic function, often create the biggest management difficulties. The standard leg ulcer bandaging applied from foot to knee can exacerbate lymphoedema of the toes and forefeet.

Wound healing and lymphangiogenesis

Effective lymph drainage is important for fluid homeostasis, as well as for the recycling of proteins and immune cells, processes essential for wound healing and prevention of infection. The growth of new lymphatic vessels (lymphangiogenesis)

Pearls and pitfalls

- Tissue fluid is drained by the lymph vessels and not by reabsorption back into the veins.
- Any chronic oedema involves a failure of lymph drainage.
- A positive Stemmer sign, where it is impossible to pinch and lift a fold of skin, is pathognomonic of lymphoedema.
- A molecular diagnosis is now possible in 25% of cases of primary lymphoedema, e.g. vascular endothelial growth factor receptor 3 in Milroy disease.
- Lipodermatosclerosis is often mistaken for cellulitis, but is not infection and does not respond to antibiotics.

SCE Questions. See question 17.

FURTHER READING AND KEY RESOURCES

Bull RH, Gane JN, Evans JE *et al*. Abnormal lymph drainage in patients with chronic venous leg ulcers. *J Am Acad Dermatol* 1993; **28**:585–90.

Lim L, Bui H, Farrelly O *et al*. Hemostasis stimulates lymphangiogenesis through release and activation of VEGFC. *Blood* 2019; **134**:1764–75.

McPherson T, Persaud S, Singh S *et al*. Interdigital lesions and frequency of acute dermatolymphangioadenitis in lymphoedema in a filariasis-endemic area. *Br J Dermatol* 2006; **154**:933–41.

Maruyama K, Asai J, Ii M *et al*. Decreased macrophage number and activation lead to reduced lymphatic vessel formation and contribute to impaired diabetic wound healing. *Am J Pathol* 2007; **170**:1178–91.

Thomas KS, Crook AM, Nunn AJ *et al*. Penicillin to prevent recurrent leg cellulitis. *N Engl J Med* 2013; **368**:1695–703.

Woodcock TE, Woodcock TM. Revised Starling equation and the glycocalyx model of transvascular fluid exchange: an improved paradigm for prescribing intravenous fluid therapy. *Br J Anaesth* 2012; **108**:384–94.

Useful website

The Lymphoedema Support Network. Cellulitis in lymphoedema. Available at: https://www.lymphoedema.org/cellulitis/cellulitis-in-lymphoedema.

27

Hair and nail diseases

Donna Cummins and Anita Takwale

Introduction

The management of hair and nail disease is a vital role of dermatologists, with few UK tertiary centres in operation. Care for these conditions is often the exclusive remit of our specialty, with little expertise offered by other medical care providers. Furthermore, information and misinformation are readily available through non-medical sectors and it is important that dermatologists have an awareness that this may add an extra layer of complexity to the consultation. For many hair and nail disorders, the evidence base for therapies is poor. Research developments are hampered by a lack of validated outcome measures, the rarity of these disorders and insufficient scientific focus on these emotionally debilitating conditions.

Hair anatomy and physiology

Hair follicles consist of four segments: the bulb, suprabulbar region, isthmus and infundibulum (Chapter 4). The bulb is found in the subcutaneous fat and is the site of the hair matrix, a group of rapidly proliferating keratinocytes responsible for the production of hair. The bulge region is found near the insertion point of the arrector pili muscle and contains hair follicle stem cells, which are required for follicular cycling and hair growth. The bulge has been identified as a site of immune privilege in human skin. Immune privilege refers to a complex combination of immunosuppressive mechanisms thought to protect tissue structures from immune-mediated injury.

The hair follicle can be found in one of three phases of the hair cycle: active growth (anagen), regression (catagen) and rest (telogen). In humans, individual follicles cycle independently. The lower region of the follicle undergoes growth and regression, whereas the upper portion remains static.

The anagen phase of human terminal scalp hair lasts between two and seven years. The duration of this phase determines final hair length. Approximately 90% of hair follicles are in the anagen phase, 10% in telogen and less than 1% in catagen. Exogen describes the exact time point at which the hair is shed. Between 50 and 150 telogen hairs are normally shed per day. Following the telogen phase, anagen resumes to produce a new hair. Kenogen describes the prolonged delay of entry into anagen after hair is shed.

History, examination and investigation

Hair loss is a common and profoundly distressing symptom for patients. By the time they are seen in clinic, they may be extremely concerned about developing complete hair loss. A detailed history is essential to establish the duration, progression and pattern of hair loss, as well as the presence of excess shedding. Other important information includes nutritional intake, medications, menstrual history, family history of hair loss, styling practices, and symptoms. The psychological and emotional impacts of hair loss should not be underestimated, and adequate support should be provided.

All hair-bearing areas should be examined, with attention given to skin type according to cultural and ethnic context, pattern of hair loss, scalp condition (scaling, inflammation), hair parting and hair density. Examination of the follicular orifices will help distinguish scarring from non-scarring hair loss, which is an important first step in delineating an accurate differential diagnosis. Obliteration of the follicular orifice and a shiny appearance of the scalp indicate scarring. Hair and scalp dermoscopy (known as trichoscopy) is helpful in determining the diagnosis, disease activity and treatment response. Standardised clinical photography at baseline and during treatment also assists in the assessment of hair loss progression and treatment response.

A hair pull test will help confirm the presence of active hair loss. Gentle traction is used, pulling away from the scalp, on 50–60 hairs gathered between the thumb and forefinger. Presence of over 10% of telogen hairs is considered abnormal. This finding may be associated with telogen effluvium and alopecia areata. The finding of anagen hairs is always abnormal (Figure 27.1).

The hair tug test can determine if hair breakage is present. A section of hair close to the scalp is grasped and the distal end is gently pulled to assess for the development of a hair shaft fracture. Light microscopy can confirm the presence of hair shaft disorders. Hairs should be trimmed and not plucked for assessment.

Where a scalp biopsy is required, a minimum of a 4-mm punch should be taken at the angle of the hair shaft, ensuring the subcutis is reached. When scarring alopecia is suspected, the biopsy should always be taken from the active edge. Vertical sections demonstrate the full thickness of the skin. However, as hair follicles grow at an angle, only a few hairs are demonstrated in each section. Transverse (horizontal) sectioning is of particular help in the assessment of non-scarring alopecia. It offers superior quantitative and qualitative parameters of follicle morphology. All follicles in a transverse specimen are counted and examined at multiple levels. Horizontal sectioning may not be within the usual scope of practice for general histopathologists and may require specialist dermatopathology input.

Figure 27.1 (a) Anagen hairs have pigmented, distorted bulbs and an attached root sheath (arrow). (b) Telogen hairs are identified with depigmented hair bulbs without an attached root sheath. Kolivras A, Thompson C. Primary scalp alopecia: new histopathological tools, new concepts and a practical guide to diagnosis. *J Cutan Pathol* 2017; **44**:53–69.

(a)

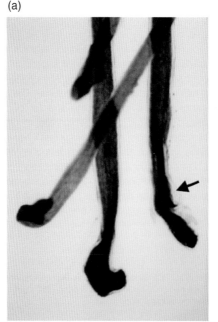

(b)

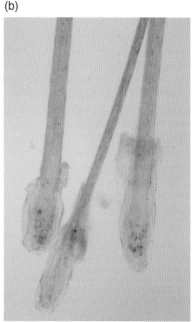

Scarring alopecia

Scarring (cicatricial) alopecia causes destruction of the hair follicle unit. Clinically, this is represented by the loss of follicular ostia. Primary cicatricial alopecia results from inflammation targeting the non-cycling portion of the follicle and/or bulge zone.

Histologically, features associated with scarring alopecia vary depending on the chronicity of the disease process and include uneven distribution of follicles, replacement of follicles with fibrous tissue, loss of sebaceous lobules and naked hair shafts within the dermis.

The North American Hair Research Society (NAHRS) developed a classification system of scarring alopecia based on the primary histological inflammatory cell present: lymphocytic, neutrophilic, mixed and non-specific (Table 27.1).

Lichen planopilaris

Lichen planopilaris (LPP) is an inflammatory scarring alopecia considered to be a follicular form of lichen planus. Clinically, it is characterised by perifollicular inflammation and follicular hyperkeratosis associated with pruritus and trichodynia (tenderness or pain). Dermoscopy may feature peripilar casts, absence of vellus hairs and broken hairs.

LPP is divided into three clinical variants:

- **Classic LPP**. Multiple irregular areas of scarring alopecia with scalp inflammation can be seen. Features of lichen planus may be present.
- **Frontal fibrosing alopecia**. This clinically distinctive variant of LPP has similar histological findings to LPP and is most often found in post-menopausal White women (Figure 27.2). Findings demonstrate frontotemporal loss of terminal and vellus hairs in a band-like distribution ('lonely hair' sign) causing progressive recession of the hairline. Loss of eyebrow and/or body hair and facial papules may be present.
- **Graham–Little–Piccardi–Lasseur syndrome** (GLPLS). GLPLS is characterised by the triad of LPP of the scalp, non-scarring alopecia affecting axillary and pubic hair, and a lichenoid follicular eruption on the trunk, limbs or face.

Treatment of LPP is challenging. Treatment goals are to slow disease progression and alleviate symptoms. Medications used include topical, intralesional and systemic corticosteroids, tetracyclines, hydroxychloroquine, pioglitazone and systemic immunosuppression (including ciclosporin, methotrexate, azathioprine and mycophenolate mofetil). From small case series, there is emerging use of mast cell stabilisers (cetirizine, fexofenadine, sodium cromoglycate) and low-dose naltrexone.

Classic pseudopelade (Brocq)

Small, skin-coloured patches of alopecia 'footprints in the snow' are found in this scarring condition, considered to result from atrophy of hair follicles rather than inflammation. Follicular hyperkeratosis with minimal or no redness is seen on dermoscopy.

Table 27.1 The North American Hair Research Society (NAHRS) classification of primary cicatricial alopecia

Inflammatory infiltrate
Lymphocytic
Chronic cutaneous lupus erythematosus
Lichen planopilaris (LPP)
Classic LPP
Frontal fibrosing alopecia (FFA)
Graham–Little–Piccardi–Lasseur syndrome
Classic pseudopelade (Brocq)
Central centrifugal cicatricial alopecia
Alopecia mucinosa
Keratosis follicularis spinulosa decalvans
Neutrophilic
Folliculitis decalvans
Dissecting cellulitis/folliculitis (perifolliculitis capitis abscedens et suffodiens)
Mixed
Folliculitis (acne) keloidalis
Folliculitis (acne) necrotica
Erosive pustular dermatosis
Non-specific

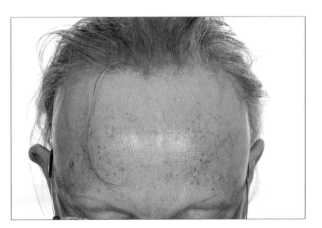

Figure 27.2 Frontal fibrosing alopecia. © Salford Royal NHS Foundation Trust.

Central centrifugal cicatricial alopecia

Central centrifugal cicatricial alopecia (CCCA) primarily affects women with afro-textured hair. Hair loss begins at the scalp vertex and gradually expands centrifugally. Clinical signs of inflammation may be present, with dermoscopy revealing irregularly distributed pinpoint white dots and white-grey halos (Figure 27.3). CCCA is usually asymptomatic. The pathogenesis is unknown; however, traumatic hair practices have been implicated.

Progression may halt spontaneously. Advice on gentle hair grooming and cosmetic camouflage is recommended, and maintenance treatment is with potent topical corticosteroids, tetracyclines and topical minoxidil.

Folliculitis decalvans

Folliculitis decalvans presents with perifollicular pustules, inflammation, scale and 'tufted' hair follicles, predominantly affecting the scalp vertex and occiput. This neutrophilic scarring alopecia is associated with pruritus and/or pain. While the cause is unknown, the presence of *Staphylococcus aureus* and subsequent abnormal response to treatment of this organism have been suggested.

Systemic antibiotics (tetracyclines, flucloxacillin, third-generation cephalosporins) offer the mainstay of treatment. Rifampicin with clindamycin, azithromycin, isotretinoin and dapsone may also result in treatment response. Tumour necrosis factor-α inhibitors, surgical excision, radiotherapy and photodynamic therapy are options in those who do not respond to standard treatment.

Dissecting cellulitis of the scalp

Dissecting cellulitis (perifolliculitis capitis abscedens et suffodiens) is part of the 'follicular occlusion tetrad' that also includes hidradenitis suppurativa, acne conglobata and pilonidal sinus. Permanent hair loss is associated with boggy fluctuant nodules and abscesses over the scalp. Commonly seen in young Black males, the condition is associated with discharge with or without pain. Treatment options include isotretinoin, oral antibiotics, tumour necrosis factor-α, intralesional corticosteroids and incision and drainage.

Non-scarring alopecia

Alopecia areata

Alopecia areata (AA) is a chronic non-scarring alopecia with an estimated prevalence of 1 in 1000 people. The mechanisms leading to AA are not clear, but AA is considered a T-cell-mediated autoimmune disease affecting genetically predisposed individuals. Patients commonly present with round patches of hair loss affecting the scalp and other hair-bearing sites, including the eyebrows, eyelashes and beard area, which are usually asymptomatic. Patterns of scalp hair loss include alopecia totalis (loss of all scalp hair), alopecia universalis (loss of all scalp and body hair) and an ophiasis pattern (a band-like pattern of hair loss across the occiput; 'ophis' means 'snake'). Dermoscopy reveals exclamation-mark hairs, and yellow and black dots. Associated

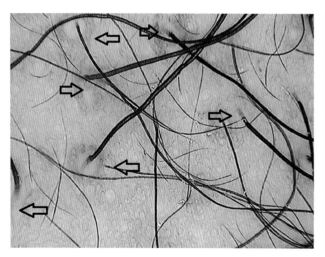
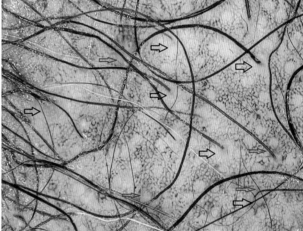

Figure 27.3 Dermoscopy of central centrifugal cicatricial alopecia. Arrows point to the peripilar white-grey halos around emerging hairs with a background of a honeycomb network. Miteva M, Tosti A. Dermatoscopic features of central centrifugal cicatricial alopecia. *J Am Acad Dermatol* 2014; **71**:443–9.

nail abnormalities include pitting, trachyonychia (rough linear ridges), brittle nails, onycholysis, koilonychia (spoon-shaped nails) and onychomadesis (periodic shedding of the nails). In limited, patchy hair loss, approximately 50% of those affected will recover within a year. Indicators of poor prognosis or high risk of relapse include childhood onset, family history, atopy, duration of over one year, distribution (totalis, universalis, ophiasis) and nail disease.

Response to medical intervention is unpredictable and it is not curative. Choice of therapy is influenced by patient age, disease duration and extent, and availability of tertiary-level services. In patchy AA, treatments include potent topical or intralesional corticosteroids, topical minoxidil, topical dithranol (to induce an irritant effect) or a combination approach. Intralesional triamcinolone can be trialled for eyebrow loss, and topical bimatoprost, a prostaglandin analogue, may be used to induce the regrowth of eyelashes and eyebrows. For extensive AA, and where available in specialist clinics, topical immunotherapy with diphencyprone or squaric acid dibutyl ester can prove an effective therapy. Systemic steroids, dosed at 40–60 mg per day in adults or 1 mg/kg per day in children and tapered slowly, may be indicated as a temporary measure where there is rapidly progressive and extensive hair loss. However, the recurrence of hair loss on discontinuation of prednisolone and adverse effects of treatment need careful consideration. There is limited efficacy data on the use of systemic immunosuppressant agents such as methotrexate, ciclosporin and azathioprine.

Patients who are unresponsive to treatment or who do not want pharmacological intervention may wish to use cosmetic options including wigs, camouflage, false eyelashes and eyebrow tattooing. Though the patient may have considered these options as a last resort, and may show initial resistance, it is important to remain positive and emphasise how effective and convenient modern appliances have become.

Cytokines that activate the JAK-STAT (signal transducer and activator of transcription) pathway are implicated in the development of AA, and inhibition of this pathway suppresses T-cell-mediated inflammatory responses in AA. Oral Janus kinase (JAK) inhibitors (tofacitinib, ruxolitinib and baricitinib) have shown regrowth of terminal hairs in AA. Early studies of topical JAK inhibitors provide promise for eyebrow and eyelash loss, but show lesser efficacy in scalp hair regrowth. JAK inhibitors are well tolerated; however, common adverse effects include increased risk of infection, increased risk of venous thromboembolism, transaminitis and lipid abnormalities. Recurrence usually occurs after cessation of treatment. JAK inhibitors are not currently licensed or available for use in the UK for alopecia.

Telogen effluvium

Telogen effluvium is a form of non-scarring hair loss resulting in the shedding of large numbers of telogen hairs simultaneously due to the premature termination of the anagen phase. Diffuse hair loss occurs 1–6 months later. Causes of telogen effluvium are listed in Table 27.2. Medications result in hair loss 2–4 months after starting treatment. A precipitating cause is not always

Table 27.2 Causes of telogen effluvium

Acute illness
Chronic illness
Hormonal changes: commencing or discontinuing the combined oral contraceptive pill
Thyroid disorders
Severe emotional stress
Nutritional deficiency
Heavy metal poisoning (arsenic, thallium)
Medications
Hormonal medications (combined oral contraceptive pill)
Beta blockers
Antihypertensives (angiotensin-converting enzyme inhibitors, angiotensin receptor blockers)
Antipsychotics and antihypertensives
Anticoagulants
Disorders of the thyroid
Anticonvulsants
Retinoids

Table 27.3 Investigations for hair fall

Full blood count
Serum iron, ferritin, B_{12}, folate
Vitamin D
Zinc
Antinuclear antibody test
Liver function tests
Renal function tests
Thyroid function tests

found. Blood tests for investigating hair fall should be performed (Table 27.3) and the hair pull test is usually positive.

Acute telogen effluvium results in diffuse hair loss and occurs 2–3 months after a triggering event. Chronic telogen effluvium occurs by chronic shedding without an underlying precipitating factor. It persists for longer than six months and hair shedding may continue for years.

A scalp biopsy may differentiate between chronic telogen effluvium and female pattern hair loss. Histology of chronic telogen effluvium shows a normal number of hair follicles with a terminal-to-vellus (T:V) hair ratio greater than 8:1.

Anagen effluvium

Anagen effluvium occurs due to an abrupt interruption of anagen without progression to catagen or telogen. Disruption of mitotic activity results in extensive hair loss, commonly occurring within 2–3 weeks of commencing antineoplastic agents.

Androgenetic alopecia

Male pattern hair loss affects up to 80% of men during their lifetime. The terminal hairs at androgen-dependent scalp regions (frontal temporal and vertex) undergo a process of follicle miniaturisation as androgen hormones activate hair follicle androgen receptors. Androgen sensitivity is genetically determined and is dependent on the production of dihydrotestosterone through 5-alpha reductase.

Female pattern hair loss (FPHL) (Figure 27.4) affects up to 50% of women and results in diffuse thinning at the crown with preservation of the frontal hairline (Ludwig pattern). The mechanism by which androgens and genetic factors contribute to the development of FPHL is less clear.

FPHL can result from underlying endocrinopathies giving rise to hyperandrogenism (polycystic ovarian syndrome, ovarian or adrenal tumours, adrenal hyperplasia). Screening tests include serum testosterone, sex hormone-binding globulin (SHBG), free androgen index (FAI), androstenedione and prolactin. An elevated concentration of free testosterone is the single most sensitive test for hyperandrogenism. Measurement of SHBG permits calculation of the FAI. FAI correlates with free testosterone in women (not in men) and is a useful surrogate for free testosterone. Most women with FPHL do not have hormonal abnormalities or endocrinopathies, and family history is very important. It may be helpful to the patient to explain that their hair follicles are more sensitive to normal levels of circulating androgens.

Dehydroepiandrosterone sulfate (DHEAS) is secreted by the adrenals, and androstenedione (secreted by ovaries) can be measured to identify an adrenal or ovarian source of hyperandrogenism. Increased serum prolactin may indicate a pituitary tumour or hypothyroidism.

Using dermoscopy, a diversity of > 20% in hair diameter is diagnostic for androgenetic alopecia. Yellow dots and vellus hairs can also be found. It may be helpful to screen for other causes of hair loss (Table 27.3), which can exacerbate FPHL. A scalp biopsy will help differentiate between AA and telogen effluvium if there is clinical doubt. Horizontal sections are required to ascertain if the T:V ratio is reduced (< 4:1), in keeping with FPHL.

Topical and oral minoxidil, oral antiandrogen therapy (spironolactone, finasteride, dutasteride, bicalutamide, flutamide) and contraceptive pills with a low FAI form the mainstay of pharmacological management. Platelet-rich plasma, low-level laser therapy, hair cosmetics and hair transplantation can also be considered in a private healthcare setting.

Tinea capitis

Tinea capitis occurs due to the presence of a dermatophyte fungus in the hair shafts. Studies in the USA have revealed that tinea capitis is most common in African American children. The reason for this is unclear. *Trichophyton* and *Microsporum* species of dermatophyte fungi are the major causative agents (Chapter 12). Children are predominantly affected, with spores spreading through contaminated hats, hairbrushes and combs, and barbers' equipment. Patients may present with scale, follicular inflammation, pustules, alopecia and lymphadenopathy. Corkscrew hairs, comma hairs, black dots, hair casts and pustules are seen on dermoscopy. A kerion is an advanced form of tinea resulting from a severe immune response and leads to boggy inflammation with crusting, abscesses and lymphadenopathy (Figure 12.7). It is most frequently caused by the zoophilic organisms *Trichophyton mentagrophytes* and *Trichophyton verrucosum*. Scarring alopecia may result.

Ectothrix pathogens, such as *Microsporum canis and Microsporum audouinii*, cover the outside of the hair shaft, resulting in scale, inflammation and green fluorescence under Wood's light. Conversely, endothrix pathogens, such as *Trichophyton tonsurans*, are found within the hair shaft and are associated with black dots and absence of fluorescence under Wood's light. Secondary staphylococcal infection may be present and swabs and plucked hairs should be sent for fungal and bacterial culture.

Ketoconazole shampoo for the patient and family is recommended, otherwise the condition will 'ping pong' back and forth between family members. Systemic therapies include griseofulvin, terbinafine and itraconazole. Griseofulvin (best absorbed with

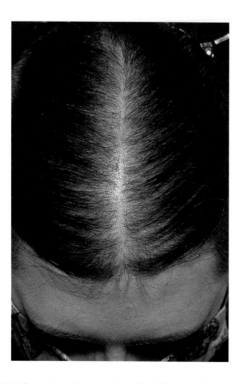

Figure 27.4 Female pattern hair loss. The Sinclair photographic classification of female pattern hair loss is based on part width (grade 1–5). © Gloucestershire Hospitals NHS Foundation Trust.

fatty food) is more effective than terbinafine in the management of the *Microsporum* species (15–20 mg/kg/day for eight weeks). Oral terbinafine (unlicensed for this indication) has been shown to have great efficacy against *Trichophyton* species and requires a shorter duration of treatment (four weeks).

Trichotillomania

Compulsive hair plucking can result in patches of alopecia affecting the scalp, eyebrows, eyelashes and other hair-bearing sites (Chapter 15). Hair pulling can begin at any age, and the frontoparietal scalp on the same side as the patient's dominant hand is more commonly affected. Clinically, irregular patches of hair loss are seen containing hairs of varying lengths. Dermoscopy typically reveals broken hairs and black dots. Where there is clinical doubt, a scalp biopsy may be helpful. A thorough psychosocial history should be taken, with consideration given to whether bullying or abusive behaviour has been experienced. Patients benefit from early psychological and/or psychiatric support.

Traction alopecia

Trauma-induced hair loss can develop from hairstyling practices causing damage by sustained or repetitive tension. It can occur in any ethnic demographic and gender; however, most cases occur in women of African descent. Marginal traction alopecia affects the frontotemporal scalp, giving rise to a 'fringe sign' with preservation of a rim of hairs. Non-marginal alopecia occurs outside of these sites, with contributing factors such as hair extensions, and is more prevalent in women with afro-textured hair. In early stages hair loss may be subtle, with inflammation, redness, papules and pustules evident at affected sites. With cessation of traumatic styling, the alopecia is reversible; however, scarring in chronic cases may occur. Evidence of hair casts on dermoscopy can be a helpful indicator of persistent traction, indicating likely progression of disease.

Stopping these traction hairstyles is important. Topical and oral minoxidil may be helpful, with intralesional corticosteroids and tetracyclines used to manage clinical inflammation. Cosmetic camouflage and hair transplantation can be considered for extensive scalp involvement.

Cosmetic camouflage

Response to treatment of hair loss can be slow and unpredictable. Cosmetic aids are a useful adjunct in patient management. Shake-on keratin fibres can provide the illusion of additional scalp coverage, and dry shampoo acts as a useful volumiser. A wig or a hair system (a wig-like covering that is attached to the scalp) is of help in more advanced cases of hair loss. Semi-permanent make-up aids in the cosmesis of lost eyebrows and eyelashes.

Hair transplantation

Hair transplantation may be considered with stable disease and where an adequate hair reservoir is present. Two surgical methods are in use: follicular unit transplantation (FUT) and follicular unit extraction (FUE). With FUT, a strip of tissue is excised from the occipital scalp. Follicular units are dissected from the tissue strip with the aid of microscopes and transplanted into areas of hair loss. This results in a linear scar from the donor site. FUE involves the removal of individual follicular units from an area of the occipital scalp, avoiding a scar.

Nail diseases

The nail unit is composed of the nail matrix, the nail bed, the proximal and lateral nail folds and the hyponychium. The nail matrix is responsible for production of the nail plate and contains a high concentration of melanocytes. The nail plate emerges from the proximal nail fold and adheres to the nail bed. The nail bed and matrix lack a granular layer, which if present likely indicates a disease state. The nail plate is surrounded by the proximal and lateral nail folds, which act to protect the plate and direct plate growth. The proximal nail fold overlies much of the nail matrix, and the distal third may be represented by a crescent-shaped structure known as the lunula, which demarcates the distal portion of the nail matrix (Figure 27.5). The hyponychium is located beneath the nail plate and forms a seal to protect the distal nail unit.

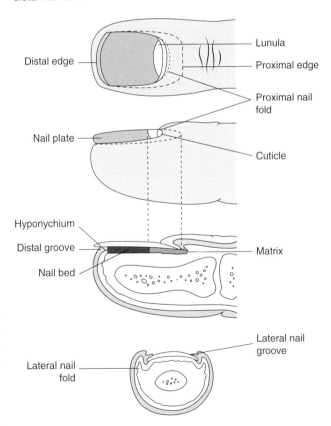

Figure 27.5 Schematic of the fingernail. Baran R *et al. Baran and Dawber's Diseases of the Nails and their Management*, 4th edn. Chichester: Wiley, 2012.

The matrix contains hair-type 'hard' keratins with a large number of sulfur-containing amino acids, providing greater resistance to chemical destruction. On average, fingernail regrowth takes approximately 6 months, whereas toenail regrowth takes 12 months (or up to 18 months for the great toenail).

Nail biopsies, in the form of a lateral longitudinal biopsy, punch, shave or excisional biopsy, are helpful to diagnose inflammatory, infective or neoplastic disorders. Be aware of the risk of scarring and permanent nail deformity. Nail biopsies may not be performed in all dermatology departments, so onward referral to surgeons specialising in nail surgery may be required, particularly if neoplasm is suspected.

Onychomycosis (tinea unguium)

Fungal nail infection is classified according to the point of fungal entry into the nail unit: distal/lateral subungual, superficial white and proximal subungual. Nail discoloration, thickening and deformity are present. Samples for mycology should include subungual debris from the proximal advancing edge of the fungus. In adults and children, oral itraconazole and terbinafine are considered first-line treatments, with fluconazole and griseofulvin considered second line if first-line treatments are not tolerated or are contraindicated. Topical treatments (amorolfine, ciclopirox, tioconazole) are useful for superficial and distal onychomycosis and for patients where oral medication is contraindicated or not tolerated. Toenail fungus may be commonly misdiagnosed in patients with psoriatic nail disease, so be sure to ask about skin disease elsewhere.

Inflammatory nail disease

Psoriasis

Psoriasis is the most encountered inflammatory condition affecting the nails, and nail involvement may be the only clinical feature of the disease. It is also associated with severe disease and psoriatic arthritis. Fingernail signs include pitting, crumbling, leuconychia and red spots in the lunula (psoriasis of the nail matrix), subungual debris, oil drops, dyschromia, splinter haemorrhages and onycholysis (psoriasis of the nail bed) (Figure 27.6). Mycology can help differentiate psoriatic nail disease from onychomycosis, particularly when affecting the toenails. The Nail Psoriasis Severity Index (NAPSI), with a maximum total score for all nails of 160, grades the severity of nail matrix and nail bed disease and can be used to monitor treatment response. Nail psoriasis is often more resistant to treatment than cutaneous psoriasis and improvement will be slow. In mild-to-moderate disease, topical treatments are recommended for a minimum of 4–6 months. When involvement is localised to the nail matrix only, local injections of steroids can be considered. For psoriasis restricted to the nail bed, topical keratolytic agents, topical steroids with or without vitamin D analogues, topical retinoids, tacrolimus 0.1% ointment or intralesional steroids can be considered. Systemic treatments, such as methotrexate, are second-line treatment options and biologic therapy may be warranted for more severe cases.

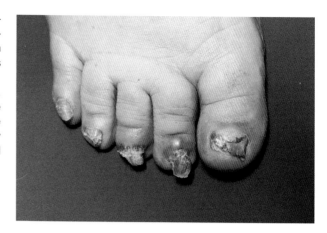

Figure 27.6 Nail psoriasis. © Gloucestershire Hospitals NHS Foundation Trust.

Eczema

Endogenous and exogenous factors relating to eczema damage to the proximal nail folds can result in nail changes manifesting as pitting, Beau's lines, onychomadesis, paronychia, subungual hyperkeratosis and onycholysis. With nail involvement, consideration should be given to an exogenous trigger, with referral to patch testing where appropriate. Management of skin disease results in gradual improvement of the nails. Advice should be given on avoidance of irritants and allergens, with use of regular emollients and topical corticosteroids.

Other inflammatory conditions

Other inflammatory conditions that can cause nail changes include AA (affecting approximately 20% of cases), lichen planus (affecting approximately 10%) (Figure 27.7 and Table 27.4) and sarcoidosis (rarely). Nail changes can also be seen associated with systemic disease or trauma, as well as with benign tumours.

Nail changes in systemic disease

Nail changes are associated with many benign tumours (Table 27.5) and systemic diseases, including

- **Clubbing**: increased curvature of the nail due to soft tissue enlargement. This may be congenital or as a result of a large number of acquired conditions, including chronic lung disease, congenital heart disease, inflammatory bowel disease, liver disorders and thyroid disease.
- **Yellow nail syndrome**: uncommon disruption of linear nail growth resulting in thickened, over-curved nails appearing yellow or green, associated with lymphoedema and pulmonary disease.
- **Autoimmune connective tissue disorders**: dermoscopy and capillaroscopy show capillary enlargement with dilated tortuous capillaries in patients with systemic lupus erythematosus, whereas in dermatomyositis and scleroderma there are avascular areas and reduced capillary density.

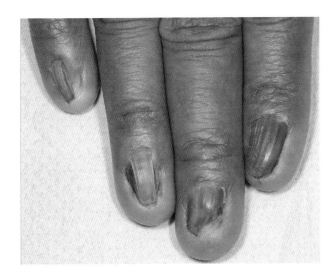

Figure 27.7 Nail dystrophy secondary to lichen planus with evidence of nail atrophy and pterygium. © Salford Royal NHS Foundation Trust.

Traumatic nail changes

Habit-tic deformity of the thumb occurs due to chronically pushing back the cuticle of the thumb with the index finger, resulting in a longitudinal central depression.

Onychophagia (nail biting) is a common habit of children and adults, involving the nail plate and the soft tissues. It may be related to stress and other habit disorders, including trichotillomania and compulsive skin picking.

Onychotillomania refers to the habit of chronic picking or manipulating the nails and may be associated with psychiatric disorders, or Tourette and Prader–Willi syndromes.

Longitudinal melanonychia

Longitudinal melanonychia refers to a pigmented, grey, brown or black, longitudinal streak of the nail plate due to increased activity of melanocytes, or melanocytic hyperplasia in the nail matrix. Ethnic melanonychia is the most common type and typically presents in skin of colour as multiple bands affecting multiple nails. It occurs more frequently on the thumbnail or the big toenail. On dermoscopy, melanonychia due to melanocytic activation appears as a grey background with thin, grey, regular, parallel lines. In chronic trauma, dark red to brown spots corresponding to extravasation of blood may also be seen (Figure 27.8).

Melanonychia of multiple nails can also be associated with genetic disorders (Peutz–Jeghers), trauma (nail biting), chemotherapy medications, endocrine disease (Addison disease), inflammatory skin disease (psoriasis, lichen planus), pregnancy or nail infection (onychomycosis). Where longitudinal melanonychia is > 3 mm in width, with variegated pigmentation or proximal widening (triangular shape), a biopsy should be considered.

Table 27.4 Common nail signs

Nail sign	Clinical findings	Affected site	Associated conditions
Beau's lines	Transverse depression in nail plate surface	Nail matrix	Systemic cause (all nails), trauma (single nail)
Koilonychia	Thin, concave nails	Nail matrix	Physiological (children), occupational, iron deficiency (severe)
Leuconychia (diffuse)	White discoloration of nail plate	Nail matrix	Chemotherapy, congenital disease
Leuconychia (punctate)	White macules on nail plate	Nail matrix	Trauma
Leuconychia (transverse)	Narrow white transverse lines along nail plate	Nail matrix	Trauma
Onychauxis	Hypertrophic nail plate	Nail bed	Psoriasis, onychomycosis, eczema
Onycholysis	Distal detachment of the nail	Nail bed	Trauma, psoriasis, onychomycosis
Onychomadesis	Proximal detachment of the nail	Nail matrix	Trauma, systemic illness, medications, drug reaction, systemic illness, autoimmune diseases
Pitting	Punctate depressions of the nail plate	Nail matrix	Eczema, psoriasis, alopecia areata
Splinter haemorrhages	Longitudinal red-brown lines along nail plate	Nail bed	Trauma, psoriasis, onychomycosis, endocarditis, vasculitis, trichinosis
Trachyonychia	Rough nails	Nail matrix	Alopecia areata, lichen planus, psoriasis, eczema

Table 27.5 Benign tumours of the nail unit

Benign nail tumours	Nail changes	Comments
Fibromas	Pedunculated lesions in proximal nail fold can result in a longitudinal groove of the nail plate	If multiple fibromas consider tuberous sclerosis
Pyogenic granuloma	Periungual or subungual rapidly evolving friable vascular lesion	Can be triggered by trauma or retinoids; for differential diagnosis, consider amelanotic melanoma
Myxoid cyst	Fluid-producing nodules, compression effects result in nail plate depression and grooves	Typically, in middle-aged women, linked with synovial fluid in the arthritic joints
Glomus tumour	Blue-red or purple nodule associated with severe pain on cold exposure	Magnetic resonance imaging and ultrasound scan helpful before surgical excision
Subungual exostoses	Slow-growing tender firm nodule: commonly on great toenail of young adults	X-ray is diagnostic
Onychomatricoma	Localised or diffuse thickening of the nail: affected nail is thickened and yellow, with features of splinter haemorrhages, prominent ridging and increased curvature of the nail plate	Rare tumour commonly misdiagnosed as onychomycosis

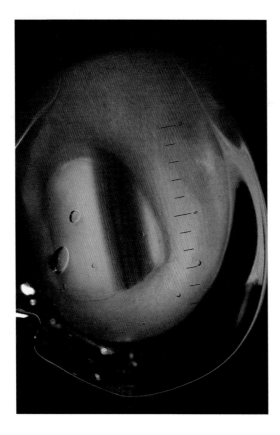

Figure 27.8 Benign melanonychia. © Gloucestershire Hospitals NHS Foundation Trust.

Malignancies of the nail unit

Squamous cell carcinoma

Squamous cell carcinoma of the nail may present as hyperkeratosis, onycholysis, longitudinal erythronychia (red discoloration of the nail), verruca, paronychia, nail plate dystrophy or a subungual mass. Squamous cell carcinoma should be suspected when a verrucous or keratotic lesion of the lateral nail is resistant to treatment for common warts. Trauma, radiation exposure, smoking and infection with human papillomavirus types 16 and 18 are predisposing factors.

Nail melanoma

Melanoma of the nail apparatus arises from the nail matrix. It accounts for 1–3% of melanomas occurring in white-skinned populations and 15–30% of melanomas occurring in dark-skinned individuals. In two-thirds of cases, a brown-to-black longitudinal band wider than 3 mm is seen. Proximal widening, blurred borders, nail dystrophy and pigmentation of the proximal or lateral nail folds (Hutchinson's sign) support clinical suspicion of a melanoma (Figure 27.9). On dermoscopy, a brown background hue may be seen with irregular longitudinal lines and micro-Hutchinson's sign (pigmentation of the cuticle visible only on dermoscopy).

A number of congenital and inherited conditions like congenital malalignment of the great toenails, nail patella syndrome, epidermolysis bullosa, pachyonychia congenita, Darier disease and ectodermal dysplasias may also show nail changes.

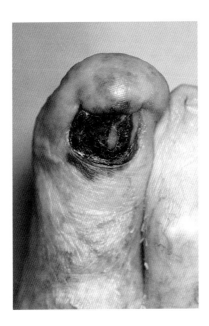

Figure 27.9 Nail melanoma. © Medical Illustration Cardiff and Vale UHB.

- Irregular patches of hair loss containing hairs of varying lengths and bizarre shapes may indicate trichotillomania.
- If multiple digits show pigmented streaks on the nails and pigmentation along the proximal nail fold, this is more likely to be associated with racial pigment and less likely to be a melanoma.
- If onycholysis along with yellowish discoloration is present only in the toenails, consider onychomycosis. If it is predominantly present in fingernails, consider the differential of psoriasis.
- Consider glomus tumour of the nail bed if pinpoint tenderness is present on a reddish area on the nail bed along with history of extreme pain following change in temperature or pressure.

SCE Questions. See questions 68 and 69.

Conclusions

The study of hair and nails is a rewarding area to develop as a specialist interest beyond core training, though all dermatologists must have skills in diagnosis and managing common conditions. A focused clinical examination with the additional practical skills of dermoscopy, microscopy, pathology and surgery can greatly enhance diagnostic yield and direct management options in the care of these patients. Understanding the psychological burden associated with these conditions must be acknowledged, particularly in light of the limited treatment options in many cases.

Pearls and pitfalls

- The pigmented scalp has unique features on dermoscopy that can make the diagnosis of scarring alopecia more difficult. As a result of hairstyling practices and the intrinsic characteristics of afro-textured hair, traction alopecia and central centrifugal cicatricial alopecia are very common. The presence of two or more different hair disorders in the same patient can be found.

FURTHER READING AND KEY RESOURCES

Bolduc C, Sperling LC, Shapiro J. Primary cicatricial alopecia: other lymphocytic primary cicatricial alopecias and neutrophilic and mixed primary cicatricial alopecias. *J Am Acad Dermatol* 2016; **75**:1101–17.

Meah N, Wall D, York K *et al.* The Alopecia Areata Consensus of Experts (ACE) study: results of an international expert opinion on treatments for alopecia areata. *J Am Acad Dermatol* 2020; **83**:123–30.

Textbooks

Baran R, de Berker DAR, Holzberg M, Thomas L, eds. *Baran & Dawber's Diseases of the Nails and Their Management*, 4th edn. Hoboken, NJ: Wiley-Blackwell, 2012.

Griffiths C, Barker J, Bleiker T, Chalmers R, Creamer D, eds. *Rook's Textbook of Dermatology*, 9th edn. Hoboken, NJ: Wiley, 2016.

Tosti A. *Dermoscopy of the Hair and Nails*, 2nd edn. Boca Raton, FL: CRC Press, 2016.

Useful website

British Hair and Nail Society. Available at: https://bhns.org.uk.

28

Genital skin diseases

Manu Shah and Karen Gibbon

Introduction

Diagnosis and management of genital dermatoses are fundamental to dermatological practice, though complex disease may require a multidisciplinary approach. This chapter will review vulval and male genital skin disease separately. However, a basic understanding of genital embryology and the development of external tissues in the anogenital region is relevant to both.

Embryology of the genitalia

In the first weeks of urogenital development, all embryos have two pairs of ducts, both ending at the cloaca. These are:

- Mesonephric (Wolffian) ducts.
- Paramesonephric (Mullerian) ducts.

Male

In the presence of testosterone (produced by the Leydig cells), the mesonephric ducts develop to form the primary male genital ducts. Meanwhile, the paramesonephric ducts degenerate in the presence of anti-Mullerian hormone – produced by Sertoli cells in the testes (Figure 28.1).

Female

In the female, there are no Leydig cells to produce testosterone. In the absence of this hormone, the mesonephric ducts degenerate, leaving behind only a vestigial remnant – Gartner's duct. Equally, the absence of anti-Mullerian hormone also allows for development of the paramesonephric ducts.

In the third week of development, mesenchyme cells, originating in the region of the primitive streak, migrate around the cloacal membrane to form a pair of slightly elevated folds – the cloacal folds. Cranial to the cloacal membrane, the folds unite to form the genital tubercle. By six weeks, the cloacal membrane is subdivided by the urorectal septum into the urogenital and anal

Dermatology Training: The Essentials. Edited by Mahbub M.U. Chowdhury, Tamara W. Griffiths and Andrew Y. Finlay.
© 2022 The British Association of Dermatologists. Published 2022 by John Wiley & Sons Ltd.
Companion website: www.wiley.com/go/chowdhury/dermatologytraining

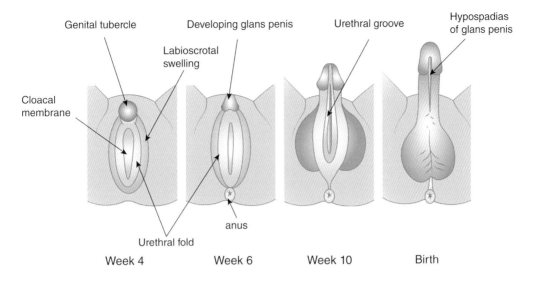

Figure 28.1 Development of the male external genitalia. Adapted from Moore KL *et al*. *The Developing Human: Clinically Orientated Embryology*, 10th edn. Philadelphia, PA: WB Saunders, 2013.

Table 28.1 Development of male and female genitals

	Female	Male
The genital tubercle forms the	clitoris	phallus
The genital folds form the	labia minora	penile urethra
The genital swellings form the	labia majora	scrotum

membranes. The cloacal folds are also subdivided into the urethral folds anteriorly and the anal fold posteriorly. The genital swellings develop on each side of the urethral folds (Table 28.1). After six weeks, development of male and female genitalia diverges: the urethral folds in males fuse forming the penile urethra, and abnormalities along the median raphe can occur as cysts, canals and sinuses.

Vulval disease

Vulval disease is common in dermatological practice and affects both girls and women. This chapter covers key points in patient assessment, vulval examination and treatment of vulval disease. Many patients with complex vulval disease will need referral to a vulval service that involves a multidisciplinary team (MDT). However, the general dermatologist should be able to assess and manage most new cases of vulval disease effectively without having to refer to an MDT, and you should aspire to meet this standard.

Anatomy and histology of the vulva

The vulva is composed of three types of epithelium and mucosa (Table 28.2). In pre-pubertal girls major differences are observed

in the skin of the mons pubis, labia majora and perineum. They appear hairless, but histologically, minute hair bulbs can be seen. Sebaceous and apocrine glands are present, but they are very rudimentary and produce no secretions. After the menopause, atrophy as a result of lower levels of oestrogen manifests as thinner epithelium, decreased vaginal glycogen content and mildly atrophic sebaceous glands. The transition of modified to glycogenated mucosa is recognised as Hart's line.

History taking

When obtaining a history, an accurate description of symptoms should be made, as this can often point to the diagnosis. Table 28.3 outlines some key questions to ask and why. An assessment of the impact on function is always revealing ('How do the symptoms affect you?' or 'What do you miss as a result of the problem?'). A psychosexual history should be explored if appropriate (see the section on male genital skin conditions). Often, the psychosexual history reveals sexual pain as the main complaint, with secondary psychosexual problems such as avoidance of sexual intercourse, phobia of touch, loss of libido and vaginismus.

Vulval examination

A full vulval examination requires sensitivity (with appropriate chaperones), time and good lighting. Each part of the vulva should be examined systematically, including the mons pubis, inguinal folds, outer and inner labia (majora and minora), clitoris (body and hood), perineum, vestibule and anus (Figure 28.2). Hart's line, the junction between the vestibule and the inner labia, marks a change in epithelium type from non-keratinised (glycogenated) to keratinised squamous epithelium. Vulval pathology may be a manifestation of a general skin condition, and therefore a complete examination, including umbilicus and natal cleft, must be considered. Examination of other

Table 28.2 Histological features of three types of skin and mucosa found at the anogenital site

	Hair-bearing skin	Modified mucosa	Glycogenated squamous mucosa
Location	Mons pubis and labia majora	Inner aspect of labia majora, interlabial sulci, outer aspect of labia minora, clitoral hood, perineum	Vestibule, including periclitoral and periurethral mucosa, introitus and vagina
Stratum corneum	Present	Present	Absent
Granular cell layer	Present	Present	Absent
Skin appendages	Hair and adnexal structures	No hair, but sebaceous glands and specialised glands	Absent

Table 28.3 History taking: key facts

Key history questions	Comments
What are the key symptoms and how severe are they? What is the impact on the patient's function?	It is important to be clear about the initial symptoms. Itch can suggest skin disease or infection. It is not the same sensation as irritation
	Pain can be secondary to itching from skin damage. As a primary symptom, pain may indicate a pain syndrome. Improvement in function (including sexual intercourse) is an important clinical outcome
How long has the woman experienced symptoms?	Acute symptoms may indicate vulvovaginal thrush or contact dermatitis. Chronic symptoms may be caused by lichen sclerosus or lichen planus
Are there any other symptoms?	For example, vaginal discharge, vulval pain or other skin disease
What treatments have been tried before?	Inappropriate topical treatments can exacerbate symptoms and potentially cause an irritant or allergic reaction. The history should explore failed treatments, e.g. topical steroid frequency and amount, as underusage is common
How does the patient clean the vulval area?	Many women feel unclean and can wash excessively, leading to skin damage and further irritation
Are there any possible contacts with irritants such as soaps, shampoos, urine and scented vaginal wipes?	These irritants can damage the skin, potentially causing inflammation. Urine is a potent skin irritant
Are symptoms stress related?	In lichen simplex, itching is classically worse during times of stress
Is there any systemic illness?	For example, diabetes, renal failure, anaemia, autoimmune conditions (including family history)
Are any other skin conditions present?	For example, eczema or psoriasis (sometimes hidden as cracking behind the ears, a scaly scalp or umbilical inflammation)

non-keratinised or mucosal surfaces, including the oral cavity, eyes and mouth, should be performed. This allows a complete assessment of disease extent and diagnosis, especially for diseases that are not restricted to the vulval region such as psoriasis, eczema, lichen sclerosus, pemphigus vulgaris, bullous or cicatricial pemphigoid and erosive lichen planus.

The vulval region is often moist, and scale is a less reliable sign than on other areas of the skin, except for the mons pubis, where scale may be a manifestation of psoriasis. On flexural sites such as the natal cleft, scale and lichenification may result in whiteness and fissuring of the skin. This can make common conditions more difficult to diagnose.

Vulval conditions

Vulval itching is often the presenting complaint of a vulval skin condition. Itch is a symptom and not a diagnosis. The causes can be separated into skin disease (vulval dermatoses), infection, and pre-malignant or malignant disease. An algorithm is useful for assessing patients (Figure 28.3). From this algorithm it follows that patients can have more than one diagnosis. It is important to remember this, as the management of vulval conditions often includes using steroid preparations of different strengths and for different durations (Table 28.4).

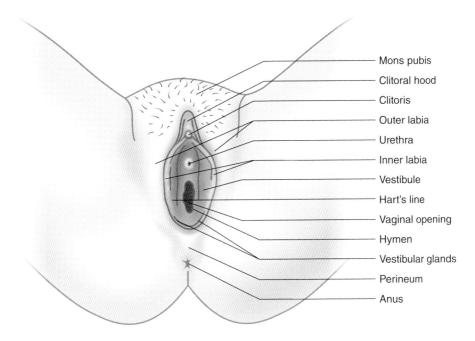

Figure 28.2 Schematic representation of the normal adult vulva.

Mons pubis
Clitoral hood
Clitoris
Outer labia
Urethra
Inner labia
Vestibule
Hart's line
Vaginal opening
Hymen
Vestibular glands
Perineum
Anus

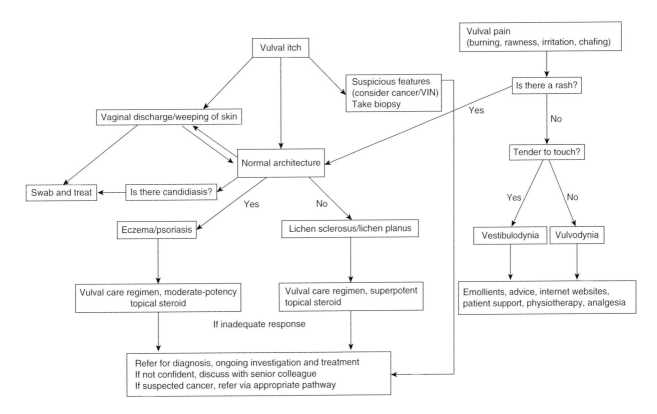

Figure 28.3 Diagnostic algorithm for vulval symptoms. VIN, vulval intraepithelial neoplasia. Adapted from Hollingworth T. *Differential Diagnosis in Obstetrics and Gynecology*, 2nd edn. Boca Raton, FL: CRC Press, 2015.

Table 28.4 Management of vulval dermatoses

Diagnosis	Clinical appearance	Diagnostic aids	Initial treatment	Subsequent management
Lichen sclerosus	Porcelain white papules and plaques, ecchymoses (subcutaneous purpura), erosions (loss of epidermis), fissures (late signs: loss of anatomy, fusion, adhesions), lichenification. This disease can have a 'figure of eight' appearance	Clinically, if confident, or a vulval biopsy may be needed. Consider biopsy if there are indurated or suspicious areas	Superpotent topical steroid and emollients	Gynaecologist, dermatologist or GP. Refer to vulval service for treatment-resistant cases and complications, and when associated with VIN
Lichen planus	Classical lichen planus: violaceous, well-demarcated plaques with overlying lacy white lines, usually affecting the labia majora and surrounding skin Erosive lichen planus: glazed redness or erosions symmetrically distributed at vaginal introitus. White, slightly raised edge to lesions. Lacy white lines (Wickham's striae) in surrounding skin May have loss of anatomy	Clinical assessment and biopsy from the edge of an erosion Lichen planus may be seen in the mouth, nails, eyes or non-mucosal skin	Superpotent topical steroid and emollients	Dermatologist or gynaecologist Refer to vulval service for treatment-resistant cases and complications, and when associated with VIN Erosive lichen planus is difficult to treat so consider referral to a vulval service
Atopic eczema	Symmetrically inflamed, red, weepy skin No loss of anatomy May be satellite lesions and have poorly defined edges	Clinical history and examination to include other skin sites for other signs of eczema	Moderate or potent topical steroid and emollients to gain control of inflammation	Dermatologist or GP
Contact dermatitis (CD)	Irritant CD: poorly defined redness and inflammation present where the irritant has been applied Allergic CD: redness and inflammation extend outside of area In both cases there may be excoriation of the skin caused by scratching	Clinical history and examination Patch testing if allergic CD suspected	Moderate or potent topical steroid and emollients to gain control of inflammation Strict avoidance of irritants and allergens	Dermatologist and GP
Seborrhoeic eczema	Glazed skin in interlabial sulci	Clinical examination of other sites, e.g. scalp, eyebrows and nasolabial folds for redness and fine scaling	Moderate or potent topical steroid and emollients to gain control of inflammation	Dermatologist and GP

Condition	Clinical features	Diagnosis	Treatment	Who manages
Psoriasis	Classically well-demarcated, scaly red, inflamed plaques, but vulval psoriatic plaques are smooth, glossy and often salmon-pink in colour. Often no scale in vulval creases but surrounding skin can have scaly lesions typically seen in psoriasis. No scarring or loss of anatomy	Clinical assessment includes examination of 'hidden sites' for other signs of psoriasis, e.g. knees, elbows, umbilicus, scalp, ears, lower back and nails. Biopsy if unsure	Moderate-potency topical steroid and emollients as recommended by NICE guidance. Consider a combination topical therapy in macerated skinfolds	Dermatologist and GP
Lichen simplex chronicus	Lichenification of the skin with erosions from chronic scratching. Usually no loss of anatomy but can give thick 'leathery' skin, often superimposed on other itchy skin disorders, e.g. eczema and lichen sclerosus	Clinical history and examination	Superpotent topical steroid and emollients. Secondary infection with candida or bacteria is common and may need treatment	Dermatologist or GP
Intertrigo	Flexural rash that may involve the groin, natal cleft, submammary region and abdominal 'apron fold'. Common in overweight patients	Infection of the flexural areas with thrush (*Candida albicans*), erythrasma (*Corynebacterium minutissimum*) and *Tinea* species	Treatment using both oral antibiotics and antifungal agents is usual. Regular use of an emollient to improve the skin barrier function at this site	Dermatologist or GP
VIN, divided into 'usual' (HPV positive) or 'differentiated' (HPV negative) types	White, red or brown patches or plaques with secondary lichenification. Differentiated VIN seen in association with LS	Multiple mapping biopsies needed to exclude 'microinvasive' SCC change	HPV positive: therapies e.g. 5% imiquimod. HPV negative associated with LS requires surgery	MDT and specialist vulval services
Vulvodynia	Often normal, but can occur with other vulval dermatoses, e.g. sebopsoriasis or lichen sclerosus (Figure 28.3)	Clinical history and examination. Listen carefully to words used to describe pain and its location	Explanation, patient information leaflets, signposting to websites. Topical and/or oral therapy, e.g. local anaesthetics, amitriptyline	GP or refer to vulval service if also has complex vulval dermatosis and other comorbidities, e.g. urogynaecological conditions

GP, general practitioner; HPV, human papillomavirus; LS, lichen sclerosus; MDT, multidisciplinary team; NICE, National Institute for Health and Care Excellence; VIN, vulval intraepithelial neoplasia.

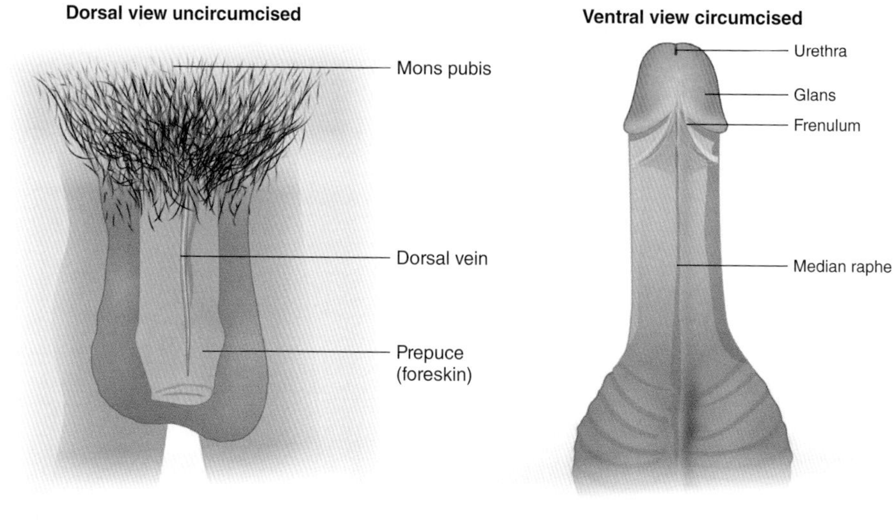

Dorsal view uncircumcised
Mons pubis
Dorsal vein
Prepuce (foreskin)
Ventral view circumcised
Urethra
Glans
Frenulum
Median raphe

Figure 28.4 Normal surface anatomy of the male genitalia.

Male genital skin disease

Male genital skin disease often requires prompt action to minimise sexual and urinary dysfunction or to reduce the risk of penile cancer. The following section is a guide to understanding some common variants and normal anatomy, taking a full history, how to examine and when to investigate, and discussion of some male genital conditions.

Anatomy

Perhaps the most important point about the anatomy of the male genitalia is the recognition of the wide variety of normality. The genitals differ in size, pigmentation and shape, and normal variations include angiokeratomas, sebaceous prominence, skin tags, pearly penile papules, long foreskin and naevi. The normal surface anatomy of the male genitalia is shown in Figure 28.4.

Knowledge of the topographical anatomy of the male genitalia is useful when describing locations of lesions. The ventral aspect of the penis is continuous with the scrotum. The penile shaft is composed of three erectile columns (two corpora cavernosa and the corpus spongiosum) enclosed by fascia with nerves, lymphatics and vessels within the penile skin (Figure 28.5).

The foreskin is a double-layered, highly innervated structure composed of skin, mucous membrane, blood vessels and smooth muscle. The outer skin is continuous with the shaft of the penis (keratinised), with the inner skin being a mucous membrane. The foreskin is incompletely separated from the glans at birth, but separation should be complete by the late teens.

Skin
Penile arteries
Vein
Corpora cavernosa
Nerve
Tunica albuginea
Corpus spongiosum
Urethra

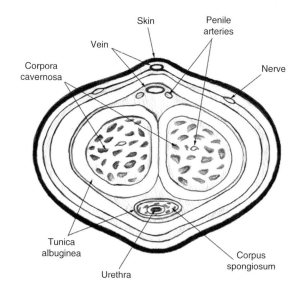

Figure 28.5 Cross-section of the penis. Source: Zachary WA Klaassen, Male Reproductive Organ Anatomy. Medscape, WebMD LLC.

History

It is essential to diagnose and manage patients with genital problems in the correct environment. Try to put the patient at ease and assure them that questions are confidential and relevant and may be sensitive or embarrassing. Explain the need for a sexual history and use terms the patient will understand. Do not make assumptions about the patient's sexuality or behaviour, and be non-judgemental when listening. The dermatological history is summarised in Table 28.5 and taking a sexual history in Table 28.6.

Examination

Men may be uncomfortable with genital examination. Therefore, explain what you intend to do before you examine the patient. Many men wrongly assume that you are going to perform an invasive procedure on them. It is best to have a systematic approach to examining the genitalia (Figure 28.6).

Table 28.5 Questions when taking a dermatological history

What are the presenting symptoms? Rash, itch, soreness

Ask specifically about discomfort on sexual intercourse (dyspareunia); this is the most common symptom, but few men will offer this as the reason for attending

Duration of symptoms

Medical history, especially skin disorders, atopy or circumcision

Previous skin conditions

Medication, including topical treatment

Does the patient smoke? (Important in several genital conditions, including penile cancer)

Family history

Occupation

Table 28.6 Questions to ask when taking a sexual history

Type of symptoms and duration (in relation to last sexual contact)

Presence of urethral symptoms such as discharge and dysuria

Pain, lumps, swellings in genital area, groin or scrotum

Ulceration or blisters. Are they painful or painless?

Recent genital or generalised rashes

Genital itching or soreness

Date of most recent sexual contact

Details of partner: male, female, regular, casual, sex worker, local, abroad

Which anatomical areas are exposed to sexual contact?

Are condoms or a barrier used? Are there other exposures?

Other sexual contacts in last 3 months

Number of contacts in last 12 months (risk assessment)

Previous sexually transmitted diseases (STDs) and risk factors for STDs such as drugs and alcohol

Examination	*Examples of conditions seen*
Examine the groins	(intertrigo, erythrasma)
Scrotal skin, testes	(lichenified eczema)
Mons pubis	(hair problems, lice)
Penile shaft	(lesions, structural and developmental abnormalities)
Glans penis: retract the foreskin noting	
any tightness	(lichen sclerosus)
meatus (abnormal shape?)	(warts, lichen sclerosus)
coronal area	(pearly penile papules)
frenulum	(loss of structure, warts)
Perineum, perianal area	
Rest of skin examination (e.g. mucous membranes)	(common dermatoses, e.g. lichen planus)

Figure 28.6 A systematic approach to male genital examination.

Male genital skin conditions

It is essential to have a knowledge of common skin diseases that affect the male genitalia, such as lichen sclerosus, lichen planus and psoriasis, and how these conditions affect the patient's life both physically and psychologically. Awareness of rare conditions such as penile cellulitis, lymphoedema and extra-mammary Paget's disease is important. It is also necessary to differentiate between malignant, pre-malignant and benign disease of the male genitalia. Table 28.7 shows examples of pre-malignant and malignant, and common and rare conditions affecting the male genitalia.

When to refer and to whom

Management of male patients with genital problems often requires a multidisciplinary approach. Patients may move between specialties depending on their clinical need (Figure 28.7). For example, a patient with lichen sclerosus may initially go to a genitourinary medicine (sexual health) clinic, then to dermatology for medical treatment, then to urology for a circumcision (Table 28.8), or they may be referred for psychosexual counselling to manage impotence.

Female and male genital disease: common management principles

Investigation of genital skin conditions

Microbiology

Vaginal swabs are indicated when the history suggests possible primary or secondary infection with bacterial, candida or viral infections. Infection is a common cause of loss of symptom control in inflammatory dermatoses, and may explain why, for example, lichen sclerosus appears initially well controlled with potent steroids and then flares. Screening for sexually transmitted disease is usually carried out by sexual health services.

The dermatologist may need to swab the skin of the penis, particularly the glans. Swab results frequently reveal commensal bacteria. Anaerobes and coliforms are often found, complicating any form of balanitis. A skin swab that shows a culture of yeast must be regarded with caution, as 'thrush' in men is actually rare, except in patients with diabetes or HIV. Mycology may be necessary to diagnose tinea cruris and other mycoses.

Biopsy

Vulval. A biopsy is usually indicated for:

- All areas of vulval melanosis and new or changing pigmented lesions.
- Persistently eroded areas.
- Indurated and suspicious ulcerated areas.

- Cases of poor response to treatment following the initial diagnosis.

The site selected for biopsy should be representative of the lesion or area of abnormality. This is usually at the edge of the lesion and should also include some normal tissue. Multiple mapping biopsies are indicated in cases of suspected multifocal vulval intraepithelial neoplasia (VIN). A 4-mm punch biopsy under local anaesthesia is adequate. If immunobullous disease is suspected, then a sample for immunofluorescence should also be sent.

Penile. The common reasons for performing a penile biopsy are:

- Diagnostic uncertainty.
- Diagnosis of pre-malignant and malignant lesions.
- Special tests needed for tissue culture, human papillomavirus typing or immunofluorescence.

Patch testing

This is indicated when allergic contact dermatitis is suspected and will help to confirm irritant contact dermatitis by exclusion. Common allergens include ingredients of contraceptives such as rubber and lubricants, preservatives, topical anaesthetics, fragrances, nail polish or gels, textile dyes and topical neomycin. Allergic contact dermatitis to the adhesive used in sanitary pads is relatively common and should be considered, particularly if the fully keratinised epithelium is affected and symptoms involve the perianal skin. Irritant dermatitis from urine or faeces is very common and often a reason for treatment failure until it is properly addressed, for example by referral for urodynamics.

The multidisciplinary team

Many chronic, rare and difficult genital problems require multidisciplinary input. Other useful services include genitourinary medicine, physiotherapy, pain management, psychosexual therapy, paediatrics and gynaecology and urology (Figure 28.7).

General treatment principles for genital skin disease

General principles for all genital disease are as follows:

- Good education, support and counselling, including leaflets, patient support websites, and diagrams showing where and how to apply topical therapies.
- Explain the importance of using emollients to maintain skin barrier function and the need to apply them regularly. Give different samples to try.
- Explain the different strengths of topical steroids and how they should be used at different anatomical areas of the anogenital skin. Emphasise the importance of achieving control, then using regular intermittent maintenance therapy.
- Safely discharge patients to their general practitioner for long-term follow-up with appropriate support information on how to re-access services, for example malignancy concerns in lichen sclerosus.

Table 28.7 Examples of pre-malignant and malignant lesions, and rashes that affect the male genitalia

Diagnosis	Typical clinical appearance	Diagnostic aids	Histology	Initial treatment	Subsequent management
Pre-malignant and malignant lesions					
Penile intraepithelial carcinoma	Wide variation from single or multiple papules to psoriasiform and verrucous papules and plaques	Skin biopsy	HPV in > 70%. Pathology confined to epidermis: dysplasia, keratinocytes with abnormal nuclei. Psoriasiform hyperplasia common	Imiquimod 5%, 5-fluorouracil, cryotherapy, surgery + circumcision	Requires follow-up in dermatology or urology
Squamous cell carcinoma	Often verrucous, may be ulcerated, fleshy and raised. Evidence of lichen sclerosus in up to 50% of cases	Skin biopsy	HPV in 20–45%. Various subtypes; commonest is keratinising. May vary from well differentiated to undifferentiated	Surgery, circumcision usually	MDT, follow-up in regional cancer service, may share care with dermatology
Common dermatoses of the genital area					
Lichen planus (LP)	Typical of the condition in circumcised men. Usually non-specific in uncircumcised patients	Diagnose clinically, but skin biopsy may occasionally be necessary. Patch tests needed for contact dermatitis	Usually typical for the condition	Moderate-to-superpotent topical steroids, emollients	GP for uncomplicated cases; dermatologist for erosive LP, investigations and cases refractory to treatment
Eczema					
Psoriasis					
Contact dermatitis					
Zoon's balanitis (the diagnosis of Zoon's is controversial as it probably represents LS or irritant dermatitis)	Typical moist red 'kissing lesions' on the glans and corresponding foreskin. May mask underlying LS or erosive LP	Diagnose clinically, but skin biopsy may be necessary to exclude LS or erosive LP	Dense inflammatory infiltrate in upper and mid-dermis with plasma cells	Attention to hygiene and cleansing, topical steroids. Circumcision is curative	No follow-up after circumcision, but many patients remain symptomatic on topical treatment alone
Lichen sclerosus (LS)	Multiple signs of acute disease, e.g. moist inflammatory plaques. Chronic disease: scarring, e.g. loss of frenulum, atrophy of foreskin, phimosis, meatal narrowing	Diagnose clinically. Skin biopsy if possibility of other conditions, e.g. erosive LP, cicatricial pemphigoid	Superficial dermal oedema, thin epidermis, vacuolar degeneration of basal layer. Homogenised collagen in superficial dermis, loss of elastic fibres	Superpotent topical steroid and emollients	Follow-up by GP or dermatologist until asymptomatic, but be aware disease may recur years later
Rare genital problems					
Extra-mammary Paget's disease	Often non-specific, may mimic intertrigo, psoriasis, eczema. May be secondary to underlying cancer	Skin biopsy	Large Paget cells, prominent pleomorphic nuclei in epidermis; may extend into dermis. Diagnosis is confirmed by immunocytochemistry	Screen for underlying cancer. Surgical excision if possible. Topical 5-fluorouracil or imiquimod is an option. Chemotherapy and radiotherapy for palliation	Follow-up by dermatologist or oncologist

GP, general practitioner; MDT, multidisciplinary team.

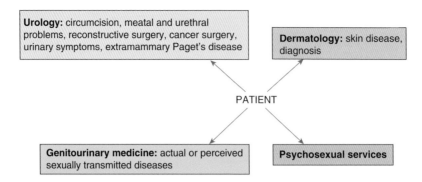

Figure 28.7 When to refer and to whom.

Table 28.8 When to refer for circumcision: medical reasons

Phimosis or paraphimosis

Recurrent inflammation of the glans and foreskin (balanoposthitis)

Unresponsive to medical therapy (especially lichen sclerosus, which is pre-cancerous)

Penile cancer and penile intraepithelial neoplasia

While there are no published core outcome measures for research in genital skin disease, suggested clinical aims include:

- A reduction in symptoms (e.g. less itch, fewer flare-ups) and improvement in quality of life.
- An improvement in function (e.g. in sexual function or mobility and urinary function).
- Increased confidence in self-management (e.g. management of flare-ups and self-examination).
- Reduction or abolition of risk of genital cancer.

Treatment of genital skin conditions with topical steroids

Topical steroids (Chapter 17) are often ineffectively used in the genitocrural areas due to concerns from patients and other healthcare professionals about side-effects, particularly skin or mucosal atrophy. Therefore, it is important to use the correct strength of steroid for the necessary length of time on the appropriate body site. In females, mucosal surfaces such as the vulval vestibule are remarkably resistant to steroid atrophy.

In contrast, keratinised surfaces such as the labiocrural folds, perineum, perianal area and thighs can develop skin thinning and striae (stretch marks) with inappropriate use of potent topical steroids. Over-usage of topical steroids presents as atrophic skin and is reversible in the early stages. Later, permanent telangiectasia and striae can develop.

Topical calcineurin inhibitors in the genital region reduce inflammation and do not cause skin atrophy. However, their role is not fully understood and there is a theoretical risk of long-term localised immunosuppression from these agents, causing skin cancers. In men, infections such as human papillomavirus or herpes simplex may be re-activated.

In lichen sclerosus and lichen planus in females and males, the use of superpotent topical steroids is recommended as first-line therapy. In general, topical steroids should be used once daily. There is no evidence to suggest that twice-daily application is superior, and twice-daily usage has greater potential to cause side-effects. Ointments are preferable to creams as they contain fewer constituents and therefore have a lower chance of causing irritation or contact allergy. Once control of inflammation and symptoms has been achieved, topical steroids should be reduced to the minimum frequency required to maintain remission. Table 28.9 provides a list of solutions in case of failure to respond to treatment.

Table 28.9 Treatment failure and solutions

Reason for treatment failure	Solution
Poor adherence	Reassurance for 'steroid-phobic' patients
	Explanation of terms like 'use sparingly' and 'sensitive areas'
Inadequate quantities of treatment used	Advise the patient on correct amounts to use, e.g. by using the 'fingertip unit'
Inaccurate placement of treatment	A mirror may be helpful. Models, diagrams and photos can be used as explanation
Continued exposure to irritants	Good hygiene measures, avoidance of wipes and non-prescribed treatments, avoid over-washing
Incorrect diagnosis	If all of the above have been tried, reconsider the diagnosis. Consider allergic contact dermatitis or pre-malignant or malignant change and investigate accordingly

Conclusions

The care of patients with genital dermatoses falls under the remit of dermatologists and also genitourinary physicians, gynaecologists, urologists, oncologists and general practitioners. This reflects the broad and sometimes complex aetiology of this type of disease. Whatever the cause, it often has a negative impact on patients' quality of life. It is essential for trainees to develop capabilities in diagnosis and management of these conditions, to understand the wider referral system and to engage in a multidisciplinary team approach for those who require tertiary-level care.

Pearls and pitfalls

- Taking a sexual history can be embarrassing for the patient and the doctor. However, it is important to get honest replies in order to help the patient.
- Regard a penile culture of yeast cautiously, as this is usually a commensal and not pathogenic.
- Diagnostic punch biopsy in male and female genital problems can be performed quickly and easily in the dermatology outpatient setting, with minimal morbidity and stress to the patient.

SCE Questions. See questions 13–16.

FURTHER READING AND KEY RESOURCES

Bunker CB, Shim TN. Male genital lichen sclerosus. *Indian J Dermatol* 2015; **60**:111–17.

Nunns D. Vulvodynia. In: *Gynecologic Dermatology: Symptom, Signs and Clinical Management* (Kirtschig G, Cooper SM, eds). London: JP Medical Publishers, 2016; 245–50.

Nunns D, Simpson R, Watson A, Murphy R. The management of vulval itching caused by benign vulval dermatoses. *Obstet Gynaecol* 2017; **19**:307–15.

Shah M, Maleki N, Edward S. Zoon's balanitis is a non-specific reactive pattern and not a clinical diagnosis. *J Am Acad Dermatol* 2015; **72** (Suppl.):AB87.

Useful websites

British Journal of Family Medicine. Skin conditions of the vulva. Available at: https://www.bjfm.co.uk/skin-conditions-of-the-vulva.

DermNet NZ. Itchy vulva. Available at: https://dermnetnz.org/topics/the-itchy-vulva.

e-Learning for Healthcare. e-dermatology. Available at: https://www.e-lfh.org.uk/programmes/dermatology.

The British Society for the Study of Vulval Disease. Available at: https://bssvd.org.

The International Society for the Study of Vulvovaginal Disease. Available at: https://www.issvd.org.

Oral medicine

Jane Setterfield

Introduction

Oral mucosal diseases present to a range of clinicians including dermatologists. In some circumstances this is part of a mucocutaneous disease, and shared care may be advisable with a local oral medicine clinician. Where the problem is confined to the oral mucosa alone and the diagnosis or treatment is unclear, then referral to oral medicine is optimal. In this chapter the most common oral mucosal disorders and oral manifestations of skin disease will be outlined. The causes of oral ulceration and distinguishing features will be discussed and the key features that suggest pre-malignant or malignant change highlighted.

Dermatologists need to acquire key skills in history taking and performing a detailed oral examination. The findings need to be recorded in a way that optimises sequential monitoring through an appropriate clinical outcome measure. The Oral Disease Severity Score (ODSS) is applicable to autoimmune blistering diseases and oral lichen planus (LP), and has been fully validated, much like the Psoriasis Area and Severity Index (PASI) score for psoriasis. Assessment of disease activity includes the use of patient-reported clinical outcomes; the Oral Health Impact Profile is another valuable tool used to track disease activity. For oral ulceration with a broad differential diagnosis, history taking is key and features to distinguish differential diagnoses will be highlighted. An ulcer diary is the optimal way to assess therapeutic efficacy in conditions such as aphthous ulceration and erythema multiforme (EM). In addition, it may be useful for the dermatologist to be able to undertake small diagnostic oral biopsies, and the optimal methodology and site will be discussed.

Many inflammatory or autoimmune oral mucosal conditions are treated initially with topical corticosteroids. These might be as mouthwashes (three-minute rinse and spit), as ointments mixed 50:50 with Orabase® (Colgate-Palmolive, New York, USA) and applied to dried mucosae, or applied directly on a cotton roll or swab for 15 minutes. Where appropriate an algorithm for treatment is shown; however, reference to updated guidelines is essential.

Further reading is recommended for the full range of conditions that might present to a dermatologist and for an in-depth guide to management. Key conditions to be aware of are presented in Table 29.1.

History taking

The oral history is similar to other site-specific histories and must include a full systems review, as the mouth is a frequent site of involvement in a wide range of systemic diseases. As oral symptoms may be a common presenting feature of many conditions, it is key to consider the following factors:

Dermatology Training: The Essentials. Edited by Mahbub M.U. Chowdhury, Tamara W. Griffiths and Andrew Y. Finlay.
© 2022 The British Association of Dermatologists. Published 2022 by John Wiley & Sons Ltd.
Companion website: www.wiley.com/go/chowdhury/dermatologytraining

- Presenting complaint.
- Timing of onset of condition and any triggers.
- Are the ulcers episodic or persistent?
- Painful or painless?
- Exacerbating and relieving factors.
- Previous treatments.
- Other affected sites, for example skin, genital, gastrointestinal tract, joints.
- Smoking: how many pack-years (packs of 20 cigarettes per day × years)?
- Alcohol intake (units per week)?
- Family history of ulcers and/or history of autoimmune disease.
- Past medical conditions, for example gastrointestinal disorders, joint pains.

It is useful for patients to keep written records, for example an ulcer diary for sequential monitoring and to assess response to treatment (see below).

Table 29.1 Differential diagnoses for key signs and symptoms

Sign or symptom	Differential diagnoses
Ulcers	Major, minor and herpetiform aphthosis
	Autoimmune blistering diseases: pemphigus vulgaris (PV), mucous membrane pemphigoid (MMP), paraneoplastic pemphigus (PNP), epidermolysis bullosa (EB)
	Ulcerative lichen planus and lupus erythematosus
	Erythema multiforme
	Stevens–Johnson syndrome and toxic epidermal necrolysis (SJS/TEN)
	Infections: herpes simplex, Coxsackie, varicella, syphilis
	Behçet's syndrome
White lesions	Lichen planus, leukoplakia
Cheilitis and/or persistent lip swelling	Exfoliative cheilitis, actinic cheilitis, oral facial granulomatosis, Crohn's disease, sarcoidosis
Other conditions	
Pain	Candida, oral dysaesthesia
Dry mouth	Drugs, Sjögren's syndrome
Mucosal lumps and bumps	Fibroepithelial polyps, viral warts
Pigmentation	Natural pigmentation, amalgam tattoos, macular pigmentation or lentigines, naevi

Examination

Trainees may be inexperienced in even basic skills and must develop the ability to undertake a systematic and thorough oral clinical examination. A consistent sequential approach (outlined below) ensures no areas are overlooked. Targeted learning opportunities and observation in a specialist clinic can also help demystify the process.

Understanding the range of 'normal' may take months to years of practice, and so examining and looking in the mouth when the opportunity arises during dermatological consultations will be valuable. The mouth contains three types of mucosae, each adapted to their function in specific sites of the mouth:

- Non-keratinised, stratified, squamous-lined mucosa protects the alveolar bone (supporting the teeth) and is the mucosa that is not tightly bound down to bone. This forms the vestibules and extends onto the buccal mucosa, inner lips, floor of mouth and ventral tongue.
- Ortho- or para-keratinised masticatory mucosa comprises the hard palate, dorsum of the tongue and the gingivae.
- Specialised mucosa comprising taste buds and structures for the perception of taste and mucus production.

Essential equipment and practice

- A bright, warm white light.
- Positioning the patient and yourself at the correct height to enable a detailed examination.
- One or two dental mirrors (to visualise sulci and palate and act as retractors), a tongue depressor and a piece of gauze to hold the tongue and move it to allow inspection of the postero-lateral borders.
- Having an assistant record findings is also ideal, so that all sites can be examined sequentially without the need to remove gloves.
- Examination sheets to record the size and location of lesions (Figure 29.1) and to record the ODSS for severity of ulcerating or blistering lesions (Table 29.2). Both of these are useful ways to ensure all sites are examined and documented.

Technique and sequence of examination

- First examine the perioral skin and then regional lymph nodes.
- Examine the lips: outer (vermillion) and then inner (labial mucosa).
- It is vital then to reflect the corner of the lips to examine the commissures.
- Using one or two dental mirrors to hold the cheeks away from the closed teeth is helpful to examine the buccal mucosa.
- Examine the gingivae buccally and lingually (with mirror). Consider the gingivae in six sections, canine to canine and then premolars backwards. The gingivae on the palatal aspect extend for approximately 5 mm from the margin of teeth.
- Hard and soft palate plus oropharynx.
- Tongue: dorsum, ventrolateral aspects, sublingual.

- Floor of mouth.
- Palpate any white or nodular areas of the mucosa: must be soft, otherwise requires a biopsy.

There are a number of published clinical outcome measures for oral diseases, but the majority are not validated. Use of a validated clinical scoring tool is highly recommended for chronic diseases to assess therapeutic outcomes, particularly when systemic immunosuppression is required. Such tools include:

- Lichen planus: ODSS.
- Autoimmune blistering disease: ODSS.

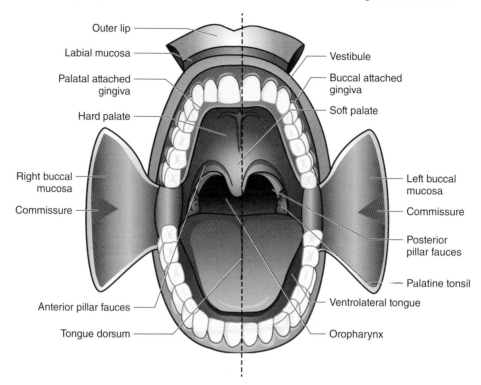

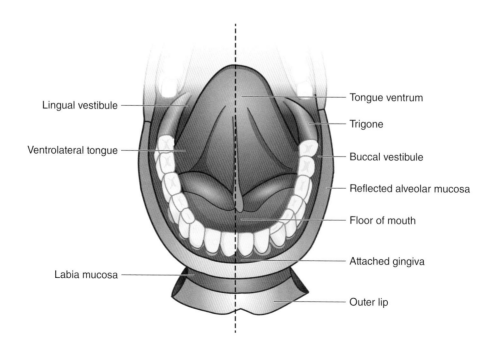

Figure 29.1 A schematic diagram to demonstrate the sites to inspect and annotate presence of lesions.

Table 29.2 Oral Disease Severity Score (ODSS)

Site	Site Score	Activity Score/unit of site (0–3)
Outer lips (1)		
Inner lips (1)		
R Buccal mucosa (1 or 2)		
L Buccal mucosa (1 or 2)		
Gingivae (1 each segment)		
Lower R (from 1st premolar)		
Lower central (canine to canine)		
Lower L (from 1st premolar)		
Upper R (from 1st premolar)		
Upper central (canine to canine)		
Upper L (from 1st premolar)		
Dorsum of tongue (1 or 2)		
R Ventral tongue (1)		
L Ventral tongue (1)		
Floor of mouth (1 or 2)		
Hard palate (1 or 2)		
Soft palate (1 or 2)		
Oropharynx (1 or 2)		
Total		

Total Score = Site Score + Activity Score + Pain Score (1–10) (maximum 106).
Site Score. 0 if no lesion. For the buccal mucosa: 1 if < 50% of area affected; 2 if > 50% of area affected. For the dorsum of tongue, floor of mouth, hard or soft palate or oropharynx: 1 if unilateral, 2 if bilateral.
Activity Score. 0 in reticular oral lichen planus – white striae that are asymptomatic are not given an activity score; 1 for mild redness or white healing lesion in pemphigus vulgaris; 2 for marked redness without erosion; 3 for erosion or ulceration. **Pain Score**. Analogue scale from 0 (no discomfort) to 10 (the most severe pain they have encountered with this condition so far). The patient is asked to provide a score reflecting their pain or discomfort as an average of the preceding week. Please note that in oral lichen planus, white striae are reflected as present with a site score but if asymptomatic are given an activity score of 0. Where a site has a score of 2, each site unit is allocated an activity score. These are then added together.

- Aphthous ulcers and recurrent EM: ulcer diary that records ulcer severity (1–3) representing mild, moderate or severe symptoms for each day in a table (calendar for 1 year on A4 paper).

Recommended patient-reported outcome measures include:

- DLQI – Dermatology Life Quality Index.
- OHIP14 – Oral Health Impact Profile.
- COMDQ – Chronic Oral Mucosal Disease Questionnaire.

Investigations

Trainees should familiarise themselves with common investigations required in various clinical presentations. If needed, do not shy away from taking a buccal mucosal biopsy, which is much less likely to result in complications such as scarring, bleeding or nerve damage compared to the vermillion lip.

The following list of investigations should be tailored to the patient's presenting complaint.

Oral swab

For microscopy, culture and sensitivity. Patients in whom topical corticosteroids are to be prescribed or have the following clinical signs or symptoms will require an oral swab for microscopy, culture and sensitivity to identify possible candida or other infections. This is important in the following scenarios:

- Angular cheilitis.
- White lesions at the commissures.
- Redness or inflammation on the palate or tongue.
- Oral dryness.
- Burning discomfort.

Viral swab

If suspicion of the following:

- Herpes simplex (needs to be taken within a few days of lesion appearing).
- Coxsackie (taken from throat).
- Varicella zoster.

Blood investigations

For an atrophic or sore tongue or oral ulceration:

- Full blood count; renal and liver function.
- Vitamins B_{12} and B_6.
- Folate.
- Ferritin.
- Zinc.
- Coeliac screen.
- Autoimmune screen.
- Indirect immunofluorescence and ELISA.

Patch testing

- Possible contact allergy to amalgam or other dental material.
- Orofacial granulomatosis.
- Exfoliative cheilitis.

Radiology

- Ultrasound scan of salivary glands or other swellings.
- MRI, CT or cone beam CT scan via multidisciplinary team for lesions of soft or hard tissues not visualised otherwise in detail.

Oral biopsy

Undertaking a simple punch biopsy (4–5 mm) from a perilesional area of the reflected alveolar mucosa is ideal for patients with an immunobullous disease confined to the gingiva (Figure 29.2).

In patients with suspected pemphigus or mucous membrane pemphigoid involving extragingival mucosae, the ideal site is normal unaffected buccal mucosa. The biopsy is undertaken with 2% lidocaine and adrenaline and the wound closed with a 4/0 Vicryl Rapide suture, which does not need to be removed. The sample is sent for direct immunofluorescence. The main indications for referral to oral medicine for biopsy are indicated in Table 29.3.

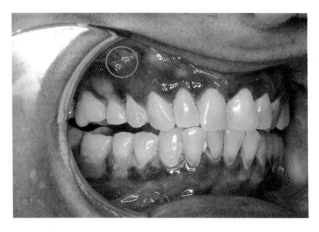

Figure 29.2 Optimal site to biopsy (green circle) in a patient with a suspected immunobullous disease (here with mucous membrane pemphigoid). Carey B *et al. Br J Dermatol* 2020; **182**:747–53.

Table 29.3 Main indications for referral to oral medicine or oral surgery for biopsy

Any lesion that is suspicious of malignancy or dysplasia
Any ulcer of unknown cause present for two weeks or longer
Any lesion failing to respond to treatment
Dry mouth and suspicion of Sjögren's syndrome
Any lesion on the lip: the risk of nerve damage and visible scarring requires experienced surgeons to operate on this site

Clinical presentations

Oral ulceration

The differential diagnosis for oral ulceration is broad, but after taking a detailed history this can be narrowed down considerably (Table 29.4). Generally, it is the severe recurrent (i.e. episodic) or widespread persistent oral ulceration subgroups that present to dermatology. However, examples of a single episode presenting more acutely, for example via accident and emergency and thus seen on call, are also discussed below.

Single episode

A single episode of oral ulceration is usually caused by an infection. The most common infection is primary herpes simplex (herpes gingivostomatitis), which manifests as widespread painful small 1–2-mm-sized yellow ulcers with prominent surrounding redness. This can affect any site in the mouth, including the gingivae and palate. It usually affects infants or young children, but can occasionally present in adulthood. It is associated with a fever. Other infections include Coxsackie (hand, foot and mouth disease), Epstein–Barr virus and varicella zoster.

Table 29.4 Presentations of oral ulceration

Single episode presents to general practitioner (GP), dentist or emergency unit

- Trauma: check for sharp tooth or dental restoration
- Infections: primary herpes simplex, varicella zoster, Coxsackie infections, syphilis (primary and secondary)
- Drug reaction: Stevens–Johnson syndrome or toxic epidermal necrolysis
- Erythema multiforme (usually secondary to infections such as herpes simplex)

Single persistent presents to GP or dentist

- Oral carcinoma: beware any unexplained ulcer, particularly on tongue or floor of mouth for > 2 weeks

Recurrent (but episodic, i.e. clears completely between attacks)

- Aphthous: major, minor and herpetiform
- Behçet's syndrome

Persistent widespread

- Autoimmune blistering diseases: pemphigus vulgaris, mucous membrane pemphigoid, epidermolysis bullosa acquisita, paraneoplastic pemphigus
- Ulcerative lichen planus and lupus erythematosus
- Inflammatory bowel disease, e.g. ulcerative colitis, Crohn's disease

(a)

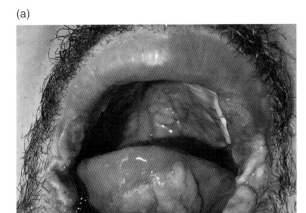

(b)

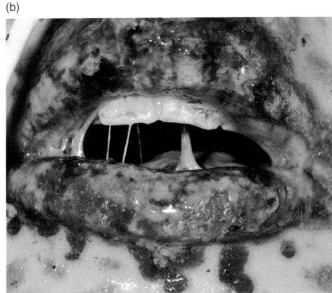

Figure 29.3 Examples of a single episode of oral ulceration. (a) Secondary syphilis with extensive mucous patches with a yellow–grey base in ulcerated areas and a serpiginous edge seen at the commissure of the lips. Thakrar P *et al.* Oral ulcers as a presentation of secondary syphilis. *Clin Exp Dermatol* 2018; **43**:868–75. (b) Stevens–Johnson syndrome/toxic epidermal necrolysis with severe exudative and erosive cheilitis is typical. Creamer D *et al.* U.K. guidelines for the management of Stevens–Johnson syndrome/toxic epidermal necrolysis in adults 2016. *Br J Dermatol* 2016; **174**:1194–227.

Where the maxillary division of the trigeminal nerve in varicella zoster is affected, unilateral ulceration of the left hard palate and left cheek is seen. Syphilis may present with a single episode of ulceration, as shown in Figure 29.3a.

A drug hypersensitivity reaction may result in severe oral ulceration and manifest as Stevens–Johnson syndrome (SJS) or toxic epidermal necrolysis (TEN) (Figure 29.3b). Rarely, less severe EM may present with a single episode of ulceration due to a drug hypersensitivity reaction. However, EM is most commonly associated with an infection such as herpes simplex or mycoplasma. It may be a single episode or recurrent (see below).

Single persistent ulcer

A single persistent ulcer lasting three weeks or more suggests a potential malignancy. It is often painless at the outset and may present late. The tissue is often firm with a raised everted margin. There is no explanation in the history for the lesion and no apparent dental cause, such as a sharp tooth or dental restoration. An urgent biopsy is mandatory through the maxillofacial or oral medicine team.

Recurrent oral ulceration

Aphthous ulcers are very common (Table 29.5 and Figure 29.4). In dermatology, patients may present with frequent episodes of recurrent oral aphthae such that there are almost continual ulcers, with or without genital ulcers. Ulcers may appear anywhere in the mouth, but have a predisposition for non-keratinised or keratinised mucosa depending upon the subtype. These may be associated with an underlying disorder such as cyclic neutropenia or inflammatory bowel disease, but they are more usually idiopathic. It is important to check haematinics and investigate as appropriate. Behçet's syndrome is a rare condition that may also show ocular and genital lesions. However, there is a group of patients who do not fulfil the criteria for Behçet's syndrome and are then given the diagnosis of 'complex aphthosis'.

Treatment is symptomatic relief with benzydamine mouthwash or spray, or topical anaesthetic gels. Avoidance of toothpastes containing sodium lauryl sulfate, and avoidance of acidic foods, chocolate and raw tomatoes, is also helpful.

Antiseptic mouthwashes (chlorhexidine 0.2%) and topical corticosteroids as a mouthwash (e.g. betamethasone 0.5 mg in 10 mL water or ointment) are also helpful. In more severe cases, colchicine 0.5 mg twice daily can be very effective. In Behçet's syndrome, patients have aphthous-like ulcers of all three morphologies, but additionally fulfil the criteria for this syndrome. Often immunosuppressive agents are required if colchicine does not control oral lesions.

Oral EM tends to affect the anterior part of the mouth, with painful, irregular, shallow ulcers involving the buccal mucosa and tongue and crusting of the lips (Figure 29.5). Other mucosal surfaces including ocular, nasal, pharyngeal, laryngeal, upper respiratory and anogenital regions may be involved. The gingivae tend to be spared. Target lesions can be found on the skin of the ears and chest, though the condition may be limited to the oral mucosa. Diagnosis is based on the history and clinical signs. Spontaneous healing of EM can be slow, taking 2–3 weeks in minor EM and up to 6 weeks in major EM. In severe cases, oral corticosteroids may be needed.

Table 29.5 Presentation and treatment of recurrent oral aphthae

Type	Approximate frequency	Age of onset	Characteristics	Treatment
Minor aphthae	> 80%	First decade	5–7 mm size	Betamethasone 0.5 mg in 10 mL water as three-minute rinse and spit twice daily
			1–5 ulcers	
			Last for 7–10 days	
			Grey with marked periulcer redness and inflammation (Figure 29.4)	Topical corticosteroids ointment ± Orabase (benzocaine) applied directly to dried mucosae
Major aphthae	< 10%	Second decade	Large, up to 2 cm	As above, but may require Flixonase nasules 400 µg in 10 mL water as a three-minute rinse and spit
			1–3 ulcers	
			Last for weeks	
			Punched-out ulcer	
			May heal with scarring	Prednisolone may be required
Herpetiform	10%	Third decade	Multiple small ulcers on non-keratinising mucosae	These typically respond to oral tetracycline mouthwashes, e.g. doxycycline 100 mg in 10 mL water as a three-minute rinse and spit four times daily
			Occur in crops that can merge	
			Resemble herpetic ulcers but *no* association (with herpes simplex virus infection)	

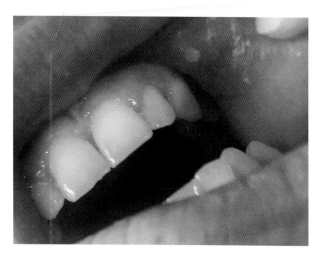

Figure 29.4 A minor aphthous ulcer demonstrating a white grey base and periulcer redness and inflammation. Courtesy Jane Setterfield.

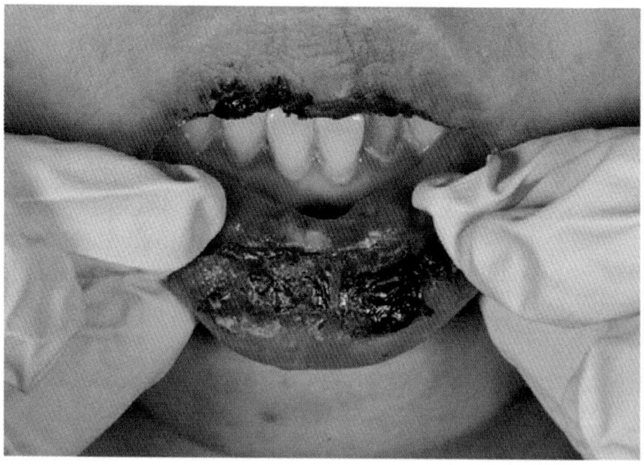

Figure 29.5 Recurrent erythema multiforme affecting the lips with sparing of the attached gingivae. Carey B, Setterfield J. *Clin Exp Dermatol* 2019; **44**:732–9.

Widespread persistent oral ulceration

This group of patients have associated disorders such as an autoimmune bullous disease (AIBD), LP (discussed under Oral white lesions) or a disorder associated with an underlying gastro-intestinal disease such as Crohn's disease (discussed under Cheilitis). The presentation and sites affected are detailed in Tables 29.6 and 29.7. While there is fluctuation in activity and severity, the ulcer location tends to be persistent, slowly remitting with treatment.

Table 29.6 Distinguishing features for autoimmune bullous disease

Condition	Oral features	Other features	Pathological features
Pemphigus vulgaris (PV)	Involves mouth in > 90% of cases (Figure 29.6). Persistent erosions and irregular ulcers seen: buccal mucosa > palatal > lingual > labial mucosa > gingivae. Scarring does not occur, but persistent depapillation of the tongue may follow ulceration	Other mucosal surfaces include conjunctiva, genitalia and upper respiratory tract. Skin lesions heal without scarring	Damage to desmosomes by predominantly IgG antibodies directed against Dsg3 and Dsg1. This leads to separation of the epithelium above the basal cell layer. Intraepithelial cleft with acantholytic cells
Paraneoplastic pemphigus (PNP)	May resemble PV, MMP, EM, GVHD or LP. Painful, severe, often recalcitrant oral ulceration. Typically hyperplastic lesions with prominent sloughing (Figure 29.7). Secondary infection frequent	Generalised polymorphous cutaneous eruption, pulmonary involvement. Frequently associated with lymphomas and haematological malignancies	Mixed pattern of intra-epidermal acantholytic bullae and keratinocyte apoptosis plus BMZ inflammation. Most common DIF features are deposition of IgG to keratinocyte cell surfaces and C3 to BMZ. Majority of patients have autoantibodies to periplakins and envoplakins
Mucous membrane pemphigoid (MMP)	Blisters leading to confluent areas of ulceration. May heal with scarring, though less frequent in mouth. Gingiva > buccal mucosa > palate > tongue > lip (Figure 29.8)	Other sites frequently scar. Second most frequent site is the conjunctiva (may affect vision), then nasopharynx, larynx, oesophagus. Skin (often face and scalp) and anogenital sites. May be generalised at outset and misdiagnosed as BP. Association with increased risk of malignancy in patients with laminin 332 antibodies	IgG and often IgA autoantibody binding predominantly to epitopes on BP180 (including NC16A domain) and laminin 332. Subepithelial separation with mixed inflammatory response. DIF: linear BMZ IgG and/or IgA. IIF: salt-split skin usually shows epidermal binding. Dermal binding may suggest laminin 332 subgroup
Bullous pemphigoid (BP)	Transient oral lesions in 10–20% of patients. Not usually associated with other mucosal sites. May affect buccal mucosa, palate, tongue or lips. In contrast to MMP, rarely affects gingivae. Lesions heal quickly. Persistence highly suggestive of MMP	A predominantly skin condition. When oral lesions persist in the context of a generalised blistering skin rash that resolves, the patient will have MMP. There can therefore be some early confusion as to the diagnosis	IgG binding to BP180 (NC16A) and BP230. Subepidermal split with eosinophil-rich inflammatory infiltrate. Rarely dermal binding, sera P200 pemphigoid (not a mucosal disease)
Epidermolysis bullosa acquisita (EBA)	Irregular ulceration anywhere in the oral mucosa including lips and tongue. Marginal gingival inflammation. Lesions often heal with scarring	Oesophagus often involved. Skin: BP type has widespread inflammatory skin lesions, or mechanobullous type with blisters on trauma-prone sites, e.g. elbows, knees, hands and feet	IgG ± IgA binding to the target antigen type VII collagen. Subepidermal separation. DIF demonstrates a dermal binding pattern with a U-serrated pattern
Linear IgA disease (LAD)	Ulcers or blisters on the tongue, palate or buccal mucosa and less frequent on the lips or gingivae	Skin lesions typically may be urticated plaques, erosions, or blisters arranged in a ring	IgA ± IgG binding to the LAD antigen (the shed ectodomain of BP180). Subepidermal separation with DIF demonstrating linear BMZ IgA ± IgG, C3. Histology typically shows a predominant neutrophilic infiltrate in the upper dermis. Neutrophilic microabscesses may be present in the papillary dermis

BMZ, basement membrane zone; DIF, direct immunofluorescence; Dsg, desmoglein; EM, erythema multiforme; GVHD, graft-versus-host disease; IIF, indirect immunofluorescence; LP, lichen planus.

Table 29.7 Diagnosis and management of autoimmune bullous disease

Condition	Diagnosis	Management
Pemphigus vulgaris (PV)	Biopsy with appropriate histopathological, DIF (intercellular fluorescence), IIF and ELISA (Dsg1, Dsg3)	Steroid mouthwashes in conjunction with systemic corticosteroids, and immunosuppressant adjuvants (azathioprine, mycophenolate mofetil, rituximab, IVIg)
Paraneoplastic pemphigus (PNP)	Biopsies for histopathology and DIF, IIF on rat bladder. May demonstrate additional lichenoid inflammation. Immunoblotting can demonstrate antibodies to Dsg3, desmoplakin 1, BP230, desmoplakin 2, envoplakin, plectin, periplakin, epiplakin	Best outcomes reported with benign neoplasms surgically excised or treatment of malignancy. First-line treatment is high-dose corticosteroids with the addition of steroid-sparing agents. Treatment failures managed with rituximab ± IVIg
Mucous membrane pemphigoid (MMP)	Mucosal disease + biopsy for histology, DIF, IIF. ELISA for BP180 NC16A (the most frequent target epitope), but additional sites on BP180 also targeted. Up to 25% of patients may demonstrate IgG and/or IgA to laminin 332 with a possible association with underlying malignancy. Consider screening	Steroid mouthwashes in conjunction with dapsone–sulfapyridine initially. Oral tetracyclines may be used in milder cases. Systemic corticosteroids and immunosuppressant adjuvants (azathioprine, mycophenolate mofetil, rituximab, IVIg) for severe cases
Bullous pemphigoid (BP)	Skin biopsy for histology, DIF, IIF. ELISA for NC16A, BP230	Treatment of BP is guided by degree of skin involvement. Mouth rarely problematic. Topical corticosteroid mouthwashes will suffice
Epidermolysis bullosa acquisita (EBA)	Combination of clinical, histological, DIF and serological investigations. Serology positive in 50% of sera. ELISA to detect antibodies against type VII collagen	Dapsone and immunosuppressive therapy similar to that described for MMP. May be recalcitrant to treatment
Linear IgA disease (LAD)	Clinical features with consistent histology and DIF. Indirect immunofluorescence may show circulating IgA anti-BMZ antibodies in 30–50% of cases. Immunoblotting studies may identify the 120 or 97 kDa antigens – shed ectodomain of BP180	Topical corticosteroids or sulfone drugs (dapsone) are first line, or sulfonamides (sulfapyridine) as second line are very effective

BMZ, basement membrane zone; DIF, direct immunofluorescence; Dsg, desmoglein; IIF, indirect immunofluorescence; IVIg, intravenous immunoglobulin.

Autoimmune blistering diseases

The distinguishing features for the AIBDs are detailed in Tables 29.6 and 29.7 and Figures 29.6–29.8. The main differential diagnoses to consider for oral immunobullous diseases are as follows:

- **Erythema multiforme** can look very similar to pemphigus vulgaris but is episodic (resolves in 2–4 weeks).
- **Angina bullosa haemorrhagica** presents as transient short-lived haemorrhagic bullae on any oral mucosal site, but often the buccal mucosa and palate. Blisters rupture in minutes and heal without scarring over a few days. This often affects those aged > 50 years. No underlying cause is identified and no treatment is required other than reassurance.
- **Bullous lichen planus** is a rare subtype of LP. Direct immunofluorescence is negative. Blisters only very occasionally present. Treatment is as for oral lichen planus.

Oral white lesions

Lichen planus

The most frequent oral disorder presenting to dermatology is oral LP, with a global prevalence of 0.5–2%. It typically presents between the fourth and seventh decades. The spectrum of clinical presentation is shown in Figure 29.9. It is a disorder of maturation of keratinocytes: where these are shed too early there is mucosal thinning associated with redness or ulceration, whereas delayed shedding results in striae, papules or plaques. The most frequent presentation is reticulated striae, seen in approximately 90% of patients and often overlapping with other features, such as atrophic LP in 44% of patients, plaque LP in 36%, papular LP in 11% and ulcerative LP in 9%.

There is a strong association with genital involvement and importantly the vulvovaginal gingival syndrome. This should be suspected in patients with generalised gingival inflammation and redness, as in Figure 29.9d. Early identification is important, as

(a)

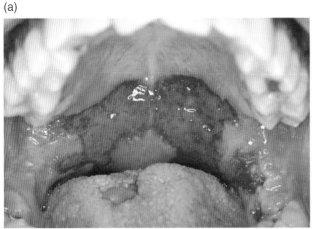

(b)

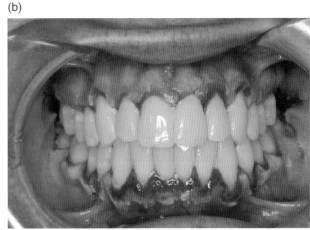

Figure 29.6 Pemphigus vulgaris. (a) Painful irregular erosion on the junction of the hard and soft palate. The lesions are red, indicating they are not 'full-thickness' ulcers. (b) Irregular ragged gingival erosions. Carey B, Setterfield J. *Clin Exp Dermatol* 2019; **44**:732–9.

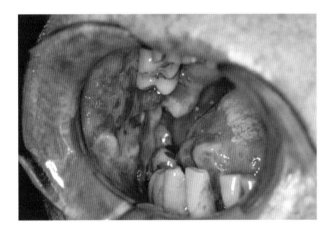

Figure 29.7 Paraneoplastic pemphigus demonstrating pansto-matitis with characteristic hyperplastic mucosae and prominent sloughing. Carey B, Setterfield J. *Clin Exp Dermatol* 2019; **44**:732–9.

this distinct subgroup has a propensity to scar mucosal sites resulting in significant morbidity, for example vulval and vaginal architectural changes and stenoses, oesophageal strictures and conduction deafness. Approximately 50% of this subgroup will require systemic therapy to reduce oral, ear or oesophageal activity. The vulvovaginal lesions are more easily controlled with topical corticosteroids.

The algorithm in Figure 29.10 outlines the management approaches for oral LP. In patients with asymptomatic reticular oral LP, follow-up under the patient's dentist is all that is required. Those with lichenoid changes only around large dental restorations should also be managed by their dentist and consider having the restoration changed. This does not apply to patients with bilateral, more generalised idiopathic oral LP, for whom dental restorations are highly unlikely to be relevant. In those with moderate or severely symptomatic, often ulcerative oral LP, a multidisciplinary

approach is recommended. Use of the validated ODSS is highly recommended for patients being managed systemically.

Risk of malignant change in oral lichen planus

Careful monitoring for potential malignant change is required, particularly in patients on immunosuppressives. The overall life-time risk is approximately 1%. Figure 29.11 shows a patient on long-term mycophenolate mofetil for ulcerative colitis who began to show proliferative verrucous change on the gingivae. This was biopsied in several sites and treated with laser therapy. The patient remains under close follow-up.

Leukoplakia

The term 'leukoplakia' comes from the Greek 'white plaque'. However, it should only be applied to those white patches without a clear diagnosis. Any patient with a white lesion of uncertain aetiology should be referred to oral medicine for an opinion and biopsy. If a biopsy shows frictional hyperkeratosis, for example due to a rough cusp on a tooth or restoration, or is plaque LP, it is not considered to be leukoplakia. Those white patches without a clear cause may have an increased risk of being dysplastic on histology and must be referred. Where lesions are mixed with redness (eryth-roleukoplakia), the risk of malignant change increases further.

Lupus erythematosus

Discoid lupus erythematosus can present in the oral mucosa and may be difficult or impossible to differentiate from oral LP. It may have a more focal distribution, typically in the buccal mucosa or tongue, and may have a characteristic brush border with white striae radiating from the margin in a sunray pattern. Often lesions are relatively asymptomatic, and treatment is usually with topical corticosteroids, or if widespread and more symptomatic with hydroxychloroquine.

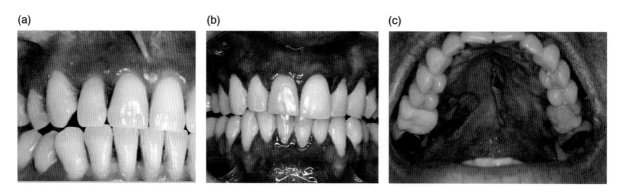

Figure 29.8 Mucous membrane pemphigoid demonstrating (a) mild gingival redness and inflammation, (b) desquamative gingivitis and (c) ulceration on the palatal gingivae and hard palate. Ormond M *et al. Br J Dermatol* 2020; **183**:78–85.

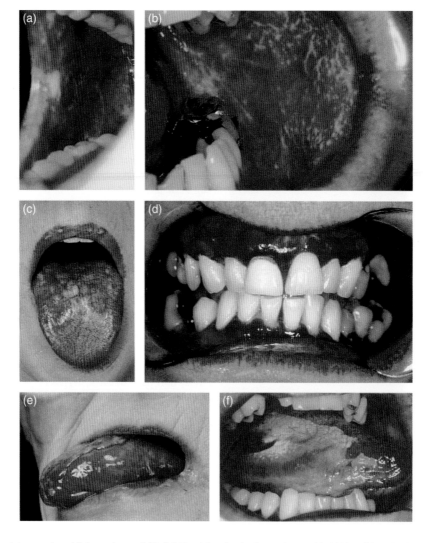

Figure 29.9 Clinical subtypes of oral lichen planus (LP). (a) Combined reticular and atrophic LP involving the buccal mucosa. (b) Combined reticulopapular LP involving the buccal mucosa. (c) Hemilunar depapillation of the lateral borders of the tongue with sparing of the lingual tip. (d) Desquamative gingivitis. (e) Ulcerative LP involving the lateral border of the tongue. (f) Dysplastic mucosa at high risk of neoplastic transformation in association with plaque-type oral LP. Setterfield JF *et al.* The management of oral lichen planus. *Clin Exp Dermatol* 2000; **25**:176–82.

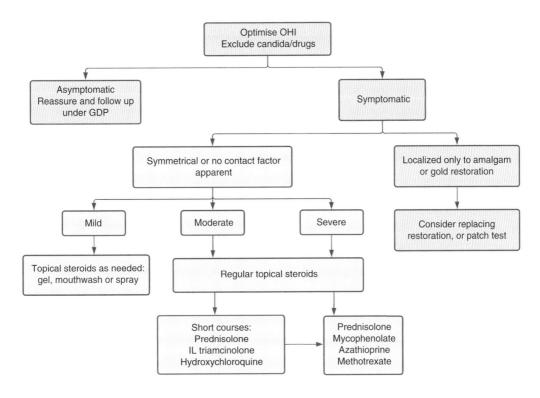

Figure 29.10 The management of oral lichen planus. GDP, general dental practitioner; IL, intralesional; OHI, oral hygiene instructions.

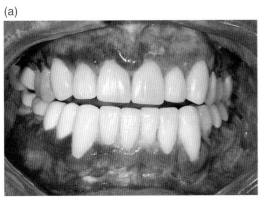

(a)

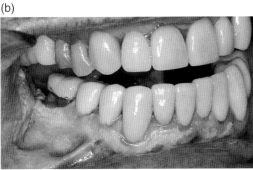

(b)

Figure 29.11 (a) Generalised desquamative gingivitis in a patient with vulvovaginal gingival lichen planus. (b) The patient has developed verrucous leukoplakia with a high risk of malignant change. Courtesy Jane Setterfield.

Cheilitis

Table 29.8 summarises the main causes of cheilitis (Figures 29.12–29.14). As the lips are richly innervated, inflammation is associated with considerable morbidity. The psychological impact is also very considerable and management of these conditions must be considered alongside psychological support.

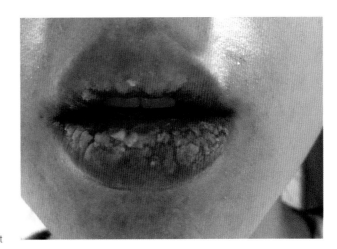

Figure 29.12 Exfoliative cheilitis showing characteristic peeling, fissuring and crusting. Courtesy Jane Setterfield.

Table 29.8 Cheilitis: clinical features and investigation

Diagnosis	Clinical features	Investigation	Treatment
Exfoliative cheilitis (Figure 29.12)	Female > male 2:1	Lip and nose swabs: approximately 70% of patients will have candida and/or *Staphylococcus aureus*	Treat infection
	Peeling and cracking of lips	Patch test	Oral antiseptics
	Associated with atopic predisposition in two-thirds of patients	No biopsy required	Light balm – *as little as possible*
	Associated with mental health disorder in approximately 40%		Tacrolimus 0.1% twice daily for six weeks and then ongoing as needed
	Concurrent infection in 70%		Psychological help
	Lip-licking habit in some		
Angular cheilitis	Redness, fissuring and pain at commissures	MC&S swab	Dependent upon swab result
	Inspect for intraoral candida	FBC, ferritin	Fucidin® H
	Check for xerostomia, which typically predisposes to candidosis	Remove dental appliances and check for candida on underlying mucosae	Nystatin oral suspension as a mouth rinse and swallow, if candida cultured
Lichenoid (oral LP, DLE)	LP cheilitis has a characteristic violaceous hue, but is not always present with other intraoral LP	Biopsy	Tacrolimus 0.1% twice daily for six weeks and as needed
		Lip swab	Sun protection
Actinic cheilitis (Figure 29.13)	Pre-malignant lesion		Sun protection. Laser therapy, 5-fluorouracil or 5% imiquimod
	Lower lip in men > 50 years		
	95% of lip SCC originates from actinic cheilitis		
	10–30% develop SCC		
Orofacial granulomatosis (Figure 29.14)	Initially intermittent swelling, then acute on chronic swelling of lips	Oral biopsy (by oral medicine specialist)	Treat infection ± topical corticosteroids, tacrolimus 0.1%
	May have buccal granulomatous inflammation resulting in 'cobblestone' appearance, sublingual rugae prominence, gingival swelling	Diet record	IL triamcinolone
	If underlying Crohn's, more likely to have fissuring or ulcers in sulci and more prominent intraoral swelling	Patch test	Cinnamon- and benzoate-free diet. May require systemic therapy
		Lip swab	
		May require GI investigations for Crohn's, or CXR and serum ACE if suspect sarcoidosis	

ACE, angiotensin-converting enzyme; CXR, chest X-ray; DLE, discoid lupus erythematosus; FBC, full blood count; GI, gastrointestinal; IL, intralesional; LP, lichen planus; MC&S, microscopy, culture and sensitivity; SCC, squamous cell carcinoma.
Fucidin®, LEO Laboratories, Hurley, UK.

(a)

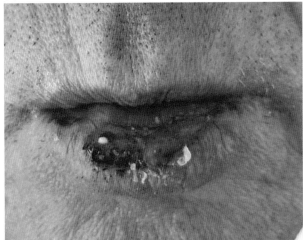

(b)

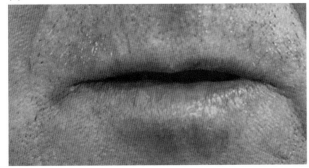

Patients may frequently develop unhelpful habits, which need to be recognised and modified, for example lip licking, peeling or picking. Similarly, allowing infected crusts to form and remain on the lips for days or weeks is unhelpful. Gentle removal of the crust following a shower each morning is advisable, which then allows treatment to reach the underlying skin.

Other oral problems

It is not within the remit of this chapter to discuss all presentations of oral disorders in detail. However, there remain four broad groups of presentations that dermatologists need to be aware of, and these are summarised in Table 29.9. Oral pain or stomatodynia may have subtle causes that are not immediately visible. These include candida, erythema migrans (geographic tongue), drug reactions and oral dysaesthesia, also known as burning mouth syndrome. Key features, investigations and therapeutic approaches are summarised in Table 29.9.

Oral dryness is poorly tolerated. Drugs are the commonest cause, but a small proportion of patients will have Sjögren's syndrome, and referral to oral medicine may be required. Mucosal lumps and swellings are generally referred to oral medicine for investigation and treatment. Pigmentation on the lips often presents to dermatologists and may require a small biopsy if this is of uncertain aetiology. Intraoral widespread pigmentation is usually genetic or post-inflammatory. In the case of any focal melanocytic pigmentation, particularly if new, it may be prudent to refer to oral medicine.

Figure 29.13 Actinic cheilitis. (a) Before treatment: a violaceous hue. Predominantly lower-lip peeling and blistering. (b) Two weeks after the second course of 5-fluorouracil. Courtesy Jane Setterfield.

(a)

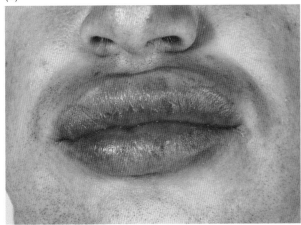

(b)

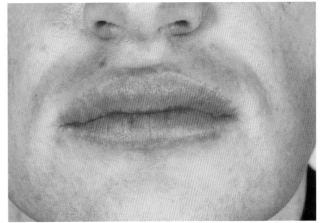

Figure 29.14 Orofacial granulomatosis. (a) Bilateral soft fluctuating swelling of the lips with mild peeling. Chaudhry SI *et al.* A swollen lip. *Clin Exp Dermatol* 2006; **31**:161–2. (b) Orofacial granulomatosis after six weeks of a cinnamon- and benzoate-free diet. Courtesy Jane Setterfield.

Table 29.9 Other oral problems

Clinical presentation	Causes	Clinical features	Investigation and treatment
Painful mouth	Candida	• Pain, burning • Predisposing factors include corticosteroid mouthwashes, dry mouth or diabetes, and dentures	• Saliva or oral swab • Treat dry mouth • May require long-term intermittent treatment with nystatin and/or fluconazole
	Oral dysaesthesia	• Burning, numbness, altered taste • Often worse as the day goes by • Fluctuates in severity • More frequent in females and in fifth decade	• Exclude diabetes, candida, haematinic deficiency and parafunctional habits, e.g. night-time teeth grinding and clenching • Counselling or cognitive behaviour therapy • Refer for treatment of anxiety and depression if appropriate • May require low-dose antidepressant treatment • Clonazepam (short term) 0.5 mg once or twice per day (two-minute suck and spit)
	Erythema migrans (geographic tongue)	• Often asymptomatic but may be painful at times, e.g. stress • Characteristic areas on dorsum tongue with thinning of the filiform papillae in the centre of the lesion and a whitish border • Typically moves over a few days • Several areas may be visible at once	• FBC, and if anaemic check ferritin, B_{12}, folate • Swab to exclude candida • Symptomatic treatment only, e.g. benzydamine hydrochloride 0.15% mouthwash
Dry mouth	Drugs	• Oral dryness (<2 mL in 10 min) • Sticky saliva • Fissured or papillated dorsum tongue • Candida	• Consider which drugs may be causative, e.g. diuretics, antihistamines, antihypertensives, anticholinergics, antidepressants, omeprazole • Discontinue if possible
	Sjögren's syndrome	As above, but potentially dry eyes and systemic features of Sjögren's syndrome	• Rheumatoid factor, ENA (Ro, La) • Labial minor salivary gland biopsy • USS salivary glands • Saliva substitutes. • Systemic treatment (after MDT)

Table 29.9 (Continued)

Clinical presentation	Causes	Clinical features	Investigation and treatment
Mucosal lumps and bumps	Fibroepithelial polyps	Common, painless, smooth firm swellings on trauma-prone sites, e.g. buccal mucosa, lip, tongue	Shave removal/excisional biopsy
	Viral warts	• Filiform lesions seen in any part of the mouth • Associated with oropharyngeal carcinoma with high-risk subtypes, e.g. HPV 16, 18, 31, 33, 45, 52, 58	Cryotherapy
	Mucocoeles	Painless translucent swelling of minor salivary glands usually within lower lip	Cryotherapy or excision. However, risk of recurrence or damage to adjacent salivary glands and ducts
Pigmentation	Natural pigmentation	• Usually fairly symmetrical brown mottled pigmentation seen on gingivae, tongue, palate, buccal mucosa and lips • Often first noticed in adulthood in patients with skin of colour	None
	Post-inflammatory	Frequent cause of focal pigmentation, e.g. following lichen planus or areas of ulceration	None
	Amalgam tattoos	Blue/grey pigmented lesion adjacent to large amalgam restoration or crown	None if clinically certain. Radiograph helpful. Excision biopsy if in doubt
	Melanotic macules	Common on lips, particularly lower lip due to sun exposure. Flat, usually small < 1 cm	Observation or photography, biopsy may be indicated if increasing in size or pigmentation
	Melanocytic naevi	Uncommon well-defined brown lesions	Excisional biopsy

ENA, extractable nuclear antigen; FBC, full blood count; HPV, human papillomavirus; MDT, multidisciplinary team; USS, ultrasound scan.

Conclusions

Oral mucosal disorders can be challenging for the dermatologist, as there is very little opportunity to have supervised training in examination of the mouth or time to acquire a thorough grasp of the wide variation in the normal oral mucosa. Thereafter it takes considerable practice to recognise the key clinical features of the main disorders presenting in dermatology clinics. The potential to miss diagnoses is therefore considerable, and having a low threshold for multidisciplinary discussions and cross-referrals is essential. In general, oral medicine will be the main team to refer to, and if oral cancer is diagnosed then patients will be referred to oral surgery teams for further management.

Pearls and pitfalls

- Beware of the single ulcer present for more than three weeks without a clear cause: this needs referral for biopsy.
- If symptoms of pain or burning persist despite objective clinical improvement, consider candida and do a swab.
- Always palpate areas of the mouth that are white or nodular, and refer if firm or gritty for urgent biopsy.
- In lichen planus, treatment is aimed at symptom relief as the clinical signs may be long lasting.
- In patients with immunobullous disease or ulcerative lichen planus, ensure that you include clinical outcome measures to document objective improvement.

SCE Questions. See questions 33–35.

FURTHER READING AND KEY RESOURCES

Carey B, Joshi S, Abdelghani A *et al*. The optimal oral biopsy site for diagnosis of mucous membrane pemphigoid and pemphigus vulgaris. *Br J Dermatol* 2020; **182**:747–53.

Carey B, Setterfield J. Mucous membrane pemphigoid and oral blistering diseases. *Clin Exp Dermatol* 2019; **44**:732–9.

Hullah EA, Escudier M. The mouth in inflammatory bowel disease and aspects of orofacial granulomatosis. *Periodontol 2000* 2019; **80**:61–76.

Lai M, Pampena R, Cornacchia L *et al*. Treatments of actinic cheilitis: a systematic review of the literature. *J Am Acad Dermatol* 2020; **83**:876–87.

Ni Riordain R, McCreary C. Validity and reliability of a newly developed quality of life questionnaire for patients with chronic oral mucosal diseases. *J Oral Pathol Med* 2011; **40**:604–9.

Ormond M, McParland H, Thakrar P *et al*. Validation of an Oral Disease Severity Score (ODSS) tool for use in oral mucous membrane pemphigoid. *Br J Dermatol* 2020; **183**:78–85.

Scully C. Dermatoses of the oral cavity and lips. In: *Rook's Textbook of Dermatology* (Griffiths C, Barker J, Bleiker T, Chalmers R, Creamer D eds), 9th edn. Hoboken, NJ: Wiley, 2016; Chapter 110.

Textbook

Lewis MAO, Jordan RCK. *A Colour Handbook of Oral Medicine*, 2nd edn. Boca Raton, FL: CRC Press, 2012.

Useful website

e-Learning for Healthcare. E-Derm 12 – Oral Medicine. Available at: https://portal.e-lfh.org.uk/Catalogue/Index?HierarchyId=0_37&programmeId=37.

Key resources and websites

Textbooks

Griffiths CEM, Barker JN, Bleiker TO, Hussain W, Simpson RC, eds. *Rook's Textbook of Dermatology*, 10th edn. Oxford: Wiley-Blackwell, 2022; in press.

Bolognia JL, Shaffer J, Cerroni L, eds. *Dermatology*, 4th edn. Amsterdam: Elsevier, 2017.

Griffiths CEM, Bleiker TO, Creamer D, Ingram JR, Simpson RC, eds. *Rook's Dermatology Handbook*. Oxford: Wiley-Blackwell, 2021.

Lebwohl M, Heymann W, Coulson I, Murrell D, eds. *Treatment of Skin Disease: Comprehensive Therapeutic Strategies*, 6th edn. Amsterdam: Elsevier, 2021.

Wakelin SH, Maibach HI, Archer CB. *Handbook of Systemic Drug Treatment in Dermatology*, 3rd edn. Boca Raton, FL: CRC Press, 2021.

Alwan W, Banerjee P, eds. *Dermatology Handbook for Registrars*. London: British Association of Dermatologists, 2020. Available at: https://www.bad.org.uk/shared/get-file.ashx?itemtype=document&id=6850.

Websites

British Association of Dermatologists. Available at: www.bad.org.uk.

British Association of Dermatologists. Patient information leaflets. Available at: https://www.bad.org.uk/patient-information-leaflets.

American Academy of Dermatology. Clinical guidelines. Available at: https://www.aad.org/member/clinical-quality/guidelines.

British National Formulary and *British National Formulary for Children*. Available at: www.bnf.org.

DermNet NZ. Available at: www.dermnet.nz.

e-Learning for Healthcare. e-dermatology. Available at: https://www.e-lfh.org.uk/programmes/dermatology. Modules are being updated in 2021–22 and new modules are being developed to complement the new curriculum, such as for teledermatology and dermoscopy.

Electronic Medicines Compendium. Available at: https://www.medicines.org.uk/emc.

European Academy of Dermatology and Venereology. Available at: www.eadv.org.

Joint Royal Colleges of Physicians Training Board (JRCPTB). Dermatology. Available at: https://www.jrcptb.org.uk/specialties/dermatology.

JRCPTB. Dermatology Syllabus Guidance. August 2021. Available at: https://www.jrcptb.org.uk/sites/default/files/Dermatology%20syllabus%20guidance%20August%202021.pdf.

JRCPTB. Dermatology Training Curriculum. Available at: https://www.jrcptb.org.uk/sites/default/files/Dermatology%202021%20Curriculum%20FINAL.pdf.

British College of Dermatology Accredited Courses

These courses are developed by experienced multiprofessional teams to deliver education based on the current training syllabus and curriculum. They are approved by the British College of Dermatology (BAD Education Board) and comply with the College's quality assurance processes.

Dermatology Training: The Essentials. Edited by Mahbub M.U. Chowdhury, Tamara W. Griffiths and Andrew Y. Finlay.
© 2022 The British Association of Dermatologists. Published 2022 by John Wiley & Sons Ltd.
Companion website: www.wiley.com/go/chowdhury/dermatologytraining

Specialty Certificate Exam (SCE): questions

Question 1

A 2-year-old child presents with a generalised red, itchy rash. On examination there is evidence of scaling and lichenification. There is hyperlinearity of the palms in the child and the parents, and a family history of atopy. You suspect the child could be predisposed to atopic dermatitis from a filaggrin mutation.

In which layer of the epidermis is profilaggrin, the precursor of filaggrin, produced?

A Stratum basale
B Stratum corneum
C Stratum granulosum
D Stratum lucidum
E Stratum spinosum

Question 2

A 55-year-old woman presents with frontal hair loss, eyebrow loss, yellow facial papules and temporal skin atrophy. You suspect a diagnosis of frontal fibrosing alopecia. The patient enquires about the chances of restoring the lost hair. You explain that the best treatment response will be prevention of further hair loss, as with the scarring hair loss the hair follicles cannot regenerate.

The regeneration of hair follicles is dependent on stem cells located in which part of the hair follicle?

A Dermal papilla
B Dermal sheath
C Hair bulge
D Hair matrix
E Inner root sheath

Question 3

A 68-year-old woman presented with a 24-hour history of feeling generally unwell, fever and an evolving rash. On examination she had small monomorphic pustules that started on her axillae and chest. She was previously fit and well, except for a diagnosis of gout for which her general practitioner had recently commenced allopurinol. A skin biopsy showed intra-epidermal pustules, focal keratinocyte necrosis and eosinophils within the pustules and/or dermis.

What is the most likely diagnosis?

A Acute generalised exanthematous pustulosis
B Folliculitis
C Impetigo
D Pustular psoriasis
E Subcorneal pustular dermatosis

Question 4

A 70-year-old previously well woman presented with a 2-day history of an evolving rash. This rash had started with some flaccid blisters, leading to erosions in the groins, extending to the medial thighs and abdominal wall (see figures). She also complained of soreness of the lips and buccal mucosa. A skin biopsy showed supra-basal acantholysis on routine haematoxylin and eosin staining and a net-like pattern of cell-surface-bound IgG in the epidermis on direct immunofluorescence.

What is the most likely diagnosis?

A Epidermolysis bullosa acquisita
B Pemphigus foliaceus
C Pemphigus vulgaris
D Stevens–Johnson syndrome
E Toxic epidermal necrolysis

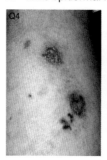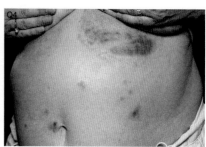

Dermatology Training: The Essentials. Edited by Mahbub M.U. Chowdhury, Tamara W. Griffiths and Andrew Y. Finlay.
© 2022 The British Association of Dermatologists. Published 2022 by John Wiley & Sons Ltd.
Companion website: www.wiley.com/go/chowdhury/dermatologytraining

Question 5

A research fellow wishes to conduct a randomised controlled trial to study psoriasis.

Which one of the following techniques is not helpful to reduce bias?

A Blinding of study personnel to the intervention allocated to participants

B Inclusion and exclusion criteria that reflect routine clinical practice

C Intention-to-treat analysis

D Randomisation

E Selective reporting of favourable outcomes

Question 6

A medical student is planning to start a clinical audit in their local department.

Which of the following is not necessary?

A Applying for ethical permission

B Defining standards for key aspects

C Designing a questionnaire for data collection

D Planning to repeat the clinical audit

E Presenting the results to colleagues

Question 7

The Mental Capacity Act states that any decision made on behalf of a person who lacks capacity must be made in their 'best interest'.

What is the definition of 'best interest'?

A Decision is made by a formal independent advocate who is trained to identify the best possible outcome for that patient

B Decision is made by a group of healthcare professionals on behalf of the patient

C Decision is made using information on what the person would have wanted (previously stated wishes or values) and on the thoughts of those who know them well

D Decision is what the next of kin feels is best for the patient

E Decision made on behalf of the person is believed to be the best possible decision in that situation

Question 8

A new trainee attended a medicolegal training session on negligence.

Which is essential in the three-part test to establish negligence?

A Claimant must have undergone a procedure for duty of care to be established

B Claimant suffered harm as a consequence of a breach of duty

C Defendant breached the duty of candour

D Defendant was contractually bound to provide long-term treatment without causing injury to the claimant

E Informed consent was obtained

Question 9

A research nurse wishes to calculate the Psoriasis Area and Severity Index (PASI) in a patient about to start biologic therapy.

Which one of the following is required to calculate PASI?

A Colour of flexural involvement

B Degree of redness in four areas

C Degree of scratch marks

D Percentage area of involvement of the face

E Severity of soreness

Question 10

A medical student was considering using the Dermatology Life Quality Index (DLQI) for an audit project on patients with psoriasis in the outpatients clinic.

Which aspect of daily life is asked about in the DLQI?

A Impact on appetite

B Impact on partner's life

C Impact on sex life

D Impact on sleep

E Impact on walking

Question 11

A 30-year-old woman presents with a recent-onset red facial rash (see figures).

Which clinical feature would help to confirm a diagnosis of rosacea?

A Absence of comedones

B Exacerbation by sunlight

C Greasy scale on eyebrows and nasolabial folds

D Improvement with moderate-potency topical steroid

E Red papules and pustules over the cheeks

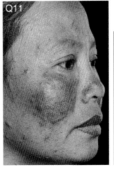
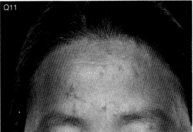

Question 12

A 45-year-old man is seen in outpatients with a 3-month history of a worsening red rash with scaling. There is a history of chronic plaque psoriasis with joint problems. The rash has spread from the elbows and knees to involve widespread confluent areas of the trunk and limbs. He is shivering and pyrexial. Close examination reveals 1-mm pustules in some areas.

What is the most likely cause for the recent deterioration?

A Change in antihypertensive medication from beta blocker to amlodipine
B Recent bereavement
C Recent streptococcal throat infection
D Weight loss resulting from recent deliberate dieting
E Withdrawal of long-term oral steroids given for arthritis

Question 13

A 24-year-old woman presented with a 6-month history of an intensely itchy rash on the labia majora, which regularly kept her awake at night. Examination revealed thick, pale white plaques of lichenified skin with otherwise normal vulval architecture. No inflammation or erosions were noted.
What is the most likely diagnosis?

A Folliculitis
B Fungal infection
C Lichen planus
D Lichen simplex chronicus
E Vaginal intra-epithelial neoplasia

Question 14

A 60-year-old woman presented with a 2-year history of an intermittent sore, itchy genital rash that had not responded to repeated mild topical and oral anti-yeast therapy. Examination revealed well-demarcated, confluent, glazed red plaques over the mons and labia majora, extending to the perineum and natal fold. There was fissuring of the plaques in the natal fold.
What is the most likely diagnosis?

A Atopic dermatitis
B Chronic vulvovaginal candidiasis
C Lichen sclerosus
D Psoriasis
E Vaginal intra-epithelial neoplasia

Question 15

A 47-year-old man presented with a 6-month history of a rash on his glans penis and dyspareunia. Examination revealed red, moist plaques on the glans and atrophic scarring of the frenulum.
What is the best initial management?

A Clobetasol propionate ointment
B Oral plus topical antibiotics
C Oral plus topical antifungal agents
D Referral to urology for circumcision
E Topical vitamin D analogue

Question 16

An 81-year-old man presented with a 3-year history of a red plaque on the glans penis. He had received multiple courses of antibiotics and antifungal agents with no benefit. Six weeks of a potent topical steroid had reduced the redness. Examination revealed a 9-mm-diameter moist, raised plaque on the dorsal aspect of the glans penis. There was some tightness of the foreskin. A skin swab grew coliform bacteria.
What is the most likely diagnosis?

A Lichen planus
B Lichen sclerosus
C Penile intra-epithelial neoplasia
D Psoriasis
E Zoon's balanitis

Question 17

An 80-year-old woman was referred to the dermatology clinic with lower-limb swelling of uncertain duration. She had no respiratory signs or symptoms.
Which of the following is least likely to be the cause for her limb swelling?

A Pharmacological causes such as amlodipine
B Primary lymphoedema
C Recurrent gynaecological malignancy
D Sarcoidosis
E Venous disease

Question 18

A 36-year-old woman presented with a history of a long-standing pigmented mole on her back that had recently become larger and darker. On examination the mole was irregular, with colour variation (see figure). It was surgically excised with a 2-mm margin. Histology showed a fully excised malignant melanoma, with Breslow thickness of 0.9 mm.
What would be your next step in management?

A No further treatment is required
B Sentinel lymph node biopsy and wide local excision with a 1-cm margin
C Sentinel lymph node biopsy and wide local excision with an 8-mm margin
D Wide local excision with a 1-cm margin without sentinel lymph node biopsy
E Wide local excision with an 8-mm margin without sentinel lymph node biopsy

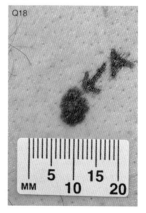

Question 19

An 88-year-old patient with a history of diabetes and ischaemic heart disease presented with a 2-year history of a slow-growing lesion on his leg. On examination he had a 2 × 2-cm flat, scaly, reddish lesion with a shiny rolled border. Histology shows multifocal nests of atypical basaloid cells arising as pods from the basal layer of the epidermis. The nests are confined to the papillary dermis.

What should be your initial management approach?

A   Cryotherapy
B   Curettage and cautery
C   Excision with 4-mm margin
D   Fluorouracil 5% cream
E   Imiquimod 5% cream

Question 20

A 67-year-old man presented with a 6-week history of a rapidly growing tender lesion on his scalp. On examination, there was a 1.5 × 1.5-cm nodular lesion with central ulceration and a red base. Histology shows a moderately differentiated squamous cell carcinoma, with 4.2-mm thickness and invasion into the dermis.

Which feature is considered high risk?

A   Invasion into the dermis
B   Moderately differentiated histology
C   Site of lesion on scalp
D   Tumour size > 1 cm
E   Tumour thickness of 4.2 mm

Question 21

A 35-year-old scientist with metastatic melanoma has been discussed at the local multidisciplinary team clinic. The decision has been made to treat her with nivolumab. She wishes to know how this drug works.

What is the mechanism of action of nivolumab?

A   Anti-CTLA-4 protein receptor monoclonal antibody
B   Anti-programmed cell death protein-1 receptor protein
C   Anti-tumour necrosis factor monoclonal antibody
D   BRAF protein inhibitor
E   Mitogen-activated protein kinase inhibitor

Question 22

A 45-year-old woman of Italian descent presents with a 12-month history of very itchy small blisters on the extensor surface of her elbows and knees. She has had some diarrhoea in the last 6 months and is awaiting endoscopy to investigate this further. You are considering starting dapsone immediately.

What blood test do you need to do prior to starting dapsone in this woman?

A   Dipyrimidine dehydrogenase (DPD)
B   Gamma-glutamyl transferase (GGT)
C   Glucose-6-phosphate dehydrogenase (G6PD)
D   Procollagen 3 peptide (P3NP)
E   Thiopurine methyltransferase (TPMT)

Question 23

A 45-year-old man who worked as a research scientist was due to start oral methotrexate for his psoriasis affecting 15% of his body surface area. He was concerned about liver problems.

How often do serum procollagen 3 peptide (P3NP) levels need to be tested?

A   Every six months
B   Every three months
C   Every two months
D   Once a month
E   Once a week

Question 24

A 12-year-old boy with atopic eczema attends clinic with his parents. The parents were extremely anxious about the treatments and expressed concerns about being able to treat him at home with the topical corticosteroid and emollients prescribed.

What is the best initial step to improve their adherence to topical therapy?

A   Explain how many times to apply the creams
B   Explain how much of the creams to apply per week
C   Refer to specialist nurses for advice
D   Write down clear detailed instructions for the parents
E   Write to their general practitioner with a detailed treatment plan

Question 25

A 32-year-old woman was attending the outpatient clinic, originally with psoriasis on her face. She had been using a potent topical corticosteroid on the face for 6 months to control the psoriasis. On examination, she had a few inflamed papules and pustules around her mouth.

What is the best initial treatment to improve her skin condition?

A   Hydrocortisone 1% cream
B   Metronidazole 0.75% cream
C   Pimecrolimus 1% cream
D   Tacrolimus 0.03% ointment
E   Tacrolimus 0.1% ointment

Question 26

A 35-year-old healthcare worker (HCW) is referred from the occupational health department with suspected immediate (type 1) latex allergy.

Which finding in your detailed history is most likely to indicate that this HCW needs to have further testing?

A   Eats bananas without any symptoms
B   Itching on hands after wearing nitrile gloves
C   Noticed lip swelling after eating apples
D   Noticed lip swelling when blowing up balloons
E   Wears gloves for 1 hour daily

Question 27

A 54-year-old man has been referred to the patch test clinic by his general practitioner to confirm possible glove allergy (see figure below). He has worked as a cleaner for 10 years. On examination, there is well-defined redness and scaling on the dorsum of both hands.

Which allergen is most likely to be the cause of his glove contact allergy?

A Linalool
B Methylisothiazolinone
C Paraben mix
D Sesquiterpene lactone mix
E Thiuram mix

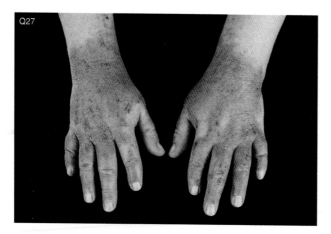

Question 28

A 45-year-old male nurse, working on the infectious disease ward, has been referred to you from the occupational health department. He thinks his surgical facial mask worn for eight hours daily has been causing moderate acne-like changes with papules and pustules on his cheeks and chin. He has experienced intermittent mild acne since his teenage years.

What is the best initial treatment for three months for his facial acne?

A Benzoyl peroxide gel
B Doxycycline orally
C Isotretinoin orally
D Metronidazole gel
E Trimethoprim orally

Question 29

A 25-year-old woman is suspected to have irritant contact dermatitis of her hands (see two figures in next column). She is on maternity leave, has two young children and works part time as a hairdresser.

What clinical finding is most likely to support the diagnosis of contact allergy in this woman?

A Dermatitis in the web spaces
B Dermatitis under her rings
C Does not wear gloves when hairdressing
D Does not wear gloves when washing dishes
E Vesicles on her fingers

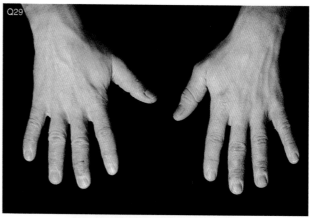

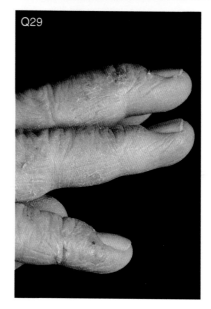

Question 30

A 48-year-old man presents with suspected contact allergy to one of his cosmetic products. You arrange patch testing to the baseline and facial (cosmetic) series and his own products to detect other potential allergies.

Which allergen is found in the British Society for Cutaneous Allergy (BSCA) facial (cosmetic) series and may be the relevant cause of his contact allergy?

A Balsam of Peru (*Myroxylon pereirae*)
B Methylisothiazolinone
C Sodium metabisulfite
D Tixocortol pivalate
E Tocopherol acetate

Question 31

A 64-year-old woman attends your surgical list for excision of a 10-mm, well-defined, infiltrative basal cell carcinoma (BCC) on her left temple. She has previously had surgery for a similar but smaller BCC on her right temple, which healed with a hypertrophic scar that causes her significant upset.

What is the most appropriate statement regarding her planned procedure?

A High risk of damage to the temporal branch of the facial nerve with any surgical procedure on the temple, resulting in ipsilateral eyebrow ptosis

B Hypertrophic scar risk bilaterally is negligible and therefore the only risks that need to be discussed are infection, bleeding and incomplete tumour excision

C Inability to raise the eyebrow immediately after the procedure indicates you have negligently damaged the facial nerve intra-operatively

D She can drive herself home after the procedure

E Surgery is the only effective option to treat her skin cancer so she must accept all the risks

Question 32

A 48-year-old lawyer presented to clinic with a small but rapidly growing lesion on his right forearm. Your colleague who saw him in clinic diagnosed a likely squamous cell carcinoma (SCC) and listed him for surgical excision. The patient presents on your theatre list 2 weeks later, but you note that the lesion has grown in that time. Even though you are confident in removing the lesion, you establish that by the time you have excised the lesion with an appropriate margin it will create a large defect that you do not feel comfortable repairing. The patient tells you he is very busy and needs to get back to work, and that he wants you just to get on with it, otherwise he will consider making a formal complaint. You happen to be the only person in the department operating that day, with no senior support due to staff illness.

What is the most appropriate course of action?

A Defer any surgical intervention and refer the patient for radiotherapy

B Discuss the situation with the patient, document everything clearly in the notes and do not proceed, but arrange an urgent senior review

C Even though the diagnosis of an SCC is very likely, you explain and do a diagnostic biopsy instead

D Go ahead with the procedure as it is the patient's choice and you do not want a complaint

E You think this represents the perfect opportunity to perform your first full-thickness skin graft repair, as you attended a surgical course recently

Question 33

A 42-year-old man was referred by his general practitioner with an itchy skin condition. On examination, he had symmetrical reticulated striae on his oral mucosal surfaces consistent with oral lichen planus (LP). He had researched LP on Google and wanted to know the long-term risk of malignancy with his oral changes.

What is the long-term risk?

A 1%
B 10%
C 20%
D 50%
E 90%

Question 34

A 35-year-old woman presented with gingival redness to her dentist (see figure) and has attended the dermatology vulval clinic regularly. She had a past history of deafness, eye problems and oesophageal strictures.

What is the most likely cause of her vulvar problems?

A Allergic contact dermatitis
B Candidiasis
C Lichen planus
D Lichen sclerosus
E Lupus erythematosus

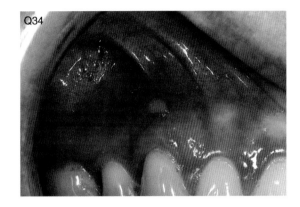

Question 35

A 23-year-old woman was referred from the general medical ward with extensive oral ulceration over the last 5 days. She had been unwell and admitted to hospital with a chest infection requiring erythromycin therapy. There was no other past medical or drug history of note. On examination, she had crusting of the lips (see figure) as well as painful, irregular, shallow ulcers involving the buccal mucosa and tongue. The rest of the skin, gingiva and genital skin were not affected.

What is the most likely cause of her oral ulceration?

A Herpes zoster virus
B HIV
C *Mycobacterium marinum*
D *Mycoplasma pneumoniae*
E *Trichophyton rubrum*

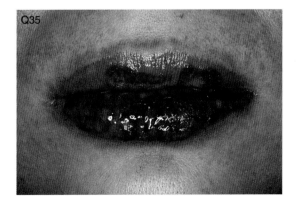

Question 36

A 73-year-old woman of Afro-Caribbean descent comes to see you as she is becoming increasingly dissatisfied with her facial appearance and asks for your treatment recommendations (see figure).

After careful facial assessment, which treatment will have the most significant impact on facial rejuvenation?

A Botulinum toxin injections to address periocular and perioral rhytids

B Broad-spectrum photoprotection and tretinoin cream

C Dermal filler injection to the cheeks to address fat atrophy of the midface

D Full-face fractionated CO_2 laser ablation for repair of photodamage

E Superficial peels to reduce risk of any pigment changes

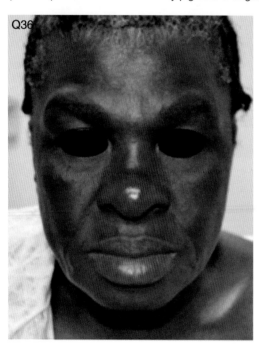

Q36

Question 37

A trainee recently achieved Dermatology Certification and is on the General Medical Council specialist register. She is keen to commence cosmetic work with injectables in her nascent private practice.

What is the most important initial consideration before commencing her new cosmetic practice?

A Be aware of procedure complications and how to manage them

B Declare the full scope of their practice to a medical indemnity insurer

C Ensure their financial model of practice is viable

D Join a voluntary register to ensure training and practice are aligned with agreed professional standards

E On-site availability of a senior colleague who can provide support at all times

Question 38

A 79-year-old woman from Somalia presents to clinic with a generalised severe bullous eruption. She can only speak a few basic words in English. She is accompanied by her daughter, who speaks English well. Her daughter tells you it is fine to speak to her, and she will go through discussions with her mother when they get back home. A face-to-face interpreter is not immediately available. A telephone interpreting service is available, and one of the dermatology secretaries speaks her language.

Which is the best course of action?

A Ask the dermatology secretary to help translate so you can speak to the patient directly

B Rearrange the consultation for when a face-to-face interpreter can be arranged

C Talk to the daughter, and let her explain the consultation to her mother when they get home

D Tell the daughter that you cannot speak to her directly as this breaches her mother's confidentiality

E Use the phone interpreting service to talk directly to the patient with her daughter in attendance, providing the patient has given her consent

Question 39

A 35-year-old man living in India has recently been diagnosed with leprosy. Since his diagnosis he has stayed at home and avoided going to the temple. He is afraid of other people's reactions to him, avoids going out to the market and asks his family to deliver food to him. He describes symptoms of low mood and anxiety.

Which option best summarises what this man is experiencing?

A He has described anticipated stigma, but you should ask further questions to assess whether he has also experienced enacted stigma or discrimination

B He is experiencing enacted stigma or discrimination and the authorities should be contacted to ensure it is safe for him to visit the temple

C He is experiencing stigma, which can lead to mental health problems such as feelings of low self-worth, anxiety and depression, which may be permanent

D He is showing signs of anticipated stigma, rather than enacted stigma or discrimination, and therefore not much can be done to help

E Social stigma is deeply ingrained in society and cannot be changed, so suggest strategies of self-help to assist the patient to live with the stigma

Question 40

A 22-year-old Ethiopian man (see figures) presented with a 3-year history of symmetrical papular and nodular lesions on his pinna and face, on a background of diffuse infiltration of the ears. Examination revealed loss of his eyelashes and early development of a saddle nose deformity. He had bilateral numbness on his fingers, with wasting over the hypothenar eminence. His ulnar nerve was palpable. Histology showed a band of normal-appearing dermis (grenz zone), which separated a normal epidermis from a dermal infiltrate consisting of Virchow cells, plasma cells and lymphocytes. Fite staining highlighted numerous bacilli and in clumps (globi).

What is the most likely diagnosis?

A Borderline leprosy
B Cutaneous leishmaniasis
C Cutaneous tuberculosis
D Lepromatous leprosy
E Tuberculoid leprosy

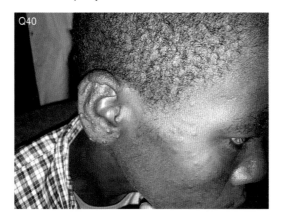

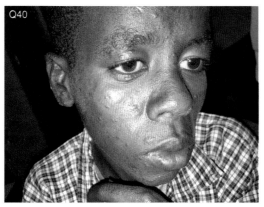

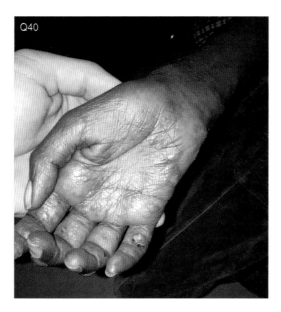

Question 41

A 62-year-old organ transplant recipient with actinic keratoses (AKs) on the arms comes to clinic with some questions about photodynamic therapy (PDT) as he had been reading about this on the internet. He wanted to know if this would be an effective and safe treatment for him.

Which of the following statements best describes the use of PDT for his AKs?

A Low-irradiance PDT may be better tolerated
B PDT is licensed for AK on the limbs
C PDT may prevent new areas of AK from developing
D PDT would be more painful due to his immunosuppression
E Photosensitivity after PDT might persist for 4 days

Question 42

A 25-year-old man has widespread psoriasis and is very keen on using the most effective light treatment. He prefers to try oral psoralen plus ultraviolet A (PUVA), but is concerned about how long he will need to wear protective glasses after each treatment.

What is the length of time you advise him to wear the protective glasses?

A 2 hours
B 24 hours
C 48 hours
D 3 days
E 5 days

Question 43

A 73-year-old man had been aware of a slowly expanding scaly patch on his cheek for over a year. The biopsy histology is shown (× 4 magnification).

What is the diagnosis?

A Adnexal tumour
B Basal cell carcinoma
C Collision tumour
D Lichenoid keratosis
E Squamous cell carcinoma

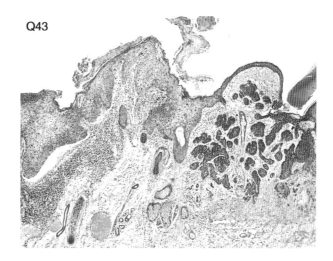

Question 44

A 42-year-old woman has been aware of a dull red, slightly swollen area on her finger for 6 weeks. A biopsy was taken and the histology at × 4 magnification is shown in the figure.
What is the most likely diagnosis?

A Chilblain
B Cutaneous T-cell lymphoma
C Granuloma annulare
D *Mycobacterium marinum* infection
E Polymorphic light eruption

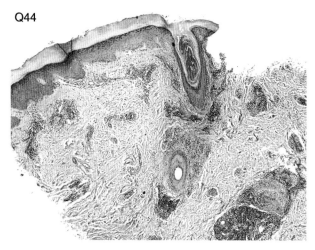
Q44

Question 45

A 70-year-old man has had a painful ulcer on the lower leg (see figure), which has been rapidly expanding over a number of weeks. Hydrocolloid dressings have been unhelpful.
What is the best initial management before commencement of systemic therapy?

A Biopsy to exclude underlying cutaneous malignancy
B Four-layer bandaging after arterial disease has been excluded
C Negative-pressure wound therapy
D Potent topical steroids under occlusive dressings
E Surgical debridement and topical antibiotics

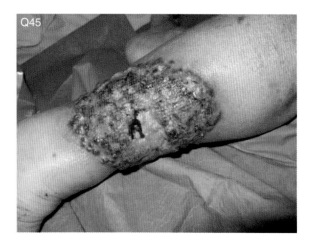
Q45

Question 46

A 61-year-old woman with Fitzpatrick phototype II skin presented with a dark lesion on the upper back of unknown duration. On examination, there was a 7-mm flat, deeply pigmented lesion (see figures).
Based on the clinical and dermoscopic findings, what is the most likely diagnosis?

A Benign compound naevus with reticular and globular pattern
B Benign junctional naevus with central hyperpigmentation
C Invasive melanoma with asymmetrical network, black blotches and irregular globules
D Lentigo maligna with polygonal structures, black blotches and grey circles
E Spitz naevus with central black blotch and peripheral streaks

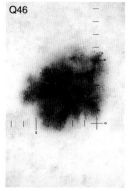
Q46 Q46

Question 47

An 82-year-old retired engineer presented with a right-cheek lesion of 2 years' duration with intermittent bleeding, usually when shaving (see figures). In the past he had a cream for 'sun damage' on the forehead, prescribed by his physician in Greece, where he spends several months every year.
Based on the history and clinical and dermoscopic findings, which of the following is the most appropriate management plan?

A Excision with a 4-mm margin
B Mohs surgery
C No treatment
D Radiotherapy
E Topical 5-fluorouracil

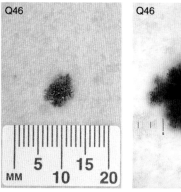
Q47 Q47

Question 48

A 70-year-old man reports a history of a rapidly growing, tender skin lesion behind the ear (see figures). You suspect a squamous cell carcinoma.

Which of the following dermoscopic findings support this diagnosis?

A Arborising blood vessels and areas of ulceration
B Irregular linear vessels and white circles
C Monomorphic hairpin vessels and keratotic surface
D Peripheral crown vessels and yellow lobules
E Uniform comma-shaped vessels in a smooth raised lesion

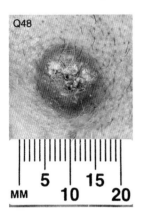 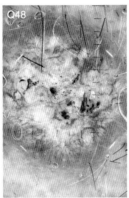

Question 49

A 45-year-old man presents with depression and anxiety linked with his moderate eczema, which is currently reasonably well controlled with topical agents.

What is the most effective strategy to help his depression?

A Arrange phototherapy
B Dupilumab therapy
C Treat with antidepressant medication alone
D Treat with both antidepressant medication and psychotherapy
E Treat with psychotherapy alone

Question 50

A 35-year-old woman presents with very itchy skin for the last 2 years. She is an intermittent recreational drug user and describes a sensation of bites on her skin. She is on beta blockers for her hypertension. She has brought in three small plastic bags containing material that she wishes you to examine.

What is the most likely primary diagnosis?

A Delusional infestation
B Depression
C Drug reaction
D Insect bites
E Obsessive compulsive disorder

Question 51

A 38-year-old woman of Middle Eastern origin presented with a 2-year history of facial pigmentation. She was extremely bothered by the pigmentation. On examination, there were irregular grey-brown patches on the cheeks and nose.

Which of the following topical treatments is unlikely to be helpful?

A Adapalene
B Azelaic acid
C Benzoyl peroxide
D Cysteamine
E Hydroquinone

Question 52

A 49-year-old Black woman presents with asymptomatic hair thinning and breakage affecting her crown. She has worn her hair in locs, where the hair is left to tangle and coil around itself into fused units, since her 20s, and generally wears them loose. Up until her 20s, she wore her hair naturally. Her mother also has hair thinning of the crown. A biopsy was taken and histology showed a lymphocytic infiltrate with premature desquamation of the inner root sheath and perifollicular fibrosis.

What is the most likely diagnosis?

A Alopecia areata
B Central cicatricial centrifugal alopecia
C Female pattern hair loss
D Traction alopecia
E Trichotillomania

Question 53

A 76-year-old woman is referred with a digital e-referral for a pigmented lesion on her back with unknown duration or history of change. It has not been painful or bled. There is no personal or family history of skin cancer. She has always lived in the UK, but has had occasional sunny holidays abroad. A blurred image of the pigmented lesion has been sent with the e-referral.

What is the most appropriate next action?

A Advise the general practitioner (GP) to refer with a high-quality image
B Arrange a face-to-face consultation
C Arrange excision urgently
D Ask the GP to arrange for the patient to send images directly to dermatology
E Discharge back to the GP

Question 54

You undertake a remote consultation with a 25-year-old man who has long-standing eczema, managed with methotrexate 10 mg once weekly as well as topical preparations. As part of the remote consultation, he has uploaded an image showing marked improvement of his eczema. After discussion with the patient, a shared decision is made to stop the methotrexate, to continue with topical preparations and to make an open follow-up appointment.

What should happen to the patient-supplied image?

A Delete the image without referring to it in the notes
B File the image on your personal desktop computer
C Save it in your personal email
D Send the image to the primary care physician
E Transfer the image to the electronic patient record, noting it was patient supplied

Question 55

A junior doctor is considering discharging a long-term follow-up patient with psoriasis from the outpatient clinic. The patient has some concerns regarding being discharged.

What is the best course of action to help the discharge process?

A Ask the general practitioner (GP) if the patient can be discharged
B Provide departmental website details
C Provide the GP with a clear management plan
D Provide verbal safety net details for re-accessing the service
E Provide a verbal treatment plan for the patient

Question 56

A senior dermatologist receives a written complaint sent to the complaints team regarding a surgical excision of a basal cell carcinoma on the central chest performed 12 months ago. The patient is unhappy with a thickened painful scar and was previously discharged.

What is the best way to proceed initially?

A Act very quickly and respond in writing to the complaints team
B Ask another consultant to review the medical notes
C Ignore the complaint as you felt the scar was acceptable at post-surgery review
D Plan to discuss at the next clinical governance meeting
E Take the criticism personally and get upset

Question 57

There has been disagreement among the dermatologists in your team about how to organise the timetable of clinics for each doctor.

What is the best next step to resolve the problem?

A Arrange a departmental meeting so all the issues can be discussed openly
B Meet individually with each colleague to try to understand their different views
C Postpone making any change until August when most staff are on leave
D Write a new timetable and ask your administrators to impose it next week
E Write and circulate a new timetable and ask for comments

Question 58

A 3-year-old child comes to your paediatric clinic with café-au-lait spots (hyperpigmented macules). You suspect the child may have neurofibromatosis type 1 (NF1).

What additional finding would help support your clinical diagnosis of NF1 in this child?

A Angiofibroma
B Granuloma annulare
C Hypopigmented macules
D Lisch nodules on slit-lamp examination
E Periungual fibroma

Question 59

A 3-year-old boy with persistent facial eczema attends your clinic. He is otherwise well and had mild flexural eczema at the age of 3 months. He has been treated by his general practitioner with hydrocortisone 1% cream intermittently. The parents are concerned about skin thinning and ask about alternative treatments.

What is the best treatment for his facial eczema?

A Clobetasone butyrate 0.05% cream
B Miconazole 2% and hydrocortisone 1% ointment
C Pimecrolimus 1% cream
D Tacrolimus 0.03% ointment
E Tacrolimus 0.1% ointment

Question 60

A 12-year-old girl presents with a 3-month history of an expanding lesion on her right ankle. She does not like the appearance, but has no symptoms. On examination, she has a 3-cm pale brown lesion that is flat in the centre but has a slightly raised palpable edge.

What is the best course of action?

A Curettage and cautery
B Localised psoralen plus ultraviolet A therapy
C Pulsed-dye laser therapy
D Punch biopsy
E Reassure and discharge

Question 61

A 9-year-old boy presents to your clinic with a 6-month history of small papules on his legs and abdomen. On examination, a few papules are umbilicated and becoming sore and inflamed. The parents are very keen for treatment as some papules are healing with slight scarring.

What is the best treatment option for the non-inflamed papules?

A Curettage and cautery
B Excision
C Hydrocortisone 1% ointment
D Liquid nitrogen cryotherapy
E Potassium hydroxide 5% solution

Question 62

A 10-year-old girl presents with a 3-month history of a rash on her forehead. She has some excoriations with scarring on her forehead and cheeks. Her parents have separated recently and both are very concerned, as she has also developed some localised hair loss on her right temple. On examination, there are very short, broken hairs with variable length on her scalp. There is no scaling, inflammation or scarring on the scalp.

What is the most likely diagnosis for the hair loss?

A Alopecia areata
B Telogen effluvium
C Tinea capitis
D Traction alopecia
E Trichotillomania

Question 63

A 28-year-old man presented to the acute medical team with a severe flare of his atopic eczema, a fever of 38 °C and lymphadenopathy. He had never experienced cold sores. However, his female partner had a history of herpes labialis. The patient had type 1 diabetes. The eczema flare is not responding to oral antibiotics. On examination, his face and neck were covered with painful monomorphic punched-out erosions.

What treatment would you recommend to start immediately?

A Aciclovir cream
B Aciclovir tablets
C Clarithromycin tablets
D Mometasone furoate cream
E Prednisolone tablets

Question 64

A 48-year-old woman presented with a 10-week history of recurrent boils affecting her legs (see figures below), upper arms and abdomen. Her general practitioner had treated her with a 2-week course of flucloxacillin. She improved initially, but then developed a new boil, which failed to respond to further flucloxacillin. Her 6-year-old daughter had also developed similar lesions.

What is your next management step?

A Prescribe clarithromycin
B Prescribe further flucloxacillin
C Skin biopsy
D Skin swab for Panton–Valentine leucocidin testing
E Treat with mupirocin ointment

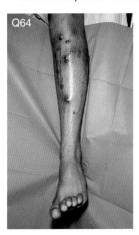
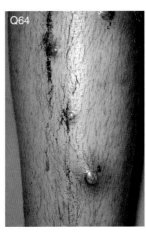

Question 65

A 45-year-old man presented with a red, tender, itchy and scaly rash on the lower legs (see figures in next column). He had regularly shaved his legs and had a history of athlete's foot, which had spread to the dorsum of both feet. His general practitioner had treated him with multiple prolonged courses of oral antibiotics and a moderate-strength topical corticosteroid for 4 weeks. There was no history of inflammatory bowel disease. On examination, he had inflamed scaly patches on the lower legs and some superficial scaling. Bacterial swabs were consistently negative and blood tests including C-reactive protein were normal.

What investigation would you arrange next?

A Colonoscopy referral
B Patch testing
C Skin biopsy
D Skin scrapings for mycology
E Skin swabs for bacterial culture

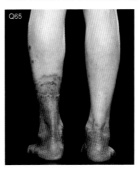
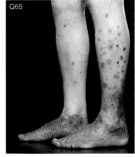

Question 66

A 37-year-old woman presents with a rash that occurs within 10 minutes of sun exposure and then usually subsides within a few hours.

What is the most appropriate first-line treatment?

A Ciclosporin
B Fexofenadine
C Hydroxychloroquine
D Methotrexate
E Thalidomide

Question 67

A 38-year-old male patient of South East Asian origin presents with suspected severe photosensitivity on the face, upper chest and dorsum of the hands. Provocation testing and the solar simulator produced a marked eczematous response, supporting the diagnosis of chronic actinic dermatitis.

What is the most likely pattern of monochromator light testing in this condition?

A Severely reduced UVA and visible light thresholds
B Severely reduced UVA thresholds
C Severely reduced UVB thresholds
D Severely reduced UVB, UVA and visible light thresholds
E Severely reduced visible light thresholds

Question 68

A 45-year-old woman presented to your clinic with female pattern hair loss.

What are the predominant dermoscopic findings in female pattern hair loss?

A Exclamation mark hairs, and black and yellow dots
B Loss of follicular openings, broken hairs, black dots and vellus hairs
C Short, regrowing hairs that may show variability
D Variability in hair shaft diameter, yellow dots and short vellus hairs
E White patches, keratotic plugs and enlarged branching vessels

Question 69

A 70-year-old farmer presents with a keratotic lesion involving his right index fingernail. He has tried over-the-counter wart paints, but the lesion is persistent and increasing in size. It is associated with nail plate changes. His grandchildren have warts on their fingers.

What is the most appropriate next step in his management?

A   Advise stronger wart paints
B   Arrange nail bed biopsy
C   Consider cryotherapy
D   Proceed with complete nail unit excision
E   Reassure the patient

Question 70

A 23-year-old woman presents with a naevus of Ota and is being considered for laser therapy.

Which of the following laser parameters determines the depth of penetration and absorption by a chromophore to treat this?

A   Fluence
B   Power
C   Site
D   Spot size
E   Wavelength

Question 71

A 45-year-old civil servant requested removal of a red tattoo on the arm because of a change in his personal circumstances.

Which laser and wavelength are most appropriate to remove red tattoo inks?

A   Alexandrite 755 nm
B CO_2 10,600 nm
C   Pulsed-dye laser 585 nm
D   Q-switch Nd:YAG 532 nm
E   Ruby 694 nm

Question 72

A 24-year-old man with Fitzpatrick phototype IV skin was referred to the laser clinic for treatment of acne scars on his face. He had completed a course of isotretinoin successfully a year ago and his acne has been well controlled since. On examination, he had moderate boxcar and ice pick scars over his cheeks and temples.

Which of the following will be the most appropriate chromophore to target with laser therapy to improve his scars?

A   Collagen
B   Eumelanin
C   Haemoglobin
D   Phaeomelanin
E   Water

The figures are copyright as follows:

Questions 4, 11, 18, 27, 29, 34, 35, 64 and 65: © Medical Illustration Cardiff and Vale UHB.

Question 36: Vashi *et al*. Aging differences in ethnic skin. *J Clin Aesthet Dermatol* 2016; **9**:31–8.

Question 40: © Thomas King.

Questions 43 and 44: © Cwm Taf Morgannwg University Health Board.

Question 45: Perricone G, Vangeli M. Pyoderma gangrenosum in ulcerative colitis. *N Engl J Med* 2018; **379**:e7.

Questions 46, 47 and 48: © Aneurin Bevan University Health Board.

Specialty Certificate Exam (SCE): answers

Question 1
Answer: C

Profilaggrin is contained within keratohyalin granules, which are produced by the stratum granulosum. Filaggrin has a key role in collapsing keratinocytes, forming the flattened cells that are characteristic of the stratum corneum. Filaggrin mutations are associated with disturbed barrier function and are the strongest known genetic risk factor for atopic dermatitis. Palmar hyperlinearity may be more common in patients with filaggrin mutations.

Question 2
Answer: C

The hair follicle has its own population of stem cells located in the hair bulge. This region is responsible for supplying progenitor cells to the hair matrix, which proliferate and differentiate to elongate hair follicles in the growth (anagen) phase. This growth is triggered by signalling from the dermal papilla.

Question 3
Answer: A

The clinical history of ingestion of allopurinol a few days prior to the onset of the rash suggests a drug reaction. The clinical features suggest acute generalised exanthematous pustulosis (AGEP), confirmed by the histological features.

Question 4
Answer: C

The clinical and histological features are characteristic of pemphigus vulgaris. Pemphigus foliaceus presents with scaly erosions rather than flaccid blisters, mucosal surfaces are generally unaffected and histology shows subcorneal acantholysis.

Question 5
Answer: E

When data from a research project is analysed, it is very tempting to focus on positive results or statistically significant differences between groups. Negative findings appear to be less interesting, but should be given equal weight in reporting of results. Selective publishing of favourable outcomes, unfortunately a very common bias, leads to a skewed message that cumulatively may have long-term negative consequences for patient care.

Question 6
Answer: A

It may seem odd that audit projects are mostly 'exempt' from the need to seek ethical permission. This is because audit is simply recording what is happening anyway, or bringing together information that is already being collected in either clinical or administrative records. So there is no need to seek additional permission for accessing this data. Clinical intervention, for which ethical permission must always be sought, does not form part of an audit. However, if you feel that an audit design is almost a 'borderline' research project, always seek advice.

Question 7
Answer: C

The overriding principle in taking decisions on behalf of someone who lacks capacity is to try to work out and follow what the person themselves would have wanted. This is not necessarily what their doctor, carer or relatives would want. It would also not necessarily lead to what the doctors or others would view as the 'best' outcome.

Question 8
Answer: B

The three-part test to establish negligence requires that (i) a duty of professional care is owed to a patient and (ii) as a consequence of a breach of that duty (iii) the patient suffers harm.

Question 9
Answer: B

Degree of redness is one of the three key signs that are assessed in PASI; the others are scaling and plaque thickness.

Dermatology Training: The Essentials. Edited by Mahbub M.U. Chowdhury, Tamara W. Griffiths and Andrew Y. Finlay.
© 2022 The British Association of Dermatologists. Published 2022 by John Wiley & Sons Ltd.
Companion website: www.wiley.com/go/chowdhury/dermatologytraining

Although excoriations may be seen in psoriasis, they are not part of PASI. The flexures are not specifically mentioned in PASI. As PASI is based on sign assessment, the subjective symptom of soreness is not included. The percentage involvement of psoriasis over the head (including the face) is a key part of PASI, but the face is not calculated separately.

Question 10
Answer: C

When the DLQI was being designed, patients were asked to write down '. . .all the ways your skin disease affects you'. The range of answers was analysed and formed the basis of the DLQI questionnaire. Although skin disease can sometimes have a major impact on sleep or walking, these items were not all included in the DLQI, as it was designed to be short and therefore practical to use. Impact on a partner's life can be measured by separate measures such as the Family DLQI.

Question 11
Answer: A

This question concerns the differential diagnosis of presentation of a red face. The absence of comedones distinguishes rosacea from acne vulgaris. Rosacea will be exacerbated by sunlight, but so will lupus erythematosus (LE). Both rosacea and acne vulgaris are characterised by papules and pustules. Rosacea will be temporarily improved with the use of topical steroids, but will ultimately be worsened by this treatment. Eczema and LE may also be improved with a topical steroid. Greasy scale and distribution on the eyebrows and nasolabial folds is a feature of seborrhoeic dermatitis, not a feature of rosacea.

Question 12
Answer: E

This question concerns the development of unstable pustular psoriasis in a patient with a long history of stable chronic plaque psoriasis. Withdrawal of oral or long-term potent topical corticosteroids can precipitate generalised pustular psoriasis. Beta blockers are known to exacerbate chronic plaque psoriasis. A bereavement may be a stressful event and may worsen psoriasis to a degree, but it would not be expected to produce such a dramatic change. Weight gain rather than loss is associated with worsening psoriasis and this would be expected to worsen plaque psoriasis, not transform it to pustular psoriasis. A streptococcal infection is known to produce a flare of guttate psoriasis, but is less likely to cause a change to pustular psoriasis.

Question 13
Answer: D

This is a case of lichen simplex chronicus. The night-time itch is very relevant in making the diagnosis. Overall, the clinical description and examination findings are less likely to suggest the other conditions listed. Folliculitis does not usually occur on mucosal surfaces. Fungal infection (dermatophyte) is likely to occur in the groin crease. Inflammation and erosions are present with lichen planus. Vaginal intra-epithelial neoplasia is usually asymptomatic.

Question 14
Answer: D

This is most likely to be a case of anogenital psoriasis. Inflammation on the mons pubis and natal cleft are characteristic of psoriasis. This requires treatment with a mild to moderately potent topical steroid with regular emollients and soap substitutes. The lack of response to topical and oral anti-yeast therapy excludes candidiasis. Vaginal intra-epithelial neoplasia is usually not itchy.

Question 15
Answer: A

This is a case of lichen sclerosus. Atrophy of the frenulum and scarring are characteristic. Superpotent topical steroids are the initial treatment.

Question 16
Answer: C

The fact that the lesion did not respond to multiple treatments suggests it is a pre-malignant lesion and should be biopsied. Look for signs of lichen sclerosus, as penile intra-epithelial neoplasia and squamous cell carcinoma are strongly associated with lichen sclerosus.

Question 17
Answer: D

The causes of lower-limb oedema may be multiple, particularly in elderly patients with many comorbidities. Obstruction of lymphatic drainage from recurrent malignancy must be excluded in a patient with a previous cancer diagnosis. Venous disease (varicose veins) is a common problem and can be the sole cause of lymphoedema, or can complicate the scenario of lymphoedema from other causes. Primary lymphoedema is not exclusive to children, and should be considered in anyone with onset of lymphoedema in their younger adult years (i.e. before the age of 40 years), especially females. Other causes of lymphoedema are much more likely in an elderly patient with swelling.

A careful drug history can reveal an association between starting calcium channel blockers (e.g. amlodipine) and the onset of lower-limb lymphoedema, typically within a few months. Prompt cessation of the causal drug can reverse the swelling, but lymphoedema is often permanent if the patient has been on the medication for more than a year. Sarcoidosis can rarely cause lymphoedema and is much less likely to be the cause without any other manifestations.

Question 18
Answer: C

The American Joint Committee on Cancer 8th edition (2018) and British Association of Dermatologists' guidelines confirm the excision margin should be 1 cm in total for a malignant melanoma of < 1 mm Breslow thickness. Another wide local excision of 8 mm is needed in addition to sentinel lymph node biopsy for patients with malignant melanoma with Breslow thickness of 0.8 mm and above.

Question 19

Answer: E

Imiquimod 5% cream 5 days per week for 6 weeks is the preferred treatment for superficial basal cell carcinomas, as it is more effective than 5-fluorouracil 5% cream daily for 4 weeks. This patient is likely to have poor peripheral circulation, so the other options are not advisable as first-line treatment due to the risk of poor wound healing.

Question 20

Answer: E

The squamous cell carcinoma British Association of Dermatologists' guidelines of 2020 confirm tumour invasion of > 4 mm is a high-risk feature; the other features are low risk. Ears, lips and hands are considered high-risk sites for tumours, but not the scalp.

Question 21

Answer: B

Nivolumab is an anti-PD1 (programmed cell death protein-1) receptor protein that downregulates T cells and the immune system. It is used for metastatic melanoma if positive BRAF V600 mutation is present. The other mechanisms of action are for other biologic drugs (Table 18.4).

Question 22

Answer: C

Care should be taken before prescribing dapsone in patients with possible G6PD deficiency, as they are likely to experience severe haemolysis. The G6PD level should be checked, especially in people of African, Asian, Middle Eastern and Mediterranean descent. Dapsone is licensed for the treatment of dermatitis herpetiformis, which is the likely diagnosis in this case. Dapsone is widely used in dermatology to treat other immunobullous diseases and neutrophilic dermatoses. The other enzymes can all be measured prior to use of other systemic drugs; for example, DPD deficiency leads to increased side effects from 5-fluorouracil chemotherapy and GGT is a liver enzyme raised with alcohol intake.

Question 23

Answer: B

Three-monthly testing of P3NP is sufficient and this does not need to be done more frequently. It is important to monitor any change in the trend of P3NP over a 12-month period, following the British Association of Dermatologists' methotrexate guidelines.

Question 24

Answer: D

Even though all the other options would be helpful, a clear detailed written plan is the best initial way to improve adherence. Verbal information on topical treatment frequency and adequate amounts to use will be forgotten quickly if not written down. Writing to the general practitioner (GP) is also important to be able to provide repeat prescriptions and for GPs to be aware of the treatments suggested. However, this will not improve the child's treatment regimen unless the instructions are clearly communicated to the parents as well. Specialist dermatology nurse input will reinforce and provide support for the parents later if the nurses are not available for advice immediately in the outpatient clinic. Often multiple strategies are required to improve adherence, but the initial best steps are to provide specific written treatment instructions for the parents and for the child to be fully aware of the recommended treatment regimen.

Question 25

Answer: B

This woman has developed perioral dermatitis, now considered to be a rosacea-like eruption induced by topical steroids. It typically presents with inflamed small papules and pustules around the mouth. This is a side-effect of the potent topical corticosteroid use over a prolonged period. She will need to stop all topical corticosteroids on her face and may need to use pimecrolimus or tacrolimus to reduce her potent corticosteroid use. However, metronidazole cream is the best option initially, and if the perioral dermatitis is unresponsive, she may need a short course of oral tetracyclines.

Question 26

Answer: D

Immediate clinical symptoms with blowing up balloons can be a sensitive indicator of possible latex allergy. Prick testing to latex could help to confirm the diagnosis and, if prick tests are negative, a use test with a latex glove may be indicated. Minor itching with nitrile gloves could occur with irritant contact dermatitis, and lip swelling with apples may indicate oral allergy (pollen food) syndrome. Bananas are the most common fruit cross-reacting with latex. Use of gloves by HCWs for over 4 hours is considered a risk factor for latex allergy.

Question 27

Answer: E

Thiuram mix is the main rubber accelerator that causes delayed (type 4) contact allergy to gloves. Carba mix is another screening agent for rubber glove accelerator allergy in the baseline series. Methylisothiazolinone is a common preservative, linalool is a perfume allergen, sesquiterpene lactone mix is a plant allergen, and allergy to the preservative paraben mix is now very uncommon.

Question 28

Answer: B

The acne in this male nurse has been caused by facial surgical masks due to a combination of occlusion, irritation, heat and sweating. As the acne changes are moderate, it is unlikely that topical agents will be sufficient, hence oral doxycycline for 3 months is probably the best initial step after considering regular rest periods and changes of mask.

Question 29

Answer: E

Vesicles indicate either likely contact allergy or pompholyx eczema of the hands. If vesicles are present and occur repeatedly, patch testing is essential to exclude contact allergy. All the other findings in the history and examination would be consistent with irritant contact dermatitis.

Question 30

Answer: E

Tocopherol acetate is vitamin E, found in many cosmetic products, and is in the BSCA facial (cosmetic) series. The other allergens listed are all in the baseline series. The criterion for inclusion in the baseline series is usually at least 1% positivity for that allergen in consecutively patch-tested patients, in data analysed with prospective allergen databases. Balsam of Peru is a fragrance allergen, methylisothiazolinone and sodium metabisulfite are preservatives, and tixocortol pivalate is a marker of hydrocortisone corticosteroid allergy.

Question 31

Answer: A

Surgical excision of any lesion in the temple region risks damaging the facial nerve, resulting in eyebrow ptosis. Radiotherapy is a non-surgical modality that may be considered if the patient is keen to avoid any surgical intervention. Adverse scarring should always be discussed during the consent process for any surgical intervention. An inability to raise the eyebrow immediately after the procedure does not necessarily indicate nerve damage during surgery, as the nerve will become paralysed as soon as local anaesthetic is administered. It is inadvisable for patients to drive home after any facial surgical procedure and, around the temple especially, patients may still experience significant periorbital swelling and bruising post-operatively.

Question 32

Answer: B

This scenario is not uncommon in clinical practice. Remember that despite pressure from patients, your over-riding duty is first to 'do no harm' as well as 'working within the level of your competence and training'. You must never feel pressurised into performing any procedure you do not feel comfortable with. In this situation, an enlarging SCC clearly requires urgent intervention, and although a biopsy would not be incorrect here, the diagnosis is not in doubt. Radiotherapy would not be considered an appropriate first-line intervention in this case. Ensure all such difficult discussions are documented clearly and fully in the medical records.

Question 33

Answer: A

The overall lifetime risk of oral cancer from oral LP is 1%. It should be suspected if there is an atypical area of ulceration not responding to treatment or if the mucosa has a gritty or firm feel. Hence palpation of the mucosa is very important. In patients with ulcerative LP, asymmetrical plaque-type LP or a non-healing ulcer lasting for 3 weeks or more, referral to oral medicine is recommended as a biopsy might be indicated. This is particularly important if the patient is on any immunosuppressive therapy.

Question 34

Answer: C

This is likely to be vulvovaginal gingival syndrome, which is a variant of mucosal lichen planus and is characterised by redness, erosions and desquamation of the vulva, vagina and gingiva. It must be considered in patients presenting with prominent gingival redness or desquamation. A high proportion of those affected may develop genital fibrosis and strictures, leading to vaginal and urethral stenosis. It can also be associated with lacrimal stenosis, oesophageal strictures and conduction deafness. The other conditions listed are unlikely to cause all these associated conditions. Lichen sclerosus does not usually affect the vagina and does not cause oral mucosal changes.

Question 35

Answer: D

Following the recent chest infection, this woman has developed erythema multiforme (EM). EM affects the anterior part of the mouth with painful, irregular, shallow ulcers involving the buccal mucosa and tongue and crusting of the lips. Ocular, nasal, pharyngeal, laryngeal, upper respiratory and anogenital mucosal surfaces may be involved. The gingivae tend to be spared. In some patients the typical target-like skin lesions are also present on the extremities. The most common causes of EM are herpes simplex infection and *Mycoplasma pneumoniae*, which is the likely cause of mucositis in this case. Many other viruses such as herpes zoster, HIV, cytomegalovirus and pox viruses can trigger EM, but are less common causes. The absence of skin lesions and of a history of drugs such as non-steroidal anti-inflammatory drugs, penicillins or anticonvulsants is against the diagnosis of Stevens–Johnson syndrome.

Question 36

Answer: C

Loss of volume is the hallmark of facial ageing and is ubiquitous across all ethnicities, therefore addressing volume loss is a fundamental strategy for most patients in their 70s. Photoageing in skin of colour manifests more commonly as pigmentation irregularity or dyschromia, compared to wrinkling and solar elastosis in white skin. Full-face fractionated CO_2 laser is not recommended due to the risk of post-inflammatory hyper- or hypopigmentation. CO_2 laser can be used to treat lax, wrinkled skin, which is less often seen in skin of colour. Superficial peels may benefit the hyperpigmentation infra-orbitally and on the lower forehead, but will have only modest impact compared to re-volumisation. The patient's eyebrows are somewhat depressed medially and will respond to botulinum toxin injections in the brow depressors located in the glabellar region, but treatment of the crow's foot lines and perioral regions will have minimal impact on her overall appearance. Sun protection is a good general recommendation, but the most significant impact will be with dermal filler injections.

Question 37

Answer: B

Although all of these factors are important, it is essential that cosmetic practice is declared to medical indemnifiers to ensure adequate cover. This is therefore the first essential step.

Question 38

Answer: E

The presentation is too urgent to rearrange the consultation for when a face-to-face interpreter might be available. It is not best practice to use relatives or non-clinical staff to help translate. It is not acceptable to carry out the consultation with the daughter then explaining things at home, as the patient is not active in the consultation and cannot ask questions or give consent to tests or treatments. If the patient does not speak fluent English, it is not acceptable to compromise, as you cannot tell whether the patient truly understands or has given valid consent to tests and treatments.

Question 39

Answer: A

Stigma is a negative response to a human difference. It can be enacted stigma (experienced or external stigma) and could lead to discrimination. It could also be anticipated stigma, which is anticipation or fear of being stigmatised or discriminated against, which may lead to similar experiences to enacted stigma. This patient has described anticipated stigma, but we do not know if there is enacted stigma as well. Stigma can be widespread in society, and can lead to mental health problems, but there are ways to reduce the impact of stigma, by reducing sources of stigma, and you can assess and manage health-related stigma and mental health wellbeing.

Question 40

Answer: D

Leprosy is an infectious and chronic contagious disease of the skin, nerves and mucous membranes, and can also affect the eyes, nose, joints, lymph nodes, internal organs and bone marrow. It is caused by *Mycobacterium leprae*. The spectrum of leprosy ranges from tuberculoid leprosy with a T-helper 1 immune response to low numbers of bacilli, through to lepromatous leprosy with a T-helper 2 immune response to high numbers of bacilli. Borderline leprosy lies in the middle of the disease spectrum. Lepromatous leprosy in early phases presents with red, oedematous, hypopigmented macules with the colour varying in pigmented skin. These progress into symmetrical disseminated papules and nodules with diffuse infiltration. There is often loss of eyebrows (madarosis). These changes can eventually lead to a 'leonine face'. There is often nerve involvement with palpable nerves, leading to weakness, wasting and sensory changes, which predispose to neuropathic ulceration. In contrast, the tuberculoid form presents with asymmetrical involvement of a small number of red or hypopigmented lesions, often with slightly elevated borders. Depending on the duration of disease the lesions can be atrophic, and hair loss might be present. Normally there is abnormal sensation to temperature, pain and touch in the affected lesions.

Question 41

Answer: C

There is evidence that repeated PDT may have a preventative role with respect to AK and even squamous cell carcinoma development in organ transplant recipients. PDT is only licensed for AK on the face and scalp, and use on the limbs is off-licence. There is no evidence that immunosuppression itself increases risk of more severe pain, but large field area, severe disease and intense fluorescence might increase risk of pain. Low-irradiance PDT is associated with lower pain scores, but there is no evidence for reduced efficacy. Photosensitivity induced by application of aminolaevulinic acid or methyl aminolaevulinate is cleared within 24 hours.

Question 42

Answer: B

Oral PUVA is the most effective light treatment available for psoriasis. Due to the risk of early development of cataracts, protective glasses should be worn during daylight hours, and advice can be given to wear eye protection for up to 24 hours including when indoors and in higher-risk patients (such as the elderly or those with diabetes).

Question 43

Answer: C

The histology shows an area of inflamed Bowen's disease on the left, and immediately adjacent micronodular basal cell carcinoma on the right. Two common skin tumours occasionally develop close to each other, described as a collision tumour.

Question 44

Answer: A

This histology of acral skin shows a fairly dense, perivascular and periadnexal lymphocytic infiltrate, compatible with perniosis (chilblain). There is little papillary oedema, which along with the length of the history makes polymorphic light eruption less likely.

Question 45

Answer: D

The clinical history of rapid expansion and pain combined with the appearance of the ulcer, with dusky purple edges and marked inflammation, points to the diagnosis of pyoderma gangrenosum (PG). Potent topical steroids would be a good initial therapy, but if they are ineffective consider systemic agents such as prednisolone or ciclosporin. Surgical debridement of PG is contraindicated due to the phenomenon of pathergy, which can cause exacerbation of disease with trauma. Skin biopsy may be indicated if there is uncertainty, but it is not diagnostic for pyoderma gangrenosum. The history of rapid onset reduces the likelihood of cutaneous malignancy. Four-layer bandaging and negative-pressure therapy are not indicated for PG.

Question 46

Answer: C

This pigmented lesion shows network and globules indicating a melanocytic origin. The other features suggest an invasive melanoma. The network here is irregular (lines and holes are not symmetrical), with areas of black blotches. The globules have different sizes and colours, and are irregularly distributed. Benign naevi with bi-component pattern (network and globules) can be seen in adolescents and young adults, where both patterns are typically symmetrical. A benign naevus with symmetrical central hyperpigmentation can be seen in individuals with skin of colour. This lesion does not show peripheral streaks radiating from a featureless black centre, a finding expected in pigmented Spitz naevus or spitzoid melanoma. In lentigo maligna, featureless dark blotches can be seen, but they are often not associated with network and globules. Instead, angulated, polygonal lines can be seen, occasionally with grey circular structures.

Question 47
Answer: A

The history of a long-standing non-healing lesion with intermittent bleeding is a common scenario for basal cell carcinoma (BCC). This is confirmed by dermoscopy, which shows arborising vessels. As the lesion is well defined, not at a tricky anatomical site (e.g. eyelid) and not a recurrent BCC, Mohs surgery is not indicated. Excision with a 4-mm clinical margin is recommended for this BCC. Excision is superior to radiotherapy, which has a higher recurrence rate and a poorer cosmetic outcome. The lesion is indurated, not keratotic, and shows no dermoscopic features of actinic keratosis. Similarly, it lacks dermoscopic features of sebaceous hyperplasia.

Question 48
Answer: B

Arborising vessels, with or without ulceration, are commonly seen in basal cell carcinoma, which is usually slow growing and non-tender. Hairpin vessels can be seen in various conditions. They are often conspicuous and monomorphic in non-pigmented seborrhoeic keratosis. They can also be seen in squamous cell carcinoma, nodular malignant melanoma and basal cell carcinoma, but there will be other features to suggest these diagnoses. In this lesion, a few hairpin vessels are seen in the lower edge, but the lesion has polymorphous vascular structures. Irregular linear vessels appear dominant with white circles (indicating a keratinising lesion), in keeping with squamous cell carcinoma. The history of rapid growth and tenderness also supports the diagnosis. Short curved (comma-shaped) vessels are often seen in benign non-pigmented compound or intradermal naevi. These are smooth, long-standing and non-symptomatic lesions. Radial (or peripheral) crown vessels and yellow lobules are typically seen in benign sebaceous hyperplasia, which often occurs on the face and is asymptomatic.

Question 49
Answer: D

While antidepressant medication and psychotherapy can be effective as solitary treatments for patients with depression and/or anxiety, the combination of antidepressant medication with psychotherapy leads to a lower chance of recurrence of the affective disease. Wherever possible, patients should be involved in choosing their treatment, making adherence more likely. Treating the primary disease alone will not address the depression, and other strategies are essential as well.

Question 50
Answer: A

The 'specimen sign' is common in patients with delusional infestation (DI). Specimens are presented by patients to try to prove the infestation is genuine. These may include skin debris and clothing or other fibres. Digital photographic and audio files may also be presented as 'evidence'. Up to 30% of patients with DI may use recreational drugs. Patients believe that the infestation is real and will often refuse psychiatric referral. Low doses of antipsychotics are effective in patients with DI. The other conditions are unlikely to present with the specimen sign.

Question 51
Answer: C

The condition described is melasma. Benzoyl peroxide has a high potential for skin irritation, which may in turn cause post-inflammatory hyperpigmentation, and this is not a standard treatment. Hydroquinone, azelaic acid, adapalene and cysteamine are all known treatments of melasma.

Question 52
Answer: B

The histological features are those of a scarring alopecia. Central cicatricial centrifugal alopecia is the most common cause of scarring alopecia in Black women. The exact cause is unknown, but it is unlikely to be fully related to hairstyling practices. Premature desquamation of the inner root sheath is a typical feature. End-stage traction alopecia may also cause scarring, but these are not the typical histological features. The other conditions all cause non-scarring alopecia.

Question 53
Answer: A

A poor-quality image for remote electronic referrals should not be accepted, and certainly no clinical advice should be offered. In order to make a confident diagnosis of a pigmented lesion, high-quality macroscopic and dermoscopic images are required. If these are not available, then return the referral, with the suggestion of resending it with macroscopic and dermoscopic images or referring for face-to-face review.

Question 54
Answer: E

It is recommended that images are retained when they have been used to make clinical judgements on patient care. Saving the image in a personal email or personal computer is not recommended, as this does not allow access by other healthcare professionals involved in the patient's current or future care. The images should not be used beyond direct clinical care, such as for teaching, without written consent from the patient.

Question 55
Answer: C

It is best to discuss possible discharge directly with the patient, preferably in advance, and to provide a clear written management plan to the GP and the patient. Giving written details on how to re-access the service if needed is useful. Vague verbal instructions are very often forgotten and cannot be accurately remembered months later.

Question 56
Answer: A

It is essential to respond quickly and efficiently to any formal written complaint. Firstly, acknowledge receipt of the complaint in writing to the complaints team, and make immediate arrangements to review the medical notes. Further discussions may be necessary with the clinical director and at clinical governance meetings to document the complaint and its outcome. The patient may need to be reviewed again, but only once this is agreed as the best way forward with the patient and the complaints team, as well as the clinical director. The patient may wish to be seen by another, new team not involved in their original care.

Question 57

Answer: B

If there is major disagreement over an issue, it is important that all staff feel that their viewpoints are understood and taken into consideration. Individual meetings to discuss the matter calmly are the best next step. A departmental meeting risks inflaming the situation further and may lead to an unsatisfactory outcome, with domination by the more outspoken staff. Circulating a timetable risks creating more aggravation, and imposing a timetable, especially during holiday time as a cover, would potentially worsen the situation.

Question 58

Answer: D

Based on the diagnostic criteria for NF1, axillary or inguinal freckles and Lisch nodules would help confirm this diagnosis. Signs such as periungual fibroma and hypomelanotic macules form some of the diagnostic criteria for tuberose sclerosis. The diagnostic criteria for NF1 require two of the following seven criteria:

1. Six or more café-au-lait spots or hyperpigmented macules > 5 mm in diameter in prepubertal and > 15 mm in postpubertal children
2. Axillary or inguinal freckles (more than two)
3. Two or more typical neurofibromas or one plexiform neurofibroma
4. Optic nerve glioma
5. Two or more iris hamartomas (Lisch nodules) – usually requires slit-lamp examination by an ophthalmologist
6. Sphenoid dysplasia or typical long-bone abnormalities such as pseudarthrosis
7. First-degree relative with NF1 (e.g. mother, father, sister, brother)

Question 59

Answer: D

Tacrolimus 0.03% ointment is licensed for facial eczema in children over the age of 2 years. This is the best option for maintenance therapy. The parents should be warned of possible side-effects such as initial skin irritation, but if tolerated well this would be a safe option for longer-term use. All the other options are not first choice and may be unlicensed (e.g. tacrolimus 0.1% for the face), be ineffective (e.g. pimecrolimus 1%) or still have potential skin-thinning corticosteroid side-effects.

Question 60

Answer: E

This scenario describes typical localised granuloma annulare in a child. The key, if the granuloma annulare is very typical, is not to biopsy, as this could cause scarring or other side-effects, and

also make the parents more anxious. The best action is to reassure the parents and discharge the child back to the general practitioner, with advice that the granuloma annulare will usually resolve spontaneously.

Question 61

Answer: E

Potassium hydroxide 5–10% solution has been shown to be effective in some cases of molluscum contagiosum. All the other treatments will either scar or not be effective against active new lesions. In most cases the papules will become inflamed and then resolve, but some may leave a scar if very inflamed. For symptomatic inflamed papules, corticosteroid creams such as hydrocortisone 1% or topical antibiotics such as fusidic acid 1% or mupirocin 2% can be useful.

Question 62

Answer: E

This is not an unusual clinical scenario in a young child with multiple stresses and recent causes for anxiety, such as parental separation and problems at school such as bullying. The excoriations on the face (acne excoriée) occur spontaneously and the hair pulling leading to non-scarring hair loss (trichotillomania) may be compulsive and severe on the scalp and the eyebrows. This is turn can lead to further distress. Treatment with cognitive behavioural therapy and careful honest discussion about the anxieties with the child and parents, coupled with support, can be useful. All the other options listed would either have different clinical presentations or have evidence of scaling and more inflammation.

Question 63

Answer: B

The clinical findings would suggest primary herpes simplex infection. Polymerase chain reaction is increasingly used as a rapid, sensitive and specific method to detect herpes simplex virus DNA. Initial treatment should be with systemic aciclovir. When intravenous aciclovir is given, adequate hydration is important to avoid crystal nephropathy in patients with type 1 diabetes.

Question 64

Answer: D

Recurrent furunculosis, carbuncles, folliculitis and cellulitis in healthy individuals and a history of close contacts with similar presentation often point to a virulent infective source such as Panton–Valentine leucocidin (PVL)-positive *Staphylococcus aureus*. Swabs should be requested and PVL test should be stated on the request form. Methicillin-resistant *Staphylococcus aureus* should also be considered and specified on the request form. Consult with local microbiologists to determine the most appropriate empirical and definitive treatment.

Question 65

Answer: D

The history suggests a non-bacterial infection such as a fungal or viral infection. A fungal infection is most likely, with the history being consistent with tinea incognito, spreading because of the use of topical corticosteroids. Skin scrapings for mycology should be the initial investigation, but skin biopsy with subsequent periodic acid–Schiff stain may be required if the skin scrapings are negative to confirm the diagnosis.

Question 66

Answer: B

This patient has solar urticaria. The clinical presentation is that of a burning sensation seconds to minutes after sun exposure, followed by redness and then usually weals. This settles within 2–24 hours. The age of onset can vary, with preponderance in the third decade, and the female-to-male ratio is 2:1. First-line treatments are antihistamines such as fexofenadine, and other treatments such as ultraviolet B or omalizumab can be considered.

Question 67

Answer: D

This patient has very severe chronic actinic dermatitis (CAD). It is classically described in older, White men, although it is now also recognised in younger, female patients with darker skin types, particularly in South East Asian and Afro-Caribbean populations. In some instances, it may develop into a pseudolymphomatous appearance (actinic reticuloid). Phototesting in most cases demonstrates very low minimal erythemal dose to UVB, UVA and sometimes visible light as well. Patch and photopatch testing may reveal sensitivity to multiple airborne allergens such as *Compositae* plants, fragrances and colophony. Management is often challenging, and may include use of immunosuppression, as well as biological therapy including dupilumab. Severely reduced UVA thresholds alone would suggest photoaggravated eczema, and CAD cannot be diagnosed without UVB involvement. Even though visible light involvement is less common, it can occur in severe cases.

Question 68

Answer: D

A variation in hair shaft diameter of over 20% is diagnostic for female pattern androgenetic alopecia. Short vellus hairs are a sign of severe miniaturisation and are frequently seen at the frontal scalp. Yellow dots also represent miniaturisation and are more numerous in patients with severe female pattern hair loss. Exclamation mark hairs with black and yellow dots are characteristic of alopecia areata; the yellow dots correspond to keratin and sebum-filled infundibula and are not visible in children before puberty. Scalp dermoscopy of discoid lupus erythematosus will reveal white patches, keratotic plugs and enlarged branching vessels. Short regrowing hairs that show variability suggest acute telogen effluvium. Hair density may be normal or reduced depending on the severity of shedding. Telogen

hairs are extracted on the pull test. Loss of follicular openings, broken hairs, black dots and vellus hairs are associated with traction alopecia. The presence of hair casts (cylindrical scale surrounding the shaft) at the periphery of the patches indicates ongoing traction.

Question 69

Answer: B

An isolated persistent hyperkeratotic or warty area on a single digit associated with nail changes in an elderly patient should raise alarm bells of a potential squamous cell carcinoma of the digit. The first step would be to confirm the diagnosis via an urgent nail bed biopsy.

Question 70

Answer: E

Naevus of Ota is also known as oculodermal melanocytosis. Histological examination shows melanocytes scattered largely in the upper dermis, with the epidermis usually normal. Besides determining depth of penetration, wavelength determines the 'colour' of the laser beam. For this indication, a longer wavelength is selected in order for the light to penetrate to a deeper depth, for it then to be selectively absorbed by the target chromophore (melanin) at that level. A wavelength of 1064 nm for Nd:YAG laser in QS (Q-switch) mode is most appropriate to produce the desired effect.

Question 71

Answer: D

The QS (Q-switch) Nd:YAG laser at 532 nm emits in the green spectrum, which is well absorbed by the red chromophore, so is best suited to treat a red tattoo. Green inks respond well to light in the red spectrum, such as QS ruby laser (694 nm) or QS alexandrite laser (755 nm). Fractionated CO_2 10,600 nm utilises water as the chromophore to eliminate skin pigmentation by non-selective vaporisation of the epidermis and superficial dermis.

Question 72

Answer: E

CO_2 and Er:YAG lasers are the main lasers used for acne scarring. The chromophore targeted in laser resurfacing of acne scars is water. Epidermal and superficial dermal destruction stimulates new collagen and elastic fibre synthesis, with subsequent improvement in appearance. Groups of boxcar scars and wide ice pick scars on a background of Fitzpatrick skin phototype I–III are best treated with ablative laser resurfacing. A laser test patch on the representative area should be done, especially when treating a patient with skin of colour.

Dermatology training and Capabilities in Practice

Capabilities in Practice (CiPs) are a new form of assessment tool aimed to identify the point at which a trainee can be entrusted to perform a high-level task independently. In the 2021 dermatology curriculum, there are six generic CiPs aligned to the Good Medical Practice guidance of the General Medical Council (GMC) and seven specialty-specific CiPs that cover the breadth and depth of dermatological practice (Table 1).

By demonstrating the ability to work unsupervised in all of the 13 CiPs, within the context of an approved training programme, the trainee can be recognised as fit for independent practice as a consultant dermatologist, and will thus meet the standard required for entry onto the GMC specialist register. Table 2 maps the 13 generic and specialty-specific CiPs to the appropriate chapters in this textbook for ease of reference.

In contrast, the previous curriculum required competency attainment for hundreds of dermatological tasks and conditions, and when this competency was met it resulted in the assumed conclusion that the standard for GMC specialist registration had been achieved. Although the detail for the entire scope of dermatological practice is still addressed in the 2021 curriculum, it is utilised in a different manner. The educational supervisor now focuses on a broader high-level skill set to determine the capability of the trainee, noting the level of supervision required in the specific areas of practice.

A decision will be made as to the level at which the trainee is allowed to perform for each of the CiPs and the progression demonstrated: from observation only, to acting under direct then indirect supervision, and finally the ability to act unsupervised.

Specific competencies in the detailed separate British Association of Dermatologists' syllabus will be used as evidence to support the decision to progress, but they will not justify, as standalone criteria, the specific level of supervision required. This decision is made by the educational supervisor with additional input from clinical supervisors and discussion with the trainee.

Overall, assessment in the 2021 dermatology curriculum moves away from the 'tick box' approach, and towards assessment frameworks that are intended to have more educational value. It underscores the importance of 'soft skills' essential to high-level practice, which are often difficult to capture when there is an exclusive focus on syllabus content. The shift in emphasis is not to the detriment of the syllabus scope, but is necessary to better recognise and assess all of the complex skills required to work effectively as a consultant dermatologist.

The changes implemented in the 2021 dermatology curriculum are a consequence of evidence-based improvements in educational assessment tools, implemented to drive forward educational standards. As practitioners of an academic specialty, dermatologists already have a fundamental appreciation for translational basic science research, which is the cornerstone for constant improvement and expansion of evidence-based clinical practice. In times of limited resource and capacity, we must also apply the same model to our educational practice, investing in high-quality educational research to inform effective and efficient dermatology training across the whole healthcare workforce, including our highly motivated trainees.

Dermatology Training: The Essentials. Edited by Mahbub M.U. Chowdhury, Tamara W. Griffiths and Andrew Y. Finlay.
© 2022 The British Association of Dermatologists. Published 2022 by John Wiley & Sons Ltd.
Companion website: www.wiley.com/go/chowdhury/dermatologytraining

Table 1 Capabilities in Practice (CiPs) for dermatology: generic and specialty specific

Generic CiPs

1. Able to successfully function within NHS organisational and management systems

2. Able to deal with ethical and legal issues related to clinical practice

3. Communicates effectively and is able to share decision making, while maintaining appropriate situational awareness, professional behaviour and professional judgement

4. Is focused on patient safety and delivers effective quality improvement in patient care

5. Carrying out research and managing data appropriately

6. Acting as a clinical teacher and clinical supervisor

Specialty CiPs

1. **Outpatient dermatology**: managing dermatology patients in the outpatient setting

2. **Acute and emergency dermatology**: managing dermatological emergencies in all environments and managing an acute dermatology service including on-call

3. **Liaison and community dermatology**: working in partnership with primary care and promoting skin health

4. **Skin tumours and skin cancer**: managing a comprehensive skin cancer and benign skin lesion service

5. **Procedural dermatology**: performing skin surgery and other dermatological procedures

6. **Paediatric dermatology**: managing paediatric dermatology patients in all settings

7. **Other specialist aspects of a comprehensive dermatological service** including:

   7A) cutaneous allergy

   7B) photobiology and phototherapy

   7C) genital and mucosal disease

   7D) hair and nail disease

Reproduced with permission from the Joint Royal Colleges of Physicians Training Board (JRCPTB). Additional information is available online.
JRCPTB Dermatology. Available at: https://www.jrcptb.org.uk/specialties/dermatology.
Dermatology Syllabus Guidance. August 2021. Available at: https://www.jrcptb.org.uk/sites/default/files/Dermatology%20syllabus%20guidance%20
August%202021.pdf.
Dermatology Training Curriculum. Available at: https://www.jrcptb.org.uk/sites/default/files/Dermatology%202021%20Curriculum%20FINAL.pdf.

Table 2 Capabilities in Practice (CiPs) for dermatology mapped to the textbook chapters

Chapter	CiPs
1. Think critically, research and publish	G5
2. How to lead and manage	G1, G3, G6, S1, S3
3. Ethical dilemmas	G2, G6
4. Basic science of the skin	G5, S1, S2
5. Dermatopathology	S1, S2, S4, S7
6. Teledermatology	S1, S2, S3
7. Dermoscopy	S1, S3, S4, S7
8. Clinical measurement methods	G5, S1, S3, S6, S7
9. Global and public health	G1, G3, G4, S3
10. Medical dermatology	S1, S2, S3
11. Paediatric dermatology	S2, S6
12. Infections and infestations	S1, S2, S3, S6, S7
13. Skin cancer	G4, S4
14. Dermatology for skin of colour	S1, S2, S3, S4, S5, S6, S7
15. Psychodermatology	S1, S2, S3, S6
16. Emergency dermatology	G3, S2
17. Topical therapy	S1, S2, S3, S6
18. Systemic therapy	S1, S2, S6, S7
19. Skin surgery	G3, S4, S5
20. Wound care and dressings	S1, S3
21. Cosmetic dermatology	G1, G2, S5
22. Laser therapy	G1, G2, S5
23. Cutaneous allergy	G3, G4, S7
24. Photosensitivity	G3, S7
25. Phototherapy and photodynamic therapy	G3, G4, S1, S7
26. Lymphoedema	G3, S1, S3
27. Hair and nail diseases	G3, S7
28. Genital skin diseases	G2, G3, S7
29. Oral medicine	G3, S7

G, generic CiP; S, specialty CiP.

Index

Dermatology Training: The Essentials. Edited by Mahbub M.U. Chowdhury, Tamara W. Griffiths and Andrew Y. Finlay.
© 2022 The British Association of Dermatologists. Published 2022 by John Wiley & Sons Ltd.
Companion website: www.wiley.com/go/chowdhury/dermatologytraining